HEAD INJURY AND POSTCONCUSSIVE SYNDROME

HEAD INJURY AND POSTCONCUSSIVE SYNDROME

Edited by

Matthew Rizzo, M.D.

Department of Neurology, College of Medicine and
College of Engineering
University of Iowa, Iowa City, Iowa

Daniel Tranel, Ph.D.

Departments of Neurology and Psychology
University of Iowa College of Medicine
Benton Neuropsychology Laboratory
University of Iowa, Iowa City, Iowa

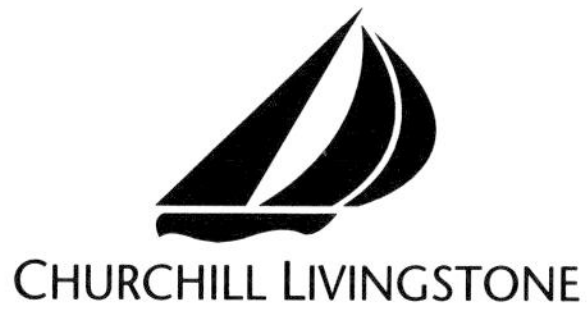

CHURCHILL LIVINGSTONE

New York, Edinburgh, London, Madrid, Melbourne, San Francisco, Tokyo

Library of Congress Cataloging-in-Publication Data

Head injury and postconcussive syndrome / edited by Matthew Rizzo, Daniel Tranel.
p. cm.
Includes bibliographical references and index.
ISBN 0–443–08964–7
1. Brain damage. 2. Brain—Concussion—Complications. I. Rizzo, Matthew. II. Tranel, Daniel D.
[DNLM: 1. Brain Concussion. 2. Head Injuries, Closed. 3. Brain Injuries—psychology. WL 354 H4326 1996]
RC387.5. H44 1996
617.4′81044—dc20
DNLM/DLC
for Library of Congress 95–37026
CIP

Distributed in the United Kingdom by Churchill Livingstone, Robert Stevenson House, 1–3 Baxter's Place, Leith Walk, Edinburgh EH1 3AF, and by associated companies, branches, and representatives throughout the world.

Acquisitions Editor: *Allan Ross*
Assistant Editor: *Marc Strauss*
Production Editor: *Gerald Feldman*
Production Supervisor: *Laura Mosberg Cohen*
Cover Design: *Paul Moran*

Printed in the United States of America

First published in 1996 7 6 5 4 3 2 1

Dedicated to Annie and Ellie
with love and gratitude
M.R.

Contributors

S. W. Anderson, Ph.D.

Adjunct Assistant Professor, Departments of Neurology and Psychology, University of Iowa College of Medicine; Director, Neuropsychological Rehabilitation Laboratory, University of Iowa Hospitals and Clinics, Iowa City, Iowa

Sue Barcellos, M.D.

Assistant Professor, Department of Neurology, University of Iowa College of Medicine, Iowa City, Iowa

S. B. Brown, M.D.

Department of Neurology, Johns Hopkins University School of Medicine, Baltimore, Maryland

Jane E. Cerhan, Ph.D.

Neuropsychologist, Benton Neuropsychology Laboratory, Division of Behavioral Neurology and Cognitive Neuroscience, Department of Neurology, University of Iowa Hospitals and Clinics, Iowa City, Iowa

T. Cole, M.A.

Research Assistant, Department of Neurology, University of Iowa College of Medicine, Iowa City, Iowa

Richard S. Cornfeld, J.D.

Partner, Coburn and Craft, St. Louis, Missouri

Kathleen B. Digre, M.D.

Associate Professor, Departments of Neurology and Ophthalmology, University of Utah School of Medicine, Salt Lake City, Utah

John T. Dunn, Ph.D.

Psychologist, Lees-Haley Psychological Corporation, Encino, California

Paul J. Eslinger, M.D.

Associate Professor Division of Neurology, The Milton S. Hershey Medical Center of The Pennsylvania State University, Hershey, Pennsylvania

John R. Gates, M.D.

Associate Professor, Departments of Neurology and Neurosurgery, University of Minnesota Medical School—Minneapolis, Minnesota; Director, Adult Service, Minnesota Epilepsy Group, St. Paul, Minnesota

Laszlo Geder, M.D., Ph.D

Assistant Professor and Director, Neurorehabilitation Department of Medicine (Division of Neurology) and University Rehabilitation Center, The Milton S. Hershey Medical Center of the Pennsylvania State University, Hershey, Pennsylvania

Barry Gordon, M.D., Ph.D.

Associate Professor of Neurology and Cognitive Science, Departments of Neurology and Cognitive Science, Johns Hopkins University; Director, Cognitive Neurology/Neuropsychology and Memory Disorders Clinics, Johns Hopkins University, Baltimore, Maryland

Mark A. Granner, M.D.

Assistant Professor, Department of Neurology, University of Iowa College of Medicine; Director, Epilespy Monitoring Unit, Department of Neurology, University of Iowa Hospitals and Clinics, Iowa City, Iowa

Lynn M. Grattan, M.D.

Department of Neurology, University of Maryland School of Medicine, Baltimore, Maryland

J. Hathaway-Nepple, M.A.

Rehabilitation Counselor, Neuropsychological Rehabiltation Laboratory, Department of Neurology, University of Iowa College of Medicine, Iowa City, Iowa

Peter Herscovitch, M.D.

Chief, Positron Emission Tomography Section, National Institutes of Health Clinical Center, Bethesda, Maryland

R. D. Jones, M.D. Ph.D.

Assistant Research Scientist, Division of Cognitive Neuroscience, University of Iowa College of Medicine, Iowa City, Iowa

Roger Kathol, M.D.

Professor of Psychiatry and Internal Medicine, Director of Medical/Psychiatry Program, Departments of Psychiatry and Medicine, University of Iowa College of Medicine, Iowa City, Iowa

Robert L. Kriel, M.D.

Professor, Departments of Neurology, Pediatrics, and Pharmacy Practice, University of Minnesota Medical School—Minneapolis, Minneapolis, Minnesota; Co-Director, Pediatric Brain Injury Services, Hennepin County Medical Center, Minneapolis, Minnesota; Co-Director, Pediatric Brain Injury Services, Gillette Children's Hospital, St. Paul, Minnesota

Paul R. Lees-Haley, M.D.

Chief Executive Officer, Lees-Haley Psychological Corporation, Encino, California

Jeffrey David Lewine, Ph.D.

Research Assistant Professor, Departments of Radiology and Psychology, University of New Mexico School of Medicine; Director, Magnetic Source Imaging and Neuroscience Divisions, New Mexico Institute of Neuroimaging, New Mexico Regional Federal Medical Center, Albuquerque, New Mexico

Maren L. Mahowald, M.D.

Department of Rheumatology, Minneapolis Veterans Administration Medical Center and University of Minnesota Medical School—Minneapolis, Minneapolis, Minnesota

Mark W. Mahowald, M.D.

Director, Minnesota Regional Sleep Disorders Center, Hennepin County Medical Center, Minneapolis, Minnesota; Department of Neurology, Hennipin County Medical Center and University of Minnesota Medical School—Minneapolis, Minneapolis, Minnesota

Daniel V. McGehee, M.S.

Associate Research Scientist, Human Factors Research Group, Iowa Driving Simulator, University of Iowa College of Engineering; Adjunct Associate Research Scientist, Visual Function Laboratory, Department of Neurology, University of Iowa College of Medicine, Iowa City, Iowa

Scott R. Millis, Ph.D., A.B.P.P.

Assistant Professor, Department of Physical Medicine and Rehabilitation, Wayne State University School of Medicine; Chief, Department of Rehabilitation Psychology and Neuropsychology, Rehabilitation Institute, Detroit, Michigan

Aditya V. Mishra, M.D.

Instructor, Department of Ophthalmology, University of Utah School of Medicine, Salt Lake City, Utah

William W. Orrison, Jr., M.D.

Professor, Department of Radiology, Associate Professor, Department of Neurology, University of New Mexico School of Medicine; Director, New Mexico Institute of Neuroimaging; Chief, Division of Neuroradiology, New Mexico Regional Federal Medical Center, Albuquerque, New Mexico

Paul J. Perry, Ph.D.

Professor, Department of Psychiatry, University of Iowa College of Medicine; Professor, Department of Clinical Pharmacy, University of Iowa College of Pharmacy, Iowa City, Iowa

Steven H. Putnam, Ph.D.

Assistant Professor, Department of Physical Medicine and Rehabilitation, Wayne State University School of Medicine; Neuropsychologist, Department of Rehabilitation Psychology and Neuropsychology, Rehabilitation Institute, Detroit, Michigan

Matthew Rizzo, M.D.

Director, Division of Cognitive Neuroscience, Visual Function Laboratory, Department of Neurology, University of Iowa College of Medicine; Attending Physician, University of Iowa Hospitals and Clinics; Director of Medical Research, Department of Industrial Engineering, Iowa Driving Simulator, University of Iowa College of Engineering, University of Iowa, Iowa City, Iowa

Warren Rizzo, M.D.

Fellow of the American College of Rheumatology; Major, U.S. Air Force, Medical Corps Flight Surgeon Chief; Internal Medicine Consultant in Rheumatology, Aviano Air Force Base, Aviano, Italy

Robert G. Robinson, M.D.

Professor and Chairman, Department of Psychiatry, University of Iowa College of Medicine, Iowa City, Iowa

Carl L. Rowley, J.D.

Partner, Coburn and Croft, St. Louis, Missouri

Mario Schootman, Ph.D.

Adjunct Professor, Department of Preventive Medicine, University of Iowa, Iowa City, Iowa; Epidemiologist, Division of Substance Abuse and Health Promotion, Iowa Department of Public Health, Des Moines, Iowa

Elsa G. Shapiro, Ph.D.

Director, Pediatric Neuropsychology, Associate Professor, Departments of Neurology and Pediatrics, University of Minnesota Medical School—Minneapolis, Minneapolis, Minnesota

Jon Tippin, M.D.

Director, Electroneurodiagnostic Laboratory, Sacred Heart Medical Center; Neurologist, Division of Neurology, Rockwood Clinic, Spokane, Washington

James C. Torner, M.D.

Professor and Director, Division of Epidemiology, Department of Preventive Medicine and Environmental Health, University of Iowa College of Medicine, Iowa City, Iowa

Daniel Tranel, Ph.D.

Professor, Departments of Neurology and Psychology, University of Iowa College of Medicine; Chief, Benton Neuropsychology Laboratory, University of Iowa, Iowa City, Iowa

Juan C. Troncoso, M.D.

Departments of Neurology and Neuropathology, Johns Hopkins University School of Medicine, Baltimore, Maryland

Ronald J. Tusa, M.D., Ph.D.

Professor of Otolaryngology, Ophthalmology, and Neurology, University of Miami School of Medicine, Miami, Florida

Michael I. Weintraub, M.D., F.A.C.P., A.C.L.M.

Professor of Neurology, New York Medical College, Valhalla, New York; Chief, Department of Neurology, Phelps Memorial Hospital, North Tarrytown, New York

Thoru Yamada, M.D.

Professor and Chief, Division of Clinical Electrophysiology, Department of Neurology, University of Iowa College of Medicine, Iowa City, Iowa

William R. Yates, M.D.

Associate Professor, Department of Psychiatry, University of Iowa College of Medicine, Iowa City, Iowa

Nathan D. Zasler, M.D.

Executive Medical Director, NeuroRehabilitation Consortium, Richmond, Virginia

Carla Zeilmann, Pharm.D.

Resident, Department of Clinical Pharmacy, University of New Mexico College of Pharmacy, Albuquerque, New Mexico

Foreword

It is a truism that mortality and morbidity associated with traumatic head injury is one of the major public health problems in Western industrialized countries. The generally accepted statistic of an incidence of about 200 cases per 100,00 means that in the United States about 500,000 persons sustain a head injury each year. The associated mortality (i.e., immediate or early death) is 50,000 to 60,000 cases. Remarkable progress in the efficacy of neurosurgical intervention in the acute stage has resulted in a considerable reduction in mortality in recent years. Unfortunately, for the most part, this has resulted in a corresponding increase in morbidity. In this respect, it is worth noting that the "Good Recovery" category of the widely employed Glasgow Outcome Scale in fact includes many patients with significant physical, cognitive, social, and economic disabilities. Similarly, although about 80 percent of traumatic head injuries are classified on the basis of initial condition as "mild" (as contrasted to "moderate" or "severe"), an appreciable proportion of the "mild" injuries do result in one or another type of disability, particularly among children who face steadily increasing demands on their cognitive abilities and social adaptability as they mature.

In recent years there have been substantial advances in our understanding of the nature, mechanisms, diagnosis, and treatment of traumatic head injuries as well as of the risk factors associated with them. However, the effect of these gratifying advances has been countered by the steady increase of motor vehicles crashes and the alarming rise of violence in Western society. Thus, the problem is as pressing today as it was 20 years ago.

It is not surprising then that professional and scientific work in all aspects of the field has burgeoned in the last decade. Experimental and clinical research has proliferated and many books summarizing the present state of our knowledge have been published. It is from the vantage point of a participant in this effort as investigator, author, and editor that I have evaluated the present volume edited by Matthew Rizzo and Daniel Tranel.

Head Injury and Postconcussive Syndrome is a distinctive and valuable contribution to the field. It is extraordinarily comprehensive, more so than any similar effort that I know. The treatment of risk factors, the review of functional neuroimaging, the analysis of driving behavior and motor vehicle crashes (the most frequent cause of head injuries), and the emphasis on prevention are particularly noteworthy. The clinical chapters provide a critical analysis of present knowledge (and ignorance) that will be useful to researchers and provide sage advice to practitioners. The still perplexing problem of the postconcussive syndrome is considered carefully and with appropriate caution. The forensic questions that are so prominent in our litigious culture receive a detailed treatment that will be of value to those who face these questions in their practice.

The editors of this volume and the contributors to it are to be congratulated on an outstanding achievement.

Arthur Benton
Professor Emeritus
Benton Neuropsychology Laboratory
Department of Neurology
University of Iowa College of Medicine
Iowa City, Iowa

Acknowledgments

We are indebted to Dr. Arthur Benton for his encouragement and advice and for writing the Foreword, and to Dr. Rob Jones for his early discussions and continuous enthusiasm for this project. We thank our colleagues in the Department of Neurology and its head, Dr. Tony Damasio, for fostering a friendly academic environment and for making available the departmental resources necessary for the completion of our work. We greatly appreciate the contributions of the authors, including their patient and timely responses to our extensive editorial advice. Finally, we thank the people at Churchill Livingstone, namely Marc Strauss, Allan Ross, and Gerald Feldman for paving the way through the road to publication, Kerry Willis for her help with the initial organization, and Nancy Mullins who first contacted us with the idea for the book.

This work was supported by NIH PO NS19632 aimed at studying the neural substrates of human behavior and CDC R49/CCR710136 aimed at the prevention of injury in motor vehicle crashes.

Contents

Section V. Forensic Issues

Overview of Head Injury and Postconcussive Syndrome 1

Matthew Rizzo
Daniel Tranel

Head trauma is a crucial public health problem. The main concern is the potential for traumatic brain injury (TBI). The associated outcomes include disability or death for the grievously injured (Marshall et al., 1991), and marked disruption of the lives of their family members (Brooks, 1991). Even patients with relatively mild impact trauma and no apparent brain injury may report a daunting array of complaints. Among these are headache, neck pain, cognitive impairment, insomnia, dizziness, mood disturbances, and "spells," often lumped together under the rubric of postconcussive syndrome or postconcussional disorder (Table 1-1). There are many possible underlying explanatory factors (Bailey, 1906; Binder and Willis, 1991; Dikmen et al., 1986, 1994; Dikmen et al., 1995a; Dikmen et al., 1995b; Miller, 1961a, 1961b; Minderhoud et al., 1980; Stuss et al., 1985; van Zomeren and van den Burg, 1985). Moreover, individual troubles are magnified by the strikingly high incidence of head trauma and its predilection for younger adults. Indeed, most persons will probably have at least one such injury in their lifetime or at least know a friend or relative who has had one. The costs to society are high in terms of lost work and wages, increased medical bills and insurance premiums, legal fees, and higher taxes. There is also the cumulative burden of human pain and suffering. Clearly, these are issues that we cannot afford to ignore.

The purpose of this book is to develop a scientifically based approach for health care professionals to the problem of head injury and postconcussive syndrome. We are especially concerned with the diagnosis and management of injuries that fall on the

TABLE 1-1. Some Principal Symptoms Associated With Postconcussive Syndrome

Memory impairment
Concentration and attention difficulty
Headache and neck discomfort
Dizziness or vertigo
Mood changes (depression, anxiety, irritability)
Insomnia
Apathy
Fatigue
Blurred vision
Anhedonia

mild to moderate side of the severity spectrum. Medical awareness of such injuries has greatly increased in recent years, with many positive effects, including renewed efforts at injury prevention. In this regard, Levin et al. (1982, 1987, 1989) deserve much credit for their efforts. However, new problems have emerged and many scientific and practical issues remain. For example, who should take charge and coordinate treatment in head-injured patients? What specialty referrals or tests are appropriate? What treatments are effective, when should they conclude, and how should we track improvement? When should patients return to work? When are they disabled and how much? Effective responses to these issues require coordinated efforts from relevant specialists, a shared body of knowledge, and better cross-fertilization of ideas. We hope our book contributes to these ends.

This opening chapter provides a brief introduction to and overview of the problem of head trauma and postconcussive syndrome. Specific topics are covered in the 26 other chapters of the book. The subject matter is far-ranging and requires the input of specialists with a variety of insights on medicine, safety engineering, public health, public policy, and the law.

EPIDEMIOLOGIC FACTORS

Head injury is a worldwide problem, and in addition to providing the best possible remedial care, we must make efforts to emphasize injury prevention. Recognizing factors that contribute to elevated risk is a key step in risk reduction (see Ch. 2). In this context one important distinction is between head injuries that are unintentional and those that are intentional.

Unintentional injury comprises a broad spectrum of incidents, which may occur at work, at home, or on the road. Children may be injured by falls while they are at play. The elderly or infirm may be unstable of gait and can often stumble to the ground, even in the course of ordinary routine. Car crashes are ubiquitous, high-energy events, which affect all age groups, with sudden and potentially disastrous results. Certain groups of drivers pose a higher road risk, men under age 25 comprising a prime example statistically. Other potential crash risks include old age, cognitive impairment, psychiatric disease, medication effects, epilepsy, vestibular disease, and even cervical arthritis with inability to check the side windows and mirrors. Of course, some collisions are unavoidable, no matter who is driving. Fortunately, there are intelligent efforts underway to mitigate the risks (see Ch. 4). Seat belts offer protection in almost every American car. Air bags are a relatively new standard and provide additional security. Similarly, motorcycle, bicycle, and horseback riders would do well to wear helmets.

Intentional injuries are usually inflicted by known assailants. Alcohol and drugs are often factors, and the victims are often the weak. The shaken baby syndrome is an example of brain damage caused by violence committed against the helpless young, usually by the parents (see Chs. 3 and 22). TBI is also a tragic outcome of domestic abuse, in which usually women are beaten by their male companions. There is also elder abuse, inflicted by hostile offspring or other caretakers. Gunshot wounds or muggings are also frequent causes of traumatic brain injury.

SPECTRUM OF INJURY

The spectrum of deficits in head injury varies widely because of the magnitude and locations of the traumatic brain lesions associated with different types of trauma. At one extreme is death or permanent coma caused by a severe blow to the head resulting in skull fracture, hemorrhage, and massive and irreversible brain damage (Leetsma, 1988). At the other extreme is "mild" head injury associated with lesser forces. In such cases there is generally no skull fracture and the cranial vault remains intact despite being hit. If there is no associated impairment of consciousness or thought content, permanent brain injury is unlikely (see definitions below). Consider how often we all bump our heads, with no sequelae except a few "stars" and a knot on the head. Fortunately, the skull, its dural coverings, and the cerebrospinal fluid (CSF) lake of support, provide a rather effective cushion for the brain.

Surprisingly, however, mild head trauma may touch a patient's life in marked ways. Affected patients may report a host of complaints even though the physical circumstances of their trauma may not seem to predict a brain injury. The ability to develop a differential diagnosis is critical, since many of the complaints arising in such patients either are nonspecific or overlap those generated by other conditions or even by medications. The neuropsychological literature provides many highly sensitive procedures for measuring subtle cognitive and behavioral deficits (see Ch. 19), and the application of such procedures should be mandatory when there are questions of TBI-related changes in cognition or personality.

TYPES OF INJURY

The head injury literature is rife with varied terminology regarding nearly every facet of the condition. It is crucial therefore to clarify our terminology at the outset in order to facilitate communication with the reader. With regard to the various types of injury, operational definitions of commonly encountered terms are (in alphabetical order) are discussed below.

Acceleration-Deceleration Injury

In acceleration-deceleration injury, the head in motion stops suddenly. Usually it has struck an immovable object, such as the dashboard of a car in a car crash or the floor in a fall to the ground. After the head stops moving, the brain continues forward owing to its inertia and may be scraped across the ridges in the bottom of the skull (e.g., the bony partitions between the middle and anterior cranial fossae). This is essentially blunt trauma with the internal surface of the skull as the weapon. In addition, other forces may act less directly, producing axonal injury. Note, however, that just because a person was exposed to acceleration-deceleration forces does not mean that a brain injury occurred (see also descriptions of coup-contrecoup injuries and whiplash below).

Axonal Injury

Axonal injury is the stretching or distraction of nerve cell filaments caused by unequal forces acting on different parts of the brain. For a crude analogy, one may think of how a fracture forms within the substance of a jiggling bowl of gelatin. Factors dictating the pattern of injury are brain shape and size and tissue strength and heterogeneity. Important stress points include the interface between the gray matter of the cortical mantle and the underlying white matter, the splenium of the corpus callosum, and areas of the brainstem. In such regions rotational or translational forces may stretch or snap nerve cell filaments. Such forces may arise with rapid accelerations and decelerations of the head, as in a car crash or a fall. In theory, a cascade of associated biochemical events begins at the time of injury (see Chs. 3 and 6).

Axonal injury is generally associated with small amounts of bleeding due to stretching of the regional microvasculature. Evidence of blood or blood products can be visualized in life by neuroimaging procedures such as computed tomography (CT) or magnetic resonance imaging (MRI) (see Ch. 5) or in tissue specimens at autopsy (see Ch. 3). However, the presence of blood does not prove axonal damage and the absence of blood may not exclude it. A hypothetical example of the latter scenario might include a temporary axonal disturbance in the acute phase of a concussion. However, most allusions to axonal injury refer, de facto, to diffuse axonal injury (Adams et al., 1982; Gennarelli et al., 1982). The typical scenario for diffuse axonal injury is a life-threatening head injury with coma; however, there can also be focal axonal injury (see the case described by Troncoso and Gordon in Ch. 3).

Concussion

A concussion (Latin *concussus,* "a shaking," from *concutio,* "I shake violently" [Skinner, 1961]) is a group of symptoms and signs that begin in the immediate aftermath of a head injury. They include loss or clouding of memory for events preceding and following the injury (i.e., retrograde and anterograde amnesia), headache, neck pain, dizziness, mood changes, insomnia, lassitude, and a variety of other complaints. The effects of an uncomplicated concussion are usually transient. In most cases they resolve over weeks or months, suggesting reversible neuronal dysfunction rather than permanent injury. According to Skinner (1961), the condition was first described by Lafranchi of Milan (who believed the safe response in severe cases was to call on the Holy Ghost). Concussio labyrinth is dizziness or vertigo due to presumed inner ear concussion (see also the section *Postconcussive Syndrome* below).

Contusion

Contusions are bruises of the brain associated with focal swelling and bleeding, typically at the crowns of the cerebral gyri. Striking the head may cause transient deformation of the skull, which transmits destructive energy to the underlying brain (Fig. 1-1). A skull fracture may be associated but is not necessary. Contusions may occur wherever the brain surface is penetrated or abraded by an object, including the inner surfaces of the skull (see also the sections *Acceleration-Deceleration Injury* and *Coup-Contrecoup Injury*).

Coup-Contrecoup Injury

Coup-contrecoup injuries generally occur in acceleration-deceleration situations. In the typical scenario the head in motion is struck in a fall of several feet or in a car crash at higher velocity. Blunt trauma to the stationary head or simply walking into an object is not an expected cause. The coup injury occurs at the site of primary impact and is generally more serious. The contrecoup injury, if it occurs, is located on the surface of the brain opposite to the side of the impact. Curiously, in certain situations the severity of the contrecoup injury may exceed that of the coup injury. A key example is a fall in which the back of the head, the occiput, is struck. The coup injury may damage the occipital lobes, affecting vision; the contrecoup injury in the frontal lobes is sometimes worse, perhaps because the inner table of the skull is rougher in the front than in the back (Fig. 1-2).

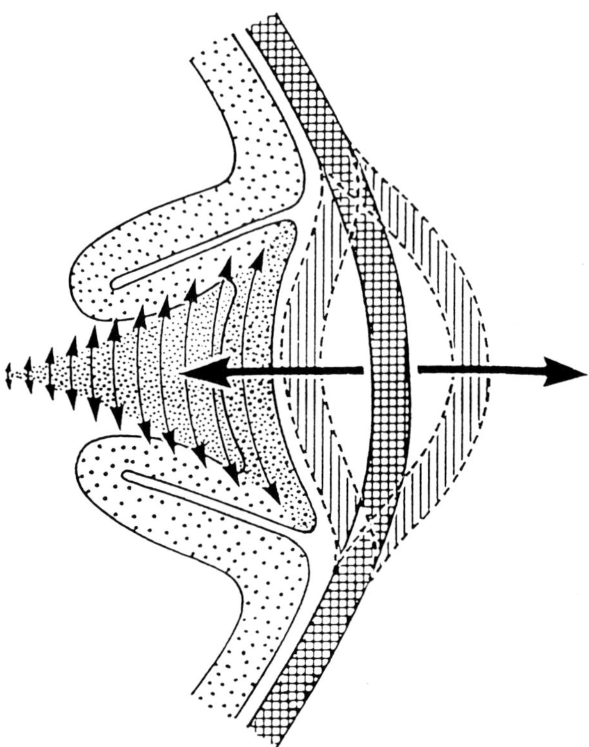

Fig. 1-1. Possible mechanism of production of contusion by mechanical deformation of the skull without fracture following a significant blow to the head. (From Leetsma, 1988, with permission.)

Edema

Injury to the brain may produce acute swelling. The swelling can be minor and focal, as in the region of a contusion. However, when there are severe injuries, the edema can be diffuse. In this case patients are generally obtunded, and their CT or MRI scans will show correlated loss of cortical surface markings and indistinct boundaries between the different tissue planes of the brain. The problem of edema is compounded when there is hemorrhage within the brain, as in an intracerebral hematoma, or around it, as in an epidural, subarachnoid, or subdural hematoma. The problem with diffuse edema is that the skull is a closed compartment and when the swelling exceeds a critical point, this elevates the intracranial pressure and can cause herniation of the brain (see the section *Herniation*).

Head Injury

A head injury can be defined as traumatic damage to any part of the head. The trauma may be exclusively extracranial; for example, it may only affect the mandible (lower jaw). Alternatively, the injury may damage the cranium or cerebral vault. There may be an associated skull fracture. Damage to the temporal bone may affect the balance mechanisms of the inner ear. An open or compound fracture exposes the cranial contents to the outside environment. There may be an associated CSF leak with infectious sequelae such as meningitis. This differs from closed head injury. It is important to note that head injury does not automatically result in brain injury or even concussion. Most individuals will receive several blows to the head during their lifetime with no resulting brain damage. Interchangeable use of the terms *head* injury and *brain* injury is unacceptable.

Hemorrhage

Head trauma may result in bleeding within the brain or around it. Within the brain, contusion and axonal injury are associated with small amounts of

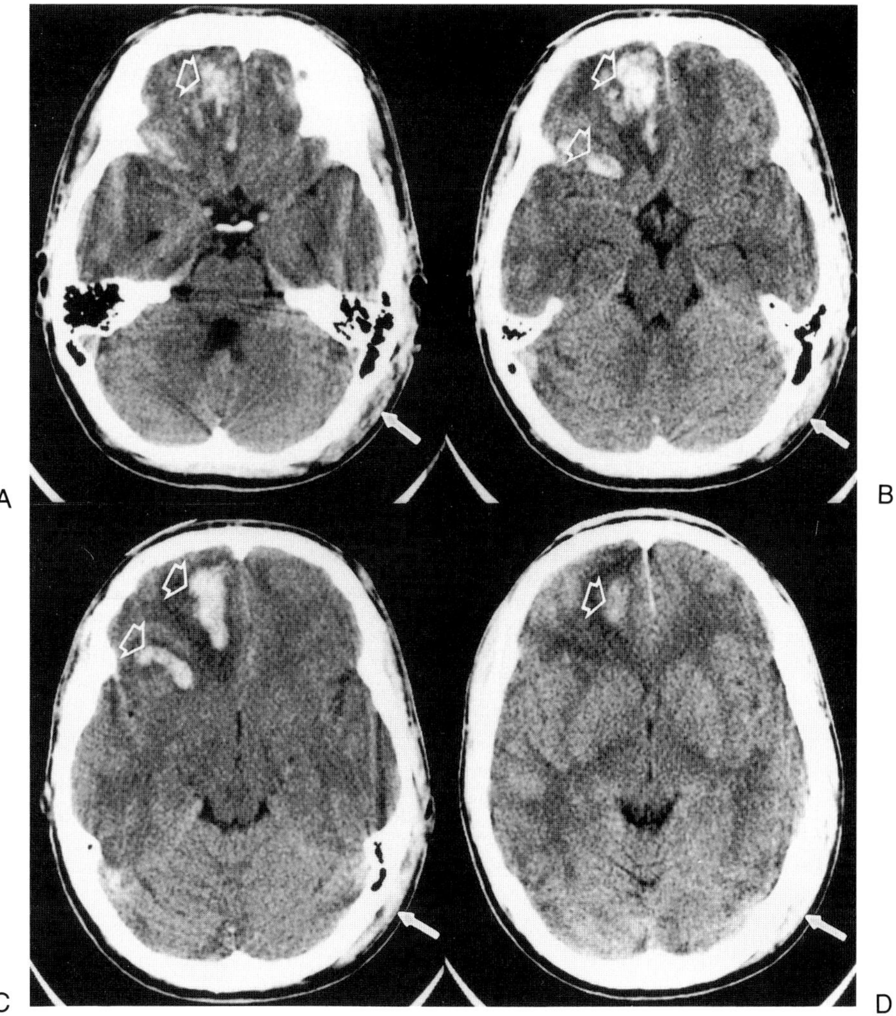

Fig. 1-2. Unenhanced CT scan of the brain of a 25-year-old man who reportedly fell off the back of a moving truck. He had a 5-minute loss of consciousness and post-traumatic amnesia lasting for several days. The CT taken the day after injury shows evidence of soft tissue swelling near the left occiput (*solid white arrows*). The underlying brain appears normal. There is a large contusion, however, on the opposite side of the brain in the right frontal lobe (*open white arrows*). The blood within the contusion appears white and the surrounding edema is dark. There is no overlying soft tissue swelling. Thus, this is probably a contrecoup injury (see text). The lesion extends from **(A)** the base of the left frontal lobe, where the brain was probably abraded by the rough inner table of the skull, in a rostral direction over several centimeters **(B–D)**. This patient had a disturbance of olfaction.

blood. Penetrating injuries can cause massive bleeding. Bleeding around the brain (i.e., extra-axial blood) can be subarachnoid, subdural, or epidural. Epidural hematoma is associated with tearing of the middle meningeal artery, usually in association with fracture of the temporal bone. This is an acute, life-threatening situation as is tearing of the dural venous sinuses. Acute traumatic subdural and subarachnoid hemorrhage in an adult are associated with severe blows to the head. Infants, however, may develop subarachnoid and subdural bleeding from being violently shaken. Older individuals may accumulate chronic subdural hematomas with minimal or even no apparent head trauma. The explanatory hypothesis is that the bridging veins between the brain and the skull are longer and more susceptible to tearing in infants and older persons. The significance of extra-axial hemorrhage is that there may be injury to the brain by secondary effects such as compression. Alternatively, there may never be symptoms.

Herniation

When the brain is swollen or bleeding, it may herniate through the rigid closed compartments of the cranium. The CSF cisterns are obliterated and the ventricles often collapse. Herniation can also lead to compression of the cerebral arteries. For example, the posterior cerebral artery may be pushed against the tentorium, producing stroke and further edema. There are several different herniation syndromes. For instance, the cingulate gyrus may herniate beneath the falx. Transtentorial herniation is more serious. Here the uncus of the temporal lobe of the swollen hemisphere pushes below the tentorial membrane and against the brainstem. This produces pupillary dilation on the side of the swelling (Hutchinson's pupil), with paralysis of the opposite limbs, deepening coma, and eventually death. Subsequent changes in the opposite pupil can provide an index of this deterioration (Ropper, 1990). Bilateral swelling over the frontal lobes or cerebral vertex may produce the central herniation syndrome, in which both hemispheres push downward through the tentorium at once, producing bilateral weakness and often demise later on. Swelling in the posterior fossa may produce herniation upward through the tentorium or downward against the brainstem and through the foramen magnum, whereupon death follows closely.

Traumatic Brain Injury

TBI is defined as damage to the brain triggered by externally acting forces. There are many causes (Leetsma, 1988). There can be direct penetration by a sharp object such as a knife or icepick. A bullet tears, lacerates, burns, and bruises the brain and produces additional damage by secondary missile fragments, skull splinters, bleeding, and infection. The brain can also be injured by a sustained force that crushes the skull. More important, however, are dynamic impacts. These include being struck on the head by a blunt object or striking one's head against a fixed object. Fragments of a displaced or open skull fracture may injure the brain; however, the edges of a nondisplaced or closed fracture may act briefly as a bevel.

Interestingly, a brain injury such as a contusion may occur in the absence of skull penetration or fracture. Somehow, transient deformation of the cranium transmits energy to the underlying tissues. Alternatively, the brain may be bruised against the inner surface of the skull when the moving head abruptly strikes a fixed object, as in a car crash or a fall (see the sections *Acceleration-Deceleration Injury* and *Coup-Contrecoup Injury*). Furthermore, there are indirect injuries caused by shearing forces between the different planes of the brain (see the section *Axonal Injury*). Dementia pugilistica in "punch drunk" boxers may reflect the accrual of axonal lesions after years of beatings.

A hallmark of traumatic brain injury is recovery, which may be partial or complete. Contusions heal, while edema and blood are reabsorbed. There are also examples of reversible axonal disturbances in both the peripheral and central nervous systems. Consider the resolution of symptoms after striking the ulnar nerve at the elbow ("funny bone") and the recovery of arm function after an axonal stretch injury of the brachial plexus. These reversible disturbances are known as *neurapraxias.* In more severe injuries, axons may grow again if axis cylinders are intact; demyelinated axons may recover in Guillain-Barré syndrome, optic neuritis, and multiple sclerosis, resulting in a range of functional residua from normal to highly impaired (see also the sections *Edema, Hemorrhage,* and *Herniation*).

Postconcussive Syndrome

Postconcussive syndrome also called Postconcussive disorder, is diagnosed when the effects of a concussion do not fully resolve (See Table 1-1). This sequela, once called "traumatic cerebrasthenia" (Bailey, 1906), may be the result of a neural injury accompanied by abnormal profiles on neurologic, neuropsychological, and other laboratory testing. However, symptoms may occur in the absence of a demonstrable neural injury, and in this case causes other than TBI must be considered. Symptoms that appear only after a significant time has elapsed following an injury raise doubts about whether they can be attributed to TBI.

Preliminary operational criteria for "postconcussional disorder" were published in the Diagnostic and Statistical Manual (1994) of the American Psychiatric Association (DSM-IV) based on the recommendation of Brown et al. (1994) (Table 1-2). The injured person must meet two of three initial criteria to be eligible for the diagnosis. The first two requirements have to do with amnesia and loss of consciousness

TABLE 1-2. DSM-IV: Proposed Criteria for Postconcussion Syndrome

A. History of head injury that includes at least two of the following:
   1. Loss of consciousness for 5 minutes or more
   2. Post-traumatic amnesia of 12 hours or more
   3. Onset of seizures (post-traumatic epilepsy) within 6 months of head injury
B. Current symptoms (either new symptoms or substantially worsening preexisting symptoms) to include
   1. At least the following two cognitive difficulties:
      a. Learning or memory (recall)
      b. Concentration
   2. At least three of the following affective or vegetative symptoms:
      a. Easy fatiguability
      b. Insomnia or sleep/wake cycle disturbances
      c. Headache (substantially worse than before injury)
      d. Vertigo/dizziness
      e. Irritability and/or aggression on little or no provocation
      f. Anxiety, depression, or lability of affect
      g. Personality change (e.g., social or sexual inappropriateness, childlike behavior)
      h. Aspontaneity/apathy
C. Symptoms associated with a significant difficulty in maintaining premorbid occupational or academic performance or with a decline in social, occupational, or academic performance

(From Brown et al., 1994, with permission.)

and the third has to do with seizures. Unfortunately, the third criterion is often not helpful in cases of mild head injury. The diagnosis of postconcussive syndrome is often at issue in this group; however the risk of an epileptic seizure is probably no greater than that of the general population (Annegers et al., 1980) (see also Ch. 11).

According to current DSM-IV criteria, individuals who meet research criteria for postconcussive syndrome would be diagnosed as having a "cognitive disorder not otherwise specified." The differential diagnosis includes somatization disorder, undifferentiated somatoform disorder, factitious disorder, and malingering.

Whiplash

Whiplash is the result of rapid movement of the head upon the neck associated with complaints of neck pain. The concept may have originated in the 1870s with "railway spine," a diagnosis made in employees of the British Railway System who rode trains that made sudden starts and stops (see Ch. 26). Nowadays, the most common cause of whiplash is a rear end vehicular collision, causing a rapid extension (hyperextension) followed by flexion of the neck. The head may simply reach its limits of excursion on the neck without having been struck. There may be soft tissue injury (i.e., a strain or sprain to the ligaments and muscles that support the spine), but the injury is typically self-limited. A protruding disc must be excluded; there is also the highly litigated morass of myofascial pain, fibromyalgia, and chronic pain, including cervicogenic headaches (see Chs. 8, 13, and 26). Cognitive complaints have also been attributed to whiplash. However, whiplash is typically self-limited, and when there is chronic pain or persistent cognitive complaints, there are often factors at play other than the injury itself (Livingston, 1993; Pearce, 1994; Radanov et al., 1993). Whiplash may be associated with head injury, traumatic brain injury, and concussion, but it is a completely different entity (see also the sections *Acceleration-Deceleration Injury* and *Axonal Injury*).

MODELS OF HEAD INJURY

Much of what we know about TBI comes from studies of brain-injured patients. The main thrust of these studies is to correlate evidence of structural brain injury with cognitive and behavioral changes. Among the many data to consider are history; coma and behavioral scales; physical examination; brain images obtained by CT, MRI, single-photon emission computed tomography (SPECT), and positron emission tomography (PET) techniques; and electrophysiologic data obtained from electroencephalographic (EEG) procedures. Tissue confirmation of injury is generally not obtained unless a patient dies of the injuries. However, long-term survivors are often lost to autopsy follow-up. It is possible to use cadavers similarly to crash test dummies to study the pattern of gross structural damage that result in different physical settings (Schneider and Nahum, 1973). However, the cascade of changes that evolves in living brain tissue following injury does not develop in tissue that was dead to start with, and obviously there is no post-traumatic behavior to evaluate. Consequently, in lieu of direct evidence in humans, inferences on the neuropathology of human brain injury survivors are sometimes made from data obtained from experiments in animals (Gennarelli, 1983).

Pathologic studies in animals have concentrated on how externally applied forces to the head are transmitted to the brain. For instance, Ommaya and Gennarelli (1974) used a helmet-piston assembly to jolt squirrel monkeys' heads over small displacements (Fig. 1-3). They reported that severe axonal injury could occur without striking the head, especially in cases of angular rotation, a finding sometimes quoted as evidence for axonal injury in simple whiplash cases. Nevertheless, the findings in such studies are difficult to translate to the human setting. One factor is the physical nature of the injury. The magnitude and direction of acceleration-deceleration forces in such experimental setups are likely to be quite different from those in any human injuries sustained in a car crash or a fall. A second factor is interspecies differences. Important factors dictating the pattern of brain injury are brain shape and size and the mobility of the head on the neck. However, the brains of monkeys are smaller by an order of magnitude or more than those of humans, and there are also differences in neck length and musculature between the species. A third factor is the outcome of the experimentally induced injury. The 12 monkeys studied in the Ommaya-Gennarelli rotational setup were comatose, all had subdural and subarachnoid hemorrhage, and death even occurred. These are hardly the typical sequelae of a mild head injury or whiplash. Similar objections obtain for other widely quoted models, such as the fluid percussion model, in which a piston is driven through a surgical window against the dura or brain of a rat (Dixon et al., 1987, 1991).

Even if the pattern of pathologic injury in experimental animals and humans were very similar, it would still be difficult to compare the behavioral outcomes in the different species. It is possible to test for memory or attentional impairments and even for increased irritability or social withdrawal, but symptoms such as headache, dizziness, depression, or post-traumatic stress disorder are virtually impossible to measure in nonhuman animals. Experiments in nonhuman species have obvious value, but the results require careful consideration and may not be transferable to humans. The growing body of research evidence in human cases is of considerable importance.

DIAGNOSTIC CONSIDERATIONS

The fair and accurate disposition in head injury cases requires a clear understanding of the relevant pathologic mechanisms and underlying science, alluded to above. It also requires a command of the historical and physical evidence. Informed practitioners will be much less likely to err and dismiss a significant brain injury as malingering or as a mere "ding" (Yarnell and Lynch, 1973). Of equal importance, they also will be less prone to invoke an unsupportable and unduly grave diagnosis in the face of low-impact circumstances and questionable laboratory results. This point cannot be overemphasized, and in our experience, the single most common source of errors in diagnosing conditions such as TBI and postconcussive syndrome is inaccurate or incomplete historical reconstruction.

History

Accurate diagnosis in cases of possible head injury and postconcussive syndrome requires a command of the historical evidence. This should include a history of present illness, past medical history, and social history. Several points warrant amplification.

Sources of Referral

Referral sources in cases of suspected TBI include colleagues (e.g., neurologists, psychiatrists, neurosurgeons, and psychologists) and other agents including insurance companies and law firms. In any case, the opinion should not depend on the source of referral.

Sources of Information

One source of information in head trauma cases is the interview with the patient. This can be supplemented by talking with the patient's family members or close friends. Such lay informants may be helpful, although they are usually untrained observers and may also have a strong point of view. On interviewing

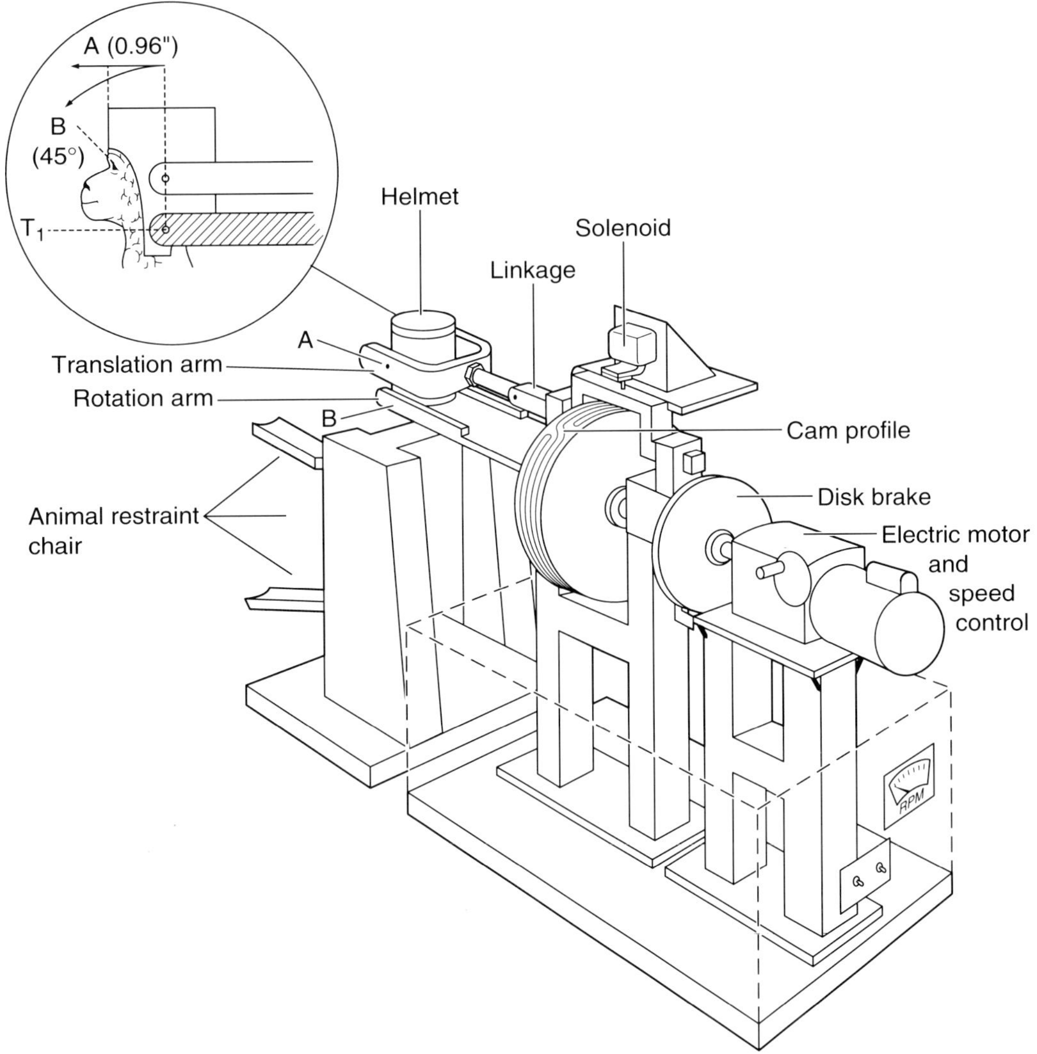

Fig. 1-3. Head-accelerating device (HAD-II). Monkeys wore a helmet (circular insert) coupled to a motor. This setup was used to jolt monkeys' heads across small displacements. Angular rotational acceleration especially produced severe injury without striking the head. (From Ommaya and Gennarelli, 1974, with permission.)

these individuals, we should gather descriptions of what they actually saw or heard, not their interpretation of those events or their diagnoses. Invested observers can sometimes misinform as much as help.

If the history as provided by informants is in doubt or unavailable, other sources may exist. These include medical records, both preceding and following an injury under evaluation, and associated laboratory studies. In cases with legal ramifications, there may be deposition testimony from the patient, defendant, and other lay or expert witnesses. These sources of information should be carefully evaluated with respect to whether they issue from disinterested or biased parties.

Reconstruction of the Incident

Weighing the likelihood or extent of TBI is aided by accurate evidence regarding the physical circumstances of trauma (Tables 1-3 and 1-4). If the incident was remote, the practitioner may want to attempt a careful reconstruction. This can take some effort, but the reward is improved accuracy of diagnosis. This best approach is to assemble as much history as is

TABLE 1-3. Factors in Evaluating the Type and Severity of a Traumatic Incident

Nature of the physical incident (e.g., blunt trauma, acceleration-deceleration in a car crash or fall)
Whether or not the head was struck
Loss of consciousness: duration
Amnesia (retrograde and anterograde) duration for the initial incident
Initial neurologic findings
Initial laboratory findings (e.g., brain CT)
Seizure occurrence in proximity to the incident
Coma scale scores

possible, especially from primary sources dating back to the incident in question. The reason that primary sources are so important is that they generally provide nonbiased accounts. Pertinent documents include the police records, ambulance report, emergency room admission and discharge summaries, nursing notes, doctors' letters and even early insurance claims. There may be a Glasgow Coma Scale score (Teasdale and Jennett, 1974) available (Table 1-5 [original version] and see Table 22-2 for pediatric version of scale), or perhaps the score can be estimated from the available descriptions of the patient's level of consciousness, verbal report, and ability to follow instructions. The Glasgow Coma Scale is one useful predictor of recovery, especially if the score is 13 to 15.

Attributing all the symptoms following a traumatic incident to brain injury can be a mistake. Seeing "stars," being "dazed," and other such colloquial descriptions do not necessarily signify a brain injury. Neither does dizziness or lack of memory for events, as described below.

Amnesia and Loss of Consciousness

Two important factors to address with respect to the acute event are amnesia and loss of consciousness (Brown et al., 1994). Amnesia is one signature of concussion. The amnesia may be retrograde, leading to an inability to relate what happened earlier in the day, before the incident. More commonly, it is anterograde, in which case the patient fails to encode what happened after the event (see Fig. 20-1). It is important to note that some patients interpret their amnesia as a loss of consciousness and mistakenly report the latter. Primary records can help to clarify this. If a patient renders in clear detail all that transpired before, during, and after an incident of head trauma, this militates against TBI.

TABLE 1-4. Factors in Evaluating Closed Head Injury in Vehicular Crashes

Relative velocities at impact
Type of impact (e.g., rear-end collision, side impact, single vehicle, multiple vehicle)
Position in the vehicle (e.g., driver, back seat)
Seat belt status (belted or unbelted)
Presence of air Bags (Front or side)
Type and size of vehicles involved (e.g., car, motorcycle, truck)

TABLE 1-5. The Glasgow Coma Scale

Eye opening	Spontaneous	4
	To sound	3
	To pain	2
	None	1
Best motor response	Obeys	6
	Localizes	5
	Withdraws	4
	Abnormal flexion	3
	Extends	2
	None	1
Verbal response	Oriented	5
	Confused	4
	Inappropriate	3
	Incomprehensible	2
	None	1
Total	Eye + motor + verbal	3–15

(From Teasdale and Jennett, 1974, with permission.)

The failure to recite details surrounding a traumatic incident does not prove amnesia, and not all amnesia is due to brain injury. Patients may not register what happened, owing to excitement, anxiety, or fear as a traumatic event such as a crash unfolds, or events may have transpired rapidly while the patients were inattentive or asleep (Loftus, 1982). Perhaps alcohol or recreational drugs was a factor, in which case the results of drug screens may be informative. Alternatively, powerful sedatives may have been administered at the scene or soon thereafter for acute musculoskeletal injuries, fractures, or other painful conditions. Also, importantly, human memory is imperfect, and normal observers may forget specific details over time (Loftus, 1982). Forgetting is not a form of post-traumatic amnesia.

Time Course of Injury

Head injury, TBI, and postconcussive syndrome, like many other acute neurologic events, tend to improve with time. The zenith of trouble is generally at the time of the acute injury and shortly thereafter. Depression or headaches that begin, for example, 3 months after a head injury are probably due to other factors. Also, the mere fact that there was a head injury does not mean that all successive troubles are related. One should avoid the logical fallacy of *post hoc, ergo propter hoc* (i.e., if one event follows another, then the former event must have caused the latter). If a patient gets worse, not better after head trauma, the culprits may be (1) medications, (2) psychological factors, (3) another medical condition, (4) legal considerations, and (5) iatrogenic effects.

Ongoing Complaints

Patients with head injury and postconcussive syndrome may report a wide range of troubles, such as cognitive and behavioral complaints, head and neck pain, and dizziness and insomnia. A diagnostic challenge presents because many of these complaints have high base rates in other conditions and in the general population. The challenge can be even greater in the setting of litigation, where the base rate of complaints is high despite no history of brain injury (Lees-Haley and Brown, 1993; Gualtieri, 1995; Youngjohn et al., 1995) (Table 1-6). Also, the level of symptoms can be falsely elevated or simulated through the use of poorly designed and leading questionnaires (Wong, 1994). Consequently, our approach with trauma patients is to have them address their complaints in order of perceived importance. Evaluators should listen carefully and try to flesh out the symptoms without leading patients or putting words in their mouth. A spontaneous complaint may carry more weight than an elicited or solicited one.

TABLE 1-6. Neuropsychological Complaint Base Rates of 170 Personal Injury Claimants[a]

Rate (%)	Symptom
93	Anxiety or nervousness
92	Sleeping problems
89	Depression
88	Headaches
80	Back pain
79	Fatigue (mental or physical)
78	Concentration problems
77	Worries about health
77	Irritability
74	Neck pain
65	Impatience
62	Restlessness
61	Feeling disorganized
60	Loss of interest
59	Confusion
56	Loss of efficiency in carrying out everyday tasks
55	Shoulder pain
53	Memory problems
44	Dizziness
41	Sexual problems
39	Numbness
38	Nausea
34	"Word finding problems, not finding the word you want, using the wrong word"
32	"Visual problems, blurring, or seeing double"
30	Trembling or tremors
29	Hearing problems
29	Constipation
24	Foot pain
24	Trouble reading
21	Bumping into things
21	Elbow pain
18	Speech problems
15	Impotence

[a] Lees-Haley and Brown (1993) found high complaint base rates in personal injury claimants who had no history of traumatic brain injury. The pattern of findings bear a striking resemblance to postconcussive symptoms (Table 1-1).

(Adapted from Lees-Haley and Brown, 1993, with permission.)

Anosognosia

Interestingly, some patients who have marked deficits due to TBI will deny they have much of a problem and fail to report it. They may have anosognosia, a pathologic failure to recognize their injury, which is due to cerebral damage. These patients are not just trying to put the best face on a bad personal situation. Anosognosics do not recognize their injury and care little to blame someone for it. We are reminded of the recent case of Reginald Denny, who was beaten senseless during the Los Angeles riots of 1992. His bland response toward his assailants, even after viewing bloody footage of their crime at their 1994 trial, bespoke TBI more likely than altruism, equanimity, or brotherly love. It is important to distinguish anosognosia from a genuine absence of defects, however, and in most cases the prudent first strategy is to accept patients' descriptions of themselves at face value.

Psychosocial History

Academic records, occupational history, social background, and psychiatric history are all quite germane to the assessment of TBI. The academic history assumes immediate relevance in head-injured children, teenagers, and young adults who are still attending school. It is also highly relevant to the issue of determining whether cognitive defects have occurred as a result of TBI (see Section IV of book, Neuropsychological Considerations). In fact, the caliber of academic performance as indicated in level of education, quality of grades, honors and awards, and standardized test scores (e.g., SAT and ACT) is probably the single best measure of premorbid cognitive status. Failure to obtain such information and reliance on patient reports that may overestimate previous ability levels can lead to serious errors in establishing acquired cognitive deficits.

Occupational history is also quite relevant. The examiner should raise several questions. Has patient held a steady job or skipped around instead? What are the demands of the patient's work? Have there been promotions or salary raises? Does the current performance deviate from the past? If so, what are the specific difficulties, and can they be reasonably explained by the patient's objective deficits? Is the patient making ends meet or seeking disability payments? There may be military records or written evaluations by job supervisors to consult as well as occupational therapy records. Multiple factors determine the patient's capability and likelihood of returning to work, as outlined by Dikmen et al. (1994).

Social life should also be investigated in the assessment of TBI. Friendships, family life, and work may suffer. Injured homemakers may fail to conduct the myriad activities that used to occupy their time, such as preparing meals, cleaning, shopping, or even doing the taxes. Husbands and wives may bicker. Children's grades may suffer. Some patients simply sit at home all day. Reading and other hobbies and even television watching may be curtailed. There are many strategies for inquiring on these issues, including detailed instruments for assessing the activities of daily life (Dikmen et al., 1995).

Premorbid or comorbid mental conditions may factor into a patient's complaints. To wit, was there a previous head injury, neurologic disease, major psychiatric condition, or personality disorder? (See Ch. 15.) Is substance abuse a factor? Is there medicine or doctor shopping? Has the patient had to take drugs with central nervous system side effects? (see Ch. 17). Are the patient's medical needs being attended to?

Internal Consistency

In practice, it is useful to compare the details told by the trauma patient with other sources. It is reassuring if they jibe, but troublesome if they differ, especially if the discrepancy favors secondary gain. Money, disability, sympathy, or even revenge can be factors. Hate may be directed toward the party perceived to have caused injury, lawyers or insurance agents provoking endless personal intrusions, or medical personnel who seem unready to recognize their trouble. Patients may embellish or falsify their reports to right these perceived wrongs. In such cases it becomes important to seek additional sources.

Trouble arises if the head that "went through a windshield" actually showed not the slightest bump or bruise in any of the primary treatment records. Equally suspicious is "retrocoma" or "retroamnesia," first appearing some time after the incident. A patient claiming former perfect health may turn out to have had a long history of migraine headaches or multiple traumas preceding the event at issue. Academic transcripts may show that the former A student was really a C student. Persons reporting severe occupational disability may have had no objective trouble at all observed at work, received raises, been promoted, or even successfully trained for an equally demanding job.

Sometimes there is absence of confirmation rather than a conflict of facts. Specifically, the number and severity of complaints may fail to match the history, physical findings, and laboratory data. For example, patients who report frequent spells diagnosed as posttraumatic epileptic seizures may never have had a single spell observed, even by their spouses, and laboratory evaluations such as EEG or MRI may produce normal or nonspecific results. Otherwise, a patient's complaints may defy expected physiology; dense amnesia with convenient islands of recall, or forgetting one's own name, are two of many possible examples (see Ch. 25).

People can, of course, forget the precise details of a remote injury. Also, recollection is moulded by rehearsal and altered by outside influences. In the case of closed head injury, repeated exposure to doctors, attorneys, and even medical literature may reshape the history and suggest symptoms that were never actually present. Patients may rationalize that they have finally become aware of a chronic deficit that they were once too confused or ignorant to recognize. Some unusual presentations of mild traumatic brain injury are listed in Table 1-7.

Physical Examination

Patients with head injury or postconcussive syndrome should have a general examination of organ systems. Usually, this has been accomplished before

TABLE 1-7. Unusual Sequelae of Mild Traumatic Brain Injury

Post-traumatic stress disorder
Repressed memory syndrome
Chronic fatigue syndrome
Complex partial seizures
Rage attacks or episodic explosive disorder
Directed violence or planned crime
Chronic pain syndromes
Dystonia
Anosmia
Late symptom onset

the patient reaches a specialist, either on an emergency basis or in subsequent follow-up appointments. It would be a grave disservice to diagnose a patient's chronic sense of reduced well-being as due to TBI when the patient actually had the treatable systemic effects of, for instance, diabetes or thyroid disease.

The neurologic examination is a cornerstone of the examination in trauma patients. A head-to-toe approach, similar to the strategy of a general medical examination is used (see Rodnitzky, 1988 and Mayo Clinic, 1981, for excellent reviews). Briefly, there is an assessment of the 12 cranial nerves. The first cranial (olfactory) nerve may be compromised by shearing off of its twiglets as it passes through the cribriform plate of the ethmoid bone. The sense of smell can also be disturbed by damage to the pyriform (olfactory) cortex at the base of the frontal lobe (Costanzo and Zasler, 1991; Doty, 1991; for testing procedures, Doty, 1983). The examiner should beware that olfactory trouble may be related to smoking, congestion, age, medications, psychiatric disorders, sinus disease, or even a deviated septum.

Evaluation of motor function should include testing of muscle strength, tone, station and gain, and ability to carry out functional maneuvers such as toe, heel, and tandem walking and hopping. Coordination assessment comprises several additional maneuvers, including rapid alternating movements of the hands (e.g., finger-on-thumb tapping and alternating pronation and supination of the hand upon the lap), finger (the patient's) to nose (the patient's) to finger (the examiner's), and heel-to-knee-to-shin testing. Tendon reflexes should be assessed in the usual manner, as should the presence of pathologic reflexes (Babinski, Glabellar, snout, root, suck).

The sensory examination requires the patient to detect, discriminate, identify, and report on different sensory stimuli (e.g., sharp, dull, vibration, and joint position); it is susceptible to error in patients without optimal cooperation. (Aspects of the neurologic examination in closed head injury are reviewed in Ch. 16 and 21.) Features of the acute examination, such as testing for CSF leaks, Battle's sign and raccoon eye (signs of basilar skull fracture) are reviewed in critical care books in neurosurgery or neurology (e.g., Ropper, 1993). The examination of the coma patient has been reviewed by Plum and Posner (1980).

Of course, the mental status screening assessment is of critical importance in the neurologic encounter with the head-injured patient (for an educational review, see Strub and Black, 1985). Pertinent impressions can be derived as soon as the examiner lays eyes on the patient and can be made throughout the interview and examination, whether or not the patient is aware of being observed. It is possible to screen for language, memory, attention, and mood, and to take note of anosognosia. The mental status of Folstein et al. (1975) is a convenient screening tool and may help direct the need for a more detailed assessment by a neuropsychologist. (See Section III of book, Specific Manifestations and Treatments.)

Depending on the pattern of complaints, the patient should also have a number of specialty evaluations. Chapter 9 reviews the neuro-otologic approach to the dizzy patient. The patient with mood, thought, or personality disorders can be referred to a psychiatrist (see Chs. 15 and 16). The evaluations of head and neck pain are reviewed in Chapters 8 and 13 and the neuro-ophthalmologic evaluation is reviewed in Chapter 10. However, it is possible for a generalist to perform a few screening maneuvers to help guide referrals to such specialists. For example, a basic neuro-ophthalmologic screen for pupillary irregularities or ocular motility or visual field defects requires only a flashlight, a Snellen card or magazine, and a few fingers. It does not take long to check visual acuity or to screen the fundi by ophthalmoscopy. These and a few other simple observations can reveal important treatable causes of headache. It takes only a few moments to check blood pressure and listen for carotid bruits to screen for hypertensive or ischemic headache. A mouthful of bad teeth is obvious, and sinusitis is easily assessed by pressing over the frontal and maxillary areas. The cervical spine is easily screened for range of motion or point tenderness. It is not difficult to learn to perform maneuvers such as the Barany maneuver to screen for a neuro-otologic disturbance.

Finally, several demonstrations on the examination may suggest that a patient's trouble is not due to traumatic neurologic injury. A few of the possible patterns are listed in Table 1-8. When such findings obtain, alternative diagnostic possibilities should be explored. These include psychological or psychiatric conditions, including somatoform, conversion or personality disorders, or malingering (see Chs. 15, 16, 25, and 26).

Laboratory Procedures

With an appropriate knowledge base, the scientist-clinician will learn to recognize the advantages, limitations, and indications of current laboratory procedures in head injury and postconcussive syndrome. The main issue is detecting the presence and gauging the severity of TBI and associated conditions. No test is 100 percent sensitive and 100 percent specific; however, skillful use of the available techniques can provide several converging lines of evidence to confirm the diagnosis.

TABLE 1-8. Suspicious Findings on the Examination of "Mild" Head Injury Patients

1. Sensory deficits that split the midline (e.g., feeling vibration only on one side of head when a tuning fork is applied to the middle of the forehead)
2. Anosmia with insensitivity to noxious trigeminal (V1) stimulants (e.g., ammonia);
3. Variable findings (e.g., the patient strolls into a room, but when leg strength is tested directly, the leg is paretic)
4. Tunnel vision that defies the laws of optics (i.e., objects just beyond view close-up remain unseen no matter how far away they are removed)
5. Monocular polyopia unexplained by abnormalities of the eye
6. Astasia-abasia (basically, the inability to stumble in a person who presents an unsteady gait, but really balances as well as a surfer)
7. Nonepileptic seizure activity
8. Lack of effort on strength testing (e.g., breakaway weakness, Hoover's [heel] sign
9. Ganser's syndrome (the patient is always slightly off [e.g., one off on counting fingers])
10. "La belle indifférence"
11. Theatrics (e.g., moaning and flinching in response to the slightest touch of the skin without specific localization)
12. MMSE scores in the range of a severely demented Alzheimer's patient in a person with an unimpressive story and otherwise normal demeanor
13. Selective memory (e.g., detailed recall of convenient facts in a person who otherwise seems to remember almost nothing or acts confused)
14. Failure to provide direct answers to direct questions

As specialty approaches to head injury have grown, so has the number of diagnostic tests (Table 1-9). Procedures employed currently include neuropsychological batteries (See Section IV of book, Neuropsychological Considerations), electrophysiologic studies, and SPECT and PET techniques (See Section II of book, Diagnostic Techniques). There are x-rays, radiographs, ophthalmologic procedures, and otolaryngologic procedures (see Section III of book, Special Manifestations and Treatments). Deciding when to apply such procedures can be difficult, and one of the objectives of this book is to provide the practitioner guidance in selecting relevant tests.

One additional consideration regards the use of nonstandard or unreliable tests. The use of neuropsychological procedures, for example, should be restricted to well standardized tests for which appropriate normative information is available (see Section IV of book, Neuropsychological Considerations). Some tests have research value (e.g., PET) but are prematurely applied in the clinical setting of head injury and postconcussive syndrome (see Ch. 6). Other tests are well accepted (e.g., EEG and nerve conduction studies) but may have technical problems or lack standards or controls for the laboratory or population in which they are being used. The American Academy of Neurology (1995) has adopted important positions on the use of certain tests, including thermography and EEG brain mapping (also called computed or quantitative EEG). Such guidelines should be carefully followed.

TREATMENT

The options for treatment in head injury and postconcussive syndrome have burgeoned. This development reflects in part the efforts of multiple specialists, all viewing the topic of head injury and postconcussive syndrome in light of their own expertise. Unfortunately, they speak somewhat different languages, often meet and publish in different places, and may have trouble keeping abreast of each other's work. As the number of potential diagnoses has grown, so have the number of treatments, including medications and rehabilitation efforts. The practical challenge is to coordinate patient care so that different specialists function together as a team. The decision as to who is in charge and how to proceed may vary in different institutions, health care plans, and areas of the country.

TABLE 1-9. Currently Available Diagnostic Procedures

Procedure	Purpose
CT	To visualize the brain, spinal cord, and bony structures
Computed or quantitative EEG (CEEG, QEEG, EEG brain mapping)	Clinical applications are questionable
EEG	To assess possible epilepsy (and also focal or diffuse brain damage and sleep disturbances). Prolonged video monitoring may improve accuracy of assessment
Electromyography and nerve conduction studies	To check for nerve or nerve root injury
Electronystagmography	To assess vestibular dysfunction
Evoked potentials	To assess the integrity of the central visual, auditory, and somatosensory pathways
Magnetoencephalography	Evaluation of epilepsy; clinical role under investigation
MRI	To assess integrity of brain, spinal cord, and soft tissues. Echoplanar techniques may show blood flow
Neuropsychological procedures	To provide a detailed profile of cognitive performance and behavioral characteristics
PET	To assess regional cerebral blood flow or metabolic activity; clinical applications under development
SPECT	To assess regional cerebral blood flow; clinical role under development
Thermography	Clinical applications are questionable
Radiography	To check for vertebral alignment, arthritis, neck and skull fractures, and sinusitis

Opinions on specific treatments of patients with head injury and postconcussive syndrome are described in the various chapters of this book. Explained are the treatment of headache and neck pain, psychiatric disorders, post-traumatic epilepsy, nonepileptic seizures, dizziness, insomnia, and visual disturbances. The roles of medication and cognitive therapy are developed, as is the assessment of disability and return to work. However, there are several general principles to observe.

Primum non noscere—that is, first of all, do no harm. Do not treat with medicines of unproven efficacy or for which there are no clear indications because the side effects may outweigh the benefits. For example, avoid anticonvulsants in patients without seizures (Smith et al., 1994) and narcotics in chronic headache patients. Remain attentive to unintended drug interactions in cases of polypharmacy (see Ch. 17).

The attitude of the caregiver is another important factor in head injury and postconcussive syndrome. A positive attitude is essential even where significant injury exists. In these cases it is critical to grade accurately and fairly the level of the newly acquired deficits, so that trauma survivors can find success within their new limitations. Every effort should be made to return patients to the mainstream even if they no longer function at premorbid levels. A return to gainful activity can offer a valuable opportunity for increased self-reliance and self-esteem. Do not unduly restrict the activity of individuals in whom the history, physical evidence, and laboratory provide little or no confirmation of injury.

LITIGATION

Head injuries and TBI have long been the subject of litigation. Medical experts are frequently called on to provide opinions about likelihood and degree of impairment, cause-and-effect relationships, and chances for recovery. Professionals who evaluate and treat head-injured patients may be called to testify. There is nearly a century of advice to draw on (Bailey, 1906).

The modus operandi of the clinician differs from that of the attorney in important ways. Clinicians assemble all the relevant facts to test a clinical hypothesis. If this proves false, an alternative hypothesis (diagnosis) is adopted. In contrast, lawyers must assume the position of their clients (the hypothesis) to be true, no matter what the facts show. There may be pressure to reject or hide important facts and to overemphasize the trivial if doing so advances the client's position (Abrams, 1994). Fee arrangements are another factor (Bailey, 1906; Stevens, 1994).

Rightly or not, in the courtroom the caregiver is often identified as an advocate while the consultant is identified as an adversary (Bailey, 1906). In either role, the clinician-scientist should display a command of the historical, physical, and laboratory data and should be prepared to offer a detailed and accurate account of their meaning. The specter of litigation tends to amplify any minor errors of omission, detail, or attribution. The clinician should review all germane records and be wary of history from individuals who are themselves invested in the case. Medical opinion must be separated from any inferences a lawyer would have the clinician draw. Clinicians should not offer testimony outside the field of their own expertise; should strive to be educators, not adversaries; should tell the truth and not trespass beyond the facts; should admit gaps in their knowledge or factual errors; and should adhere to basic accepted scientific and ethical principles such as those of American Psychological Association (1992).

Head trauma and postconcussive syndrome seem to provide a fertile substrate for unconventional "science" and opinions (Scheinberg, 1994). For example, the EEG finding in migraine or drowsiness may be interpreted as post-traumatic epilepsy (Epstein, 1994) and nonspecific white matter signals or Virchow-Robin spaces on MRI (see Ch. 5) as diffuse axonal injury. Minor deviations in neuropsychological tests may become "severe cognitive deficits" (Matarazzo, 1990), and fright or other transient disturbances may become "post-traumatic stress disorder" (Lees-Haley, 1986; Silvain, 1986). We have seen all manner of manifestly unsupportable claims of closed head injury, ranging from the bizarre (e.g., post-traumatic headaches caused by a popping balloon) to the ridiculous (e.g., traumatic brain injury from contact with a Nerf ball). We have also seen claims of minor whiplash or closed head injury triggering repressed memories and even robbery and murder—the "medicalization" of crime. While the expert defense testimony in civil cases is generally more accurate that the plaintiff's (Safran et al., 1992), we know one case of a traumatic frontal lobotomy and another of a missile wound to the left parietal lobe, in which the defense experts apparently felt the affected brain bits were quite dispensable. Unfortunately, some expert witnesses seem willing to endorse anything an attorney places before them (Bailey, 1906; Huber, 1991; Cornfeld, 1993). Tort reform is much needed (Howard, 1994).

CONCLUSION

Head trauma is a crucial public health problem, with a predilection for younger adults and a wide range of possible outcomes from full recovery to death. Interestingly, even patients with relatively mild impact trauma and no apparent brain injury may report a daunting array of complaints, often lumped together under the rubric of postconcussive syndrome. There are many underlying factors to consider.

Accurate diagnosis in trauma cases requires a clear understanding of the various terms that may be encountered. For instance, the terms *head* injury and *brain* injury should not be confused. An appreciation of the relevant neuropathologic models is also necessary. Models derived from experiments in nonhuman species are important; however, they may not transfer to the human situation. A command of the historical evidence is also essential and should take into account the sources of referral and information. Primary records are most helpful in determinations of amnesia, loss of consciousness, and the physical circumstances of a potential injury. Together with the patient's verbal account and other factors, including premorbid psychosocial, occupational, and educational history, these data help predict the potential for recovery and return to work.

The neurologic examination is a cornerstone in the evaluation of patients with continuing complaints. A general medical examination will help identify any treatable systemic factors. Mental status screening for disturbances of perception, attention, language, memory, decision making, mood, or self-awareness may help direct the need for a more detailed neuropsychological assessment. The results are susceptible to depression, fatigue, drugs, and chronic pain and require expert interpretation. Also, depending on the pattern of complaints, the patient may warrant an evaluation by a specialist in psychiatry, otolaryngology, neuro-ophthalmology, or head and neck pain. The practical challenge is to coordinate patient care in such a manner that different specialists function together as a team.

As specialty approaches to head injury and postconcussive disorder have grown, so have the variety of diagnostic tests and treatment options. Laboratory assessment often includes plain radiographs and CT or MRI procedures to image the head and neck. Electrophysiologic studies are commonly used. The roles of SPECT and PET are under active investigation. Skillful use of the available techniques can provide several converging lines of evidence to confirm the diagnosis. There is no place for nonstandard and unreliable tests.

The most important principle of treatment is to do no harm. For example, medicines with unproven efficacy or unclear indications should be avoided, since the side effects may outweigh the benefits. The attitude of the caregiver is another important factor; a positive attitude is essential, even where significant injury exists. Every possible effort should be made to return patients to the mainstream even if they no longer function at premorbid levels. A return to gainful activity can offer a valuable opportunity for increased self-reliance and self-esteem.

Finally, the clinician-scientist who sees head injury patients may be called upon as a witness to educate the court. A command of facts is necessary, and so is the ability to provide a detailed and accurate account of their meaning. It is essential to adhere to basic accepted scientific principles.

REFERENCES

Abrams F: Why lawyers lie. The New York Times Magazine (Oct. 9):54–55, 1994

Adams JH, Graham DI, Murray LS, Scott G: Diffuse axonal injury due to nonmissile head injury in humans: an analysis of 45 cases. Ann Neurol 12:557–563, 1982

American Academy of Neurology: AAN Practice Handbook. Minneapolis, 1995

American Psychiatric Association, DSM IV. Washington, 1994

American Psychological Association: Ethical Principles of Psychologists and Code of Conduct. Am Psychol, 1992

Annegers JF, Grabow JD, Groover RV et al: Seizures after head trauma: a population study. Neurology 30:683–689, 1980

Bailey P: Diseases of the Nervous System Resulting from Accident and Injury. D. Appleton, New York, 1906

Binder LM: Persisting symptoms after mild head injury: a review of the postconcussive syndrome. J Clin Exp Neuropsychol 8:323–346, 1986

Binder LM, Willis SC: Assessment of motivation after financially compensable minor head trauma. Psychol Assessment: J Consulting Clin Psychol 3:175–181, 1991

Brooks DN: The head-injured family. J Clin Exp Neuropsychol 13:155–188, 1991

Brown SJ, Fann JR, Grant I: Postconcussional disorder: Time to acknowledge a common source of neurobehavioral morbidity. J Neuropsychiatry Clin Neurosci 6:15–22, 1994

Cornfeld RS: Help stamp out junk science: a practical approach. For the Defense (Apr):27–29, 1993

Costanzo RM, Zasler ND: Head trauma. pp. 711–730. In Getchell TV, Doty RL, Bartoshuk LM, Snow JB (eds): Smell and Taste in Health and Disease. Raven Press, New York, 1991

Dikmen SS, Machamer JE, Winn HR, Temkin NR: Neuropsychological outcome at 1-year post head injury. Neuropsychology 9:80–90, 1995a

Dikmen SS, McLean A, Temkin N: Neuropsychological and psychosocial consequences of minor head injury. J Neurol Neurosurg Psychiatry 49:1227–1232, 1986

Dikmen SS, Ross BL, Machamer JE, Temkin NR: One year psychosocial outcome in head injury. J Int Neuropsychol Soc 1:67–77, 1995b

Dikmen SS, Temkin NR, Machamer JE et al: Employment following traumatic head injuries. Arch Neurol 51:177–186, 1994

Dixon CE, Clifton GL, Lighthall JW et al: A controlled cortical impact model of traumatic brain injury in the rat. J Neurosci Methods 39:253–262, 1991

Dixon CE, Lyeth BG, Povlishock JT et al: A fluid percussion model of experimental brain injury in the rat. J Neurosurg 67:110–119, 1987

Doty RL: The Smell Identification Test. Sensonics, Haddon Heights, NJ, 1983

Doty RL: Olfactory system. pp. 175–203. In Getchell TV, Doty RL, Bartoshuk LM, Snow JB (eds): Smell and Taste in Health and Disease. Raven Press, New York, 1991

Epstein CM: Computerized EEG in the courtroom [editorial]. Neurology 44:1566–1569, 1994

Folstein MF, Folstein SE, McHugh PR: "Mini-mental state." J Psychiatr Res 12:189–198, 1975

Gennarelli TA: Head injury in man and experimental animals: clinical aspects. Acta Neurochir Suppl (Wien) 32:1–13, 1983

Gennarelli TA: Mechanisms of brain injury. J Emerg Med 11:50–11, 1993

Gennarelli TA, Thibault LE, Adams JH et al: Diffuse axonal injury and traumatic coma in the primate. Ann Neurol 12:564–574, 1982

Gualtieri CT: The problem of mild brain injury. Neuropsychiatry, Neuropsychology, and Behavioral Neurology 8:127–136, 1995

Howard P: Death of Common Sense. Random House, New York, 1994

Huber P: Galileo's Revenge. Harper Collins, New York, 1991

Lees-Haley PR: Pseudo post-traumatic stress disorder. Trial Diplomacy J 17–20, 1986

Lees-Haley PR, Brown RS: Neuropsychological complaint base rates in 170 personal injury claimants. Arch Clin Neuropsychol 8:203–209, 1993

Leetsma JE: Forensic Neuropathology. Raven Press, New York, 1988

Levin HS, Benton AL, Grossman RG: Neurobehavioral Consequences of Closed Head Injury. Oxford University Press, New York, 1982

Levin HS, Eisenberg HM, Benton AL: Mild Head Injury. Oxford University Press, New York, 1989

Levin HS, Grafman J, Eisenberg HM: Neurobehavioral Recovery from Head Injury. Oxford University Press, New York, 1987

Livingston M: Whiplash injury and peer copying. J R Soc Med 86:535–536, 1993

Loftus EF: Memory and its distortions. pp. 123–154. In Kraut AG (Ed): The G. Stanley Hall Lecture Series. American Psychological Association, Washington, 1982

Marshall LF, Gautille T, Klauber MR et al: The outcome of severe closed head injury. J Neurosurg 75:S28–S36, 1991

Matarazzo JD: Psychological assessment versus psychological testing: validation from Binet to the school, clinic, and courtroom. Am Psychol 45:999–1017, 1990

Mayo Clinic and Mayo Foundation for Research: Clinical Examinations in Neurology. WB Saunders, Philadelphia, 1981

Miller H: Accident neurosis: Lecture I. Br Med J 919–925, 1961a

Miller H: Accident neurosis: Lecture II. Br Med J 992–998, 1961b

Minderhoud JM, Boelens MEM, Huizenga J, Saan RJ: Treatment of minor head injuries. Clin Neurol Neurosurg 82:127–140, 1980

Ommaya AK, Gennarelli TA: Cerebral concussion and traumatic unconsciousness. Brain 97:633–654, 1974

Pearce JMS: Polemics of chronic whiplash injury. Neurology 44:1993–1997, 1994

Plum F, Posner JB: The Diagnosis of Stupor and Coma. FA Davis, Philadelphia, 1980

Radanov BP, Stefano GD, Schnidrig A et al: Cognitive functioning after common whiplash: a controlled follow-up study. Arch Neurol 50:87–91, 1993

Rodnitzky R: Van Allen's Pictorial Manual of Neurologic Tests. Year Book Medical Publishers, Chicago, 1988

Ropper AH: The opposite pupil in herniation. Neurology 40:1707–1709, 1990

Ropper AH: Neurological and Neurosurgical Intensive Care. Raven Press, New York, 1993

Safran A, Skydell B, Ropper S: Expert witness testimony in neurology: Massachusetts experience 1980–1990. Neurol Chronicle 2(7):1–6, 1992

Scheinberg P: The hidden costs of medicolegal abuses in neurology. Arch Neurol 51:650–652, 1994

Schneider DC, Nahum AM: Impact studies of facial bones and skull. Proc Staap Car Crash Conference, Society of Automotive Engineers:186–202, 1973

Silvain PB: Psychological injury claims: a primer for defense counsel. For the Defense (July):7–11, 1986

Skinner HA: The Origin of Medical Terms. Williams & Wilkins, Baltimore, 1961

Smith KR Jr, Goulding PM, Wilderman D et al: Neurobehavioral effects of phenytoin and carbamazepine in patients recovering from brain trauma: a comparative study. Arch Neurol 51:653–660, 1994

Stevens A: Firms try more lucrative ways of charging for legal services. The Wall Street Journal (Nov. 25): pp. 1, 3, 1994

Strub RL, Black FW: The Mental Status Examination in Neurology. FA Davis, Philadelphia, 1985

Stuss DT, Ely P, Hugenholtz H et al: Subtle neuropsychological deficits in patients with good recovery after closed head injury. Neurosurgery 17:41–47, 1985

Teasdale G, Jennett B: Assessment of coma and impaired consciousness: a practical scale. Lancet 2:81–83, 1974

Van Zomeren AH, van Den Burg W: Residual complaints of patients two years after severe head injury. J Neurol Neurosurg Psychiatry 48:21–28, 1985

Weintraub MI: Medicolegal perspectives: litigation—chronic pain syndrome—a distinct entity: analysis of 210 cases. Am J Pain Management 2:198–204, 1992

Wong JL, Regennitter RP, Barrios F: Base rate and simulated symptoms of mild head injury among normals. Arch Clin Neuropsychol 9:411–425, 1994

Yarnell PR, Lynch S: The "ding": amnestic states in football trauma. Neurology 23:196–197, 1973

Youngjohn JR, Burrows L, Erdal K: Brain damage or compensation neurosis? The controversial post-concussion syndrome. The Clinical Neuropsychologist 9:112–123, 1995

Epidemiology of Closed Head Injury

2

James C. Torner
Mario Schootman

Traumatic head injury accounts for a quarter of injury-related deaths (Sosin et al., 1989; Sosin et al., 1992), and 22 out of 100,000 people will die of a head injury-related death each year. The peak age for head injury-related mortality is in the 15- to 24-year range. However, traumatic brain injury not only accounts for the death of persons early in their productive life but also is a major cause of lifelong disability and impairment. The cost to the individual and society is great because of the consequences of injury to the young. Transportation is the major cause of head injury, with highest rates in the young. Interpersonal violence causing penetrating injuries has been an increasing component of urban head injuries, particularly in young males.

Closed head injury accounts for 95 percent of head trauma events and 60 to 80 percent of head injury-related deaths (Frankowski et al., 1985). Closed head injury and penetrating head injury are often grouped together in descriptive studies. However, outcome from penetrating injuries, particularly gunshot wounds, is worse.

It is difficult to separate penetrating from closed head injuries in incidence studies. Hence this chapter describes the epidemiology in terms of the nature and magnitude of closed and penetrating head trauma in populations, the common causes of injury, and the prognosis of patients with brain injuries.

DEFINITION AND CLASSIFICATION

Diagnosis

The definition of what is a head injury is important for epidemiologic assessment and outcome evaluation. Does head trauma equate with head injury, and does head injury mean brain injury as verified by pathology? Does it include lacerations, skull fractures, and those injuries not causing loss of consciousness? There is a spectrum of head trauma ranging from minor bumps or lacerations not seen by medical professionals to injuries causing death at the scene. *Differences in definitions can lead to differences in morbidity and mortality estimates,* particularly at the mild end of the spectrum. The epidemiology of head injuries is dependent on measurement criteria involving not only the definition of head trauma but also the severity of the injury. Rates of incidence and outcome vary with differences in diagnostic criteria for case selection. Uniform diagnostic criteria are essential for comparison.

Pathology from head trauma can be categorized into five main types: extracranial injuries (face, scalp), skull fractures, focal brain injuries, diffuse brain injuries, and penetrating injuries. Classification based on symptoms is broad and could include amnesia, loss of consciousness or coma, headache, nausea, dizziness, tinnitus, retrobulbar pain, ophthalmic changes, motor deficits, inability to remember, inability to concentrate, and behavioral changes. Only some of these are evident at first medical attention; others may be evident in the recovery phase. Hence the type of clinical facility and expertise in head injury diagnosis and assessment can yield diagnostic differences in head trauma classification.

Changes in diagnostic patterns over time have led to changes in admission practices and degree of diagnosis. Skull radiographs were and are the standard of diagnosis for skull fractures. In the review by Masters et al. (1987) of 22,058 skull radiographic examinations for head trauma, 3 percent were positive for skull fracture and 0.6 percent were positive for intracranial injury. Criteria for management were established based on low-, moderate- and high-risk groups. Low-risk patients were those with minimal abnormal findings. Moderate-risk patients were those with neurologic findings, progressing neurologic status, multiple trauma, unreliable history of injury, or age less than 2 years, as well as other indicating factors. High-risk patients were those with depressed level of consciousness, focal neurologic signs, decreasing level of consciousness or a penetrating head injury. In the clinical series reported for the low-risk group the fracture rate was 0.4 percent, for the moderate-risk group it was 4.2 percent, and for the high-risk group it was 21.5 percent. Skull radiographs were recommended in those patients at highest risk for intracranial hematomas. Conversely, the presence of a skull fracture on skull radiography increases the odds that a patient has a hematoma (Miller, 1991). Patients with an altered state of consciousness or coma also have increased odds of a hematoma.

Definitive diagnosis for the presence of a hematoma is by computed tomographic (CT) scanning or magnetic resonance imaging (MRI), which are techniques that became widely available in the late 1970s. CT scans for detection of hematomas are recommended by Masters et al. (1987) for moderate-risk patients and considered necessary for high-risk patients. CT scans can be used for emergent diagnosis of hematomas but can also be used to diagnose the type of head injury and the presence of swelling and ischemic lesions. Not all pathology can be visualized on admission, and secondary lesions can develop. Ischemic lesions and accumulating hematomas make take days to be present on CT scans.

The presence of CT abnormalities is correlated with the magnitude of trauma and the presence of neurologic findings on examination. Unenhanced admission CT scans were investigated by Schynoll et al. (1993). In 264 patients, age, mechanism of injury, loss of consciousness, coma, headache, cranial nerve deficit, Babinski sign, skull fracture, abnormal pupils, antegrade amnesia, motor paralysis, raccoon eyes, and abnormal motor and reflex examination were associated with CT abnormalities (hematoma, contusion, edema, pneumocephalus). Even in patients with minimal risk or with mild head injury with normal level of consciousness (Glasgow Coma Scale [GCS] score of 15), several recent studies have found 10 to 16 percent of these patients to have abnormal CT scans (Livingston et al., 1991; Servadei et al., 1988; Stein and Ross, 1990). Of patients with abnormal scans in mild head injury, 20 percent required surgery in the study by Stein and Ross (1990). The importance of complete diagnostic studies in ascertainment of head injury type is crucial in comparing frequency of head injury occurrence as well as prognosis by type.

As mentioned earlier, MRI can also play a role in enhancing head injury diagnosis. Jenkins et al. (1986) performed MRI within 1 week of injury in 50 patients of whom 46 (92 percent) had an abnormality on MRI while 25 (50 percent) had findings on CT. Six of eight patients who were fully conscious had cortical lesions on MRI. Approximately 90 percent of those who were impaired or in coma had MRI lesions. MRI lesions were found in 24 patients with severe head injury and a normal CT scan (Wilberger et al., 1987). Levin et al. (1988) also found lesions on MRI, and the presence of a lesion was related to level of consciousness. MRI is likely to be more sensitive for detecting cortical contusions, small subdural hematomas, and diffuse axonal injuries than CT and may be better than CT in childhood head injury (Sklar et al., 1992).

Classification Methods

Epidemiologic studies that utilize death certificate records or hospital discharge records have found cases by using The International Classification of Diseases (ICD) (National Center for Health Statistics, 1978). This classification is based on the nature of the injury. Codes N800-N804 and N850-N854 are based on the pathologic diagnosis (Table 2-1). The subcodes that reflect digits to the right of the decimal point allow further subclassification by either location or severity. For example, N850 has subcodes relating to concussion that categorize loss of consciousness as brief, moderate (1 to 24 hours) or prolonged (more than 24 hours). Multiple codes for trauma are possible, and with multiple trauma, particularly in motor vehicle collisions, the N code for intracranial injury may be the primary or a contributing code. N codes on death certificates allow also for case finding for patients with a prehospital or unwitnessed death. Use of the ICD9 code for discharge records or death certificates also allow for more complete diagnoses that result from serial diagnostic examinations during hospitalization and/or autopsy. Also, secondary complications from the clinical course of head and multiple trauma are detected. Codes N905.0 and N907.0 represent late effects of intracranial injury and may identify cases that escaped detection because the patients were not hospitalized but have lingering problems or complications. The recent use of CT scanning and MRI has also enhanced diagnosis of pathology and thereby enhanced classification. A more complete evaluation of pathologic damage by radiologic examination is possible, which thereby affects diagnostic accuracy and completeness. This contributes to the changing of the type of injuries recorded through ICD codes over time.

Another scale used to classify pathology and severity is the Abbreviated Injury Scale (AIS) (American Association for Automotive Medicine, 1990). Extra digits correspond to severity of the injury in terms of its likelihood of causing morbidity and mortality. An AIS code of XXXXXX.1 would correspond to minor injury and XXXXXX.6 to a maximum, fatal injury. For the head the AIS codes are separated into several areas of injury (e.g., the whole area, the intracranial vessels, the cranial nerves, the internal organs, and the skeletal tissue) and also consider length of unconsciousness. As many codes as necessary may be used. With multiple trauma this scale allows for coding severity of all injuries, not just those of the head. The Injury Severity Score is calculated by summing the squared value of the three most severely injured body regions and is strongly related to prediction of mortality (Baker et al., 1992). Few studies have strictly used the AIS for case finding owing to its complexity and the need by most facilities to collect ICD9 coding for medical and financial records. MacKenzie et al. (1989) have developed an algorithm for transforming ICD9 codes to AIS codes. The method has been used in the 1985 version of the AIS.

The National Institute of Neurological Disorders and Stroke established a registry of patients with severe head injury known as the Traumatic Coma Data Bank (Foulkes et al., 1991). Four medical centers participated, in which the investigators developed the protocol and measures of injury. Patients who were in coma within 48 hours of their injury were included. Classification of the pathology of head injury was made by using available clinical and radiologic data that were obtained after patient admission. The Traumatic Coma Data Bank Intracranial Diagnosis Classification separated patients with mass lesions from those with diffuse injury (Marshall et al., 1991b) (Ta-

TABLE 2-1. International Classification of Diseases for Head Injury (9th Edition, Clinical Modification)

N800	Fracture of the vault of the skull
N801	Fracture of the base of the skull
N802	Fracture of the face bones
N803	Other and unqualified skull fractures
N804	Multiple fractures involving skull or face with other bones
N850	Concussion
N851	Cerebral laceration and contusion
N852	Subarachnoid, subdural, and extradural hemorrhage following injury
N853	Other and unspecified intracranial hemorrhage following injury
N854	Intracranial injury of other and unspecified nature
N905.0	Late effect of fracture of skull and face bones
N907.0	Late effect of intracranial injury without mention of skull fracture

(From National Center for Health Statistics, 1978.)

ble 2-2). Severity of diffuse injury was based on CT findings of swelling and shift. Mass lesions were classified on the basis of size (i.e. > 25 mm) and not separated by type. Mass lesions were also categorized by surgical evacuation or nonevacuation.

Not all head trauma can be classified on the basis of pathology alone. The full spectrum of head trauma included in epidemiologic studies depends on the classification of mild head trauma. For example, Jennett et al. (1977) conducted a survey of Scottish hospitals, in which they used head injury to mean: (1) a definite history of a blow to the head; (2) a laceration of the scalp or forehead; or (3) altered consciousness without a time specification. Excluded were facial lacerations and jaw fractures. In another study, Kraus et al. (1984) restricted cases to those involving brain injury (i.e., physical damage or functional impairment from acute head trauma diagnosed by a physician). Excluded were patients with fractures without functional change. Persons with autopsy-confirmed brain injury were included.

Teasdale and Jennett in 1974 proposed and evaluated the GCS, which is a classification based on the depth of coma (Teasdale et al., 1992). The scale is the sum of three components: the best eye response, the best motor response, and the best verbal response (see Table 1-5). The verbal response may be missing or untestable in patients who are intubated. The eye response may be untestable in patients with facial trauma. Use of sedatives or alcohol intoxication may yield lower or untestable scores. This scale has been widely adopted and used in classification of severity. Patients with a GCS between 3 and 8 are classified as severe, while 9 to 12 is considered moderate and 13 to 15 mild. The GCS has been included in the trauma score and has been shown to have high reliability in various settings (Champion et al., 1981). It is likely to be found in most emergency system records as well as in the hospital record.

A classification of head injury severity which combined symptoms and pathology has been described by Frankowski et al. (1985). Patients could be classified on the basis of pathology and loss of consciousness or post-traumatic amnesia (Table 2-3). This classification covered the spectrum of head trauma, allowing for inclusion of those with "trivial" injury.

Further classification of mild closed head injury has been proposed and validated (Williams et al., 1990). In 215 patients, comparisons in baseline and outcome measures suggested that mild head injuries could be classified as (1) mild (initial lowest GCS score of 13 to 15, a normal CT scan, and a normal skull radiograph or only a linear or basilar skull fracture) and (2) mild with complications (initial lowest GCS score of 13 to 15, and CT or radiographic evidence of a focal brain lesion and/or depressed skull fracture).

Elson and Ward (1994) proposed another definition for mild head injury, in which those with an acute mild injury are those who do not have CT or MRI parenchymal or vascular abnormalities; may or may not have had a loss of consciousness; may or may not have had amnesia; have a GCS score of 13 to 15 with normal motor and eye scores; and do not deteriorate neurologically. Cases classified also as mild brain injury are those of patients who suffer from postconcussive syndrome.

TABLE 2-2. Traumatic Coma Data Bank Intracranial Diagnosis Classification

Injury Classification	Indications
Diffuse injury I	No visible intracranial pathology on CT
Diffuse injury II	Cisterns present with shift ≤5 mm and/or lesion densities ≤25 ml
Diffuse injury III	Cisterns compressed or absent with shift ≤5 mm and/or lesion densities ≤25 ml
Diffuse injury IV	Shift >5 mm and/or lesion densities ≤25 ml
Evacuated mass lesion	Any surgically evacuated lesion
Nonevacuated mass lesion	High or mixed density lesion >25 ml, not surgically evacuated
Brain death	No brainstem reflexes Flaccidity Fixed and nonreactive pupils No spontaneous respirations with a normal $PaCO_2$

(From Marshall et al., 1991b, with permission.)

TABLE 2-3. Classification of Head Injuries by Severity

1. *Fatal*
2. *Severe:* where loss of consciousness (LOC) and/or post-traumatic amnesia (PTA) occurred for more than 24 hours or a cerebral contusion, laceration, or intracranial hematoma was present
3. *Moderate:* where LOC and/or PTA occurred for more than 30 minutes but less than 24 hours and/or a skull fracture occurred
4. *Mild:* without LOC or PTA, with no skull fracture, cerebral contusion, laceration, or intracranial hematoma
5. *Trivial:* without LOC or PTA, with no skull fracture, cerebral contusion, laceration, or intracranial hematoma

(From Frankowski et al., 1985.)

MAGNITUDE OF HEAD INJURY

Population-Based Studies

The case definition of head injury and severity can vary according to the definition used and the completeness of diagnosis. Kraus et al. (1994) have reviewed the definitions used in several population-based studies and cautioned against direct comparison of rates because of varying definitions. It therefore is important that the definition and case ascertainment method be considered when the rates are compared. Case finding is an important aspect of epidemiologic estimates. The inclusion of out-of-hospital deaths, those cases observed in emergency rooms or physician's offices, and late sequelae cases as well as patients admitted to hospitals affect estimates. Deaths at the scene or during transport to a hospital may account for two-thirds of the total number of fatal head injury cases. Fatal injuries account for 5 to 10 percent of all head injuries (Frankowski et al., 1985). Patients not seeking medical care may be as many as 20 to 40 percent, and those not admitted may account for another 20 to 30 percent. Triage and transfer of patients to level I trauma centers can also lead to double counting of cases. A comprehensive record system with appropriate patient identifiers is necessary to estimate the true incidence of head injury.

Several states have established statewide registries (Harrison and Dijkers, 1992). In 11 of 12 states in 1992 there was a legislative requirement for reporting. Variations in case definitions, severities to be included, and case-finding methods exist between the states. The purpose of the registries is to (1) identify injured persons to facilitate rehabilitation; (2) gather data for prevention; (3) gather data for health planning; and (4) evaluate services provided for injured persons. The usefulness of these registries in documenting incidence, trends, and outcome related to services provided has yet to be determined.

Incidence Rate

The occurrence of head injury in a population is not easy to measure. As described before, diagnosis, classification, and severity are determinants of use of emergency services and of hospital admission as well as location and completeness of medical records. Factors such as urbanization, age of the population, time of the year, and environmental conditions, as well as the availability of medical services, may all influence rates.

Estimates of incidence have come from surveys, medical record reviews, and prospective registries. The estimates are from heterogeneous populations representing urban and rural areas and differing climates reflecting different exposure patterns. Most of the studies were conducted in the 1970s and 1980s. An incidence estimate of 200 per 100,000 is the rough average of the population-based studies in the United States (Fig. 2-1). No population-based studies from the early 1990s are yet available.

National data were first available through the National Head and Spinal Cord Survey (Kalsbeek et al., 1980). In 305 hospitals included in the survey between 1970 and 1974, 1,210 inpatients from head injury were found. A rate of 200 hospitalized cases per 100,000 population was estimated in these hospitals.

Individual populations have also been studied for incidence. A rate of 295 per 100,000 was found by

Klauber et al. (1981a and 1981b) for 1978 in San Diego County. Three years later Kraus et al. (1984) found a rate of 180 per 100,000. Differences between the two rates might be due to case finding of fatal cases, changes in admission policies of hospitals, differences in resident definitions, and denominators used. Studies of rural Olmstead County, Minnesota for a 40-year period showed a rate of 193 per 100,000 (Annegers et al., 1980), and Charlottesville, Virginia, which excluded prehospital deaths, had a rate of 208 per 100,000 (Jagger et al., 1984). Higher rates have been observed in urban studies. In the Bronx, New York, a rate of 249 per 100,000 was observed (Cooper et al., 1983). This study included head injuries diagnosed at local hospitals within 24 hours of injury for Bronx residents. Prehospital deaths were included. Rates of nearly 400 per 100,000 were found by Whitman et al. (1984) in their study of three areas of Chicago. Cases were determined from participating hospital records of head-injured patients with neurologic effects. Coroner cases were included. The rates in these urban studies were influenced by the etiology of urban trauma, which included interpersonal violence. Hence, the differences in U.S. rates might be explainable by methods of case ascertainment and cause of injury in the studied population.

Outside the United States several population-based studies have also been conducted. Studies in England, Wales, and Scotland in 1974 showed rates of 270 and 313 per 100,000 (Jennett and MacMillan, 1981). A study in Norway found a rate of 89 per 100,000 of hospitalized or dead-on-arrival cases (Edna and Cappelen, 1985). A prospective study in Aquitaine, France in 1986 showed an overall rate of 281 per 100,000 (Tiret et al., 1990). Fatalities prior to hospitalization as well as hospitalized cases were included. Facial injuries without loss of consciousness were not included. A study in Cantabria, Spain collected cases in 1988 and included only hospitalized patients for the calculation of incidence (Vasquez-Barquero A et al., 1992). A rate of 91 per 100,000 was observed. A study of Amerika Samoa found a rate of 165 per 100,000 (Wallace, 1993). A survey of six regions in China was made in 1983 (Wang et al., 1986). Questions were asked regarding the occurrence of unconsciousness following head injury or evidence of brain dysfunction from a past head injury. Medical records were examined to verify cases. The age-adjusted incidence rate was estimated to be 56 per 100,000. A study of Johannesburg, South Africa revealed a rate of 316 per 100,000 based on sampling of cases from eight hospitals (Nell and Brown, 1991). Cases were counted if they had an appropriate ICD9 code and the patients exhibited a loss of consciousness, seizures, headaches, vomiting, or cerebrospinal fluid rhinorrhea within 5 days of admission.

Prevalence Rate

Few studies have determined the prevalence of head injury in a population. With the majority of injuries being nonfatal (i.e., mild) the prevalence is expected to be large but is still undocumented. Of hospitalized patients in the National Head and Spinal Cord Injury Survey, 439 per 100,000 were estimated to still have head injury in 1974, with a ratio of prevalence to incidence was 2.2 (Kalsbeek et al., 1980). Kraus (1993) estimated the disability rate based on hospital admissions, survival rates, and variable disability proportions. Based on a residual deficit rate of 10 percent in mild, 67 percent in moderate, and 100 percent in severe injuries, a population-based rate of 33 per 100,000, or nearly 83,000 persons in the United States in 1990, has been calculated. Another calculation using 18 percent of mild head injuries with deficits yield 45 per 100,000, or 111,614 individuals. A practical method for assessing the prevalence would be those currently institutionalized, those in rehabilitation, and those collecting disability payments for head injury. Long-term effects on behavioral, cognitive, and physical function in terms of school performance, employment, and social activities probably also could be classified as a prevalent condition. This might be obtained through the National Health Interview Survey.

Mortality Rate

Population-based mortality rates in the United States have ranged from 14 per 100,000 in central Virginia to 30 per 100,000 in San Diego in 1981 (Jagger et al., 1984; Kraus et al., 1984) (Table 2-4). The estimate from death certificate analysis using head injury ICD9 codes for the United States for the period 1979 to 1986 was 16.9 per 100,000 (Sosin et al., 1989). However, when further analysis was done accounting for penetrating injuries, the rate approximated 22 per 100,000 (Sosin et al., 1992). Mortality rates from other populations are comparable, with the exception of South Africa, where a rate of 80 per 100,000 has been reported (Nell and Brown, 1991).

TABLE 2-4. Incidence, Mortality, and Severity Rates in Population-Based Studies

Population	Year	Method	Population	Rate per 100,000	Mortality Rate per 100,000	Mortality (%)	Mild (%)	Moderate (%)	Severe (%)
Olmstead County, MN	1965–1974	R	Pop	193	22	11	63	29	7
San Diego, CA	1978	R	Pop	295	22	7	|—91—|		9
San Diego, CA	1981	R	Pop	180	25	14	82	9	9
Charlottesville, VA	1978	R	H	208	14	7	49	26	25
Chicago, IL	1979–1980						86	9	5
Inner city black		R	H	403	32	8	88	9	4
Suburban black		R	H	394	19	5	89	2	9
Suburban white		R	H	196	22	11	77	13	10
Maryland	1986	R	H	134			70	17	13
Aquitaine, France	1986	Pr	Pop	281	22	8	80	11	9
Cantabria, Spain	1988	Pr	H	91	19.7	22	88	7	5
Johannesburg, South Africa	1986–1987	R	H	316	80	25	88	8	5

Abbreviations: R, retrospective; Pr, prospective; Pop, population-based; H, hospital-based.

(Data from Annegers et al., 1980; Jagger et al., 1984; Klauber et al., 1981a; Klauber et al., 1981b; Kraus et al., 1984; Mackenzie et al., 1990; Nell and Brown, 1991; Tiret et al., 1990; Vasquez-Barquero A et al., 1992; Whitman et al., 1984.)

Severity of Injuries

Since most population-based studies are based on hospital admissions, the distribution of severity of head trauma can be different (e.g., mechanism, triage criteria, and referral patterns). Also, the definition of mild, moderate, and severe can affect the proportions. The mild head injury patients are more likely not to be admitted or referred to hospitals but may include patients with varying lengths of loss of consciousness. The reported percentage of mild head injury ranges from 49 percent in central Virginia to 91 percent in 1978 in San Diego County (Table 2-5). Since the study in Virginia included patients from several counties, this referral for neurosurgical evaluation may have an effect on the number of mild injury patients admitted. The percentage of severe injury patients ranges from 4 to 25 percent, with most estimates clustering near 10 percent.

Risk Factors

Mechanism

The cause of brain trauma varies by population and method of case ascertainment. As an external cause of death, motor vehicles account for the largest proportion of head injury fatalities (Sosin et al., 1989). This percentage varies by race, sex, and geographic location. Whites have a higher percentage of motor vehicle deaths (59 percent versus 42 percent in blacks). Blacks have a higher percentage of head injury deaths from firearms (19 versus 14 percent in whites) and from other causes (28 versus 16 percent in whites). Men suffer a motor vehicle-related head injury mortality rate of 14.5 per 100,000 (56 percent of head injury deaths), while the rate in women is 5.1 per 100,000, or 60 percent of deaths. Falls cause twice as many deaths in men as in women but represent only 10 percent of total deaths in men versus 15 percent in women. Deaths from firearms are six times more likely in men, and other causes of death are three times more likely in men than in women.

In the National Head and Spinal Cord Injury Survey, the major cause of head injury was motor vehicle accidents (51 percent) followed by falls (42 percent) (Kalsbeek et al., 1980). More patients presented with concussion from motor vehicle crashes, while in patients presenting with hematomas, most were from falls.

In population-based studies the largest percentage of head injuries are from transportation (Fig. 2-1). In the San Diego study in 1981, 48 percent of the injuries were due to transportation-related events (Kraus et al., 1984), and 92 percent of these were due to traffic crashes. There is a reasonable consistency across population-based studies of a rate between 80 and 120 per 100,000. Of all brain injuries, 7 percent involved bicycles, with 33 percent of those occurring in collisions with motor vehicles (Kraus JF et al., 1987). Males had a higher rate than females. Bicycle-related head injuries are the highest for ages 5 to 9 years (283 per 100,000) (Thompson et al., 1990).

Falls account for between 20 and 30 percent of head injuries in population-based studies. Rates are highest in the very young and elderly and exceed those of motor vehicle crashes in these age groups (Kraus et al., 1984). Assaults range from 7 to 45 percent depending on the population studied. Injuries from firearms accounted for 6 percent of head injuries in San Diego County in 1981 (Kraus et al., 1984). In Johannesburg assaults accounted for 45 percent of the injuries and 44 percent of the deaths, with 12 percent of deaths due to firearms (Nell and Brown, 1991). Few studies have categorized trauma from sports and recreation. In San Diego County it was observed that 10 percent of the injuries were due to these causes in 1981 (Kraus et al., 1984).

Work-related causes may account for 4 to 5 percent of head injuries (Annegers, 1980). Kraus and Fife (1985) found a rate of 20 per 100,000 for work-related brain injuries. The rates were 37 per 100,000 for military and 15 per 100,000 for civilian employees. In the civilian population half of the work-related brain injuries were due to falls. In the military 57 percent were related to transportation. Heyer and Franklin (1994) used the Workers' Compensation Data System for the state of Washington to determine the number of work-related traumatic head injuries. They found 301 incidents, or a rate of 9.4 per 100,000 workers. The incidence was higher in the 16 to 34 and 55 to 64 year age groups. Men had a higher rate than women (15.1 per 100,000 versus 2.4 per 100,000). The majority of injuries (48.5 percent) were from falls, and 26 percent were from being struck by an object. Motor vehicle accidents accounted for 18 percent of work-related injuries. Of work-injured patients, 40 percent suffered concussion, 36 percent suffered stupor of varying duration, and 23 percent required craniotomy. Eight industrial occupations accounted for one-third of the cases: logging, roofing, garbage collecting, street and road

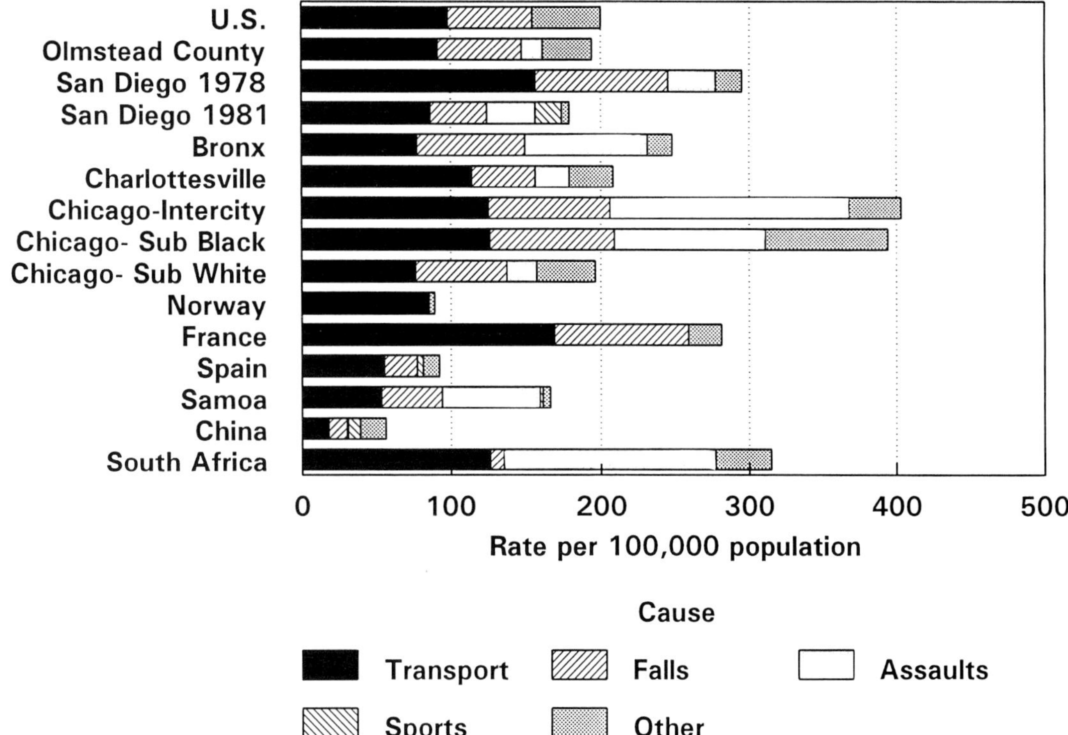

Fig. 2-1. Population-based rates of head injury by mechanism. (Data from Annegers et al., 1980; Edna and Lappelen, 1985; Jagger et al., 1984; Klauber et al., 1981a; Klauber et al., 1981b; Kraus et al., 1984; Nell and Brown, 1991; Tiret et al., 1990; Vasquez-Barquero et al., 1992; Wallace, 1993; Wang et al., 1986; Whitman et al., 1984.)

construction, trucking, dairy farming, interior carpentry, and wood-frame construction.

Age

The peak risk of head injury occurs between the ages of 15 and 30 (Fig. 2-2). Although population-based studies have varied in overall rates, the peak age is the same. Motor vehicle crashes and interpersonal violence are the major contributors to these high rates. Rates are above average for infants and young children and for the elderly. The rate for pediatric head injury was 219 per 100,000 in San Diego in 1981. The rates rise in the teenage years with driving and motor vehicle crashes. The ratio of mortality to injury is highest in the elderly (Fig. 2-3).

Sex

The head injury rate of males to females is approximately 2:1 (Frankowski et al., 1985). Both sexes peak in the young adult ages. The ratio of males to females decreases to nearly equivalency at older ages because of the large contribution of falls to head injury.

Race and Socioeconomic Status

Rates of head injuries in blacks are higher than in whites in the Chicago and Bronx studies and in central Virginia (Cooper et al., 1983; Jagger et al., 1984; Whitman et al., 1984). A threefold difference was observed in nonfatal head injuries for nonwhites in Johannesburg (Nell and Brown, 1991). Two studies have examined the effect of income on incidence of head injury (Cooper et al., 1983; Kraus JF et al., 1986). The rate of injury was inversely correlated with family income. Rates were highest in the lowest income strata and were more often caused by motor vehicles and assaults.

Prevention

Prevention of head trauma can be accomplished through behavioral change, by providing through technology a barrier, or through legislative laws. The

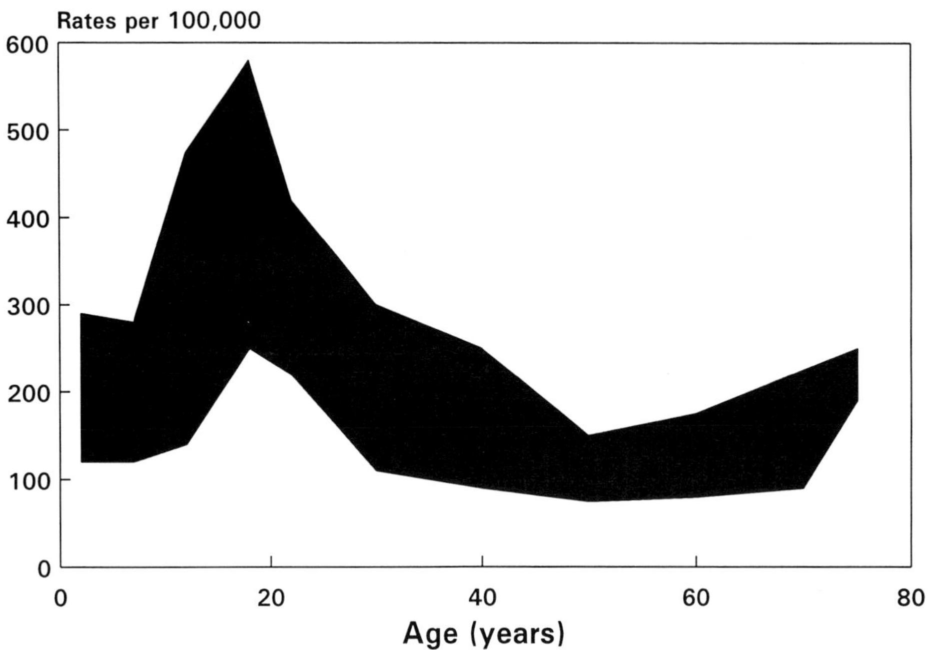

Fig. 2-2. Age-specific incidence rates in U.S. population-based studies. (From Kraus, 1993, with permission.)

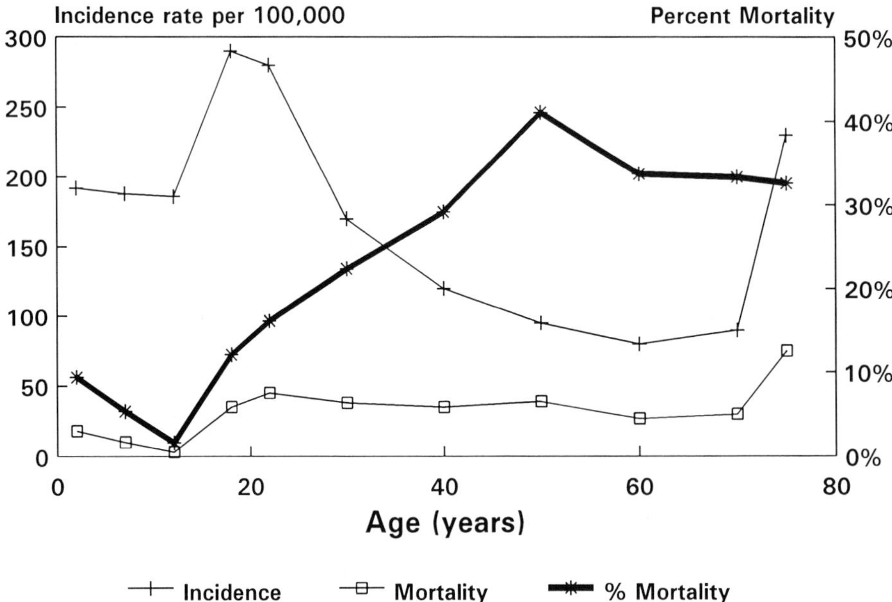

Fig. 2-3. Age-specific incidence rates, mortality rates, and mortality percent of incidence in San Diego (1981). (From Kraus et al., 1984, with permission.)

legislation and use of helmets by motorcyclists and bicyclists is one strategy in head injury prevention that has been associated with reduction in injury rates, decreased severity, and lower mortality rates. Several studies have shown an average 30 percent reduction in motorcycle fatalities associated with the introduction of helmet laws. Sosin and Sacks (1992) found that in states that had a full helmet law there was a lower rate, with 9.0 head injury deaths per 1,000 motorcycle crashes as compared with 12.4 per 1,000 in states without such a law. In a comparison of motorcycle crashes and outcomes from 1991 and 1992 in California, Kraus et al. (1994) found a decrease in fatalities by 37.5 percent and a decrease in fatal and nonfatal head injuries of approximately 30 percent. The severity of the head injuries was also decreased.

Bicycle helmets can also reduce the head injury rates. The effectiveness of bicycle helmets in a case control study in Seattle, Washington showed that head injuries with associated brain pathology or symptoms were reduced by 88 percent in individuals wearing helmets as compared with controls involved in bicycle crashes (Thompson et al., 1989). In Australia, a case control study showed a reduction of 63 percent in head injury occurrence (Thomas et al., 1994). Reduction in loss of consciousness was 86 percent.

Seat belt use and child restraints are also associated with a reduction in deaths and head injuries (Baker et al., 1992). Air bags offer further protection, but the percentage of cars without air bags is still high, and so effects will be seen at some time in the future.

Trends

Few studies have examined trends in head injury rates. The changes in incidence and mortality rates are not consistent between studies and may reflect methods of case ascertainment as well as changes in cause of and management of head trauma.

In Olmstead County, Minnesota, Annegers et al. (1980) studied hospitalizations for head injuries from 1935 to 1974 and observed an increase over the four decades in hospital admissions for head trauma. The largest increase was in cases of mild injury. Increases were observed in both men and women. The greatest increase was in admissions for persons between 15 and 24 years of age.

In the National Head and Spinal Cord Injury Survey, the rate for head injury admissions was 177 per 100,000 in 1970 and 233 per 100,000 in 1973, an increase of 32 percent (Kalsbeek et al., 1980). However, the rate declined in 1974 to 204 per 100,000. This may have been attributable to a decrease in motor vehicle fatalities associated with speed reduction and increased seat belt use.

Mackenzie et al. (1990) examined hospital discharge abstracts for the state of Maryland from 1979 to 1986. Cases were determined from ICD-9 codes at discharge. An assumption was made that the observed number and characteristics of cases were the same as would be expected from Maryland residents—that is, it was assumed that the numbers and frequency of head injury treatments given to patients who were nonresidents would equal those of residents going outside the state (e.g., to Washington, D.C.). They found an increase in head injury discharge rates, which climbed from a rate of 113.7 per 100,000 in 1979 population to 134.2 per 100,000 in 1986. This increase was noted for all severities. Patients 4 years of age and younger had a decrease in rates, while persons between 50 and 70 years of age showed little change. The increase was noted for men and women and for whites and nonwhites, with nonwhites increasing at a faster rate. A decline in case fatality rate was found across all severities. An increase in patients entering rehabilitation or extended care facilities was observed.

The U.S. data can be serially examined from the National Hospital Discharge Survey (National Center for Health Statistics, 1994a). These data are from discharge abstracts sampled from nonfederal, short-term hospitals in the United States. The number of discharges decreased from 364,000 in 1979 to 194,000 in 1992 for acute head injury codes listed as the first diagnosis (Fig. 2-4). Examination of all-listed head injury diagnoses showed a similar decline from 483,000 to 279,000 discharges (Fig. 2-5). The greatest decrease in discharges was in ICD-9 code 850 (concussion) (Fig. 2-6). There was also a decline in discharges associated with other skull fractures (803). However, there was an almost doubling of cases in patients with hematoma (codes 852 and 853), from 15,000 to 29,000. The trends were similar for men and women and across age groups where sufficient data were available. These changes over time probably do not entirely reflect changes in coding but may reflect changes in admission policies for patients with mild head injury coupled with improvements in diagnosis by use of CT. The contribution of preventive interventions such as helmets, drunk driving and seat belt laws and programs, and speed limit changes may

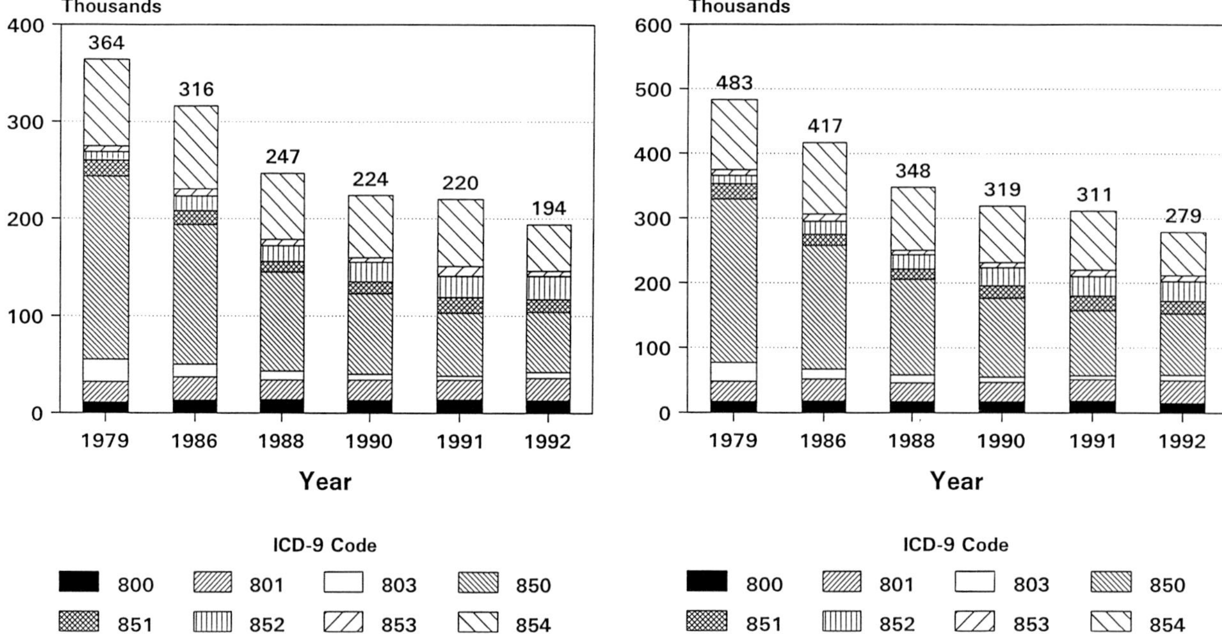

Fig. 2-4. First-listed diagnosis for head injury hospital admissions on National Hospital Discharge Survey. (From National Center for Health Statistics, 1994b.)

Fig. 2-5. All-listed diagnosis for head injury hospital admissions on National Hospital Discharge Survey. (From National Center for Health Statistics, 1994b.)

also have an effect but the magnitude is difficult to estimate. The effect may be also observed at a higher or lower rate within localities.

The Injury Mortality Atlas of the United States, 1979–1987, presents data from the National Center for Health Statistics (1994b) by etiology from death certificates. Figure 2-7 presents the change in age-adjusted rates by cause. Motor vehicle deaths declined from 23.2 per 100,000 in 1979 to 19.4 per 100,000 in 1987. The decline was 20 percent for men and 8 percent for women. The decrease was observed for persons under 75 years of age and for all races. Deaths related to falls declined from 3.6 per 100,000 to 2.7 per 100,000. The decrease was found in both men and women and mostly in the elderly. The homicide death rate declined from 10.0 to 8.5, with decrease observed in men 25 to 74 years. An approximately 20 percent decrease was observed in both white and black males, with the rates changing from 9.7 to 7.6 and 68.8 to 53.2, respectively. No change in suicide rates were observed over the time periods under study.

Sosin et al. (1989) examined data from death certificates for head injury-associated deaths utilizing the Nature of Injury Codes (N803.0 to N804.9, N850.0 to N854.9, N905.0, N907.0). They required that the death certificate also have a corresponding External Cause of Death Code (E800–E999). They observed a decline in head injury mortality rates, particularly in the early 1980s. There was a 21 percent decline in head injury deaths due to motor vehicles. Firearm deaths declined by 18 percent and deaths from falls by 14 percent. The decline was observed for all age groups except those over 75 years. Blacks were similar to whites and males had a greater decline than females, 22 versus 15 percent, respectively. There was a difference in decline related to geographic location, with the greatest percent change in the West (26 percent) and the lowest in the South (19 percent).

An unpublished analysis (1994) by M. Schootman of the Iowa Department of Public Health demonstrated a decline in head injury mortality. The age-adjusted rate was 11.0 per 100,000 in 1989 and decreased to 9.4 per 100,000 in 1993 (Fig. 2-8). The decline was noted for motor vehicle deaths, bicycle-related deaths, and motorcycle-related deaths. No change was noted for falls, suicides, or homicides.

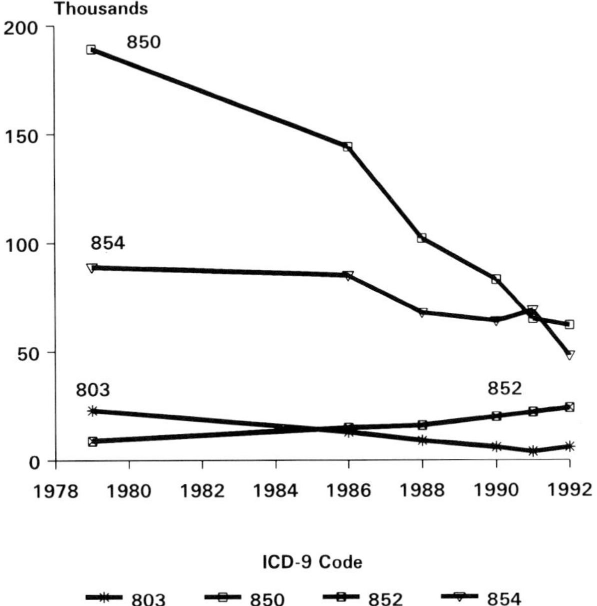

Fig. 2-6. Trends in first-listed diagnosis for head injury hospital admissions on National Hospital Discharge Survey. (From National Center for Health Statistics, 1994b.)

Costs

The cost of brain injury is not only measured in the direct medical costs of emergency medical services, hospitalization, and rehabilitation but also in the loss of productivity and lifetime earnings. The National Head and Spinal Cord Injury Survey estimated the direct cost in 1970 at $1.14 billion annually. Indirect costs (which include lost income, home care, transportation, etc.) were estimated at $2.76 billion annually. Grabow et al. (1984) conducted a study of Olmstead County, Minnesota. The cost was related to severity of injury, with an overall estimate of $1 billion for direct costs and $11.5 billion for indirect costs per year. Max et al. (1991) estimated the total lifetime costs of traumatic brain injury survivors at $24 billion for 1985. The direct cost per person in the United States was $1,031 for mild, $1,872 for moderate, $16,260 for severe, and $2,335 for fatal head injury. Indirect costs per person were estimated as $558, $1,063, $11,145, and $265,087, respectively.

Johnston (1989) has reviewed the current literature on cost of head injuries. The estimated cost in 1986 dollars was $2.79 billion in direct and $25.9 to $34.4 billion in indirect costs annually, with severe

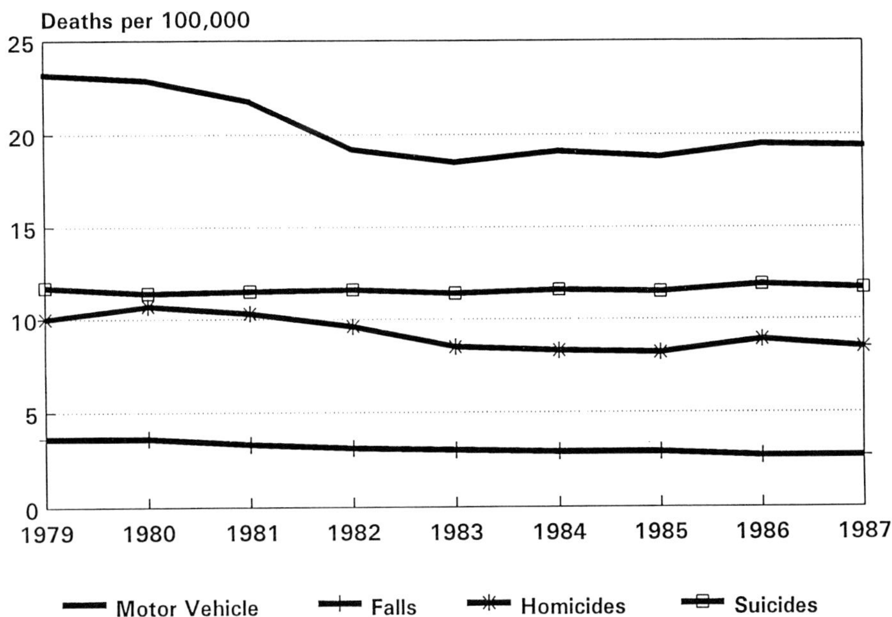

Fig. 2-7. Trends in cause-specific injury deaths in the United States (age-adjusted to 1940 U.S. population.) (From National Center for Health Statistics, 1994a.)

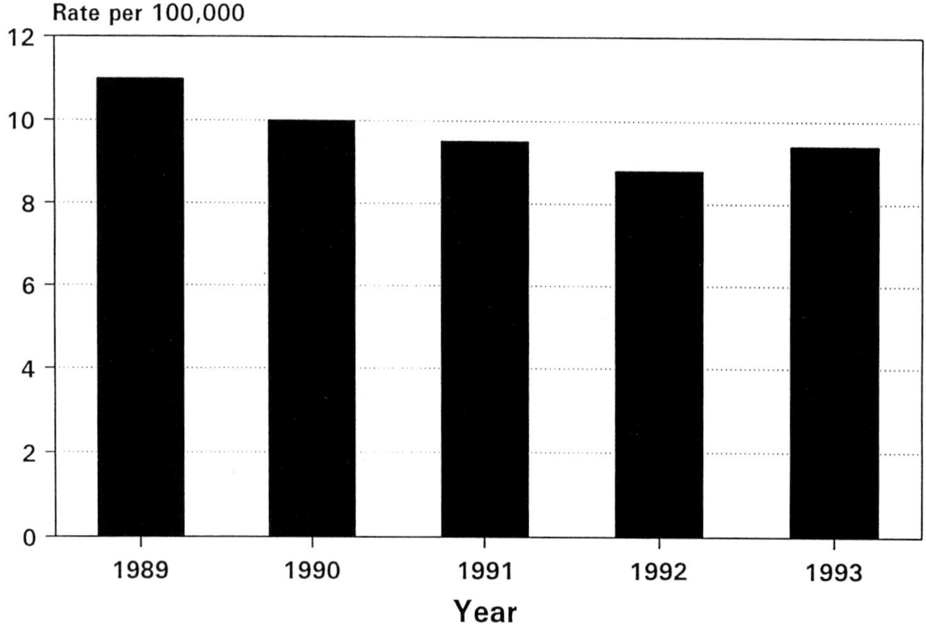

Fig. 2-8. Trends in head injury mortality in Iowa (age-adjusted mortality rates). (Schootman, 1994.)

injuries accounting for the major direct and indirect costs of brain trauma. Today the cost may be as high as $50 billion annually.

OUTCOME FROM HEAD INJURY

There are residual deficits from head trauma and primary intracranial damage, and the course of recovery is variable, a rapid phase occurring after the acute injury being followed a slower phase, with maximum recovery taking several years. The pattern of survival and recovery is important in determining the utilization of medical services and outcome. Much attention has been focused on mortality and its prognostic factors. Recent attention has focused on the magnitude of disability via functional and neuropsychological testing. Minor and moderate head injury outcome remains difficult to predict, and more research is needed to determine prognostic factors for outcome.

Mortality

Approximately 45,000 deaths are attributed to head injury each year. The cause of death is primarily intracranial but there are variations in time from injury to death and in method used to determine the cause. Of the head injury-related death certificates, 87 percent reported an intracranial injury as the cause of death and 27 percent reported a skull fracture (Sosin et al., 1989). Deaths that occur from systemic complications and those of patients who are in vegetative status until death may be underrepresented.

Kraus et al. (1985) observed that 69 percent of the deaths occurred outside of the hospital at the scene or in route. Most of the deaths occurred within 20 minutes of the injury (Conroy and Kraus, 1988). Of patients dead at the scene, 59 percent had a cause of death specified as skull fractures (22.8 percent) or cerebral lacerations or contusions (36.8 percent). Internal injuries other than intracranial were listed as the underlying cause of death in 35.2 percent.

Case-fatality rates of population-based series range from 3 to 7 percent, with most including only in-hospital deaths (Kraus JF, 1993). Six percent of hospitalized patients died, with the underlying cause reported as skull fractures (55 percent), cerebral lacerations or contusions (15.4 percent), intracranial hemorrhage (7.9 percent), and internal injuries (15.3 percent) (Conroy and Kraus, 1988).

The overall mortality rate depends on the type of cases included (e.g., prehospital [community rate] or just admitted cases). Conroy and Kraus (1988) report a 4-year mortality rate of 20 percent for the population-based cohort, 10 percent mortality rate for the admitted cohort, and 4 percent mortality for the discharged cohort, which matched the 4 percent total for the unselected age- and sex-matched population-based rate.

In clinical series the mortality rates have been stratified by head injury severity at admission. In Maryland, using hospital discharge cases of head injury, approximately 5 percent of the patients died in 1986 (Mackenzie et al., 1990). The mortality rates varied by severity as measured by the AIS score: minor injury had a 1 percent, moderate a 5 percent, serious a 13 percent, and severe a 48 percent mortality. Mortality was lower in every severity stratum than in 1976.

Mortality in patients with moderate head injury is low. Rimel et al. (1982) evaluated the outcome at discharge for patients referred from central Virginia. The overall mortality rate was 2.5 percent (5/199), with two (40 percent) of the deaths due to nonintracranial causes. All the deaths occurred in patients with a GCS score of 9 or 10.

In the Traumatic Coma Data Bank the mortality rate at discharge was 33 percent and that at last contact (up to 2 years) was 36.3 percent (Foulkes et al., 1991; Marshall et al., 1991a). In 70 percent of these cases death was primarily due to the head injury. Medical causes of death were pneumonia, coagulopathy, and cardiovascular events.

Disability

Disability can be measured as disposition rates, symptom abnormality rates, and functional outcome rates. In Rhode Island in 1979 and 1980, of all patients hospitalized for head injury, 86 percent went home, 2 percent went home with home health care nursing services, 3 percent were transferred to another acute care facility, and 4 percent went to a chronic care facility (Fife et al., 1986). Age was an important factor in patients returning home. Older patients were more likely to require institutionalization. In Maryland the discharge status of hospitalized head injury patients showed that 9 percent were transferred to another acute care facility or a rehabilitation/extended care facility in 1986 (Mackenzie et al., 1990). The transfer rates varied by severity: minor cases had a 5 percent, moderate a 14 percent, serious a 21 percent, and severe a 29 percent rate. The rates of transfer to rehabilitation or extended care facilities increased in every severity stratum as compared with 1976.

Of 424 mild head injury patients followed in Virginia, 84 percent had complaints at 3 months and 50 percent had memory difficulties (Rimel et al., 1981). Only 34 percent had returned to work at 3 months postinjury. For moderate head injuries (GCS 9 to 12), Rimel et al. (1982) found that transfer to another facility occurred in 12 percent, but the proportion transferred ranged from 24 percent in GCS-9 to 8 percent in GCS-12. Complaints at 3 months postinjury were reported by 96 percent of patients: 90 percent reported headaches, 90 percent had memory difficulties, and 87 percent had problems in activities of daily living. Of these patients with a moderate injury, 69 percent remained unemployed at 3 months.

One measure of function is the Glasgow Outcome Scale (GOS), which was developed to measure neurologic and social dependence, with a gradation based on function (Teasdale and Jennett 1974). The GOS measures the degree that the patient is self-sufficient, ranging down to vegetative survival and death. Assessment is subjective but based on the patient's mental and neurologic function. The term *severe disability* refers to a patient who is conscious but dependent on some other person for some daily activities. *Moderate disability* is used to classify patients who are independent but have some disability in residential living, transportation, or ability to work. A patient with a *good recovery* may not have to make a complete recovery but may be independent and capable of a normal life and of employment. For persons with head injury in San Diego County, 90 percent had a good recovery at discharge and 4 percent were moderately or severely disabled (Kraus et al., 1984). Discharge time is variable and may not be the best time to assess future function. Assessment at 6 months, 1 year, or longer postdischarge may be necessary to assess the recovery and future functional capabilities of those with deficits. Figure 2-9 shows the pattern from the International Data Bank of change in recovery from severe injury in survivors (Jennett and Teasdale, 1981).

Rappaport et al. (1982) expanded the GOS with the Disability Rating Scale with eight items to assess at a high reliability. The scale has 30 points and is designed to assess progress to recovery in the rehabilitation setting. The Cognitive Function Scale has been developed to measure cognitive performance and has been shown to have better reliability and validity (Gouvier et al., 1987). The Karnofsky Performance Status Scale and the Functional Assessment Inventory

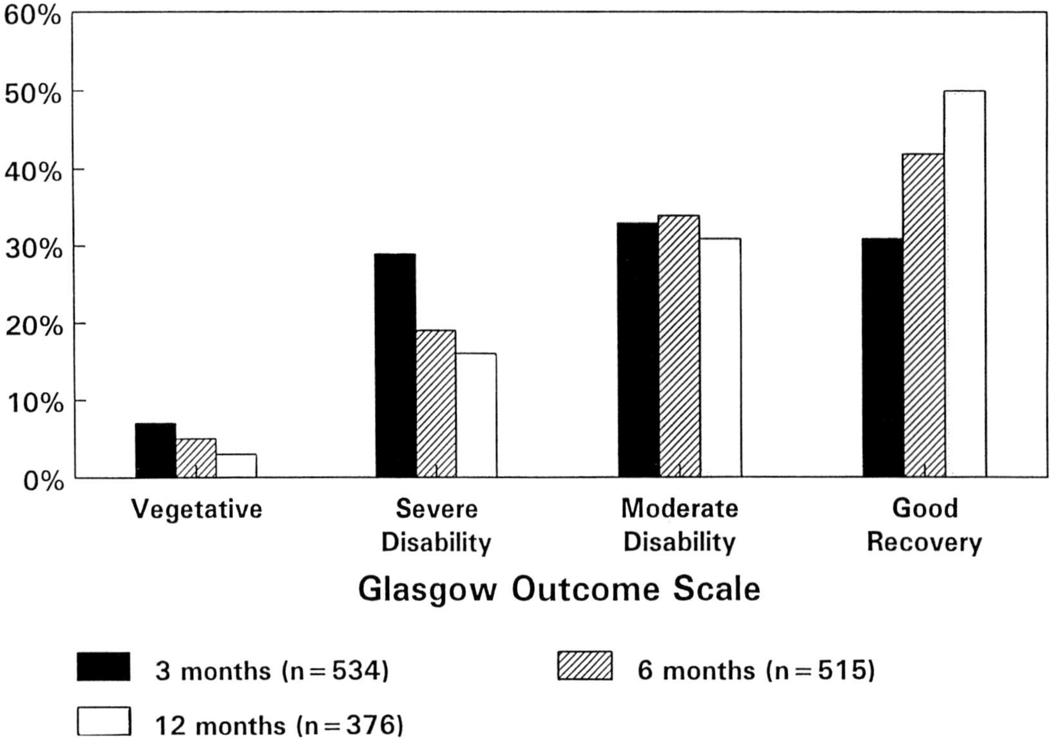

Fig. 2-9. Time-related outcome in severe head injury patients using the Glasgow Outcome Scale (From Jennett and Teasdale, 1981, with permission.)

have also been used to measure outcome (Sakata et al., 1991).

Another relatively recent scale is the Functional Independence Measure (FIM) (Hamilton et al., 1987). This scale has 18 items in the areas of self-care, mobility, communication, sphincter control, locomotion, and social cognition. The patient is evaluated on performance and is assessed at one of seven levels (7 = complete independence, 1 = total assistance) for each item. The total score ranges from 18 to 126. The FIM has been shown to have high interobserver reliability (0.86 to 0.88). Granger and Hamilton (1993) reported on their experience with the FIM in 139 rehabilitation hospitals in 35 states. For 1991, 2,054 patients with "traumatic brain dysfunction" were evaluated. The mean time from onset of the injury was 39 days. The mean score at admission to the facilities was 62.9 (sd 20.9) and at discharge (an average of 41 days) was 96.6 (sd 25.7). Of these patients 82 percent were discharged to home or community placement, 8 percent were discharged to long-term care facilities, and 4 percent were discharged to acute care facilities.

Chronic pathophysiologic measures may be useful as outcome measures and in determining whether patients may have a structural or physiologic cause of their deficits. Their advantage as outcome measures is that they may reflect the actual mechanism of primary and secondary intracranial injury. Routine follow-up of radiologic and physiologic measures is not routinely done but may provide diagnostic and mechanistic information. Patients with a head injury may have hydrocephalus, infarction, abscess or cyst formation, atrophy, or white matter lesions, which may be detected on follow-up CT and MRI scans (Lipper and Kishore, 1989). Levin (1992) has described the results of using MRI at 2-month follow-up. The presence of lesions in subcortical white matter and deep central gray matter and brainstem were associated with disability. Cerebral blood flow measured at follow-up was found to be related to cognitive performance. (Terayama et al., 1991). Brain performance may be assessed by using evoked potentials and electroencephalographic (EEG) analysis. Use of evoked potentials at follow-up was reported by Rappaport et al. (1991) for 75 patients. Cortical auditory evoked potentials were related to level of dysfunction on the Disability Rating Scale.

Deficits from brain injury also include limitations in cognitive and behavioral function. Jennett et al. (1981) demonstrated a relationship of the GOS to cognitive and psychosocial deficits. Patients with a severe disability were also likely to have severe deficits in personality, cognition, verbal capability, performance, verbal memory, and nonverbal memory.

Cognitive function was assessed in patients from the Traumatic Coma Data Bank who completed neuropsychological testing at baseline, 6 months, and 1 year. Three patterns of verbal learning were determined: no change, an improved response, and a rise and fall (Ruff et al., 1991). Factors possibly related to differential performance were education and hypoxia. In another analysis four tests showed relationships to the GOS in 110 patients. These tests evaluated fine motor functioning, verbal fluency, and visual memory (Clifton et al., 1993). Cognitive tests that have been recommended by a conference of head injury experts for evaluation in clinical trials are the Digital Symbol Substitution, the Paced Auditory Serial Addition Test, Rey Complex Figure, Selective Reminding, Controlled Oral Word Association, Trail Making B, Wisconsin Card Sorting, Grooved Peg Board, and Neurobehavioral Rating Scale (Clifton et al., 1992).

Neurobehavioral recovery has been studied by Levin (1992). Early recovery can be measured by restoration of consciousness and post-traumatic amnesia. Long-term recovery measures focus on verbal memory, visual memory, selective deficits, organization of memory, information processing, hemispheric disconnection, and behavioral changes.

Prognostic Factors of Outcome

Mechanism of Injury

The cause of a head injury is associated with its severity and pathology. The biomechanics of the distribution of traumatic force is correlated with the amount of damage. Patients with penetrating injuries have the most serious damage with very poor prognosis. In patients with closed head injuries, falls are more likely to produce intracranial hematomas and are associated with poor neurologic grade. Rapid acceleration and deacceleration injuries can cause diffuse axonal injury with swelling, which can cause significant permanent deficits.

In the Traumatic Coma Data Bank, etiology was examined in relation to outcome of severe head injuries (Foulkes et al., 1991). Gunshot wounds represented 16 percent of the population and were 88 percent fatal. Closed head injuries accounted for 72 percent of the cases, with a mortality rate of 33 percent and a good recovery rate of 7 percent. The distribution of cases by mechanism of injury showed that 64 percent were from motor vehicles, 16 percent from a fall or jump, 11 percent pedestrian, 5 percent from assault, and 4 percent from other causes. Patients who suffered a severe head injury in this series from a fall or jump or who were pedestrians had a higher mortality than those with other causes of injury (Marshall et al., 1991a).

Age

Age is an important factor for survival, disposition, and recovery from head injury. In the population-based study of San Diego County, age had a significant, independent effect on survival of admitted and discharged cases (Conroy and Kraus, 1988). Survival decreased with increasing age stratum, but only for those 50 to 69 years old (odds ratio 3.8) and those 70 and over (odds ratio 5.2) was the correlation statistically significant. Several clinical studies have demonstrated that age is one of the most significant risk factors. Vollmer et al. (1991) examined the independence of age as a prognostic factor in closed head injury patients. Age was linearly related to outcome (Fig. 2-10), and there appeared to be no threshold for age effects. The survival distributions by age demonstrated that older persons continued to die postinjury over a longer time period than younger patients.

Age was related to mechanism of injury, type of injury, and extracranial (systemic) events. Older patients were more likely to have a mass lesion, particularly a subdural hematoma, than younger persons. Vollmer et al. (1991) determined that despite the other age-related factors, age was a major independent predictor of outcome.

Coma Assessment

The GCS was demonstrated as predictor of outcome by Teasdale and Jennett (1974). An example of the relationship of GCS at admission and mortality is displayed in Figure 2-11. Other scales have been proposed, but the GCS has been most widely adopted. (Starmark et al., 1988). Its predictive power was further demonstrated in the Traumatic Coma Data Bank

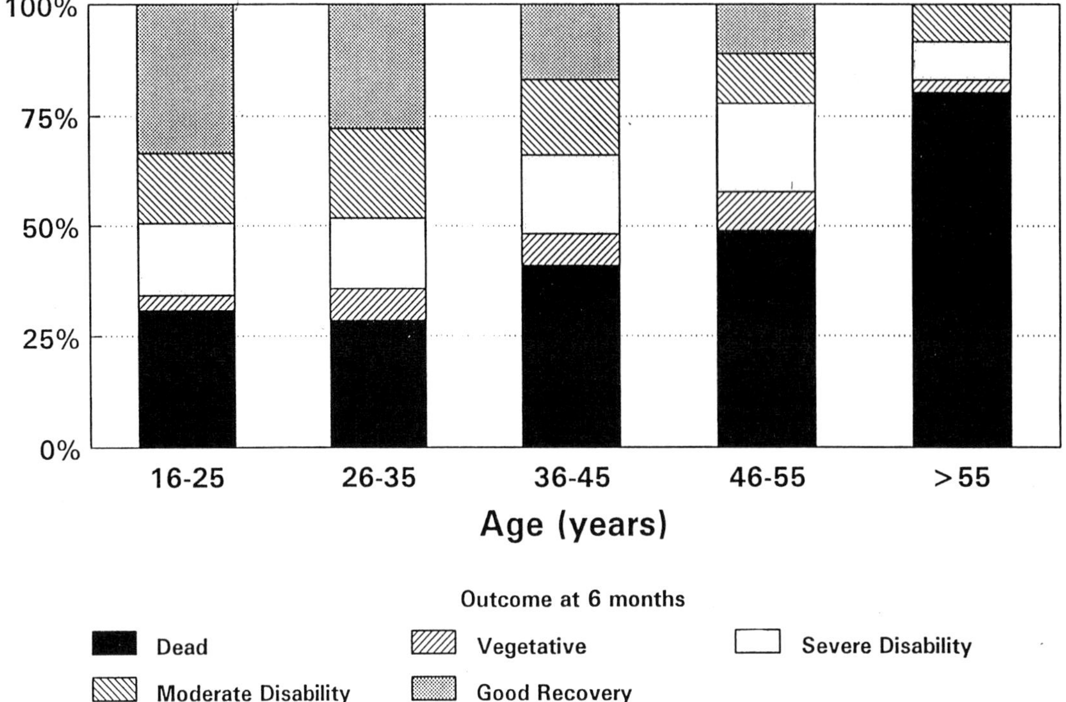

Fig. 2-10. Age-specific distribution of the Glasgow Outcome Scale in severe head injury patients. (From Vollmer et al., 1992, with permission.)

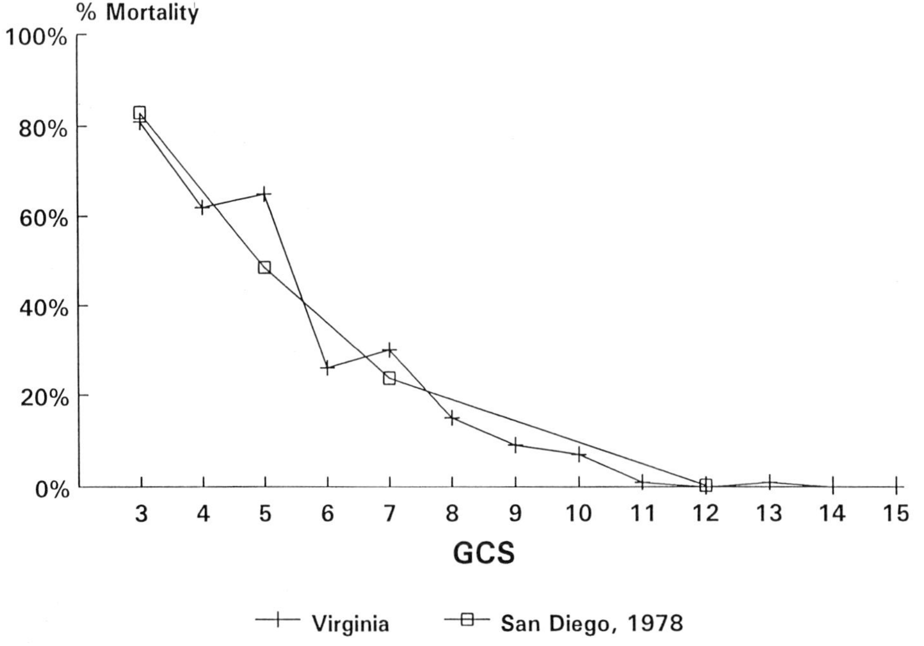

Fig. 2-11. Mortality by level of the Glasgow Coma Scale. (Data from Jane and Rimel 1982; Klauber et al., 1981.)

analysis of outcome following severe head injury. The population included patients with traumatic coma (GCS < 9) within 48 hours of injury (Marshall et al., 1991a), and the scoring system was adapted for missing GCS components. Postresuscitation levels were better predictors than initial GCS scores. The postresuscitation GCS measurement showed a gradation in recovery, disability, and death (Fig. 2-12). Levin et al. (1990) also evaluated the postresuscitation GCS ability to predict neuropsychological outcome. The worst postresuscitation GCS was related to ability to complete the neuropsychological examination and to performance; however, this was observed to have a significant interaction with pupillary status.

In a subset of patients who deteriorated to coma from initial scores of GCS above 8, there was a higher mortality than in patients with initial GCS levels 6 to 8. This indicates the dynamic nature of head injury and that serial evaluation of coma status is necessary in determining prognosis.

The GCS has been problematic for use in children, particularly small children, who may not understand commands. The Paediatric Coma Scale was studied in 66 children less than 72 months of age (Simpson et al., 1991). There was an association with outcome but there were few children in coma in this study. Replication of the results in larger studies is necessary.

Pupil Response

Abnormal pupil response is a poor prognostic indicator. In the International Data Bank almost all the patients with nonreactive pupils had a poor outcome (Jennett et al., 1979). There is also an increased risk of death with two nonreactive pupils versus one. Pupil response was associated with age in the Traumatic Coma Data Bank but was independently related to outcome (Vollmer et al., 1991).

Pathology

The degree of pathologic damage is related to prognosis. Among admitted patients in San Diego County, brain hemorrhage was associated with poorer survival than nonhemorrhage cases (Conroy and Kraus, 1988). Ribas and Jane (1992) reviewed the literature to determine risk factors for traumatic intracerebral

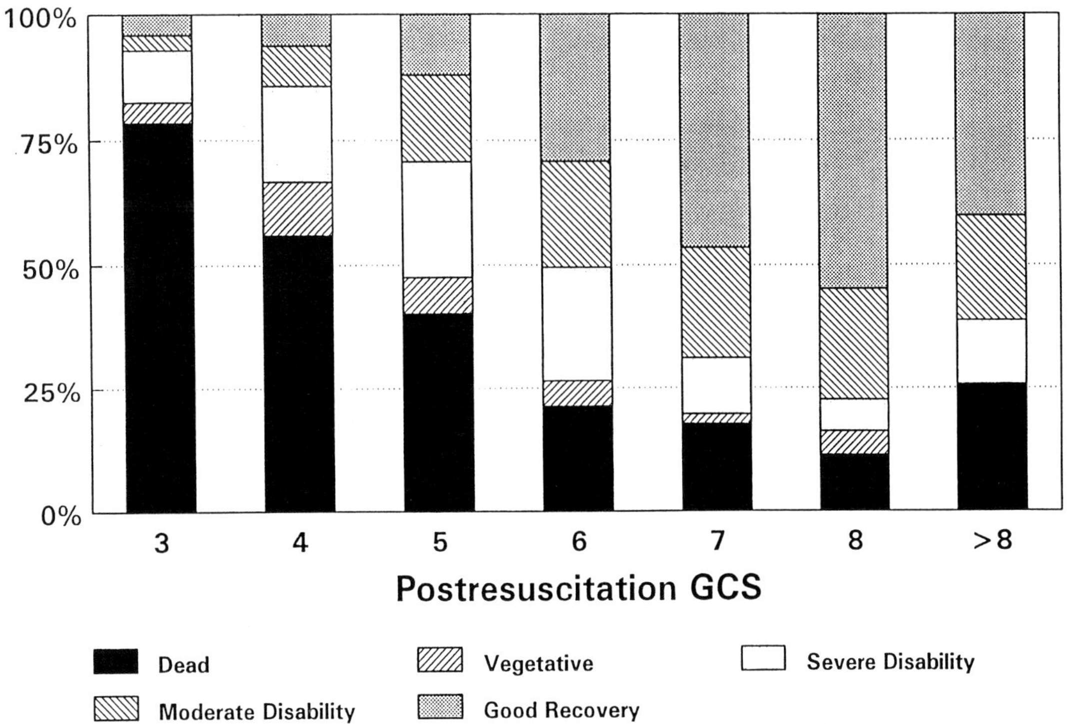

Fig. 2-12. Postresuscitation GCS-specific distribution of the Glasgow Outcome Scale in severe head injury patients. (From Marshall et al., 1992, with permission.)

hemorrhages and contusions and their relationship to outcome. Factors that contributed to hemorrhage and outcome were intracranial pressure, midline shift, presence of other lesions, admission GCS, and age. Jamjoom et al. (1992) evaluated determinants of outcome in patients who were 65 years or older and who had surgical evacuation of an intracranial hematoma. Factors related to outcome in this population were age, time of surgery post-trauma, admission and preoperation GCS, and pupillary response.

In a series of 211 patients who were initially lucid and then deteriorated into coma, Lobato et al. (1991) evaluated factors relating to deterioration and outcome. Deterioration was associated with the presence of a mass lesion and with age. Overall outcome was related to GCS following deterioration, highest mean intracranial pressure, degree of midline shift, type of intracranial lesion, and age. Early deterioration (< 6 hours) correlated with type of mass lesion (subdural > epidural > diffuse > brain contusion/hematoma). Late deterioration (>24 hours) was related to lesion in an opposite fashion. Mortality was higher in patients with early deterioration.

Cerebral edema is an important prognostic factor. A study of 53 patients with clinical signs of transtentorial herniation was made to determine factors related to the GOS (Andrews and Pitts, 1991). Good recovery was related to age, anisocoria, bilateral pupil reactivity, hemiparesis, motor response, and GCS. No difference was found for the effect of the presence or absence of intracranial hematomas on functional outcome.

The prognosis of patients remaining in coma is important in the determining the course of therapy and resource utilization. Levin et al. (1991) evaluated patients in the Traumatic Coma Data Bank who were discharged in a vegetative state. Factors related to the occurrence of a persistent vegetative state were lower GCS, abnormal pupil responses, and diffuse injury with swelling or shift on CT.

Radiologic Findings

As described earlier, CT allows rapid diagnosis of hematomas and classification of the intracranial pathology. Teasdale et al. (1992) reviewed the status of CT and MRI classification of head injury. The number and distribution of CT findings were associated with differential outcome. Patients with deep white matter lesions and brainstem or cerebellar lesions had poor outcome. CT has also been useful to predict patients with increased intracranial pressure. Ischemic lesions may be frequent in head injury but are only detectable with serial CT examinations.

The predictiveness of CT has been also evaluated by Kido et al. (1992) in 72 patients. Lesion size was associated with outcome measured by the GOS. Patients whose lesions had a volumetric measurement of 4,100 mm^3 had a poor prognosis. Patients with normal scans had only mild dysfunction.

Eisenberg et al. (1990) evaluated the effect of CT findings on prognosis in severe head injury patients in the Traumatic Coma Data Bank. Patients with an abnormal CT scan had poorer prognosis. For patients with abnormal scans, the order of risk was mass lesions > swelling with shift > swelling with no shift > other abnormalities. The compression of cisterns was also a poor prognostic sign. The presence of subarachnoid blood resulted in a doubling of risk for mortality.

Marshall et al. (1991*b*, 1992) described the classification used in the Traumatic Coma Data Bank, as discussed above, and its importance in prognosis of outcome from severe head injury. The differentiation of size of mass lesions, evacuation of mass lesions, and subcategorization of diffuse injury were demonstrated to be in relationship to GOS (Fig. 2-13). The gradation of swelling and shift for diffuse injury indicates the severity of brain damage and secondary pathophysiology. The equivalence of evacuated mass lesions and diffuse injury may be important, since removal of the hematoma allows reevaluation of prognosis.

CT allows for stratification of injuries based on pathology. Marshall et al. (1992) examined the factors determining outcome for patients with diffuse head injury with swelling. Factors related to outcome were highest intracranial pressure (ICP) in the first 72 hours, pupil reactivity, and lowest ICP in the first 72 hours. In an analysis of children under age 17 years with diffuse injury and swelling in the Traumatic Coma Data Bank, Aldrich et al. (1992) observed that there was a higher occurrence of early hypoxia and hypotension and a higher mean percentage of the time that ICP was greater than 20 mmHg. Children with diffuse injury with swelling had higher mortality rates in the acute period at 6 days, and long term 3 years from injury, than children in other categories.

The increased sensitivity of MRI has also increased the number of lesions visualized. MRI has been shown to be more likely than CT to detect lesions of the cortex, small subdural hematomas, and diffuse axo-

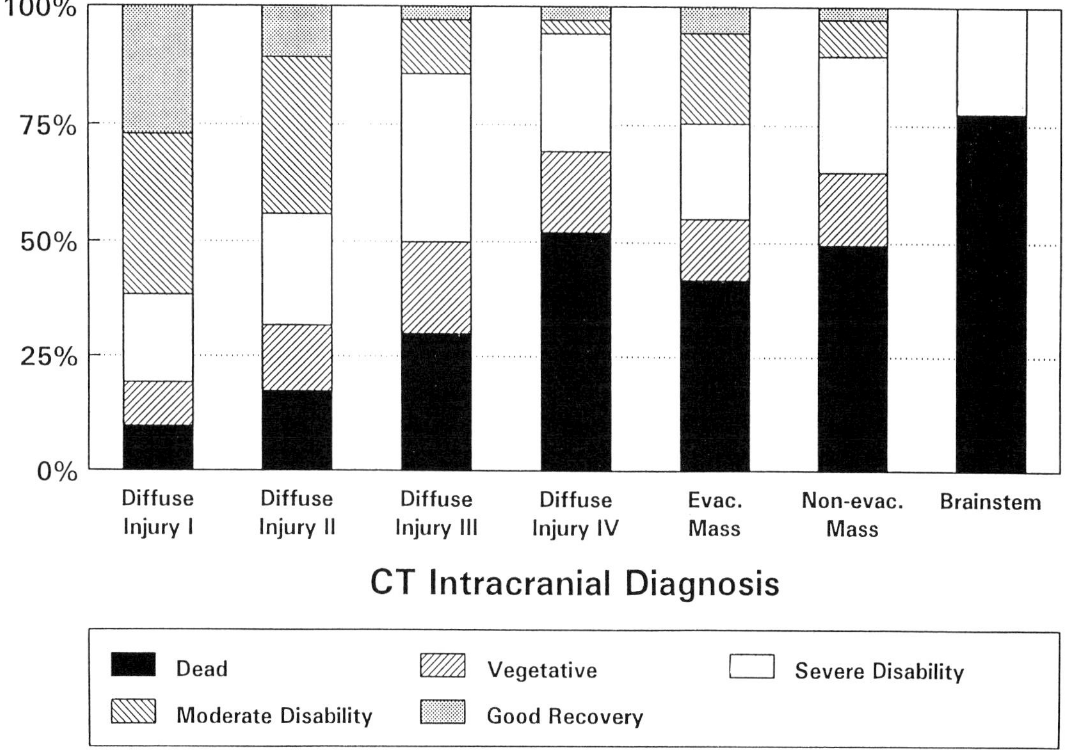

Fig. 2-13. Distribution of the Glasgow Outcome Scale in severe head injury patients by intracranial diagnosis. (From Marshall et al., 1992, with permission.)

nal injuries (Sklar EML et al., 1992). Also, vascular abnormalities may be diagnosed with newer magnetic resonance angiography methods. CT and MRI can be used to complement each other to determine the intracranial pathology, but the prognostic utility of MRI still needs to be demonstrated (see Ch. 5).

Analysis of head injury victims by single-photon emission computed tomography (SPECT) also may be of diagnostic and prognostic importance. Newton et al. (1992) compared MRI and CT but also included SPECT. In 19 patients they found evidence of more lesions with SPECT than with MRI or CT. Cerebral atrophy was more apparent on CT. There was an association of lesions on SPECT and of global cerebral blood flow with GOS score (see Ch. 6).

Evoked Potentials and Electroencephalography

Serial assessment using somatosensory evoked potentials (SEPs) may yield a measure of brain activity. The prognostic utility of evoked potential measurement of brain stimuli has been studied. Dauch (1991) evaluated deterioration in 75 comatose patients, in whom SEP demonstrated a high association with neurologic decline. Barelli et al. (1991) used serial measurement of brainstem auditory evoked potentials (BAEPs) and SEPs in 73 patients with severe head injury. The evoked potentials were measured between 1 and 21 days post-trauma and graded according to the pattern exhibited. Patients with high BAEP scores had a 100 percent mortality rate, but BAEP grades did not show an association with GCS. SEP grades did not show a clear pattern with outcome or GCS (see Ch. 7).

Specific components of the evoked potential measurements have demonstrated prognostic significance. Gott et al. (1991) found that the P300 ERP component of auditory evoked potentials was related to the likelihood of awakening from coma and to the Keren et al. (1991), using early and late evoked potentials, observed that recovery was related to differences in central conduction time. In patients with only frontal lesions, Wirsen et al. (1992) compared reduction in the P300 amplitude in the anterior electrodes with controls. Quantified electroencephalographic (EEG) analysis was also performed and the modal frequency of EEG was found to be associated with lesion volume and injury severity. Rae-Grant et al. (1991) developed an EEG rating scale by classifying EEG findings into dichotomous categories. The classification was tested in 57 patients with head injury and found to have high reliability and to predict outcome at discharge as measured by the GOS. Thatcher et al. (1991) evaluated EEG and evoked potentials with a 1-year follow-up using the Disability Rating Scale. They found that the EEG-phase along with late GCS were the best predictors of function.

Marshall (1991) has questioned the usefulness of evoked potentials in patient management. Their relationship to outcome may be the result of neurologic changes caused by alterations in cerebral perfusion; hence they are a surrogate measure for outcome. Whether or not they independently predict outcome above other factors needs to be evaluated. Their use in subgroups such as patients with diffuse axonal injury may be important to clarify their utility.

Cerebral Blood Flow and Oxygenation

Changes in cerebral blood flow (CBF) measured by xenon inhalation techniques, have been demonstrated in association with severe head injury (Muizelaar 1989). Studies have correlated CBF and arteriovenous oxygen difference with GCS and outcome. Bouma et al. (1991) measured both in 186 adult patients with severe head injury. An association between motor response and CBF was observed during the first 8 hours. Arteriovenous oxygen difference was highest shortly after admission and decreased over time. CBF was also associated with the GOS at follow-up.

Robertson et al. (1992) studied 102 patients with severe head trauma, making serial measurements of CBF, arteriovenous oxygen difference ($AVDO_2$), cerebral metabolic rate of oxygen and of lactate, and ICP. Factors related to CBF were age of the patient, $AVDO_2$, and cerebral metabolic rate. GCS level and intracranial hypertension were not different in CBF groups. Mortality was highest in the patients with low CBF. Good recovery was highest in patients with high CBF and lowest in the low CBF group. Low CBF was related to outcome independently of age, GCS, cerebral metabolic rate of oxygen, cerebral perfusion pressure, and hemoglobin. Also, within levels of CBF, $AVDO_2$ was related to poor outcome. The relationship of low CBF and outcome might be explained by differences in metabolic rate and resulting reduced oxygen availability or increased oxygen demand. Continuous oxygen saturation was also studied in a subgroup of 33 patients. A trend of low oxygen saturation was found in the reduced CBF group. These findings indicate that patients with reduced CBF may develop transient hypoxia and ischemia.

Intracranial Pressure

Marmarou et al. (1991a, 1991b) of the Traumatic Coma Data Bank have studied increased ICP and prognosis. For severe head injury patients, 65 percent had ICP monitoring, with 72 percent of those patients having an elevated ICP higher than 20 mmHg. The level of ICP and the time that ICP remains elevated are related to outcome. The interaction with hypotension is important as it relates to cerebral perfusion pressure. The proportion of time ICP was greater than 20 mmHg and the proportion of time systolic blood pressure was below 80 mmHg were related to outcome at 6 months even after controlling for age, motor response, and pupil response in the model. Factors observed on CT that may predict elevated ICP are brain swelling with midline shift and compressed or absent mesencephalic cisterns (Eisenberg et al., 1990).

Multiple Trauma

Brain trauma generally does not occur in isolation. The role of multiple trauma in severity measures and in relation to outcome is important for prognosis. In a study of patients seen at the University of Virginia it was found that brain AIS scores accounted for most of the variation in total score (Fife and Jagger, 1984). The contribution of head injury to outcome in patients with multiple trauma has been assessed in the Major Trauma Outcome Study (Gennarelli et al., 1989). Mortality associated with head injury was three times that of patients without head trauma. Of the deaths in head-injured patients, two-thirds were attributed to the head injury, 7 percent to extracranial injury, and 26 percent to both. Patients with a minor or moderate head injury were more likely to die if there was a severe extracranial injury.

Extracranial Complications

Secondary systemic complications are frequent in hospitalized patients with severe head injury. Changes in metabolism, pulmonary function, cardiac function, hematologic and immunologic parameters, gastrointestinal function, and endocrine levels occur following head injury.

Hypoxia and Hypotension

In the prehospital phase of head injury, the patient may suffer hypoxia and hypotension. Subsequently these patients may develop ischemic lesions. In the Traumatic Coma Data Bank, hypotension (systolic blood pressure <90 mmHg) occurred 35 percent of the time (Piek et al., 1992}. Hypotensive episodes may also occur during hospitalization. Diffuse swelling has been associated with the occurrence of early hypotension or hypoxia.

Metabolic Changes

Young et al. (1992) reviewed the metabolic response to injury. The response may be hypermetabolism, hypercatabolism, an acute-phase response, decreased immunocompetence, hyperglycemia, increased hormone levels, increased ventricular fluid and cytokine levels, and altered gastric functions. Hypermetabolism is increased with injury and with injury severity. In the acute-phase response patients with severe injury suffer hypoalbuminemia, which may be mediated by cytokines. Whether this is a protective mechanism has yet to be determined.

Hyperglycemia is a stress response to trauma. Hyperglycemia may be related to poor outcome through the possibility of further brain cell damage by lactate accumulation. Lam et al. (1991) evaluated serum glucose levels in 169 patients with all grades of head injury. Glucose levels were found to be higher in comatose patients and were associated with poorer outcomes when measured at 10 days postinjury.

Other Systemic Complications

Electrolyte changes are the most frequent in head-injured patients, occurring in nearly 60 percent of cases (Piek et al., 1992). Electrocardiographic (ECG) changes have been documented to occur frequently in patients with head injury. These changes are probably due to catecholamine release associated with the cerebral damage. Most result in subendocardial damage without major consequence (Miner, 1985). Elderly patients with severe cardiac complications appear to be at highest risk for poor outcome. (Vollmer et al., 1991). Pneumonia also occurs frequently (40 percent of cases) in patients with severe head injury. The necessity of intubation coupled with altered pulmonary function may allow colonization of bacteria. This complication occurs most frequently in days 5 through 10 after injury (Piek et al., 1992). Septicemia occurs in approximately 10 percent of head-injured patients. Owing to the invasive nature of monitoring and treatment, this complication is difficult to prevent. Septic shock can further add to hypotension in causing ischemic damage. Coagulopathies are known to occur and are associated with severity of the brain injury. Disseminated intravascular coagulation in particular may not be independent of severity of the head injury.

Multivariate Analyses

Several analyses have included multiple predictors of coma outcome. In a population-based study of San Diego County, the prognostic factors for mortality that showed importance were severity of the brain injury (GCS), nature of injury (hemorrhage and fracture), cause of injury (firearms), and age (Conroy and Kraus, 1988). In a large clinical series of head-injured patients in 1980 and 1981 in 41 hospitals, Klauber et al. (1981b) found that predictors for death were motor score, pupil response, systolic blood pressure, abdominal injury, chest injury, age and hospital (combined variable).

In clinical-based studies with severe head injury patients, various factors have historically shown importance: age, pupillary reaction, GCS, surgical lesion, ICP, midline shift on CT, and multimodality evoked potentials (Braakman et al., 1980; Choi et al., 1988; Narayan et al., 1981; Stablein et al., 1980; Young et al., 1981). Marshall et al. (1991a) from the Traumatic Coma Data Bank found that factors related to outcome were age, postresuscitation GCS, and pupil reactivity. Warme et al. (1991) evaluated patients in a historical control study to assess the effectiveness of a neurologic intensive care unit. They found that factors related to outcome were age, mechanism of injury, GCS, pupil response, CT diagnosis, and the occurrence of complications of hypotension, hypoxia, hyperthermia, and epilepsy. Vollmer et al. (1991) also studied patients with closed head injury from the Traumatic Coma Data Bank to determine if age was an independent predictor of outcome. No variable replaced age as an independent predictor. The resulting logistic regression for vegetative survival or death at 6 months included (in order of importance) number of serious complications, motor response, age, absence of mesencephalic cisterns on CT, subarachnoid hemorrhage on CT, shock, the presence of an extracerebral lesions, intracerebral hematoma evacuation, and pupil response. Thatcher et al. (1991) evaluated 162 patients, using comprehensive examinations including GCS, CT scan, EEG, and evoked potentials. EEG and GCS at the time of the evoked potentials (not admission) were the strongest predictors of outcome. EEG phase and coherence measures explained the greatest variance in the Disability Rating Scale score. Piek et al. (1992) evaluated the contribution of extracranial complications to prognosis. Poor outcome was related to age, preresuscitation GCS motor score, prehospital shock, shock during hospitalization, pneumonia, coagulopathy, and septicemia.

The multivariate models have demonstrated correct predictions in approximately 90 percent of cases. Models have focused on mortality, and a few have included vegetative survival along with death as an outcome. Since the models have been developed in severe head injury, mortality dominates the estimation. Models that focused on recovery might be useful in differentiating patterns of recovery associated with, for example, nature of injury, length of coma, and age. A recent article by Horn et al. (1992), describes the recovery of a patient with severe head trauma who, on the basis of our current prognostic variables, would have been expected to have a poor outcome. However, the patient made a good recovery.

Prognostic models need to focus on phases of the head injury (i.e., prehospital, hospital, and recovery). They also need to be time-sensitive. Prognostic factors change and need to be reassessed periodically to alter the prediction for death or disability for a given patient. Many of the models are focused on the status at the time of injury. Recent models have shown that inclusion of secondary intracranial and extracranial events is important in determining a final intracranial diagnosis, the occurrence of complications, and brain function (EEG, SEP). They may play a role in long-term prognosis. By use of CT, MRI, and SPECT, new classification systems have been and can be developed. Newer methods such as magnetic resonance angiography, transcranial Doppler ultrasound, and laser Doppler flowmetry offer further ability to classify the type and degree of brain impairment (Meyerson et al., 1991). Evoked potentials and EEG recordings have added to the measurement spectrum. These measurements may predict recovery potential, and with serial recordings for monitoring, their effectiveness in reflecting change in brain activity will be important.

CONCLUSION

The epidemiology of head injury shows that the rates of head injury vary by population. This is a reflection of the causes of the injuries as well as of classification and inclusion criteria. Motor vehicle crashes account for nearly half the injuries and falls for approximately 20 percent. Falls are an important cause in the young and elderly. Inclusion of prehospital deaths, classification of cases with CT or MRI, and referral patterns and admission practices affect the rates. Although the rates of head injury mortality appears to be declining, there still remains a great deal to be done in prevention, since the majority of deaths occur prior to hospitalization. The majority of head injuries are not severe, and head injury appears to be a declining cause of hospital admissions.

Whether decline in head injury mortality is due to changes in classification, prevention programs, referral patterns, or effectiveness of treatment is difficult to determine. Ongoing population-based surveillance that would provide incidence and outcome data does not exist. Populations such as that of Olmstead County, Minnesota that are well documented are useful, but small numbers are not very sensitive to particular time points or changes in case ascertainment or interventions. The need for emergency room surveillance and population surveys is evident in order to determine the changing epidemiology of head injury.

The prevalence of head injury is also an unanswered question. The unrecognized prevalence of cognitive deficit and the need for cognitive rehabilitation still need to be assessed.

Measurements of injury severity measured by depth of coma, duration of coma, and intracranial pathology are important advances in determining prognosis and outcome of head trauma. Prognostic factors have shown that there are important subgroups that may be keys for recovery prediction and medical and rehabilitation intervention. Advances in knowledge of biochemical and physiologic changes have contributed and need to further contribute to the etiology of secondary complications and consequences of primary brain injury. These advances may lead to the development of neuroprotective drugs or regimens that can limit the damage and promote recovery.

However, the cost of acute treatment and rehabilitation to promote recovery is enormous. The investment in prevention programs to decrease the incidence and severity of head injury not only saves lives but cuts the cost of disability. Continuous appraisal of incidence, causes, and outcome of head trauma is needed to mark changes that are made.

REFERENCES

Aldrich EF, Eisenberg HM, Saydjari C et al: Diffuse brain swelling in severely head-injured children. J Neurosurg 76:450–454, 1992

American Association for Automotive Medicine: The Abbreviated Injury Scale. Des Plaines, IL, 1990

Andrews BT, Pitts LH: Functional recovery after traumatic transtentorial herniation. Neurosurgery 29:227–231, 1991

Annegers JF, Grabow JD, Kurland LT, Laws ED Jr: The incidence causes, and secular trends of head trauma in Olmstead County, Minnesota, 1935–1974. Neurology 30:912–919, 1980

Baker SP, O'Neill B, Ginsburg MJ, Guohua L: The Injury Fact Book. Oxford University Press, New York, 1992

Barelli A, Valente MR, Clemente A et al: Serial Multimodality-evoked potentials in severely head-injured patients: diagnostic and prognostic implications. Crit Care Med 19:1374–1381, 1991

Bouma GJ, Muizelaar JP, Choi SC et al: Cerebral Circulation and metabolism after severe traumatic brain injury: the elusive role of ischemia. J Neurosurg 75:685–693, 1991

Braakman R, Glepke GJ, Habbema JDF et al: Systematic selection of prognosis features in patients with severe head injury. Neurosurgery 6:362–370, 1980

Champion HR, Sacco WJ, Carnazzo AJ et al: Trauma Score. Crit Care Med 9:672–676, 1981

Choi SC, Narayan RK, Anderson RL et al: Enhanced specificity of prognosis in severe head injury. J Neurosurg 69:381–385, 1988

Clifton GL, Hayes RL, Levin HS et al: Outcome measures for clinical trials involving traumatically brain-injured patients: report of a conference. Neurosurgery 31: 975–978, 1992

Clifton GL, Kreutzer JS, Choi SC et al: Relationship between Glasgow Outcome Scale and neuropsychological measures after brain injury. Neurosurgery 33:34–39, 1993

Conroy C, Kraus JF: Survival after brain injury. Cause of death, length of survival, and prognostic variables in a cohort of brain-injured people. Neuroepidemiology 7:13–22, 1988

Cooper JD, Tabaddor K, Hauser WA: The epidemiology of head injury in the Bronx. Neuroepidemiology 2:70–88, 1983

Dauch WA: Prediction of secondary deterioration in comatose neurosurgical patients by serial recording of multimodality evoked potentials. Acta Neurochir (Wien) 111:84–91, 1991

Edna TH, Cappelen J: Head injury on road traffic accidents. A prospective study in Trondela, Norway, Scand J Soc Med 13:23–27, 1985

Eisenberg HM, Gary HE, Aldrich EF et al: Initial CT findings in 753 patients with severe head injury. A report from the NIH Traumatic Coma Data Bank. J Neurosurg 73:688–698, 1990

Elson LM, Ward CC: Mechanisms and pathophysiology of mild head injury. Semin Neurol 14:8–18, 1994

Fife D, Faich G, Hollinshead W, Boynton W: Incidence and outcome of hospital-treated head injury in Rhode Island. Am J Public Health 76:773–778, 1986

Fife D, Jagger J: The contribution of brain injury to the overall injury severity of brain-injured patients. J Neurosurg 60:697–699, 1984

Foulkes MA, Eisenberg HM, Jane JA et al. (Traumatic Coma Data Bank Research Group): The traumatic coma data bank: design, methods and baseline characteristics. J Neurosurg 75:S8–S13, 1991

Frankowski RF, Annegers JF, Whitman S: Epidemiological and descriptive studies. Part I: The descriptive epidemiology of head trauma in the United States. pp. 33–43. In Becker DP, Povlishock JT (eds): Central Nervous System Trauma Status Report 1985. National Institute of Neurological Disorders and Stroke. Bethesda, 1985

Gennarelli TA, Champion HR, Sacco WJ et al: Mortality of patients with head injury and extracranial injury treated in trauma centers. J Trauma 29:1193–1202, 1989

Gott PS, Rabinowicz AL, Degiorgio CM: P300 Auditory event-related potentials in nontraumatic coma. Association with Glasgow Coma Score and awakening. Arch Neurol 48:1267–1270, 1991

Gouvier WD, Blanton PD, Laporte KK: Reliability and validity of the Disability Rating Scale and the Levels of Cognitive Functioning Scale in monitoring recovery from severe head injury. Arch Phys Med Rehabil 68:94–97, 1987

Grabow JD, Oxford KP, Rieder ME: The cost of head trauma in Olmstead County Minnesota, 1970–74. Am J Pub Health 74:710–712, 1984

Granger CV, Hamilton BB: The uniform data system for medical rehabilitation report of first admissions for 1991. Am J Phys Med Rehabil 72:33–38, 1993

Hamilton BB, Granger CV, Sherwin FS: A uniform national system for medical rehabilitation. pp. 137–147. In Fuhrer MJ (ed): Rehabilitation Outcomes: Analysis and Measurement. Brooks, Baltimore, 1987

Harrison CL, Dijkers M: Traumatic brain injury registries in the United States: an overview. Brain Inj 6:203–212, 1992

Heyer NJ, Franklin GM: Work-related traumatic brain injury in Washington State, 1988 through 1990. Am J Public Health 84:1106–1109, 1994

Horn S, Watson M, Wilson BA, McLellan DL: The development of new techniques in the assessment and monitoring of recovery from severe head injury: a preliminary report and case history. Brain Inj 6:321–325, 1992

Jagger J, Levine J, Jane J et al: Epidemiologic features of head injury in a predominantly rural population. J Trauma 24:40–44, 1984

Jamjoom A, Nelson R, Stranjalis G et al: Outcome following surgical intervention of traumatic intracranial haematomas in the elderly. Br J Neurosurg 6:27–32, 1992

Jane J, Rimel R: Prognosis in head injury. Clin Neurosurg 29:346, 1982

Jenkins A, Teasdale G, Hadley MDM et al: Brain lesions detected by magnetic resonance imaging in mild and severe head injuries. Lancet, 2:445–446, 1986

Jennett B, MacMillan R: Epidemiology of head injury. Br Med J 282:101–104, 1981

Jennett B, Murray A, MacMillan R: Head injuries in Scottish hospitals. Lancet 2:696–698, 1977

Jennett B, Snoek J, Bond MR, Brooks N: Disability after severe head injury observations on the use of the Glasgow Outcome Scale. J Neurol Neurosurg Psychiatry 44:285–293, 1981

Jennett B, Teasdale G: Management of Head Injuries. FA Davis, Philadelphia, 1981, p. 309

Jennett B, Teasdale G, Braakman R et al: Prognosis of patients with severe head injury. Neurosurgery 4: 283–289, 1979

Johnston MV: The economics of brain injury: a preface. pp. 163–186. In Miner ME, Wagner KA (eds): Neurotrauma. Treatment, Rehabilitation and Related Issues. No. 3. Butterworths, Boston, 1989

Kalsbeek WD, McLaurin RL, Harris BSH, Miller JD: The National Head and Spinal Cord Injury Survey: major findings. J Neurosurg 53:s19–s31, 1980

Keren O, Groswasser Z, Sazbon L, Ring C: Somatosensory evoked potentials in prolonged postcomatose unawareness state following traumatic brain injury. Brain Inj 5:233–240, 1991

Kido DK, Cox C, Hamill RW et al: Traumatic brain injuries: predictive usefulness of CT. Radiology 182:777–781, 1992

Klauber MR, Barrett-Connor E, Marshall LF et al: The epidemiology of head injury. A prospective study of an entire community: San Diego, California, 1978. Am J Epidemiol 113:500–509, 1981a

Klauber MR, Marshall LF, Barrett-Connor E, Bowers SA: Prospective study of patients hospitalized with head injury in San Diego County, 1978. Neurosurgery 9:236–241, 1981b

Kraus JF: Epidemiology of head injury. p. 1–26. In Cooper PR (ed): Head Injury. Williams & Wilkins, Baltimore, 1993

Kraus JF, Black MA, Hessol N et al: The incidence of acute brain injury and serious impairment in a defined population. Am J Epidemiol 119:186–201, 1984

Kraus JF, Conroy C, Cox P et al: Survival times and case fatality rates of brain-injured persons. J Neurosurg 63:537–543, 1985

Kraus JF, Fife D: Incidence, external causes, and outcomes of work-related brain injuries in males. J Occup Med 27:757–760, 1985

Kraus JF, Fife D, Conroy C: Incidence, severity, and outcomes of brain injuries involving bicycles. Am J Public Health 77:76–78, 1987

Kraus JF, Fife D, Ramstein K et al: The relationship of family income to the incidence, external causes and outcomes of serious brain injury, San Diego, California. Am J Public Health 76:1345–1347, 1986

Kraus JF, McArthur DL, Silberman TA: Epidemiology of mild brain injury. Semin Neurol 14:1–7, 1994

Kraus JF, Peek C, McArthur DL, Williams A: The effect of the 1992 California motorcycle helmet use law on motorcycle crash fatalities and injuries. JAMA 272: 1506–1511, 1994

Lam AM, Winn HR, Cullen BF, Sundling N: Hyperglycemia and neurological outcome in patient with head injury. J Neurosurg 75:545–551, 1991

Levin HS: Neurobehavioral recovery. J Neurotrauma suppl. 1, 9:S359–S373, 1992

Levin HS, Gary HE, Eisenberg HM et al: Neurobehavioral outcome 1 year after severe head injury. Experience of the Traumatic Coma Data Bank. J Neurosurg 73:699–709, 1990

Levin HS, Saydjari C, Eisenberg HM et al: Vegetative state after closed-head injury. A Traumatic Coma Data Bank report. Arch Neurol 48:580–585, 1991

Levin HS, Williams D, Crofford MJ et al: Relationship of depth of brain lesions to consciousness and outcome after closed head injury. J Neurosurg 69:861–866, 1988

Lipper MH, Kishore PRS: Radiologic investigation of acute head trauma. pp. 102–137. In Becker DP, Gudeman SK (eds): Textbook of Head Injury. WB Saunders, Philadelphia, 1989

Livingston DH, Loder PA, Koziol J, Hunt CD: The use of CT scanning to triage patients requiring admission following minimal head injury. J Trauma 31:483–489, 1991

Lobato RD, Rivas JJ, Gomez PA et al: Head-injured patients who talk and deteriorate into coma. Analysis of 211 case studies with computerized tomography. J Neurosurg 75:256–261, 1991

Mackenzie EJ, Edelstein SL, Flynn JP: Trends in hospitalized discharge rates for head injury in Maryland, 1979–1986. Am J Public Health 80:217–219, 1990

Mackenzie EJ, Steinwachs DM, Shankar B: Classifying trauma severity based on hospital discharge diagnoses: validation of an ICD-9CM to AIS'95 conversion table. Med Care 27:412–422, 1989

Marmarou A, Anderson RL, Ward JD et al: NINDS Traumatic Coma Data Bank: intracranial pressure monitoring methodology. J Neurosurg 75:S21–S27, 1991a

Marmarou A, Anderson RL, Ward JD et al: Impact of ICP instability and hypotension in patients with severe head trauma. J Neurosurg 75:S59–S66, 1991b

Marshall LF: Evoked potentials: a decade later. Crit Care Med 19:1337, 1991

Marshall LF, Gautille T, Klauber MR et al: The outcome of severe closed head injury. J Neurosurg 75:S28–S36, 1991a

Marshall LF, Marshall SB, Klauber MR et al: A new classification of head injury based on computerized tomography. J Neurosurg 75:S14–S20, 1991b

Marshall LF, Marshall SB, Klauber MR et al: The diagnosis of head injury requires a classification based on computed axial tomography. J Neurotrauma suppl. 1, 9:S287–S292, 1992

Masters SJ, McClean PM, Aracarese JS et al: Skull x-ray examinations after head trauma. Recommendations by a multidisciplinary panel and validation study. N Engl J Med 316:84–91, 1987

Max W, Mackenzie EJ, Rice DP: Head injuries: cost and consequences. J Head Trauma Rehabil 6:76–91, 1991

Meyerson BA, Gunasekera L, Linderoth B, Gazelius B: Bedside monitoring of regional cortical blood flow in comatose patients using laser Doppler flowmetry. Neurosurgery 29:750–755, 1991

Miller JD: Changing patterns in acute management of head injury. J Neurol Sci 103:S33–S37, 1991

Miner ME: Systemic effects of brain injury. Trauma 2:75–83, 1985

Muizelaar JP: Cerebral blood flow, cerebral blood volume, and cerebral metabolism after severe head injury. pp. 221–240. In Becker DP, Gudeman SK (eds): Textbook of Head Injury. WB Saunders, 1989

Narayan RK, Greenberg RP, Miller JD: Improved outcome prediction in severe head injury. A comparative analysis of clinical examination, multimodality evoked potentials, CT scanning, and intracranial pressure. J Neurosurg 54:751–762, 1981

National Center for Health Statistics: International Classification of Diseases. 9th Revision, Clinical Modification. Commission on Professional and Hospital Activities, Ann Arbor, MI, 1978

National Center for Health Statistics: Detailed Diagnosis and Procedures. National Hospital Discharge Survey, 1991. U.S. Department of Health and Human Services, Hyattsville, MD, 1994a

National Center for Health Statistics: Injury Mortality Atlas of the United States, 1979–1987. U.S. Department of Health and Human Services, Hyattsville, MD, 1994b

Nell V, Brown DSO: Epidemiology of traumatic brain injury in Johannesburg. II. Morbidity, mortality and etiology. Soc Sci Med 33:289–296, 1991

Newton MR, Greenwood RJ, Britton KE et al: A study comparing SPECT with CT and MRI after closed head injury. J Neurol Neurosurg Psychiatry 55:92–94, 1992

Piek J, Chesnut RM, Marshall LF et al: Extracranial complications of severe head injury. J Neurosurg 77:901–907, 1992

Rae-Grant AD, Barbour PJ, Reed J: Development of a novel EEG rating scale for head injury using dichotomous variables. Electroencephalogr Clin Neurophysiol 79:349–357, 1991

Rappaport M, Hall K, Hopkins HK et al: Disability rating scale for severe head trauma: coma to community. Arch Phys Med Rehabil 63:118–123, 1982

Rappaport M, Hemmerle AV, Rappaport ML: Short and long latency auditory evoked potentials in traumatic brain injury patients. Clin Electroencephalogr 22: 199–202, 1991

Ribas G, Jane JA: Traumatic contusions and intracerebral hematomas. J Neurotrauma suppl. 1, 9:S265–S278, 1992

Rimel RW, Giordani B, Barth JT et al: Disability caused by minor head injury. Neurosurgery 9:221–228, 1981

Rimel RW, Giordani B, Barth JT, Jane JA: Moderate head injury: completing the clinical spectrum of brain trauma. Neurosurgery 11:344–351, 1982

Roberston CS, Contant CF, Narayan RK, Grossman RG: Cerebral blood flow, $AVDO_2$ and neurologic outcome in head-injured patients. J Neurotrauma suppl. 1, 9:S349–S358, 1992

Ruff RM, Young D, Gautille T et al: Verbal learning deficits following severe head injury: heterogeneity in recovery over 1 Year. J Neurosurg 75:S50–S58, 1991

Sakata R, Ostby S, Leung P: Functional status, referral and cost of treatment for persons with traumatic head injury. Brain Injury 5:411–419, 1991

Schnyoll W, Overton D, Krome R et al: A prospective study to identify high-yield criteria associated with acute intracranial computed tomography findings in head-injured patients. Am J Emerg Med 11:321–326, 1993

Servadei F, Ciucci G, Pagano F et al: Skull fracture as a risk factor of intracranial complications in minor head injuries: a prospective CT study in a series of 98 adult patients. J Neurol Neurosurg Psychiatry 51:526–528, 1988

Simpson DA, Cockington DA, Hanieh A et al: Head injuries in infants and young children: the value of the Paediatric Coma Scale. Childs Nerv Syst 7:183–190, 1991

Sklar EML, Quencer RM, Bowen BC et al: Magnetic resonance applications in cerebral injury. Radiol Clin North Am 30:353–366, 1992

Sosin DM, Nelson DE, Sacks JJ: Head injury deaths: the enormity of firearms. JAMA 268:791, 1992

Sosin DM, Sacks JJ: Motorcycle helmet-use laws and head injury prevention. JAMA 267:1649–1651, 1992

Sosin DM, Sacks JJ, Smith SM: Head injury-associated deaths in the United States from 1979 to 1986. JAMA 262:2251–2255, 1989

Stablein DM, Miller JD, Choi SC et al: Statistical methods for determining prognosis in severe head injury. Neurosurgery 6:243–248, 1980

Starmark JE, Holmgren E, Stalhammar D: Current reporting of responsiveness in acute cerebral disorders. J Neurosurg 69:692–698, 1988

Stein SC, Ross SE: The value of computed tomographic scans in patients with low-risk head injuries. Neurosurgery 16:638–640, 1988

Teasdale G, Jennett B: Assessment of coma and impaired consciousness. A practical scale. Lancet 2:81–83, 1974

Teasdale G, Teasdale E, Hadley D: Computed tomographic and magnetic resonance imaging classification of head injury. J Neurotrauma suppl. 1, 9:S249–S257, 1992

Terayama Y, Meyer JS, Kawamura J: Cognitive recovery correlates with long-term increases of cerebral perfusion after head injury. Surg Neurol 36:335–342, 1991

Thatcher RW, Cantor DS, McAlaster R et al: Comprehensive predictions of outcome in closed head-injured patients. The development of prognostic equations. Ann N Y Acad Sci 620:82–101, 1991

Thomas S, Acton C, Nixon J et al: Effectiveness of bicycle helmets in preventing head injury in children: case-control study. Br Med J 308:173–176, 1994

Thompson DC, Thompson RS, Rivara FP: Incidence of bicycle-related injuries in a defined population. Am J Public Health 80:188–1390, 1990

Thompson RS, Rivara FP, Thompson DC: A case-control study of the effectiveness of bicycle safety helmets. N Engl J Med 320:1361–1367, 1989

Tiret L, Haysherr E, Thicoipe M et al: The epidemiology of head trauma in Aquitaine (France), 1986: a community-based study of hospital admissions and deaths. Int J Epidemiol 19:133–140, 1990

Vasquez-Barquero A, Vasquez-Barquero JL, Austin O et al: The epidemiology of head trauma in Cantabria. Eur J Epidemiol 8:832–837, 1992

Vollmer DG, Torner JC, Jane JA et al: Age and outcome following traumatic coma: why do older patients fare worse? J Neurosurg 75:S37–S49, 1991

Wallace GL: Stroke and traumatic brain injury in Amerika Samoa. Hawaii Med J 52:234–250, 1993

Wang CC, Schoenberg BS, Li SC et al: Brain injury due to head trauma. Epidemiology in urban areas of the People's Republic of China. Arch Neurol 43:570–572, 1986

Warme PE, Bergstrom R, Persson L: Neurosurgical intensive care improves outcome after severe head injury. Acta Neurochir 110:57–64, 1991

Whitman S, Coonley-Hoganson R, Desai BT: Comparative head trauma in two socioeconomically different Chicago-area communities. A population study. Am J Epidemiol 119:570–580, 1984

Wilberger JE, Deeb Z, Rothfus W: Magnetic resonance imaging in cases of severe head injury. Neurosurgery 20:571–576, 1987

Williams DH, Levin HS, Eisenberg HM: Mild head injury classification. Neurosurgery 27:422–428, 1990

Wirsen A, Stenberg G, Rosen I, Ingvar DH: Quantified EEG and cortical evoked responses in patient with chronic traumatic frontal lesions. Electroencephalogr Clin Neurophysiol 84:127–138, 1992

Young B, Ott L, Yingling B, McClain C: Nutrition and brain injury. J Neurotrauma suppl. 1, 9:S375–S383, 1992

Young B, Rapp RP, Norton JA et al: Early prediction of outcome in head-injured patients. J Neurosurg 54: 300–303, 1981

Neuropathology of Closed Head Injury 3

Juan C. Troncoso
Barry Gordon

Trauma of the head accounts for significant mortality and morbidity in contemporary society. Trauma of the nervous system occurs most frequently as a consequence of traffic accidents, falls, and blows to the head. Each of these modalities results in different types or patterns of lesions. The brain is well protected from trauma by the skull and by the cerebrospinal fluid, which acts as a shock absorber, providing additional protection. However, bony structures may also become the source of injury, and we will discuss the mechanisms of fracture/contusions and the role of the topography of the anterior fossa of the skull in contrecoup injuries of the frontal and temporal lobes.

The pathogenesis of neural injury in trauma is complex and to a large extent remains to be elucidated. Mechanical stress and mass effects are two major mechanisms of neural tissue injury, frequently accompanied by vascular perturbations and cerebral edema.

This chapter reviews the neuropathology of head trauma in general but with particular emphasis on the pathogenesis of diffuse axonal injury and its role in mild head trauma and the postconcussive syndrome.

TOPOGRAPHY OF LESIONS IN TRAUMATIC HEAD INJURY

Lesions of the scalp consist of abrasions, contusions, lacerations, and hematomas. A thorough examination of the scalp is important because it allows the physician to locate the site of impact. However, an important caveat is that severe brain injury may exist in the absence of scalp lesions. Examples of this situation include victims of automobile collisions and "shaken babies." It is also important to underscore the frequent injuries of cervical spine and cord that accompany severe head trauma.

Fractures of the Skull

Nondepressed fractures that involve the calvarium are common in falls and may have a linear or more complex pattern. In cases of severe trauma, these fractures of the calvarium often extend downward to involve the base of the skull. Depressed fractures are more commonly seen in cases of blunt trauma to the head. As one would expect, depressed skull fractures are frequently the cause of brain contusions and lacerations. However, linear fractures may cause similar lesions, although the magnitude of the parenchymal lesions is milder. It is important to bear in mind that at the time of impact edges of the fracture may actually become depressed, with an internal bevel, for a fraction of a second, before becoming realigned. Fractures of the base of the skull are usually the consequence of severe trauma. These fractures may constitute a challenge to detection because of the complexity of radiologic images of the base of the skull. A fracture that traverses the entire width of the base of the skull is known as a *hinge fracture.*

Hemorrhages of the Dura Mater

Epidural and subdural hemorrhages constitute mass-occupying lesions and have the potential to cause marked displacement and herniation of brain structures. Important differences exist between these two types of hemorrhages. Epidural hemorrhages are commonly associated with fracture of the squamous portion of the temporal bone and laceration of the middle meningeal artery. Frequently, epidural hematoma occurs in the absence of a parenchymal lesion of the brain (e.g., cortical contusion or laceration), and thus, there is an excellent potential for clinical recovery. Epidural hemorrhages, however, are not chronic lesions; instead they are characterized by rapid accumulation and mass effect leading to shifts and herniations of brain parenchyma, which are often fatal if untreated.

Subdural hematomas, very common in all types of trauma, originate in cortical contusions and/or tears of bridging vessels. This latter mechanism is frequent in individuals with severe brain atrophy, in whom the vessels bridging the dura and the brain become stretched and therefore more susceptible to tears, even with minor trauma. The majority of subdural hematomas occur over the frontal, parietal, or temporal convexity, and they are uncommon in the posterior fossa. In our experience, about 50 percent of acute subdural hematomas recognized at autopsy are associated with severe injury of brain parenchyma (e.g., contusions and/or lacerations), which explains the frequent and early neurologic manifestations that characterize this type of hematoma. In contrast to epidural hemorrhages, subdural hemorrhages accumulate at a slower rate and thus allow compensatory mechanisms for increased intracranial pressure to operate, decreasing the magnitude of potential shifts of brain parenchyma. Thus, at times subdural hematomas may not be evacuated and become chronic lesions. However, these chronic hematomas represent an important threat because they are prone to rebleed spontaneously or with minimal head trauma. Another speculative mechanism is expansion of blood products through osmotic pressure gradient.

Hemorrhages of the Subarachnoid Space

Subarachnoid hemorrhage (SAH) is the most common pathologic consequence of head trauma seen at autopsy. Its distribution is variable, but generally it is more prominent over the convexity of the hemispheres, in contrast to the hemorrhage from an aneurysm, which is more abundant at the base of the brain. However, the pattern of SAH is not specific for different mechanisms of head trauma. In severe head injuries, SAH is usually diffuse. However, SAH is not uncommon as an incidental finding in individuals who died of causes other than head trauma (e.g., someone who collapses from myocardial infarction and hits the head against the ground).

Contusions of the Brain

Brain contusions represent bruising of the brain, most frequently the cerebral cortex, because of impact against the skull. Most but not all contusions are hemorrhagic. The pattern and distribution of cortical contusions are very important in determining the mechanism of injury (i.e., fall versus blow to the head). Briefly, in blows to the head, the brain contusion is found at the site of impact, frequently underlying a scalp lesion and skull fracture. In falls, however, contusions located opposite to the site of impact tend to dominate the pathologic picture. Cortical contusions of any origin may give rise to focal neurologic manifestations and/or seizures.

Lacerations of the Brain

Wounds or cuts in the parenchyma of the brain result from high mechanical stress. Such lesions frequently accompany and are the result of skull fracture.

Hemorrhages and Hematomas of the Brain

Traumatic hemorrhages can be single or multiple, and their distribution is different from that of hemorrhages associated with high blood pressure. A site of predilection for traumatic hemorrhages is the subcortical cerebral white matter, particularly in the frontal lobes. Amyloid deposition in the cerebral blood vessels makes older individuals more prone to traumatic hemorrhages.

Axonal Shearing

Invisible to the naked eye, axonal shearing is a common lesion of the cerebral white matter and occurs particularly in acceleration/deceleration injuries (e.g., automobile collisions) (see Fig. 3-4). In our experience with postmortem examination of vehicular accident victims, at least 75 percent of individuals with fatal head trauma show evidence of axonal shearing. Axonal injury is one of the major lesions responsible for the cognitive and motor deficits that characterize the aftermath of severe head trauma. Axonal shearing is common in subjects who suffer severe head injury and present with low Glasgow Coma Scale (GCS) scores (<12). Because axonal shearing can only be ascertained at autopsy, there are very limited observations of this type of lesion in individuals who suffer mild or moderate head trauma, among whom mortality is low. However, anecdotal reports on human cases and observations in experimental animals indicate that axonal shearing may occur even in head trauma with mild impairment of consciousness (i.e., GCS scores of 13 to 15 (Williams et al., 1990). This type of lesion is discussed in detail below (Adams et al., 1982; Adams et al., 1985; Blumbergs et al., 1989); Povlishock et al., 1985; Strich, 1956).

Brain Edema

Brain edema or swelling is a frequent complication of severe head trauma. At times edema is localized surrounding a contusion or laceration or it can be generalized, as seen in cases of diffuse axonal injury associated with acceleration/deceleration mechanisms. Brain edema is characterized pathologically by flattening of the cortical gyri, collapse of the ventricular system, and in severe cases, cerebral herniations.

Herniations

Because of edema and/or a mass-occupying lesion, the parenchyma of the brain can extrude through natural or surgical openings in the skull. For example, unilateral supratentorial lesions are commonly the cause of herniation of the uncus (the mesial portion) of the temporal lobe through the tentorial notch (transtentorial herniation) and/or the cingulate gyrus under the dural falx (cingulate or subfalcial herniation). Bilateral supratentorial mass lesions have the potential to push the diencephalon and hypothalamus downward (central herniation). Lesions of the posterior fossa may result in herniation of the tonsils of the cerebellum through the foramen magnum, an ominous event caused by the potential for compression and impairment of cardiovascular and respiratory regulatory centers in the medulla. Following neurosurgery, the swollen brain parenchyma may herniate through the craniotomy.

Vascular complications arise from the stretching or compression of blood vessels during herniation. The best examples are the midline hemorrhage of the upper pons (Duret's hemorrhage) and occipital lobe ischemia/hemorrhagic infarct caused by compression of the posterior cerebral artery in uncal herniation.

MECHANISMS OF HEAD INJURY AND PATTERNS OF LESIONS

Although brain lesions in head trauma are usually the consequence of a combination of mechanisms, for the sake of simplicity the three most common mechanisms of traumatic brain injury—blows to the head, falls (coup/contrecoup), and acceleration/deceleration injuries—are discussed separately.

Blows to the Head

Blows to the head are characterized by scalp contusion/laceration, skull fracture, and underlying contusion or laceration of the parenchyma of the brain, which may also be accompanied by epi- or subdural hemorrhage. Edema surrounding the contusion or laceration, involving a lobe or an entire hemisphere, is the rule in individuals who survive the injury for more than 6 to 8 hours.

Falls (Coup/Contrecoup)

In falls the point of contact of the head against the ground is marked by a scalp contusion or laceration. The skull may or may not be fractured; if there is an underlying brain lesion (coup injury), it is relatively small. In contrast, in the opposite side of the brain, extensive cortical contusions are present (contrecoup injuries). A common example of this pattern of lesions is that of an individual who falls backward and hits the back of the head. At the site of impact, there is a scalp contusion and subgaleal hematoma, no skull fracture, and no lesion of the cerebellum or occipital lobes; however, large cortical contusions of the frontal and temporal poles and orbitofrontal regions are encountered (Figs. 3-1 and 3-2).

This pattern of injury, which is the rule in cases of falls, is counterintuitive and thus has been the source of long-standing debate among neuropathologists. The experiments of Ommaya et al. (1971) on the mechanics of visible brain injuries in the rhesus monkey suggest that skull distortion and head rotation are important determinants of coup/contrecoup injuries. The combination of translation of the brain and impact against the skull appears to be responsible for focal cortical injuries (Ommaya and Gennarelli, 1975). Because the frontal poles, orbitofrontal cortex, and temporal poles lie against the very irregular surfaces of the anterior and middle cranial fossae, these cortices are more susceptible to contusion than the occipital lobes, which rest on the tent of the cerebellum, a supple and smooth support. However, it is fair to admit that a comprehensive explanation for coup/contrecoup brain injuries does not exist.

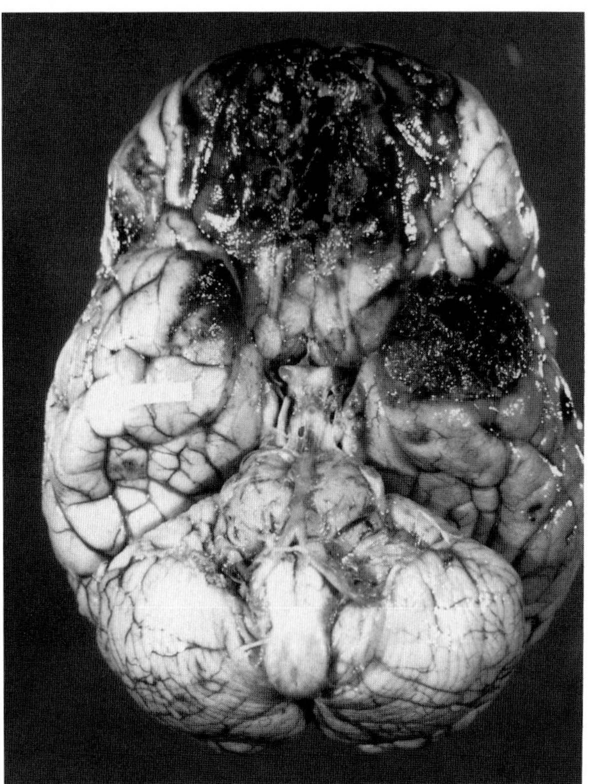

Fig. 3-1. *Contrecoup:* Basal view of the brain of a subject who fell down and hit the back of the head. No fracture was found at autopsy. Cerebellum and occipital lobes were free of injury, but extensive hemorrhagic contusions involved frontal poles, orbitofrontal regions, and temporal poles. These contusions constitute typical contrecoup injury.

Acceleration/Deceleration: Diffuse Axonal Injury

Acceleration/deceleration injuries are most frequently encountered with loss of consciousness in automobile crashes and sports accidents. Patients are generally rendered unconscious, the scalp and skull are intact, and at autopsy external examination of the brain may be unremarkable except for a variable degree of edema. Diffuse SAH over the convexity is common. Macroscopic examination of brain slices reveals hemorrhages (frequently linear) of the frontal and temporal white matter, corpus callosum, and periaqueductal region (Fig. 3-3). These hemorrhages are known as gliding contusions (Adams et al., 1986; (Lindenberg and Freytag, 1960). Diffuse axonal injury affects preferentially the white matter of the superior frontal gyrus and of the isthmus of the temporal lobe. Moreover, under the microscope hemorrhages are seen to be accompanied by signs of extensive axonal shearing, hence, the name diffuse axonal injury (Fig. 3-4). Because diffuse axonal injury may be extensive and not accompanied by hemorrhages, patients with "closed head trauma" may occasionally have devastating neurologic impairment (e.g., coma), and neuroimaging studies can be unrevealing except for localized or diffuse brain edema.

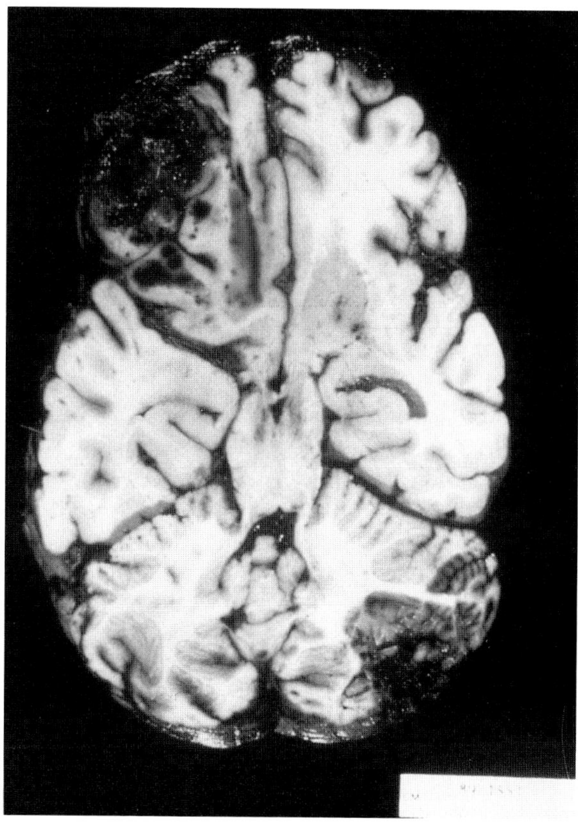

Fig. 3-2. *Coup-contrecoup:* Horizontal section through the brain of individual who suffered a fall with impact in the right occipital region. A linear fracture is present in the occipital bone. A small hemorrhagic contusion is noted in the right cerebellar hemisphere at the site of impact (coup lesion). Very extensive hemorrhagic contusions involve gray and white matter of the left frontal lobe (contrecoup lesion).

CLINICAL AND NEUROIMAGING CONSIDERATIONS

In head injuries caused by blows or falls, it is usually possible to identify a site of impact by a scalp lesion and at times a skull fracture. Intracranial lesions associated with these mechanisms (e.g., meningeal hemorrhages and brain contusions and lacerations) are frequently easily detectable by neuroimaging. In contrast, lesions caused by an acceleration/deceleration mechanism can be insidious and difficult to demonstrate, both to the clinician and to the neuroradiologist. First, these lesions may occur without actual head impact (e.g., in the case of a shaken infant of a restrained driver in a high-speed collision), and therefore no scalp or skull injury will exist. Furthermore, although white matter hemorrhages should be readily demonstrated by magnetic resonance imaging (MRI), scattered axonal damage (not associated with hemorrhage) may easily remain undetected. These circumstances explain why at times victims of closed head injury who eventually come to autopsy may have suffered profound neurologic impairment (e.g., coma) despite a paucity of demonstrable focal anatomic lesions of the head and brain. Neuroradiologic correlates of lesions responsible for neurologic impairment that are beyond the resolution threshold of current neuroimaging techniques are covered in Chapter 5.

PATHOLOGY OF POSTCONCUSSIVE SYNDROME

Acceleration/Deceleration

The pathologic hallmark of acceleration/deceleration is diffuse axonal injury as first reported by Strich (1961), who examined the brains of 20 subjects with a history of severe brain trauma and emphasized the importance of shearing of nerve fibers in the pathogenesis of brain damage, a concept reaffirmed by subsequent investigations (Adams et al., 1982; Gennarelli et al., 1982). Depending on the force of the injury, clinical manifestations and pathological lesions cover a spectrum from mild to severe (Williams et al., 1990). Although the division is arbitrary, for the sake of this exposition we will discuss the two extremes of this spectrum of brain injuries separately.

Diffuse Axonal Injury

Mild Head Trauma

The clinical and neurobehavioral abnormalities that follow mild head injury are fairly well established, but the neuropathology and pathogenesis of this entity are less well defined because for obvious reasons there are a very limited number of pathologic examinations in this type of case. Thus, a comprehensive understanding of the pathology of mild head trauma is only possible by combining the few autopsy observations with neuroimaging data and observations in experimental animal models.

For the purpose of this discussion, we define mild head injury by an initial and lowest GCS score of 13 to 15 (Askanas et al., 1992). Individuals within this category may have no detectable structural abnormality or may harbor linear or depressed skull fractures, focal parenchymal brain lesions, or dural hemorrhages.

Severe Head Trauma

The settings for severe head injury include vehicular accidents at high rates of speed, frequently against a stationary object, with rollovers and/or ejection from the vehicle, and falls from heights (i.e., more than 5 feet) or rolling downstairs. In our experience we also frequently encounter severe diffuse axonal injury in individuals with impaired postural reflexes who fall to the ground or roll downstairs. These individuals include very elderly persons, parkinsonian patients, and alcoholics. At autopsy, the scalp may demonstrate contusions and lacerations and the skull may show fractures. However, these structures are frequently intact, and external examination of the brain can be unremarkable, except for variable degrees of edema and diffuse subarachnoid hemorrhage over the convexity of the cerebrum. However, gross examination of brain slices consistently reveals hemorrhages, usually linear, of the frontal and temporal white matter, corpus callosum, and periaqueductal gray matter. (Fig. 3-3). Other structures frequently involved are the septum pellucidum and putamen. These hemorrhages of the white matter are also known as *gliding contusions* (Adams et al., 1986; Lindenberg and Freytag, 1960) and characteristically involve the subcortical white matter and the gray-white matter junction. Microscopically, these hemorrhages are accompanied by extensive axonal shearing, hence the name diffuse axonal injury. Moreover, foci of axonal injury

A
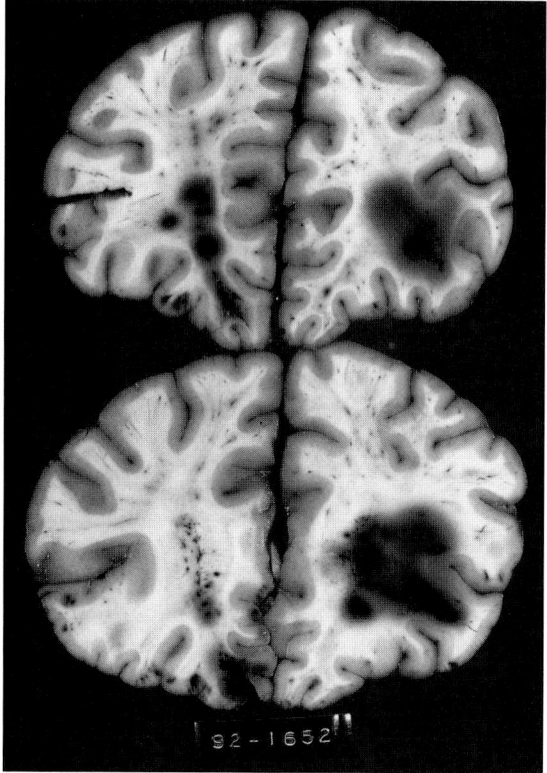

B
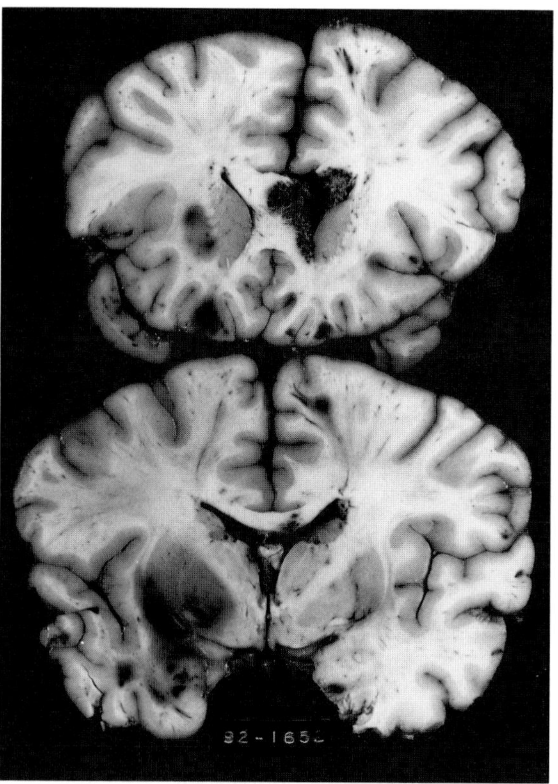

Fig. 3-3. **(A & B)** *Acceleration-deceleration injuries:* Coronal sections of the brain of an individual who suffered acceleration-deceleration injury as consequence of motor vehicle accident. The external surface of the brain was free of contusion and had moderate subarachnoid hemorrhage over the convexity. Hemorrhagic lesions are present in the white matter of the frontal and temporal lobes (gliding contusion), left internal capsule-putamen, and corpus callosum. The genu of the callosum appears torn.

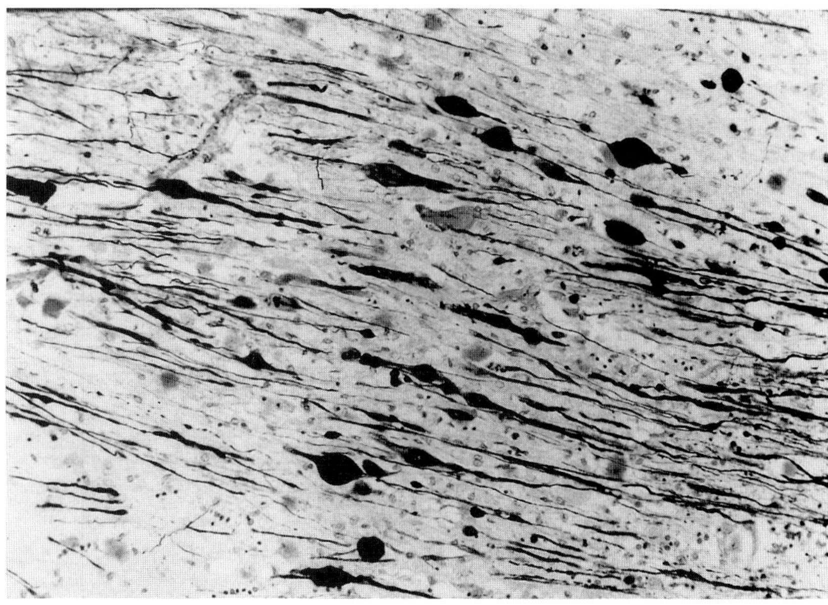

Fig. 3-4. *Axonal shearing:* Microscopic section of corpus callosum in a subject who suffered acceleration-deceleration injury to the brain and survived for 10 days. Immunocytochemical staining with antibodies for neurofilaments shows multiple axonal balloons or swellings, the hallmark of traumatic axonal injury.

are also frequently present independently of hemorrhages. Axonal injury consists of focal swellings and axonal balloons, which can be seen on hematoxylin and eosin or silver stains but are best demonstrated by immunostaining for neurofilament proteins (Grady et al., 1993) (Fig. 3-4).

Autopsy Observations

As mentioned before, reported neuropathologic observations in mild head injury are scant. Oppenheimer (1968) reported microglial clusters in the brainstems of patients with minor head injury, and Nevin (1967) described white matter changes. In a more recent study, Blumbergs et al. (1989) reviewed the neuropathology of 11 head injury victims who were rendered unconscious initially for an undetermined period of time but subsequently regained awareness and were able to communicate before dying from systemic and neurologic complications. None of these subjects had macroscopic lesions of the corpus callosum or brainstem, but all had mild diffuse axonal injury microscopically.

A recent case examined by us illustrates the potential neuropathologic changes present in head trauma not associated with loss of consciousness. A 77-year-old male driver crashed head on at about 25 miles per hour against a stationary vehicle. He was not restrained, and he hit and broke the windshield with his forehead. His wife, who was in the passenger seat and was wearing the safety belt, recalls that her husband did not lose consciousness but got out of the car and behaved erratically. He was examined at a local emergency room and released after skull films, which were normal were obtained. Although no record of his GCS rating is available, in view of the description of erratic behavior, it is possible that he might have had a score of 13 or 14. The patient remained behaviorally abnormal for approximately 1 month and 18 months following the accident died from an unrelated cause. Examination of the brain showed a 2-cm cavitary lesion confined to the white matter of the right superior frontal gyrus. Microscopically, the cavity contained few hemosiderin-laden macrophages and was surrounded by reactive astrocytes and axonal balloons. In our view, this man suffered an acceleration/deceleration injury of the head in the automobile accident and developed a gliding contusion of the right frontal lobe that involved axons and capillaries. It is important to remark that this lesion caused significant behavioral abnormalities but no loss of consciousness. Given its size (2 cm) and hemorrhagic nature, this lesion would have been detected by computed tomography (CT) or MRI of the head. In terms of clinicopathologic correlation, the right frontal lesion constituted a focal injury and was not part of a diffuse axonal injury.

This vignette illustrates the potential for development of significant parenchymal injuries of the brain in individuals with head injuries that can be classified as mild, as judged by the reported lack of unconsciousness and the prompt release from the emergency room.

PATHOGENESIS OF DIFFUSE AXONAL INJURY

Autopsy Observations

Immunostaining with antibodies against neurofilament subunits is useful to detect the early stages of axonal shearing in human autopsy material. Using this technique, Grady et al. (1993) showed that in the brains of humans who suffered head injuries caused by vehicular collisions, vehicle-pedestrian accidents, or falls, focally swollen axons appear as early as 6 hours postinjury. By 12 hours the focal swelling progresses to disconnection, and the immunoreactive proximal stump continues to expand over the ensuing weeks. In an extension of this study, Christman et al. (1994) examined diffuse axonal injury ultrastructurally. At 6 hours postinjury, axons with immunoreactive focal swellings revealed axolemmal infolding or perturbations of the neurofilament network, without disruption of the myelin sheath and within a field of normal axons. Changes were enhanced by 12 hours, with more pronounced disorganization of the cytoskeleton, vacuolation, and occasional interruption of the nerve fiber. Finally, by 30 and 60 hours postinjury, clearly disconnected axonal swellings or balloons were noted, filled with a core of disordered neurofilaments capped by organelles.

Experimental Studies in Animal Models

Experimental models of traumatic brain injury fall into three general categories: mechanical impact to the head; head acceleration; and direct brain deformation (Lighthall et al., 1989). The latter two experimental paradigms are used preferentially for the study of diffuse axonal injury and have also been useful to explore the pathogenesis of injury to blood vessels and specific neuronal populations in head trauma. A caveat is that these models may not replicate the biomechanics of human head injury. For example, an important difference between humans and animals is the size, shape, and mass of the head in addition to its mobility on the neck. The role of these factors is poorly understood.

Mild Head Trauma

Jane et al (1985) used the *Macaca fascicularis* monkey as a model for minor acceleration/deceleration nonimpact injury of the head in the sagittal plane (60 degrees for 5 to 25 ms). The animals sustained a brief loss of consciousness, and no neurologic sequelae were observed. The brains were examined 7 days postinjury and showed degenerating axons in the inferior colliculus, pons, and dorsolateral medulla. Degeneration was not seen in the subcortical white matter, which suggests that lesions of the brainstem were the substrate of concussion.

Povlishock et al. (1983) examined anterograde axonal transport of horseradish peroxidase in cerebral and cerebellar nerve fibers in cats following minor head trauma. Cats were anesthetized at the time of fluid-percussion injury over the parasagittal dura mater, which caused vascular, respiratory, pupillary, and electroencephalographic changes characteristic of a concussive response. All animals were normal after recovering from anesthesia. Morphologic observations at various times between 1-24 hours postinjury showed intra-axonal pooling initially, followed by lobulation and finally formation of axonal balls or clubs with separation from distal axonal segment. An important observation in this experiment was that axonal injury occurred in the absence of vascular changes or parenchymal damage.

Severe Head Trauma

Studies in monkeys have shown that acceleration forces the head to produce consistent functional and structural perturbations. Gennarelli et al. (1982) showed that in *Macaca mulatta* and *Papio nubis,* angular acceleration of the head, without impact, through a 60-degree arc in time periods ranging from 11 to 22 ms in the sagittal, oblique, and lateral planes produces loss of consciousness and brain injuries comparable with those in the brain of humans involved in vehicular accidents. These injuries were characterized grossly by hemorrhages of the white matter (the gliding contusions described by Lindenberg and Freytag (1960) and microscopically by shearing of axons. The length of coma and severity of pathologic lesions were greatest for acceleration in the lateral plane and least in the sagittal plane. Neuropathologic lesions were not observed in monkeys with unconsciousness for less than 16 minutes. No hemorrhage was detected without loss of consciousness.

Evolution of Axonal Lesions

Taken in concert, morphologic observations of diffuse axonal injury in humans and experimental animals suggest that trauma causes disorganization of neurofilament cytoskeleton and axolemma, pivotal pathologic events that evolve over several hours to culminate in axonal disconnection (Christman et al., 1994).

VASCULAR LESIONS

Hemorrhages of cerebral white matter following head trauma are usually the harbinger of diffuse axonal injury. For this reason, one may think that shearing of capillaries and axons takes place concomitantly. However, there is growing evidence that axonal injury may occur independently of vascular abnormality (Povlishock et al., 1983). Thus, the absence of hemorrhage does not rule out shearing of nerve fibers. The size of traumatic hemorrhages is related to the magnitude of acceleration/deceleration and also to the preinjury status. In our experience, older subjects and alcoholics tend to develop larger hematomas than other individuals.

INJURY OF SPECIFIC NEURONAL POPULATIONS

To unravel the pathologic substrate of memory dysfunction that follows mild head trauma in humans, investigators have begun to examine the hippocampus in animal models of head trauma. Kotapka et al. (1991) have reported loss of neurons in CA_1 region in an acceleration model of brain injury in nonhuman primates. Hicks et al. (1993) examined the effects of a mild lateral fluid percussion injury to the brains of rats, which were sacrificed following assessment of memory with the Morris water maze paradigm. Injured animals developed significant memory deficits that correlated with neuronal cell loss in the hippocampus. Extension of these conclusions to humans appears premature.

CLINICOPATHOLOGIC CORRELATIONS

Many of the symptoms of postconcussive syndrome can be plausibly related to organic pathology. This concept has been established by animal studies, occasional human clinicopathologic correlations, and human clinical research. Although exact correlations are uncertain, it does appear that different types of injury give rise to different types of lesions, which in turn give rise to more specific symptom complexes. High-force acceleration/deceleration, particularly when it is rotational, is likely to cause diffuse axonal injury (axonal shearing or tears), especially in the midbrain, superior cerebellar peduncles, corpus callosum, and central white matter. Such lesions are likely to be responsible for loss of consciousness and contribute to impaired concentration, dizziness, and ataxia. Acceleration/deceleration of the head may also damage the labyrinth, the mechanoreceptor in the neck, or the central vestibular connections. Such lesions may cause dizziness, vertigo, or a sense of unsteadiness in space. In addition, blood vessels and their associated vasoregulatory systems may be stretched and injured. Impairment of vascular contractility and autoregulation is frequently seen, either as a direct result of vascular damage or as a response to tissue injury. Headache in postconcussive syndrome is thought to arise from this injury. Acceleration/deceleration may also stretch and strain the cervical ligaments, muscles, and supporting bones. Neck fatigue, aches, and pains are the frequent result. Blows or falls are likely to cause focal cortical contusions, directly at the site of impact as well as more broadly distributed with a predilection for the frontopolar and orbitofrontal regions and the anterior, lateral, and inferior portions of the temporal lobes. The involvement of these brain regions may contribute to the attention and concentration difficulties, loss of mental flexibility, memory loss, distractibility, and change in personality that these patients can suffer (Gordon, 1990).

CONCLUSION

The neuropathology of severe head trauma (i.e., cortical contusions and axonal shearing) is well established, although the precise mechanisms responsible for the patterns of these lesions are not fully understood. We know less about the pathologic changes associated with milder forms of head trauma and its aftermath, the postconcussive syndrome. Observations in humans and in experimental animals suggest that axonal injury and the ensuing disconnection of nerve cells are important anatomic substrates of this syndrome. A better understanding of the factors that cause and modulate axonal damage following head trauma can help us to develop novel therapeutic approaches to traumatic brain injury.

ACKNOWLEDGMENTS

This work was supported by grants from the U.S. Public Health Service (NIH AG 01546), the Alzheimer's and Related Diseases Association, and the Charles Dana Foundation.

REFERENCES

Adams JH, Doyle D, Graham DI et al: Microscopic diffuse axonal injury in cases of head injury. Med Sci Law 25:265–269, 1985

Adams JH, Doyle D, Graham DI et al: Gliding contusions in nonmissile head injury in humans. Arch Pathol Lab Med 110:485–488, 1986

Adams JH, Graham DI, Murray LS, Scott G: Diffuse axonal injury due to nonmissile head injury in humans: an analysis of 45 cases. Ann Neurol 12:557–563, 1982

Askanas V, Engel WK, Alvarez RB: Light and electron microscopic localization of β-amyloid protein in muscle biopsies of patients with inclusion-body myositis. Am J Pathol 141:31–36, 1992

Blumbergs PC, Jones NR, North JB: Diffuse axonal injury in head trauma. J Neurol Neurosurg Psychiatry 52: 838–841, 1989

Christman CW, Grady MS, Walker SA et al: Ultrastructural studies of diffuse axonal injury in humans. J Neurotrauma 11:173–186, 1994

Gennarelli TA, Thibault LE, Adams JH et al: Diffuse axonal injury and traumatic coma in the primate. Ann Neurol 12:564–574, 1982

Gordon B: Postconcussional syndrome. pp. 208–213. In Johnson RT (ed): Current Therapy in Neurologic Disease. BC Decker, Philadelphia, 1990

Grady MS, McLaughlin MR, Christman CW et al: The use of antibodies targeted against the neurofilament subunits for the detection of diffuse axonal injury in humans. J Neuropathol Exp Neurol 52:143–152, 1993

Hicks RR, Smith DH, Lowenstein DH et al: Mild experimental brain injury in the rat induces cognitive deficits associated with regional neuronal loss in the hippocampus. J Neurotrauma 10:405–414, 1993

Jane JA, Steward O, Gennarelli T: Axonal degeneration induced by experimental noninvasive minor head injury. J Neurosurg 62:96–100, 1985

Kotapka MJ, Gennarelli TA, Graham DI et al: Selective vulnerability of hippocampal neurons in acceleration-induced experimental head injury. J Neurotrauma 8:247–258, 1991

Lighthall JW, Dixon CE, Anderson TE: Experimental models of brain injury. J Neurotrauma 6:83–97, 1989

Lindenberg R, Freytag E: The mechanism of cerebral contusions. A pathologic-anatomic study. Arch Pathol Lab Med 92:440–469, 1960

Nevin NC: Neuropathological changes in the white matter following head injury. J Neuropathol Exp Neurol 26: 77–84, 1967

Ommaya AK, Grubb RL Jr, Naumann RA: Coup and contrecoup injury: observations on the mechanisms of visible brain injuries in the rhesus monkey. J Neurosurg 35:503–516, 1971

Ommaya AK, Gennarelli TA: Experimental head injury. pp. 67–107. In Vinken PJ, Bruyn GW (eds): Injuries of the Brain and Skull, Part I. North-Holland, Amsterdam, 1975

Oppenheimer DR: Microscopic lesions in the brain following head injury. J Neurol Neurosurg Psychiatry 31:299–306, 1968

Povlishock JT, Becker DP, Cheng CLY, Vaughan GW: Axonal change in minor head injury. J Neuropathol Exp Neurol 42:225–242, 1983

Strich SJ: Diffuse degeneration of the cerebral white matter in severe dementia following head injury. J Neurol Neurosurg Psychiatry 19:163–185, 1956

Strich SJ: Shearing of nerve fibres as a cause of brain damage due to head injury. A pathological study of twenty cases. Lancet 2:443–448, 1961

Williams DH, Levin HS, Eisenberg HM: Mild head injury classification. Neurosurgery 27:422–428, 1990

Head Injury in Motor Vehicle Crashes: Human Factors, Effects, and Prevention

4

Daniel V. McGehee

The first section of this book details the epidemiology of head injury and presents regional and national case studies of head injury causation. We see that head injuries are generally caused by motor vehicle crashes, falls, violence, sports, and recreation. Now that these areas are identified, what factors go into the major cause of head injury, the automobile crash? Can any of these injuries be prevented? What is the direction of automotive transportation research? Although grasping the importance of the physics behind head injury is important, the events that lead to impact should also be understood. Since automobile crashes cause the majority of head injuries, pre-crash factors will be analyzed in this chapter. By better understanding the complex cognitive and visual aspects of the pre-crash factors that produce head injury, medical practitioners and researchers may be able to develop a more complete mental model of the most frequent causes of automobile crashes.

DIRECT INJURY CAUSES AND PREVENTIVE EQUIPMENT

Causes of Head Injury

To summarize the direct causes of head injury, half of all traumatic brain injuries (Fig. 4-1) are caused by motor vehicle crashes, 21 percent by falls, 12 percent by assaults and violence, and 10 percent by injuries from sports and recreation (National Head Injury Foundation, 1993). The percentage of head injuries due to motor vehicle crashes seems to be fairly consistent from state to state. However, large urban areas see more head injuries relating to violence (Kraus, 1984).

While comparisons among populations require variables that are easy to categorize and tabulate, such as gender or age, it is much more complicated to evaluate specific causes by using such categorical

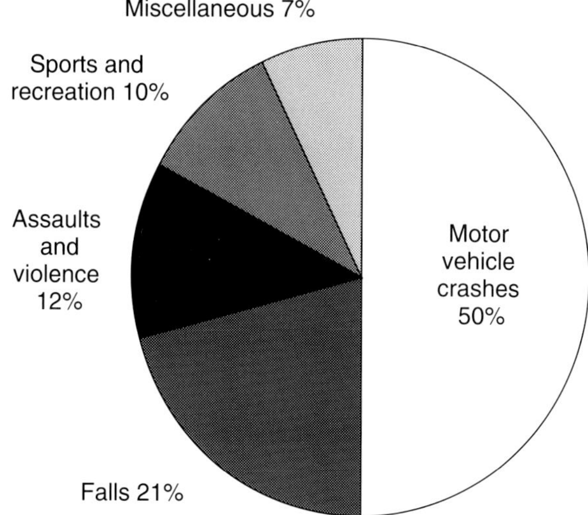

Fig. 4-1. Head injury causes.

variables as "motor vehicle crashes," "falls," "sports and recreation," or "assaults and violence." Using broad categories does little to identify risk or provide insight into specific factors that cause head injury. For more detail on head injury epidemiology, see Chapter 2.

This chapter focuses on analyzing the most prevalent cause of head injury, the motor vehicle crash. Although head injury is just a subset of all injuries that can be received in a motor vehicle crash, it is often the most debilitating. Besides causing over half of all head injuries in the United States, motor vehicle crashes are one of the leading causes of death and injury in the United States and many other countries. More than 40,000 people die on U.S. roadways every year, and another 3.5 million are injured (Evans, 1991). This high rate of mortality and injury makes motor vehicle crashes one of the areas most heavily studied by transportation researchers. One problem that researchers face, however, is that police crash records vary greatly from state to state and often lack sufficient detail to evaluate specific events such as head injuries by crash type. Figure 4-2 illustrates the frequency and distribution of police-reported automobile crashes (Knipling et al., 1993) in the United States. It should also be noted that each crash type generally has a different alcohol involvement. Alcohol is involved in approximately 55 percent of single-vehicle crashes and in 45 percent of multiple-vehicle crashes (Evans, 1991).

The types of automobile crashes that have the greatest potential for causing head injury account for nearly three-quarters of all crashes. These are front-to-rear-end, crossing path or intersection incursion, single-vehicle roadway departures, and head-on crashes.

Although head-on crashes may seem to be the most catastrophic, lateral collisions have a significantly higher mortality rate. Drivers involved in head-on collisions are more likely to have been drinking and less likely to use seat belts (Dischinger et al., 1993).

It should be noted that in nearly two-thirds of front-to-rear-end crashes, the lead vehicle is stationary, which generally causes severe injury to the striking vehicle's driver and occupants. Severe head injury often results from the worst type of rear-end crash, in which a vehicle collides with a tractor-trailer truck and underrides the trailer (Mortimer, 1988).

As mentioned previously, intersection incursion crashes that produce lateral impacts can result in severe injuries. Little protection is afforded by a vehicle's door. There is also a significantly higher proportion of lateral crashes among drivers over 55 years of age (Dischinger et al., 1993). This increase in crash rate is discussed further in the section *Driver Attention and Vision.*

Single-vehicle roadway departures, also known as "run off the road" crashes, are the most frequent motor vehicle crashes. Because they often involve striking stationary objects such as trees and terrain, these types of crashes can be particularly severe. Head-on collisions can also be classified as single-vehicle roadway departures. Instead of striking a stationary target, a driver drifts into the oncoming lane of traffic.

Current Automotive Safety Equipment

During the past several years, automotive safety technology has proved to be an important selling point for new automobiles. The installation of driver's and passenger-side air bag technology is predicted to reduce driver fatalities by about 20 percent (Evans, 1991). It is still too early to tabulate valid estimates of true injury and fatality reductions. As air bags become standard equipment on all vehicles, more valid estimates will be available. Air bag technology is one of the most important technologies in the reduction of head injury since it significantly reduces the impact force of the face and head into protruding objects within the vehicle. It is important to point

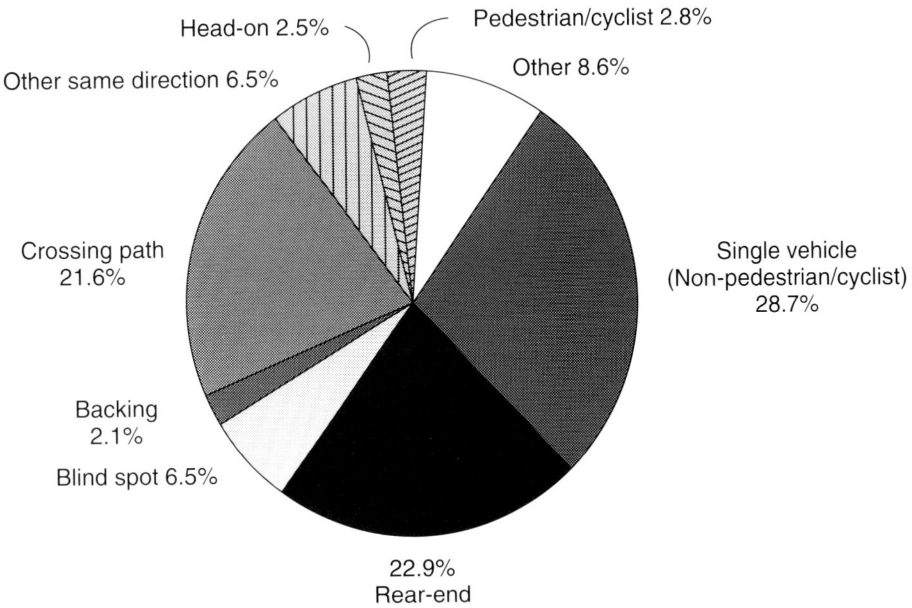

Fig. 4-2. Police-reported crashes.

out that the inflation of an air bag is quite literally an explosion, not the soft pillow sequence that is seen in superslow motion on television and print advertising.

In addition to driver and passenger air bags for frontal collisions, the automotive industry is also investigating air bags for side-impact crashes. The 1995 model year will see its first implementation of side-impact air bags by Volvo. Sensor technology used for side-impact collisions is different from that for frontal collisions, which utilizes the large volume of the engine compartment to sense the magnitude of a collision. The large volume of the engine compartment during the compression of a crash also allows enough time for the air bag to inflate and protect the driver. Side impacts, however, compromise the structural integrity of a vehicle very quickly since there is no engine compartment crumple zone to protect the driver. Side-impact air bags are built into the door side of the seat back and inflate vertically, so that both short and tall drivers are protected.

The complete deployment sequence of frontal air bags generally takes about 0.1 second. The deployment sequence begins at about 10 ms, when the computer initiates the inflation sequence. This is started after multiple sensors located around the vehicle detect a negative acceleration. The threshold of inflation is generally around 7 g's (g is the acceleration of gravity). At 30 ms the igniter fires; at 50 ms a high-pressure release of nitrogen inflates the air bag; at 80 ms the air bag explodes outward; and at 0.11 seconds the air bag is taut and is impacted by the vehicle occupant. At the time of complete inflation, the driver or passenger has moved only about 8 inches. Air bags generally will contain a volume of 50 to 60 L of air, which greatly enlarges the impact area of the driver.

Antilock brake systems also have the potential of reducing the severity of some types of automobile crashes by preventing drivers from locking up their brakes, thereby allowing controlled steering. Like air bags, this technology is still too young to evaluate its overall effects.

The percentage of motor vehicle occupants who use safety belts has also increased since the mid-1970s. Motorized safety belts, state laws, and overall safety awareness enhance the rate at which drivers wear their seat belts. Seat belt laws have done more to increase safety belt use than any other campaign.

While automotive manufacturers are including more salient safety features in their products, more and more vehicles are built with reinforced side impact protection, rollover ceiling panel protection, crumple zones, and interiors designed to protect the driver and other occupants from impact with vehicles. As with other new technologies, the effectiveness of these additions seem intuitive but has not yet been proved in crash data.

Given that all these safety improvements are likely to reduce the probability of injury and death in a motor vehicle crash, the next step in future automotive safety is to fully understand driver behavior and performance and the root causes of automobile crashes. By understanding the complex visual and cognitive factors that are required to operate a motor vehicle, researches can gain insight into further preventing injuries and mortality. The following sections detail the driver/human factors that contribute to car crashes and describe current and future trends in driver performance and automotive design research.

MOTOR VEHICLE PRE-CRASH HUMAN FACTORS

Driving is a complex behavior, which requires simultaneous use of sensory, perceptual, cognitive, and physical factors. The driver must scan the environment constantly and respond properly in order to maintain control, avoid obstacles, and properly interact with vehicles. Because driving is highly overlearned, automatic, and often taken for granted, driver performance problems can occur during its execution. Several driver performance factors contribute to motor vehicle crashes: perception/reaction time, driver inattention, and limitations in the human visual system.

Driver Attention and Vision

Driver inattention is generally one of the largest causal factors in motor vehicle crashes. In one sampling (National Highway Traffic Safety Administration, 1993) by the National Accident Safety System (1991), 63 percent of rear end crashes were caused by driver inattention. Although it is possible for a driver to "look but not see," attention in driving is generally directly related to where a driver is looking at any given time. The driver is constantly scanning the environment—looking out the forward windshield and side windows, scanning mirrors, and attending to stimuli in the vehicle. Since the capacity of human visual attention is limited, drivers experience intervals when they are not processing any information from the forward roadway. Operating in-vehicle controls, navigating to a destination, and carrying on conversations require drivers to take their eyes off the roadway and attend to other stimuli. Often, drivers return their point of gaze repeatedly "head down" to the dashboard or to others in the vehicle. It is these repeated non-forward-looking glances that create the potential for a crash.

Visual sampling both in and out of the vehicle has been modeled previously (Wierwille, 1993). Figure 4-3 illustrates this normative, deterministic model. The model starts when the driver begins to perform an in-vehicle task by glancing to an appropriate location. Information extraction begins as time elapses. If the information can be obtained or chunked within about 1 second, the driver will comfortably return to the forward scene. However, when experiencing time pressure, the driver will take up to 1.5 seconds to glance and retrieve information. If the information cannot be chunked within 1.5 seconds, the driver will return the glance to the forward scene and try again later. The driver continues to extract other information in the same way until all required visual information has been obtained. This model breaks down when a driver has difficulty with sensation, perception, attention, decision making, and implementation. Motor control failure due to head injury or neurologic diseases will also occur at several levels of this model.

Wierwille (1993) also states that manual tasks requiring in-vehicle glances can be separated into five categories, based largely on the driver resources they require. Some tasks, such as operating light switches, turn signals, and other simple controls are learned quickly after only a few glances and are quickly and manually mapped out by the driver. The driver can then perform these tasks automatically.

A subset of this control mapping (manually only) occurs when a driver looks at a control to obtain position or status information, then adjusts the control without looking. For example, the driver might check to see where the climate control system is set and then manipulate the controls without looking at them. Wierwille classifies this type of action as *manual primarily.*

Visual only tasks are those that require no manual input and are information gathering in nature. These tasks include monitoring the speedometer or checking the radio station frequency and time of day.

Wierwille categorizes tasks that rely heavily on vision but also require a degree of manual input as *visual primarily.* An example of this type of task is determining the radio station frequency when the initial display reads like a clock.

The last classification that Wierwille describes is that of *visual-manual.* This type of task is related to

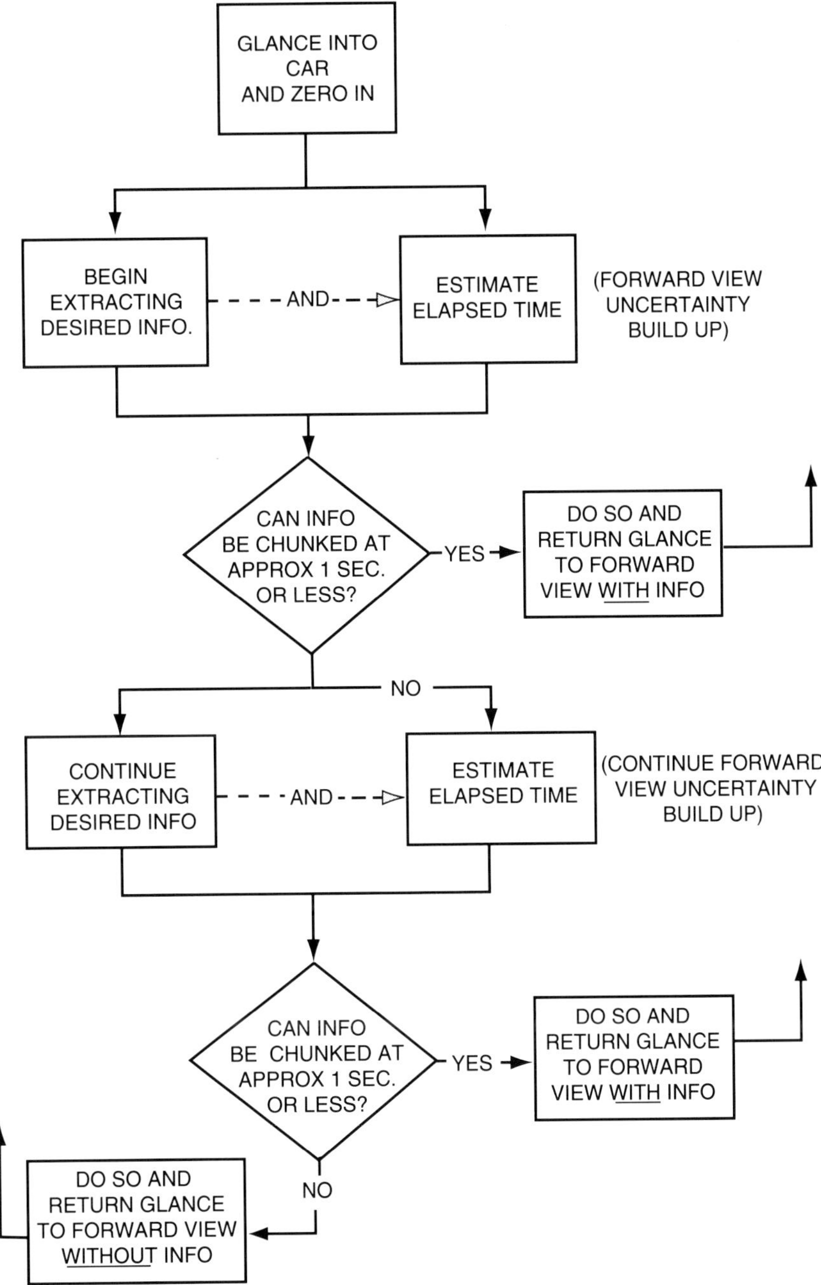

Fig. 4-3. Model of visual sampling for in-vehicle tasks.

interactive activities inside the vehicle, activities that require repeated input and visual attention. Some examples are manually tuning a radio to a specific frequency, operating a cellular phone, and adjusting an outside rearview mirror.

Most glances in-vehicle require more than 1.2 seconds (Bhise et al., 1986; Dingus et al., 1990). This relatively long glance duration time is one of the key factors contributing to a driver's loss of situation awareness with respect to surrounding vehicles. Scanning behavior resulting in the head-down factor in normal driving leads to reduced out-the-window glance times. Wierwille et al. (1988) have calculated probabilities of a driver's eyes being on the forward

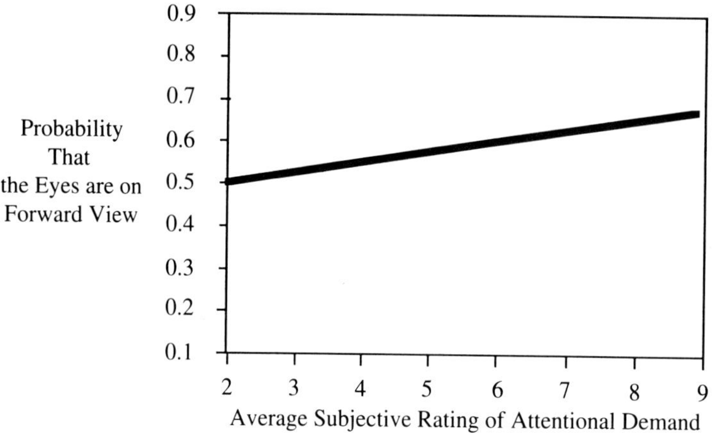

Fig. 4-4. Probability that the eyes are on the forward view as a function of attention demand.

roadway under varying degress of attentional demand (Fig. 4-4). They found that as the driver's subjective rating of attention demand increases, so does the probability that the driver's eyes will be on the forward view. Wierwille et al. (1988) surmised that when drivers experience increased visual loading from the primary task of driving, they adapt their visual sampling strategy. They are under greater pressure to return their glance to the forward view sooner and to maintain it a greater proportion of the total time.

Wierwille et al. (1988) also found that traffic density increases the driver's glance time in the forward view and thus decreases the number of glances to other areas of the roadway (Fig. 4-5).

Driver age also has a bearing on glance duration. Hayes et al. (1989) found that middle-aged and older drivers had significantly longer in-vehicle glance times than did younger drivers. This age effect is generally caused by deterioration of vision and slowing of cognitive processes (Fig. 4-6).

As vision deteriorates with age, risk factors and crash frequency increase. By the year 2024, 25 percent of the drivers in the United States will be over the age of 65. Older drivers have more crashes and fatalities per vehicle-mile than any other adult age group. Poor vision in and of itself is not a good predictor of crashes. However, Owsley et al. (1991) have found that the useful field of view (UFOV) and MOMSEE scores are the only variables that significantly predict crash frequency in their model. Although this model acknowledges that eye health is related to visual sensory function and visual sensory function is related to visual attention, neither eye health nor visual sensory function has a direct effect on the prediction of crashes. However, it is important to emphasize that visual sensory function is critical to driving. In addition, Ball et al. (1993a, 1993b) have also found that an individual's ability to complete a central target identifier task coupled with a peripheral target localization task provides a measure of the UFOV. The size of the UFOV is a function of at least three factors that are varied during a vision test: the duration of the target presentation, the competing

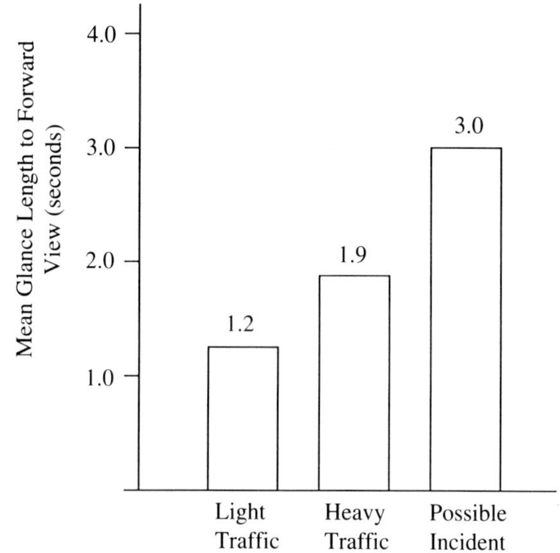

Fig. 4-5. Glance length to forward view as a function of traffic type.

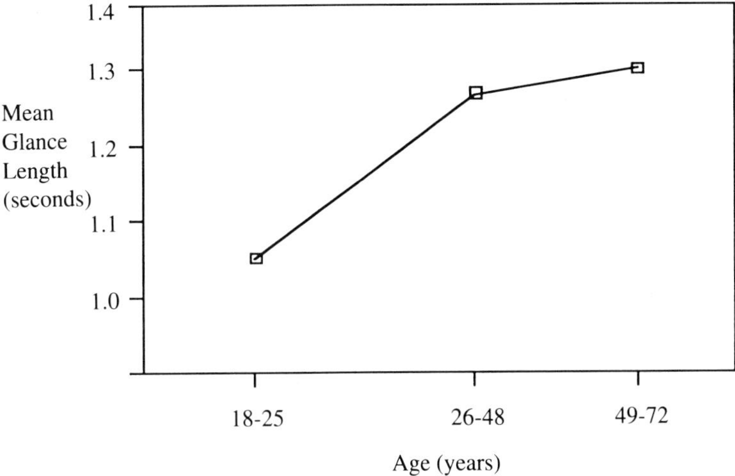

Fig. 4-6. Mean in-vehicle glance length as a function of age.

attentional demand of central and peripheral tasks, and the salience of the peripheral target. Thus, the UFOV incorporates stimulus and task features that reflect key components of driving. It becomes an important factor when evaluating crash causation of older drivers.

All types of head injury-producing crashes increase with age (front-to-rear-end, intersection incursion, head-on, and single-vehicle roadway departures). Ball et al. (1993b) found that drivers with reduced UFOVs had significantly higher crash rates than those with a lower percentage reduction of (larger) UFOVs. Figures 4-7 and 4-8 illustrate these differences. These findings are consistent with the finding of Dischinger et al. (1993) that drivers over the age of 55 had a significantly larger proportion of lateral crashes. This increase is most likely due to these drivers' reduced UFOVs.

Driver Perception/Decision/Reaction Time

The usual driver reaction to a potential collision is sudden braking and/or steering. As a major consequence, the driver's perception reaction time is a factor in determining whether a collision will be avoided and is crucial to identifying vehicles or objects that may pose a threat. A delay in either recognizing or reacting may cause a driver to crash. For unexpected events, driver reaction time estimates vary from 0.9 seconds with athletes as drivers (Davis et al., 1990), to 1.6 seconds for drivers drawn from a more representative population (Olson and Sivak, 1986).

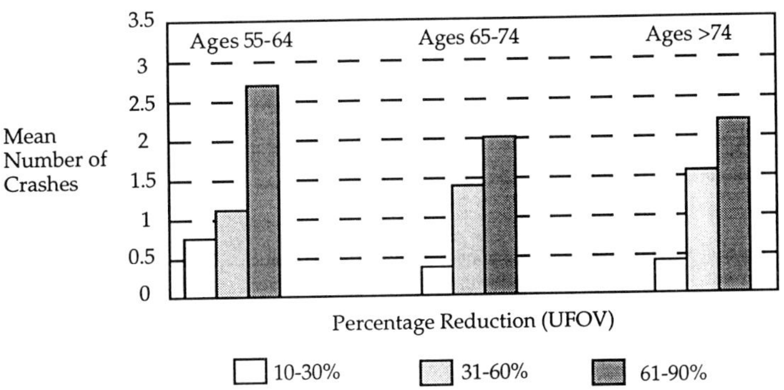

Fig. 4-7. Crash frequency as a function of age and UFOV.

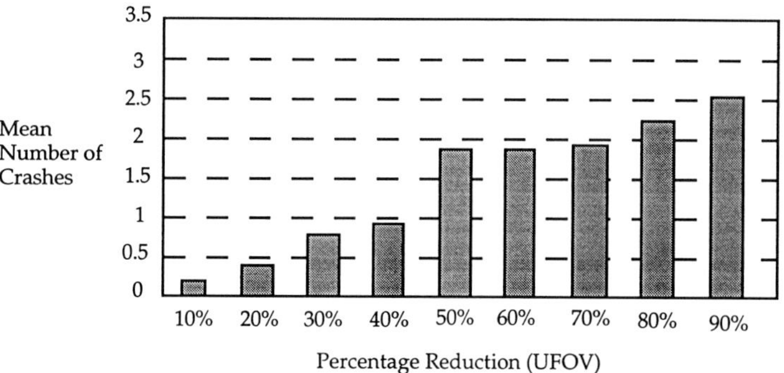

Fig. 4-8. Crash frequency as a function of UFOV.

In perhaps one of the most ecologically valid studies on brake perception-reaction time, Lerner (1993) instrumented over 116 personal vehicles to conduct "roadway quality" drives in older and younger drivers. After about 1 hour of evaluating roadways, the drivers were directed onto a new section of deserted freeway. After they had driven 0.7 mile on the new freeway section, a bright yellow barrel was launched from behind a bridge abutment, and reaction times in the form of braking and/or steering were recorded. Lerner found that 87 percent of the 116 drivers made some overt vehicle maneuver. About 43 percent of the 116 both braked and steered, 36 percent steered only, and 8 percent braked only. The mean perception-reaction time for all subjects was 1.5 seconds with a standard deviation of 0.4 second.

In reviewing studies on perception-reaction time, a wide range of values was found. Davis et al. (1990) commented that in certain situations, the reaction may be simple or complex, depending on test procedures. They found that perception-reaction time increased with following distance and explained this effect of short times for short headways by the increased attention drivers gave toward the lead vehicle. This is consistent with the claim of Wierwille et al. (1993) that as traffic increases (i.e., following distances decrease), more time is spent looking out the forward windshield.

Most studies found no significant effect of driver gender or age on brake reaction times. A study by Wilson (1987) found that older subjects had a longer perception time but compensated with a shorter reaction time. There is some indication that younger drivers have longer decision times and therefore longer overall reaction time than do older drivers. Lerner (1993) found that older drivers react very quickly to roadway hazards even if they pose no danger, while younger drivers have a longer decision time while they evaluate potentially dangerous situations.

Summary of Driver/Human Factors Relating to Injury

To review the contributing variables that make up the collision scenario, some of the factors that influence driver/vehicle behavior are presented along a time line in Figure 4-9.

The first component involves the development of a collision situation. In a normal driving environment, the driving condition is safe with little potential for a collision to occur. As the condition (e.g., traffic, intersections, lead vehicle behavior) surrounding the driving environment change, the potential for a collision also changes. This component includes the potential collision precursor events requiring immediate driver/vehicle action to avoid an impending collision. Under everyday driving circumstances, drivers must rely solely on their own attentional and sensory abilities to detect the presence of a collision situation. Several variables listed for this component can directly affect how efficiently the driver detects a problem.

The next portion of the collision scenario pertains to the drivers' evaluation of the lead vehicle's behavior. Drivers attempt to gather information about the behavior of the vehicle ahead to determine the situation's criticality. At this point the drivers are aware of potential collision situations through their own abilities. After evaluating the information gathered about a potentially threatening vehicle, drivers must decide on the appropriate action to be taken, which will ultimately determine whether or not a crash will be avoided.

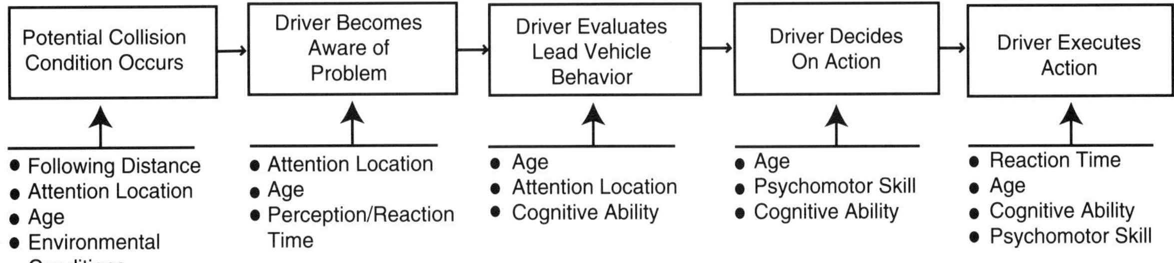

Fig. 4-9. Collision scenario and contributing variables.

The final step in the model is to execute the action that has been decided. This step will often consist of moving the foot from the accelerator to the brake pedal and pressing it and/or initiating a steering change. If any portion of this model is delayed, either by poor attention or by poor cognitive abilities, a crash may result. It is important to emphasize that driving is a highly automatic task. Driving becomes so automatic that over the course of a drive, a driver avoids many crashes and does not necessarily know it.

HEAD INJURY IMPACT SITES CAUSED BY MOTOR VEHICLE CRASHES

Head injuries occur through contacts between the head and the interior part of a vehicle. One countermeasure that has demonstrated effectiveness against head injury is the safety belt, one of the main effects of which is to reduce the likelihood of this type of impact. Hartmen et al. (1977) concluded that the safety belt is very effective as a head protector up to a certain speed, but that at higher speed levels the head becomes one of the body regions most exposed to injury.

In an in-depth investigation of car crashes in New South Wales, Herbert et al. (1975) showed that head impacts against the interior walls of cars are the principal cause of death of belt wearers. In tests of three 1975 car models, they measured the space available for the head and found it to be inadequate. These results indicate the value of increased head space in reducing the incidence of head impacts. Although this research was conducted nearly 20 years earlier, it should be noted that this research was conducted in Australia, where the vehicles at that time, like those in Europe, were similar in size to those in the United States in the mid-1990s.

The distribution of impact direction of skull/brain injuries among drivers with and without safety belts were examined in a series of studies conducted by Nygren (1985). Figure 4-10 describes this distribution.

For *belted drivers,* the most frequent direction of impact was frontal (59.3 percent of cases), which was also associated with highest frequency of fatal injuries (5.7 percent fatally injured). In rollover crashes, 15.7 percent were injured (1.9 percent fatally injured). In lateral impacts from the left 11 percent were injured, and in those from the right 4.4 percent. For unbelted drivers, in frontal crashes 55.4 percent were injured (13.5 percent fatally), while in rollover crashes 26.6 percent were injured (13.1 percent fatally), in left lateral crashes 6.8 percent were injured (1.3 percent fatally), and in right lateral crashes 8.1 percent were injured (2.7 percent fatally injured). Rear-end crashes accounted for 3.2 percent of the injuries and 0.5 percent of the fatalities.

When *front-seat passenger* injuries and fatalities were examined by the same criteria, belted passengers received 58.3 percent of the injuries (5.3 percent fatally); 16.2 percent were involved in rollovers and 1.3 percent of these were fatally injured (Fig. 4-11). In left lateral collisions the injury frequency was 6.0 percent, with no fatal injuries, and in right lateral collision this figure was 7.3 percent, with 1.7 percent of the injuries fatal.

In rollover crashes the frequency of injured/fatally injured drivers with skull/brain injuries was lower among those wearing safety belts than among those who were not (15.7 versus 26.6 percent). Rollover crashes were more frequent among unbelted than among belted passengers (26.9 versus 16.2 percent), and in such crashes among fatally injured front-seat passengers the proportion of unbelted persons was seven times that of belted ones (9.3 and 1.3 percent respectively).

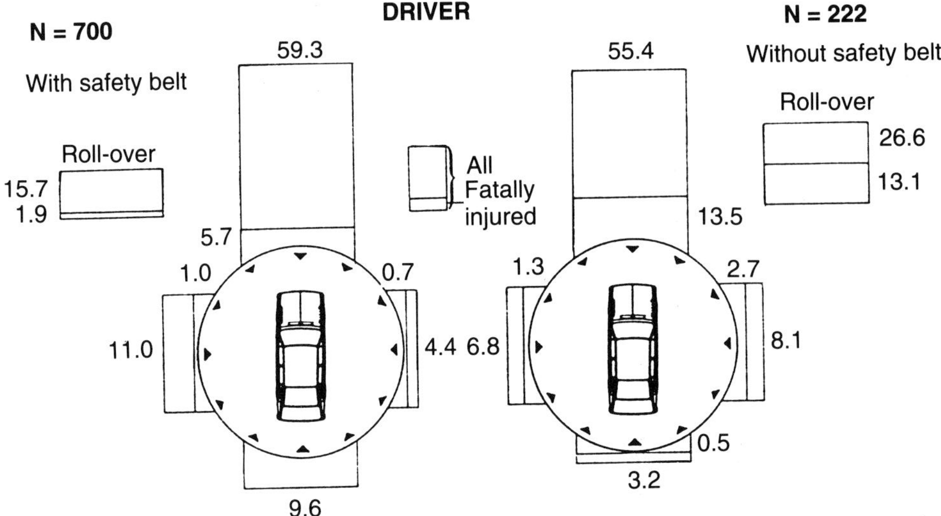

Fig. 4-10. Distribution of impact directions among drivers with skull/brain injuries with known belt usage.

Classification of Automobile Head Injury

There are three major types of mechanical effects causing head injury—sharp impacts, blunt impacts, and nonimpact inertial loading. The head is subject to inertial loading when a person is restrained by a safety belt in a frontal crash. The body is held back by the safety belt and the head tries to continue forward but is prevented from doing so by the neck. However, a head injury very seldom occurs unless the head strikes something.

In a study examining the physical causes of head injury resulting from car crashes, Tarriere et al. (1981) found that head-against-steering wheel impact occurred in 18 percent of cases (70 percent involved velocities above 40 km/h), the face was involved in 92 percent of the cases, and combined facial injury and brain lesion occurred in 26 to 32 percent of the cases and constituted virtually all the extremely serious injuries. Tarriere et al. also found that the head of the unbelted driver strikes part of the vehicle in 40 percent of the cases.

After reviewing the literature on head injury, it becomes more and more apparent that safety belts combined with air bags can contribute to the reduction of injuries and fatalities in general and head injuries specifically. Although air bags can cause injuries themselves, the impact injury is often much more severe. Air bags have the potential to break ribs and cause facial bruising and abrasions. Eye irritation has also been reported from the powder used to preserve the air bag (personal communication from T. Wright, Johnson County Paramedics, Iowa City, IA, 1994). It is important to note the difficulty in determining which injuries are caused by air bags and which are caused by the impact itself.

One difficulty in assessing head injury in motor vehicle crashes is due to the reporting systems used. Federal, state, and regional authorities all place different values on each aspect of a motor vehicle crash. Police officers are not trained to conduct thorough, scientific crash investigations. Only if there is litigation or suspicious circumstances surrounding a crash is it thoroughly investigated. Skid marks, if any, are measured and photographs taken, but no analysis of the force of impact is generally made. Insurance companies will complete their own analyses; however, their interest is primarily in the costs involved in the crash.

This lack of standardized data poses significant problems for transportation safety researchers in many fields. Individual case studies are required rather than statistical comparisons of large samples on common issues. Case studies are often lacking owing to the detail required in crash and injury reconstruction. For head injuries due to vehicular crashes, careful and tedious analyses are the only method to obtain accurate force estimation. Since each motor vehicle crash has its own unique combination of causal factors, it is difficult to generalize many types of crashes outside the standard "rear-end",

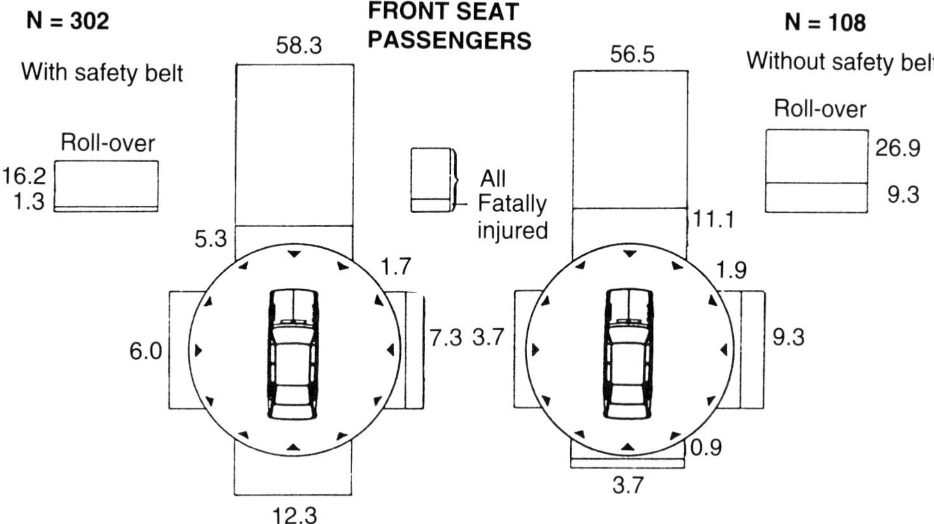

Fig. 4-11. Distribution of impact directions among front-seat passengers with skull/brain injuries with known belt usage.

''run-off-the-road'', ''head-on'', ''intersection incursion,'' and ''backing'' crash categories.

FUTURE TRENDS IN AUTOMOBILE SAFETY RESEARCH: PREVENTING CRASHES THAT PRODUCE INJURY AND MORTALITY

Now that factors in the production of head injury have been globally introduced, future trends in automotive safety and related technologies are discussed in this section. As described at the beginning of this chapter, since the mid-1970s the automotive industry has concentrated on making vehicles that can withstand crashes and reducing impact injuries through the increased use of safety belts, air bags, side impact protection, and several other vehicle safety technologies. Government and industry are now developing a variety of new technologies that could markedly reduce crashes altogether. Toward this end, the National Highway and Traffic Safety Administration (NHTSA) has created an Office of Crash Avoidance Research, which has in turn developed a multidisciplinary program to identify crash-causing factors and applicable countermeasure concepts. Under this program researchers are examining major target crash types. Research and development programs on the following crash types directly reflect the incidence of injury and mortality in the motor vehicle domain:

Front-to-rear-end
Backing
Single-vehicle roadway departure
Lane change/merge
Intersections with traffic signals
Intersections without traffic signals

Most of these crash countermeasure programs bear directly on head injury. For instance, lateral impact crashes (at intersections both with and without signals) are currently being investigated to provide the driver with enhanced situation awareness. This could be done via a display informing the driver that an intersection is approaching and that the traffic light will be red when the vehicle arrives. Older drivers may benefit greatly from such a display, which could also provide other in-vehicle signing capabilities (e.g., road signs).

Also under development are rear-end crash technologies that provide the driver with information about following distance and closure rates. It is anticipated that some form of automatic vehicle deceleration in the form of down-shifting or braking may be included in such systems. Several automobile manufacturers are currently investigating the feasibility of such systems.

Single-vehicle roadway departures, another large cause of head injury, are also being investigated. Systems that automatically track the driver's current lane, as well as in-vehicle signing displays that provide the driver with enhanced roadway information, are being investigated.

In addition to these technologies, which focus on providing the driver with enhanced situation awareness, the U.S. Department of Transportation is conducting research on driver drowsiness and alcohol impairment. Sophisticated in-vehicle sensors may detect when a driver is impaired either by fatigue or by alcohol. The system may inform drivers of their poor driving performance and even could prevent a driver from crossing a lane marker or striking the rear end of the vehicle ahead.

Quite possibly, the most promising of all of the automotive technologies is the driver and passenger air bag. During the crash sequence, the combination of an exploding air bag and safety belt holds the driver away from the impacting areas of the vehicle for a split second—long enough to reduce the catastrophic impact of some crashes. Air bags are by no means a panacea; however, they provide much needed protection for the driver.

CONCLUSIONS

The focus of this chapter has been on the events leading to car crashes that produce head injury. A more thorough understanding of the events that lead to head injury should help medical practitioners and researchers understand the most frequent cause of head injury. Practitioners should also be aware of visual sensory function and the importance of attention to driving, since many of their patients who have already experienced head injury or neurologic diseases might suffer from side effects that diminish their driving abilities.

ACKNOWLEDGMENT

This work was supported by CDC R49/CCR710136.

REFERENCES

Ball K, Owsley C, Roenker D, Sloan M: Isolating risk factors for crash frequency among older drivers. pp. 211–214. Proceedings of the Human Factors and Ergonomics Society, 37th Annual Meeting. Vol. 1. 1993a

Ball K, Owsley C, Sloan M et al: Visual attention problems as a predictor of vehicle accidents among older drivers. Invest Ophthalmol Vis Sci 34:3110–3123, 1993b

Bhise V, Forbes L, Farber E: Driver behavioral data and considerations in evaluating in-vehicle controls and displays. Paper presented at the Transportation Research Board, National Academy of Sciences, 65th Annual Meeting, 1986

Davis G, Schweitzer N, Parosh A et al: Measurement of the Minimum Reaction Time for Braking of Vehicles. Wingate Institute Technical Report. Wingate, Israel, 1990

Dingus T, Antin J, Hulse M, Wierwille W: Attentional demand requirements of an automotive moving map navigation system. Transportation Res A23 (4):301–315, 1989

Dischinger PC, Cushing BM, Kerns TJ: Injury patterns associated with direction of impact: drivers admitted to trauma centers. J Trauma 35 (3):371–383, 1993

Evans L: Traffic Safety and the Driver. Van Nostrand-Reinhold, New York, 1991

Hartman F, Thomas C, Henry C: Belted or not belted: the only difference between two matched samples of 200 car occupants. 21st Stapp Car Crash Conference, New Orleans. Society of Automotive Engineers Paper 770917, 1977

Hayes B, Kurokowa K, Wierwille W: Age related decrements in automobile instrument panel task performance, Proceedings of the Human Factors Society 3rd Annual Meeting, 1989

Herbert DC, Stott JD, Corben CW: Head space requirements for seat belt wearers. Stapp Car Crash Conference 19, San Diego. Society of Automotive Engineers, Paper 711164, 1975

Knipling R, Mironer M, Hendricks D et al: Assessment of IVHS countermeasure for rear-end collision avoidance: rear-end crashes. National Highway and Traffic Safety Administration Technical Report, 1993

Kraus JF, Black MA, Hessol N: The incidence of acute brain injury and serious impairment in a defined population. Am J Epidemiol 119:186–201, 1984

Lerner ND: Brake reaction times of older and younger drivers. Proceedings of the Human Factors and Ergonomics Society 37th Annual Meeting, 1993

Mortimer RG: Rear-end crashes. pp. 275–303. In Automotive Engineering and Litigation. John Wiley & Sons, New York, 1988

National Accident Safety System: National Accident Safety System Annual Report. Centers for Disease Control, Washington, 1991

National Head Injury Foundation: Interagency Head Injury Task Force Reports, National Institute of Neurological Disorders and Stroke, National Institutes of Health, Bethesda, MD, 1993

National Highway and Traffic Safety Administration: Frontier Engineering Task 1 report. 1993

Nygren A: Injuries to Car Occupants—Some Aspects of the Interior Safety of Cars. ISSN 0365-5237. The Almqvist and Wiksell Periodical Co., Stockholm, 1984

Olson PL: Driver Perception Response Time. Society of Automotive Engineers Report No. 890731, 1989

Olson PL, Sivak M: Perception-response time to unexpected roadway hazards. Hum Factors 28:91–96, 1986

Owsley C, Ball K, Sloan M et al: Visual/cognitive correlates of vehicle accidents in older drivers. Psychol and Aging 6:403–415, 1991

Tarriere C, Leung YC, Fayon A et al: Field facial injuries and study of their simulation with a crash dummy. 25th Stapp Car Crash Conference San Francisco. Society of Automotive Engineers Paper 811013.

Wierwille W: In-car controls and displays. In Peacock, Karwoski (eds) Automotive Ergonomics. Taylor Francis, NY, London

Wierwille W, Hulse M, Fischer T, Dingus T: Strategic use of visual resources by the driver while navigating with an in-car navigation display system. 22nd FISITA Congress Technical Papers; Automotive Systems Technology: The Future. Vol. 2. Society of Automotive Engineers P-211, Paper number 885180, 1988

Wilson FR: Measurement of collision avoidance times. pp. 41–64. In Proceedings of the Roads and Transportation Association of Canada, 1987

Neuroimaging in Closed Head Injury

5

William W. Orrison, Jr.
Jeffrey David Lewine

Neuroimaging studies often provide the basis for differential treatment and intervention with head-injured patients, and they play an integral role in guiding the management of head trauma victims. Traumatic events that can lead to neuroimaging abnormalities range from penetrating wounds caused by projectiles or sharp objects to more common types of traumatic injuries such as those associated with the impact of blunt objects on the head. Neuroimaging abnormalities may also result from whiplash or rotational injuries such as those often seen in nonaccidental head trauma (particularly in cases of child abuse).

The extent of brain injury varies with the force and direction of the blow, the nature of the impacting object, and the age of the patient, but even relatively mild trauma, such as in patients with no loss of consciousness, can cause significant neuropathologic changes visible by modern imaging techniques. In addition to direct injury of the brain, significant trauma may also cause damage to the scalp, skull, sinuses, face, and neck.

Both neuroanatomic and neurophysiologic techniques are of interest in the study of head trauma because subtle dysfunction may be present in the absence of gross structural pathology. Computed tomography (CT), a technique to assess brain structure, is the most frequently used imaging technique in the clinical evaluation of head trauma patients, but other techniques such as magnetic resonance imaging (MRI) and more physiologic techniques (positron emission tomography [PET], single-photon emission computed tomography [SPECT], and magnetic source imaging [MSI]) are beginning to be evaluated, especially in the assessment of mild traumatic brain injury.

MRI is increasingly being used as a primary imaging modality in traumatic brain injury. Its use in head trauma requires some understanding of the methods of image acquisition, and it is important to remember that abnormalities on MRI will vary greatly in appearance depending on the specific imaging techniques employed. Standard MRI sequences used in most imaging centers include some type of T_1- and T_2-weighted sequences. T_1 is also called the *relaxation time* or the *spin-lattice relaxation* and refers to the time required for nuclei, predominantly protons (the alignment of which has been altered by the process of MRI) to return to their original alignment. T_1-weighted images typically have limited contrast changes when pathology is present but show tremendous anatomic detail. On these images cerebrospinal fluid (CSF) is dark or black, and most pathology will be seen as an area of slight darkening (decreased signal intensity) on the images.

T_2, also called *spin-spin relaxation,* refers to a measurement of decreasing transverse activity or phase coherence of, again, predominantly protons that have been altered by the process of MRI. CSF is generally white on T_2-weighted images but does not have to be in order for heavy T_2-weighting to be present. T_2-weighted sequences and partially T_2-weighted sequences, called *proton density-weighted* will usually demonstrate less anatomic detail than T_1-weighted images but improved contrast, particularly for pathology. On T_2- or proton density-weighted sequences, most pathology will be seen as areas of whiteness or increased signal on the images. The exception to this rule and virtually every other "rule" in MRI occurs in the case of hemorrhage, which is discussed below in detail.

Although not currently widely employed in cases of trauma, MRI contrast agents are also available to improve the definition of pathologic changes in the brain. Agents such as gadolinium diethylenetriamine pentaacetic acid (Gd-DTPA) can be administered intravenously, and these relatively nontoxic paramagnetic contrast agents provide an "enhanced" image similar to that of contrast-enhanced CT. These paramagnetic substances provide local magnetic fields, which can act as relaxation centers for other nuclei. The distribution and excretion of these agents is similar to that of radiographic contrast substances but requires lower doses for improved contrast effects.

The first several sections of this chapter are concerned with structural consequences of head trauma in adults, after which special considerations in pediatric head injury are discussed briefly.

SKULL FRACTURES

Skull fractures are a common finding in structural neuroimaging studies of moderate (Glasgow Coma Scale [GCS] score 9 to 12) and severe (GCS score 3 to 8) head trauma, although one-third of these patients do not show fractures. It is important to note that the lack of a fracture does not imply a lack of intracranial damage. On the other hand, the presence of a skull fracture on a neuroimaging study is not necessarily indicative of underlying intracranial pathology. In some cases of fracture, the skull absorbs much of the impact force and the brain may remain without significant insult. The identification of a skull fracture does not correlate well with the amount of intracranial injury (Fong et al., 1984; Orrison, 1989). Nevertheless, the finding of a fracture may have clinical and management significance, particularly in instances of depressed skull fracture, displaced fracture fragments, and child abuse.

Plain radiographic films are somewhat better than CT in identifying skull fractures per se, but CT is vastly superior in determining the significance of displaced fragments (Feverman et al., 1988; Fong et al., 1984; Hackney, 1991; Macpherson et al., 1990; Orrison 1989; Osborn, 1994). The characterization of displaced fragments is of far greater clinical import than the simple identification of a fracture line; therefore CT or MRI examination of head injured patients should not be delayed pending prior plain film examination. It is often the case that CT or MRI examination identifies surgical emergencies that plain films cannot. In the absence of CT or MRI, it is probably most important to be able to identify evidence of mass effect on plain films. A shifted pineal gland is a good indicator of this, and patients with this sign should be transferred to a facility with CT and/or MRI capabilities.

Classification of Fractures

Skull fractures are classified as linear, depressed, or diastatic. Linear fractures are particularly difficult to identify by neuroimaging methods. MRI is especially poor, and even CT identifies only about 20 percent of linear skull fractures. Plain films are best, but in determining the first line of diagnosis for a trauma patient, this observation is of little import because CT and MRI are able to diagnose a far greater range of critical clinical conditions (Feverman et al., 1988; Macpherson et al., 1990; Orrison, 1989). Linear skull fractures on plain film are generally thin, straight, and sharp. They are more radiolucent than adjacent vascular markings but nevertheless difficult to identify. When in doubt about the diagnosis, linear fractures will show evidence of healing on repeat examinations (Fong et al., 1984; Orrison, 1989).

Depressed skull fractures often have a stellate or spoke-wheel pattern on plain films, and the fracture line may appear denser than adjacent bone. These fractures are frequently associated with underlying brain injury; therefore, CT is most valuable in diagnosing the degree of depression and the need for surgical intervention (Fong et al., 1984; Macpherson et al., 1990; Orrison et al., 1989) (Fig. 5-1).

Diastatic fractures are linear fractures that extend into a suture. Separation of the suture can be identified without demonstration of an accompanying linear fracture in some cases. Suture separation of more than 2 mm is generally indicative of a diastatic fracture. A CT examination is the best method for confirming this diagnosis (Orrison, 1989; Osborn, 1994).

Basilar skull fractures can be linear, depressed, or diastatic. These fractures are frequently accompanied by air-fluid levels in the sinuses or middle ear cavity. In patients with symptoms such as dizziness or hearing loss following head trauma, high-resolution thin-section CT may demonstrate fractures involving the temporal bone. Pneumocephalus may be encountered whenever a fracture communicates with an open wound; however, this finding is frequently seen in basilar skull fractures involving air-filled sinuses. Large amounts of pneumocephalus can be identified by either MRI or CT. However, small areas of pneumocephalus may be difficult to see on MRI, regardless of technique, and on CT when only soft tissue windows are reviewed. Bone windows make the finding of even minimal pneumocephalus relatively easy to identify. The face may provide some element of protection in head trauma, and in addition to basilar skull fractures, complex facial fractures are frequently encountered in patients with head injury.

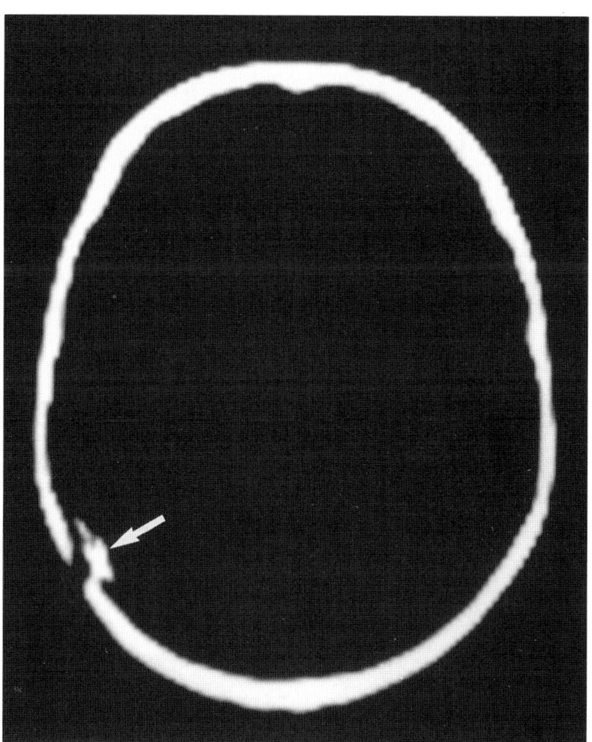

Fig. 5-1. CT scan with bone windows demonstrating the depressed skull fracture and clearly defining the amount of displacement (*arrow*).

EXTRA-AXIAL HEMORRHAGE

CT and MRI are both valuable in the evaluation of extra-axial hemorrhages. CT is particularly useful in the acute setting, where it is important to identify extra-axial fluid collections that cause significant pressure effects. However, a negative CT examination does not completely rule out the possibility of an extra-axial fluid collection. Additional MRI examination may be required to exclude the presence of extra-axial fluid in the acute trauma setting. In general, MRI is advisable for all patients with unexplained neurologic symptoms following head injury (Gentry et al., 1988a; Gentry et al., 1988b; Orrison et al., 1994).

Subdural Hematomas

Subdural hematoma (SDH) resulting from head trauma can be a life-threatening injury, with mortality rates as high as 85 percent (Osborn, 1994; Wilberger et al., 1991). SDH commonly results from an insult to bridging cortical veins that cross the subdural space. Since this space may be significantly enlarged during infancy or in old age, these groups of patients are particularly susceptible to SDH following head trauma. Up to 20 percent of all head trauma patients will be found to have an SDH, and more than one-fourth of all head trauma deaths will include the finding of SDH (Osborn, 1994; Wilberger et al., 1991). The clinical condition of the patient with SDH will frequently be related to the amount of direct cerebral injury accompanying the SDH. When the clinical status changes relative to the SDH, it is at a time when the SDH has expanded beyond the compliance for the individual patient. Clinical symptoms will vary widely, particularly in elderly patients, who may have markedly increased cerebral compliance. Acute SDHs are usually identified as extra-axial fluid collections of increased density on CT. These areas of abnormal increased density will typically be noted to be crescent-shaped, following the normal contour of the brain surface with a "concave" inner margin and a "convex" outer margin. SDHs may be quite extensive, occupying most of a cerebral cortical surface (Fig. 5-2). It is important to remember that bilateral SDHs, isolated interhemispheric SDHs, and parafalcine SDHs are relatively uncommon injuries in the general trauma population. In contrast, these types of findings are frequently seen in child abuse (Orrison, 1989; Osborn, 1994).

Although the anticipated appearance of an acute SDH on CT is that of a homogeneously "white" crescent-shaped extra-axial collection, this is not always the case. Up to 30 percent of SDHs have evidence of rebleeding, and up to 40 percent have mixed density on CT. This is due in part to combinations of blood and CSF, unclotted blood, and extruded serum (Hashimoto et al., 1991; Orrison, 1989; Osborn, 1994; Reed et al., 1991). In some instances even an acute SDH may be isodense with adjacent brain tissue (Fig. 5-3). Isodense SDHs can be associated with severe anemia or coagulopathies, and in these circumstances finding on CT may be limited to secondary signs. Important secondary signs include indications of mass effect, such as effacement of adjacent cortical sulci, deviation of the lateral ventricle, and midline shift. Varying the window level on CT may improve the definition of an SDH. Intravenous contrast administration can reveal enhancement of the margins of an SDH that is isodense on the noncontrasted scans. MRI may be particularly useful in identifying CT-isodense SDHs regardless of the age of the bleed (Amendola and Ostrum, 1977; Boyko et al., 1991; Orrison, 1989; Orrison et al., 1994; Osborn, 1994; Smith et al., 1981; Wilms et al., 1992) (Fig. 5-4).

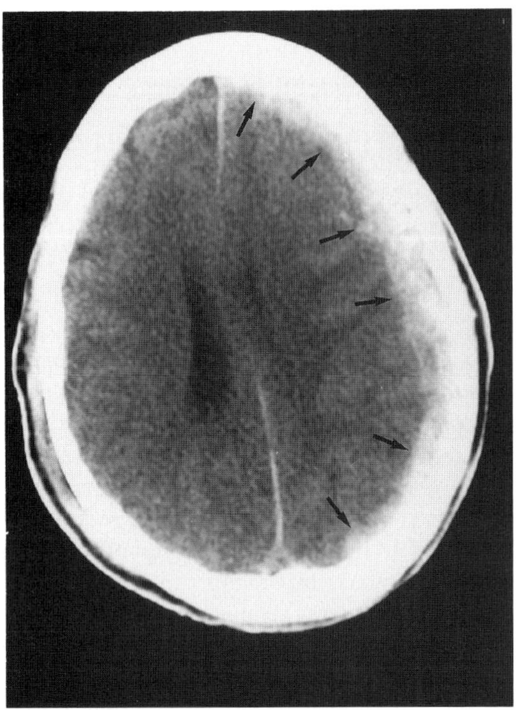

Fig. 5-2. CT scan demonstrating a large left-sided subdural hematoma with midline shift. Note that the subdural hematoma extends from the falx anteriorly to nearly the midline posteriorly (*arrows*).

Age and CT density are often used to classify SDHs as acute, subacute, or chronic. Acute SDHs are less than 7 days old, with the general appearance of a region of increased density relative to surrounding areas (Fig. 5-2). Between 7 and 21 days, the subacute phase, the hematoma usually shows regions of isodensity (Fig. 5-4). Chronic SDHs, more than 21 days old, typically appear as a region of decreased density on CT (Fig. 5-5). These imaging guidelines, defining the age of an SDH, cannot be considered absolute, and consideration must be given to extenuating circumstances, such as a rebleed or low hematocrit (Amendola and Ostrum, 1977; Orrison, 1989; Osborn, 1994; Reed et al., 1991; Smith et al., 1981).

Epidural Hematomas

An epidural hematomas (EDH), in contrast to an SDH, can be identified as a biconvex or lentiform extra-axial fluid collection, which is commonly accompanied by an adjacent skull fracture. Approximately 90 percent of EDHs are associated with a skull fracture that lacerates the middle meningeal artery or a dural sinus, although EDHs may also occur as a result of arterial or venous bleeding without an adjacent fracture (Orrison, 1989; Osborn, 1994). EDHs are much less common than SDHs. They are found in only 5 percent of patients with cerebral trauma but in 10 percent of fatal cases. Patients with EDHs are often quite lucid for several hours after the trauma, with subsequent impairment of consciousness reflecting continued enlargement of the EDH during the first 24 to 48 hours postinjury (Hamilton and Wallace, 1992; Orrison, 1989; Osborn 1994; Poon et al., 1992).

Acute EDHs may be isointense on T_1-weighted MRI images and of decreased signal on T_2-weighted sequences (because of rapid clot formation) (Fig. 5-

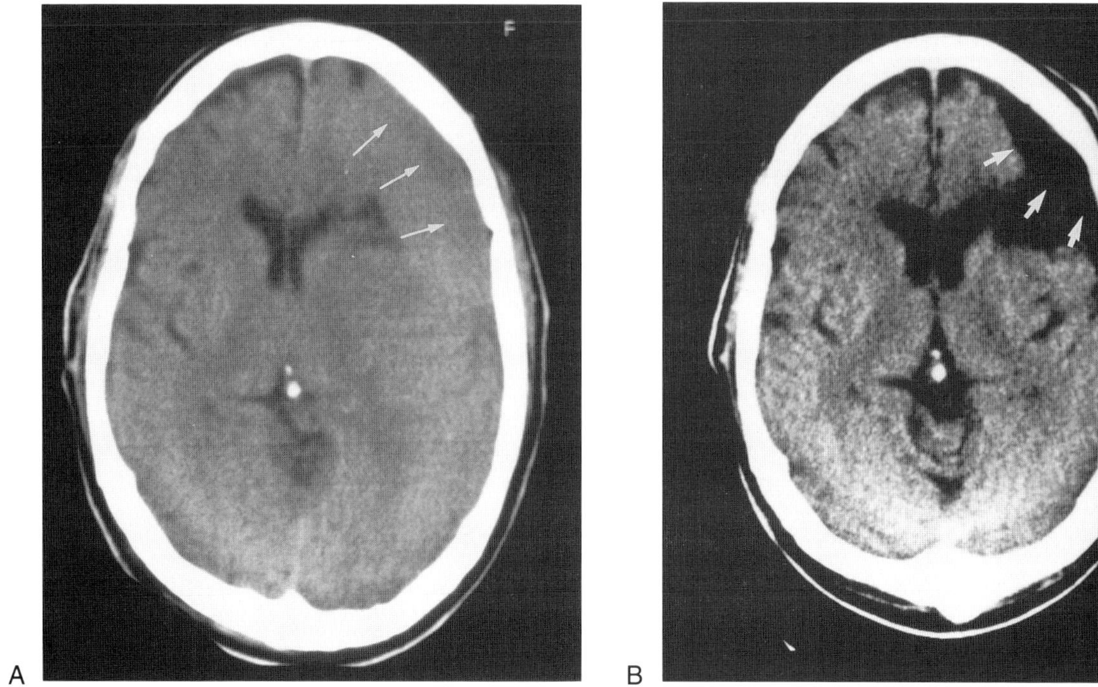

Fig. 5-3. (A) CT scan demonstrating an isodense subdural hematoma (*arrows*). **(B)** Postoperative CT scan demonstrating chronic subdural fluid collection (*arrows*) in the region where the previous isodense subdural hematoma was identified (see Fig. A). Note that there is a focal area of decreased density in the underlying brain cortex, consistent with post-traumatic encephalomalacia.

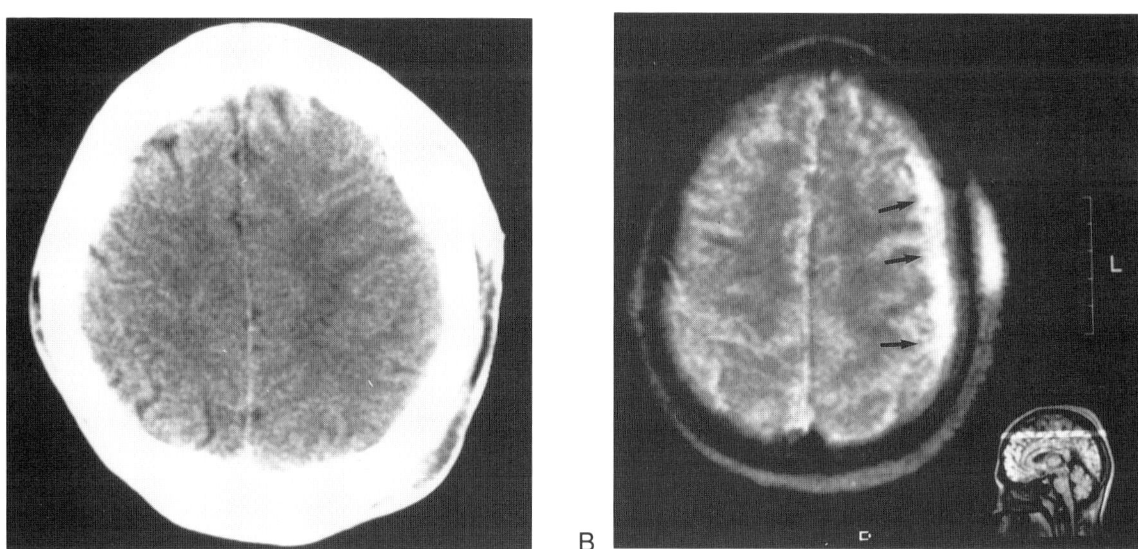

Fig. 5-4. (A) CT scan demonstrating minimal effacement of the cortical sulci on the left and adjacent superficial soft tissue injury. **(B)** Axial MRI (TR2000, TE45) obtained at the same time as Fig. 5-9A. Note the subdural hematoma on the left (*arrows*), which is isodense on the CT scan.

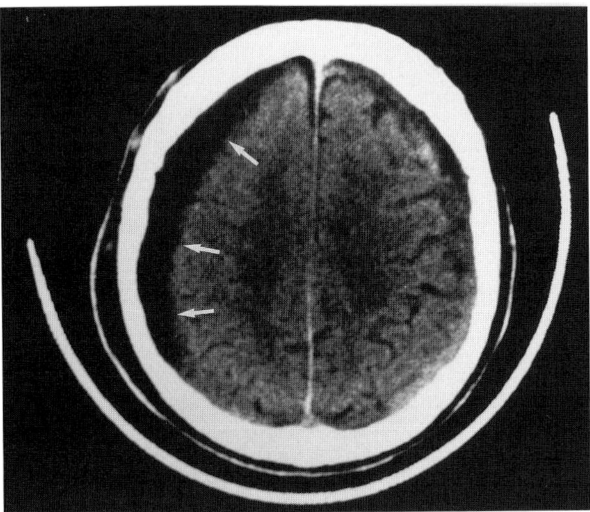

Fig. 5-5. CT scan demonstrating a large right-sided chronic subdural hematoma (*arrows*). Note that there is effacement of the adjacent cortical sulci.

6). While methemoglobin is present, more chronic EDHs generally show increased signal on all pulse sequences. In some cases acute arterial hemorrhage may cause rapid expansion of the EDH, with accompanying mass effect and midline shift. Identification of venous epidural bleeding located over the convexities can be problematic on CT; therefore MRI may be necessary to establish the diagnosis. When an extra-axial hematoma bridges the interhemispheric fissure, it is most likely epidural in location, since the superior sagittal sinus and falx represent a barrier to SDHs. It is important to remember that follow-up CT or MRI evaluation of an EDH or SDH is indicated, because removal of the mass effect from one side may allow accumulation of fluid on the other side. Additional reasons to consider a repeat scan include residual hematoma, expanding size of remaining hemorrhage, and associated hemorrhage or infarction. An apparent EDH or SDH may actually represent both EDH and SDH, since a tear in the dura can allow dissection of blood into both spaces simultaneously (Nelson et al., 1982; Orrison, 1989; Osborn, 1994; Sipponen et al., 1984; Sweet et al., 1978).

Subarachnoid Hemorrhages

Subarachnoid hemorrhage (SAH) is often present in patients who have suffered significant head injury. An SAH manifests as an area of increased density in the basal cisterns, sylvian fissures, superior cerebellar cistern, and the sulci over the cerebral convexities. These narrow, high-density collections of fluid are occasionally overlooked, especially when they are diffuse and symmetrical (Fig. 5-7). SAH may be the only abnormal finding on a scan, or it may be associated with single or multiple areas of intracerebral hemorrhage.

There are several conditions that mimic SAH, and these false signs or misleading appearances are important to note. Pseudo-SAH may be seen when there is severe cerebral edema. Edema causes the brain to have dereased attenuation on CT, with the dura and superficial vasculature appearing dense, as in true SAH. Parafalcine or interhemispheric SAH may produce an appearance similar to the so-called empty delta sign of superior sagittal sinus thrombosis. An isolated CT finding of increased density in the interhemispheric fissure may be a false sign for SAH, and it must be evaluated carefully (Modesti and Binet, 1978; Orrison, 1989; Osborn, 1994; Yeakley et al., 1988).

INTRAPARENCHYMAL HEMORRHAGE

Intraparenchymal hemorrhage represents one of the most commonly encountered sequelae of significant brain injury. It is found in most forms of trauma, including contusions, shearing type injuries, and direct arterial or venous insult. Acute intraparenchymal hemorrhage has a characteristic appearance on CT, with focal areas of increased density readily identified in most cases. This high density decreases over time as the hemorrhage resolves. Following the initial injury, there is a gradual decrease in density on CT, until the hemorrhage becomes isodense with surrounding brain about 2 to 3 weeks after the acute event. At this stage of a brain hematoma, contrast enhancement surrounding the hematoma is common. In many cases, contrast injection may be necessary in order to demonstrate an abnormality by CT. This ring enhancement can typically be seen after approximately 1 week on CT studies. As the intraparenchymal hemorrhage continues to age, it becomes a focal area of decreased density. The final density may take as long as 6 months to be achieved. A delay in the formation of an intracerebral hematoma can occur following head injury, and this may be for as long as several weeks after the initial insult. The overall size and

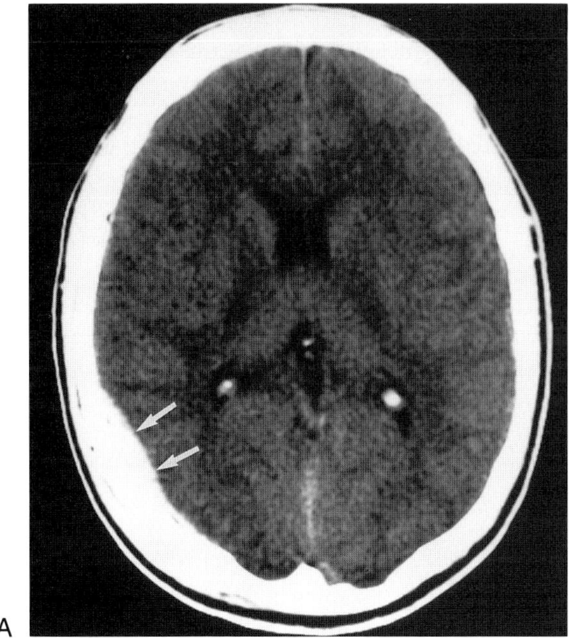

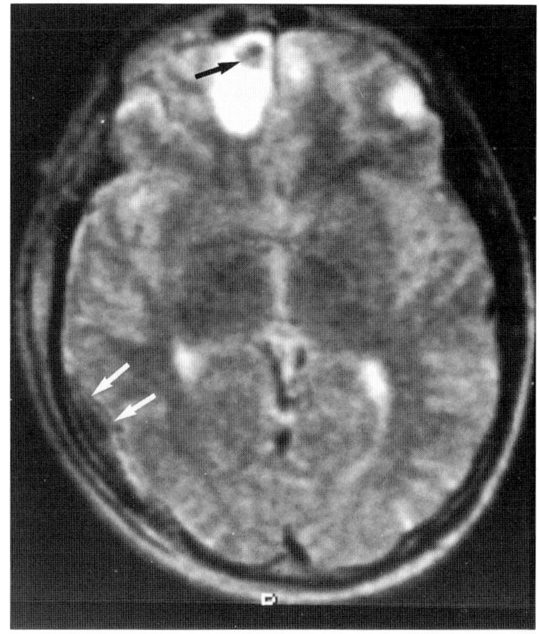

Fig. 5-6. **(A)** CT scan demonstrating a focal epidural hematoma (*arrows*). **(B)** Axial T_2-weighted MRI (TR2000, TE105) obtained at the same time as the CT scan in Fig. A. Note the appearance of the epidural hematoma (*white arrows*), which is of decreased signal intensity. There is also a focal acute right frontal hematoma (*black arrow*) with adjacent edema. A smaller left frontal contusion is also present. This was not identified by CT.

number of areas of intraparenchymal hemorrhage may also increase with time following the injury. This delayed intraparenchymal hemorrhage formation is often indicative of a poor prognosis (Kishore et al., 1981; Orrison, 1989; Osborn, 1994; Tsai et al., 1978; Weisberg, 1979; Zimmerman et al., 1977).

Intraparenchymal hemorrhages tend to lose peripheral density first. Their high density which is initially seen by CT, decreases by approximately 1 to 2 Hounsfield units per day with variations based on the size and location of the hemorrhage. For example, an intraparenchymal hemorrhage that is contiguous with a CSF space may lose density at a more rapid rate than deeper regions of hemorrhage, and larger bleeds may take longer to become hypodense than smaller ones (Dolinskas et al., 1977a; Dolinskas et al., 1977b; Orrison, 1989; Osborn, 1994; Weisberg, 1979).

Diagnosis on MRI

It is important to be able to recognize intraparenchymal hemorrhage on MRI, since the management of patients may be directly affected; in some cases MRI may provide a diagnosis of intraparenchymal hemorrhage when CT is negative for hemorrhage. As the hemorrhage resolves, its MRI appearance changes dramatically; therefore, a detailed understanding of the appearance of blood and of intraparenchymal hemorrhage on MRI is important for the proper identification and treatment of patients. The appearance of blood on MRI has been the subject of numerous reports, but the data are disturbingly conflicting, (Atlas et al., 1987; Atlas et al., 1988; Barkovich and Atlas, 1988; Brooks et al., 1989; Bydder et al., 1988; Chaney et al., 1992; Clark et al., 1990; dela Paz et al., 1984; Dooms et al., 1986; Edelman et al., 1986; Gomori and Grossman, 1988; Gomori et al., 1985; Hardy et al., 1990; Hayman et al., 1991). The MRI features of intraparenchymal hemorrhage are extremely variable. This reflects time from ictus, hemorrhage source, hemorrhage location, and field strength, as well as variations in hematocrit, clotting times, blood oxygenation, intracellular protein concentrations, and rates of red blood cell settling or packing (Brooks et al., 1989; Bydder et al., 1988; Clark et al., 1990; Gomori and Grossman, 1988; Go-

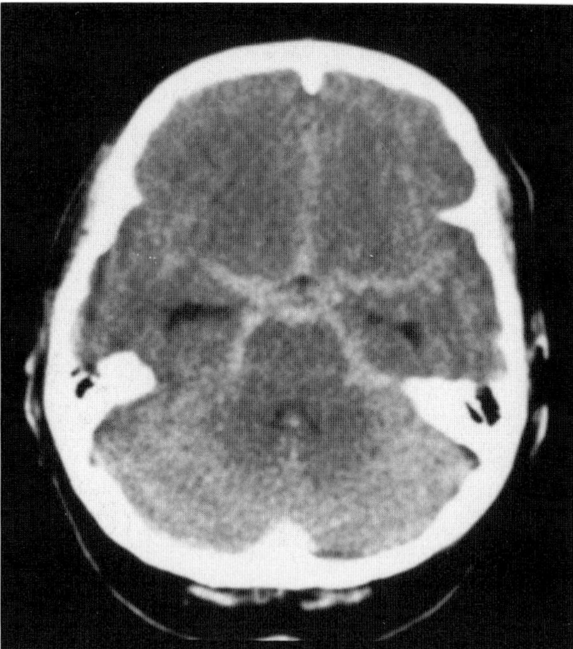

Fig. 5-7. CT scan demonstrating abnormal increased density in the basal cisterns and interhemispheric fissure, as well as a small amount of abnormal increased density in the fourth ventricle from subarachnoid hemorrhage. Note there is early ventricular dilation of the temporal horns from obstructive hydrocephalus, which frequently accompanies diffuse subarachnoid hemorrhage.

mori et al., 1985). As a result the MRI image of intraparenchymal hemorrhage is heterogeneous and subject to frequent change. The best imaging sequences to use for the MRI evaluation are not well agreed upon (Atlas et al., 1987; Atlas et al., 1988; Barkovich and Atlas, 1988; Chaney et al., 1992; Dooms et al., 1986; Hardy et al., 1990; Hayman et al., 1991).

In order to simplify this extraordinarily complicated area of trauma imaging, it is useful to note that there are some features of intraparenchymal hemorrhage on MRI that are relatively consistent and reliable across various conditions. These provide a foundation from which to form a diagnostic reference. In general, on T_1-weighted images, an intraparenchymal hemorrhage begins as a region of subtle hyperintensity or isointensity, which becomes hypointense within the first 12 to 24 hours. During this hyperacute (<24-hour) time period, T_2-weighted sequences demonstrate an initial hyperintensity, which rapidly changes to marked hypointensity. This hypointense T_1- and T_2-weighted sequence change persists throughout the acute phase of the hemorrhage (Fig. 5-8). This very early hyperintensity, identifiable on MRI images, probably reflects the longer T_2 of oxygenated blood (when compared with the normal brain parenchyma) and the effect of increased proton density on the T_1-weighted sequences (Brooks et al., 1989; Chaney et al., 1992; Dichiro et al., 1986; Zimmerman et al., 1988).

The hypointensity of the acute phase of intraparenchymal hemorrhage is characteristic of all pulse sequences although it is most notable on T_2-weighted images. This is probably due to the presence of a combination of deoxyhemoglobin, red blood cell dehydration, and clot matrix formation (Chaney et al., 1992; Gomori et al., 1985).

The subacute (1 week to 1 month) time period postictus gives a fairly consistent intensity pattern on both T_1- and T_2-weighted sequences. T_1-weighted images demonstrate an increasing signal intensity, which begins as a hyperintense rim converging centrally to encompass the entire lesion. This T_1-weighted shortening is believed to represent the paramagnetic effect on the formation of methemoglobin, the oxidative breakdown product of deoxyhemoglobin (Chaney et al., 1992; Gomori and Grossman, 1988; Gomori et al., 1985).

The marked hypointensity of intraparenchymal hemorrhage on T_2-weighted sequences begins to disappear at about the same time that this hyperintensity is seen on T_1-weighted images. The paramagnetic effect of intracellular methemoglobin results in a persistent reduction of the signal on T_2-weighted sequences. However, as red blood cells begin to lyse, the heterogeneous magnetic fields and local magnetic gradients caused by the intracellular paramagnetic methemoglobin are lost. This leaves the hemorrhage appearing hyperintense on T_2-weighted sequences. Because the hemolysis does not affect T_1, the T_1-weighted images also remain hyperintense. This situation accounts for the so-called "bright-bright" appearance of subacute intraparenchymal hemorrhage on MRI (Brooks et al., 1989; Chaney et al., 1992; Zimmerman et al., 1988) (Fig. 5-9).

In the chronic (>1 month) phase of intraparenchymal hemorrhage there is the gradual appearance of a thin rim of hypointensity around the area of hemorrhage that is most marked on T_2-weighted sequences (Fig. 5-10). This surrounding "dark" rim thickens over time, and the central area of methemoglobin may be resorbed or replaced by CSF. When

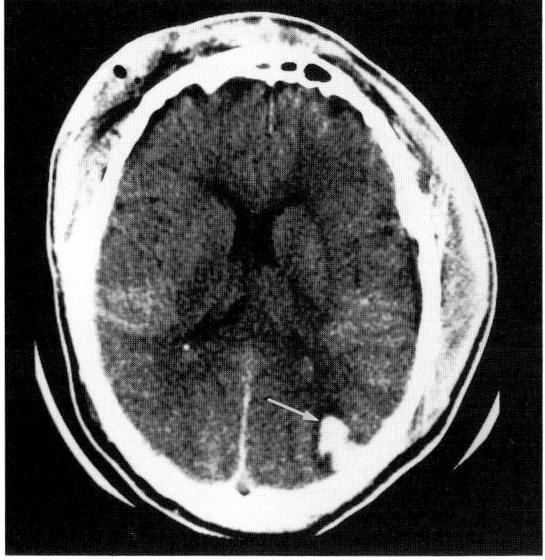

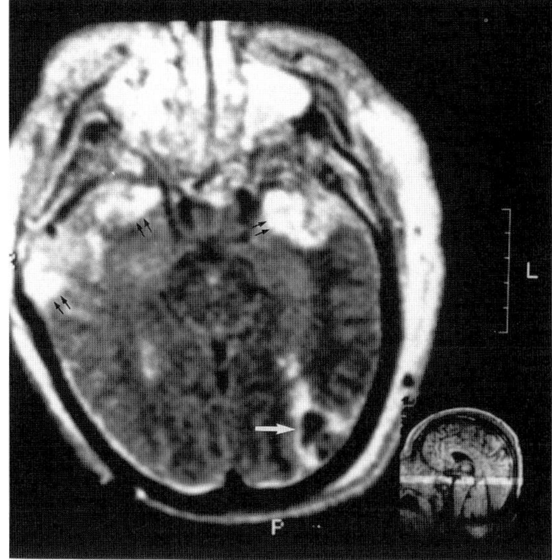

Fig. 5-8. **(A)** CT scan demonstrating a left posterior intraparenchymal hematoma (*arrow*) with massive severe bilateral superficial soft tissue swelling and scalp edema. There is also increased density over both inferior parietal regions consistent with subarachnoid hemorrhage. **(B)** Axial T_2-weighted MRI (TR1800, TE105) obtained at the same time as Fig. A. Note the decreased signal intensity of the acute intraparenchymal hemorrhage with surrounding increased signal from edema (*white arrow*). There is also markedly abnormal increased signal intensity in the temporal lobes bilaterally from severe contusions, which were not identified on the CT scan (*double arrows*). In addition, there is significant abnormal increased signal intensity in the sinuses and superficial soft tissues.

replaced by CSF, the central core of the lesion will be of decreased signal on T_1 and of increased signal on T_2 (following the signal intensity of CSF). The hypointense rim is believed to reflect the magnetic susceptibility effects of iron in methemoglobin breakdown products. This is thought to be predominantly an effect of hemosiderin, which accumulates in the lysosomes of macrophages that have converged on the region of hemorrhage. These hemosiderin-laden macrophages are also seen as a less hypointense rim on T_1 sequences, since the degradation of methemoglobin into its breakdown products causes a loss of T_1 shortening (Barkovich and Atlas, 1988; Chaney et al., 1992; Gomori et al., 1985).

Gradient-Recalled Echo Sequences

Gradient-recalled echo (GRE) sequences have been advocated as a means of improving the identification of IPH on MRI (Atlas et al., 1988; Mills et al., 1987). Available data suggest that GRE sequences are superior to spin-echo sequences in characterizing some of the stages of intracranial parenchymal hemorrhage, particularly at higher field strengths. The lack of a 180-degree pulse in GRE scans leads to a greater sensitivity to paramagnetic substances. This results in part from shortened T_2 and T_{2*} decay times due to the local magnetic field susceptibility differences between hemosiderin, ferritin, and intracellular deoxyhemoglobin and methemoglobin (Atlas et al., 1988; Edelman et al., 1986; Unger et al., 1981).

Although GRE sequences are more sensitive to susceptibility variations than are standard spin-echo sequences, this improved sensitivity does not give rise to a similar improvement in specificity. In addition to hemorrhage, other substances such as calcification, air, normal brain iron, and paramagnetic contrast agents also show decreased signal intensity on short flip-angle, long-TE, gradient-echo sequences. Because most of the various forms of intraparenchymal hemorrhage and associated blood products (deoxyhemoglobin, methemoglobin, and hemosiderin) all demonstrate hypointensity on gradient-echo sequences, this type of imaging can be used to assist in the identification and verification of hemorrhagic foci within the brain (Fig. 5-11).

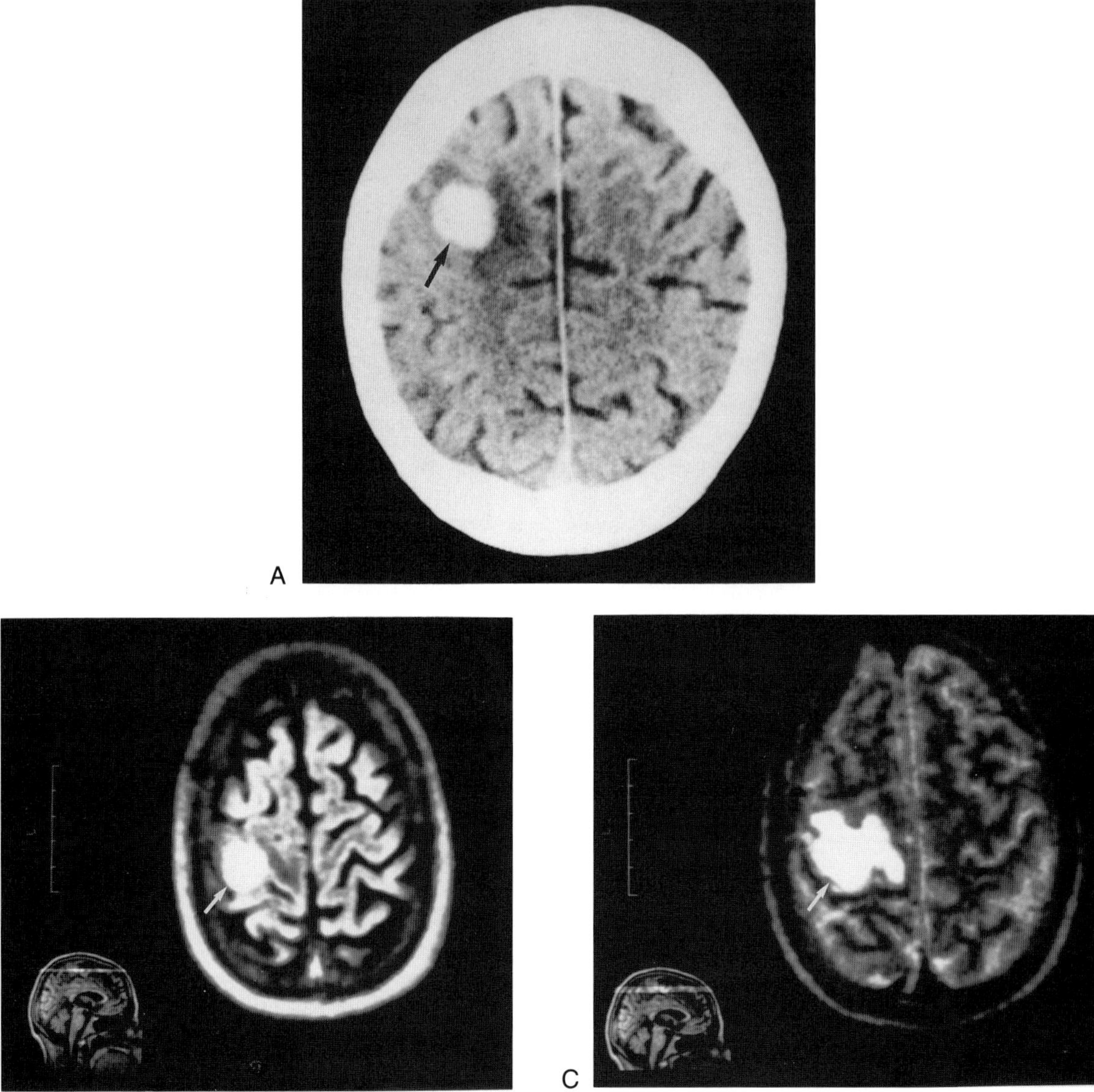

Fig. 5-9. (A) CT scan demonstrating increased density from a hematoma (*arrow*). **(B)** Axial T_1-weighted MRI (TR68, TE24, FA60) demonstrating increased signal intensity during the subacute phase of this focal hematoma (*arrow*). The MRI examination was obtained approximately 3 weeks after the initial CT scan. **(C)** Axial T_2-weighted MRI (TR2000, TE105) demonstrating abnormal increased intensity in this subacute hematoma (*arrow*). The "bright-bright" appearance on T_1- and T_2-weighted sequences is typical of subacute hemorrhage on MRI.

CONTUSIONS

Cortical contusions are a frequently encountered form of primary neuronal injury. These lesions consist of punctate parenchymal hemorrhages (microhemorrhages) or linear zones of hemorrhage that tend to be found along the cortical gyri. Contusions are often centered about the gyral crests under the calvarium, and they are particularly common to regions of the anterior temporal and frontal lobes as

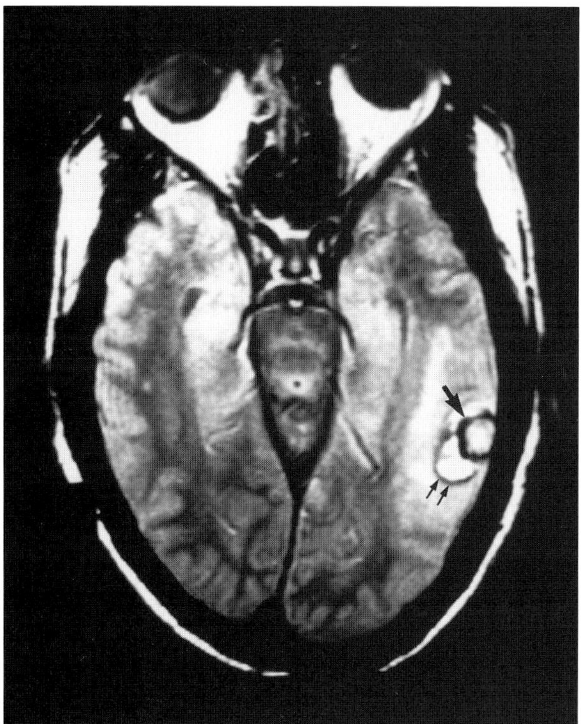

Fig. 5-10. Axial proton density-weighted MRI (TR2500, TE22) demonstrating a dark hemosiderin rim around an area of more chronic hematoma (*arrow*), with an adjacent area of less chronic hemorrhage having a thinner, less hypodense rim (*double arrows*).

well as to the occipital poles (Gentry et al., 1988a; Gentry et al., 1988b; Orrison, 1989; Orrison et al., 1994; Osborn, 1994).

The imaging findings in cortical contusions are variable, as these lesions typically go through several stages of evolution. Initially the CT may be negative or minimally abnormal, whereas MRI usually shows the abnormality from the onset of injury (Gentry et al., 1988a; Gentry et al., 1988b; Orrison et al., 1994) (Fig. 5-12). CT is capable of demonstrating progression over time in the size and number of contusions and amount of hemorrhage within them. These changes are particularly evident over the first 24 to 48 hours. It is noteworthy that nearly one-fourth of patients can show a delayed hemorrhage in regions that were previously nonhemorrhagic (Gentry et al., 1988a; Osborn, 1994).

EDEMA

Cerebral edema is an easily missed but common abnormality in post-traumatic brain imaging. Mild edema may be seen in patients with minimal injury (GCS scores 13 to 15), but it is more often found in patients with a GCS score below 12. The CT appearance of edema can be limited to regions of hypodensity, which are sometimes acompanied by mass effect. However, at times mass effect may be subtle or even absent, particularly when the edema is diffuse. Severe diffuse cerebral edema may be accompanied by the decreased identifiability of basal cisterns, the fourth ventricle, or cortical sulci. Advanced stages of diffuse cerebral edema can result in a lack of visibility of the lateral ventricles and are often associated with GCS scores below 8. Focal edematous changes may present with displacement of the ventricular system, localized effacement of the cortical sulci, and/or midline shift. When identifiable on CT, focal edema is seen as an area of decreased density (Kishore et al., 1981; Koo and LaRouge, 1977; Orrison, 1989; Tsai et al., 1978).

Although MRI is relatively insensitive to the changes of diffuse cerebral edema, it is exquisitely sensitive to changes of focal edema. Edema is seen as decreased signal on T_1-weighted images and increased signal on T_2- and proton density-weighted sequences (Gentry et al., 1988a; Gentry et al., 1988b; Orrison, 1989; Orrison et al., 1994; Osborn, 1994; Zimmerman et al., 1986).

SHEARING

Rotational and/or rapid deceleration/acceleration types of insults may cause shearing injuries, also known as diffuse axonal injuries or deep white matter injuries. These injuries are often associated with a tear at nonuniform brain regions such as the gray-white matter interfaces of the cerebral cortex, the internal capsule, the deep gray matter, the upper brainstem, and the corpus callosum (Gentry et al., 1988a; Gentry et al., 1988b; Orrison, 1989; Orrison et al., 1994; Osborn, 1994). These patients are frequently among the most severely neurologically impaired (GCS score 8 or below), particularly when the diffuse axonal injury involves deep cerebral or brainstem regions.

The initial CT scan in shearing injury is often normal in spite of marked clinical impairment. Less than

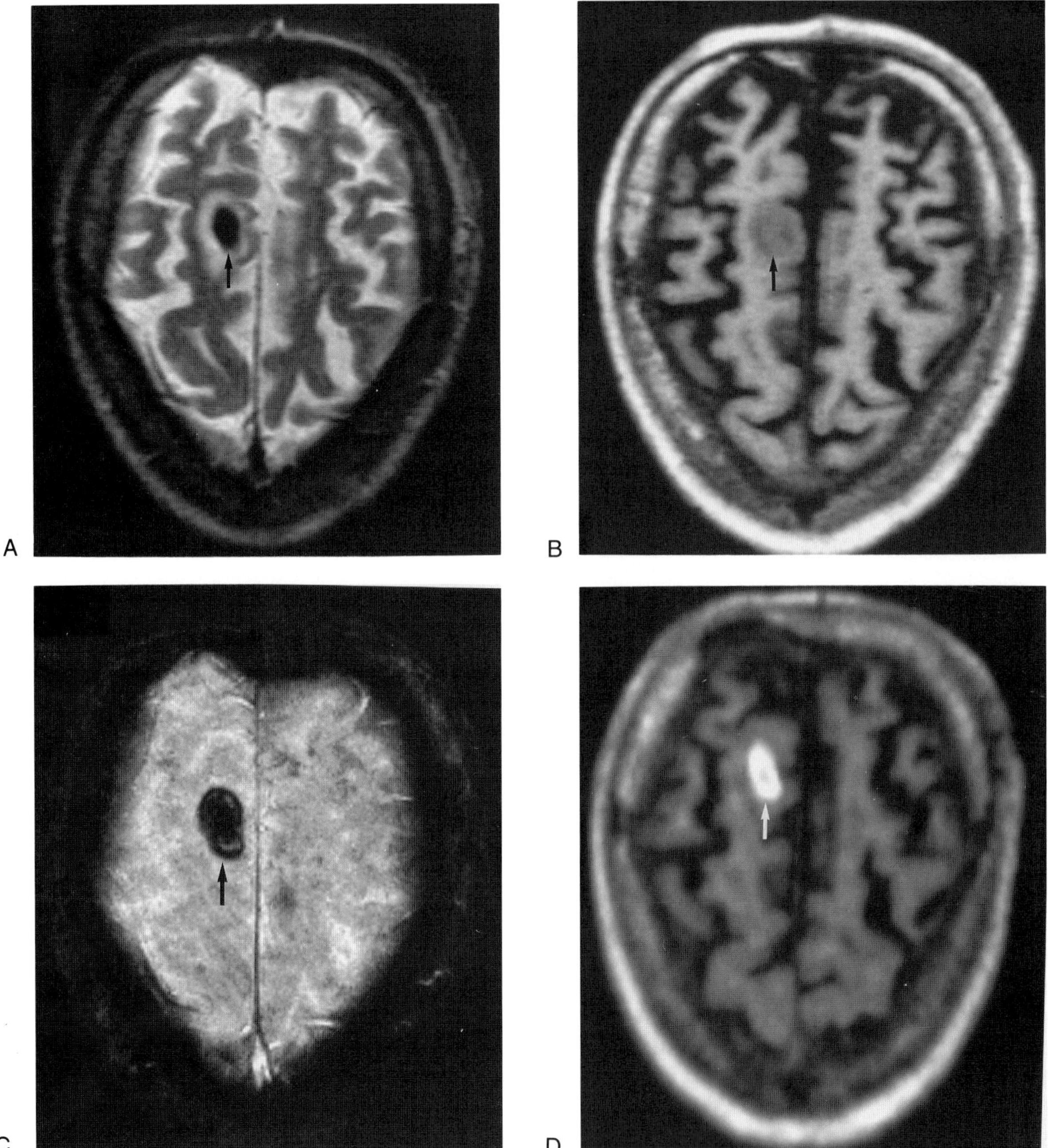

Fig. 5-11. **(A)** Axial T_2-weighted MRI (TR2500, TE90) demonstrating a focal area of decreased signal intensity with surrounding rim of edema consistent with acute hemorrhage (*arrow*). **(B)** Axial T_1-weighted MRI (TR10, TE4, FA10) demonstrating relative isointensity to slightly decreased signal intensity in the region of abnormality identified on the T_2 image (*arrow*). (**C**) Gradient recalled echo (GRE) sequence (TR70, TE30, FA40) demonstrating decreased signal intensity consistent with a paramagnetic effect, as would be expected with deoxyhemoglobin in an acute hemorrhage (*arrow*). (**D**) Axial T_1-weighted MRI (TR10, TE4, FA10) obtained 4 days after the initial scan demonstrating progression to intracellular methemoglobin (*arrow*) with increased signal intensity (cf. Fig. B) (*Figure continues.*)

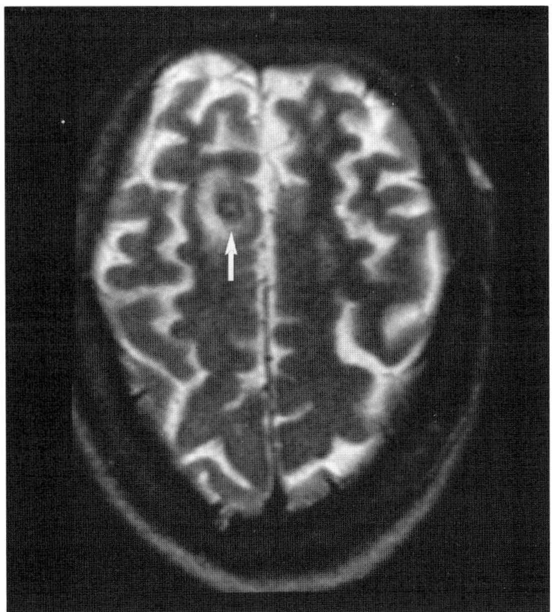

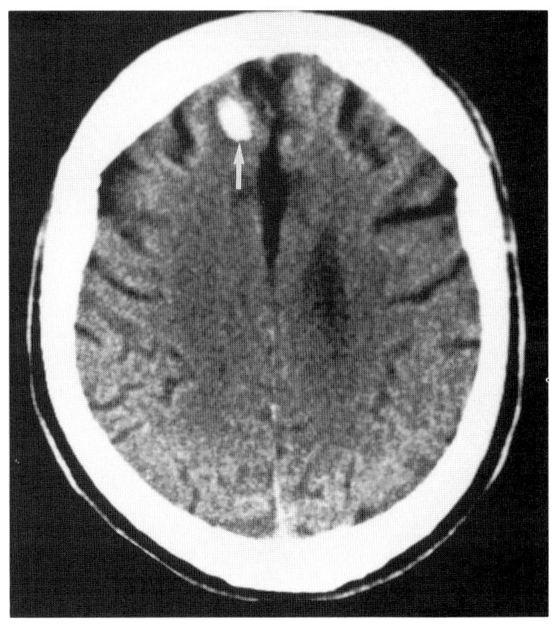

Fig. 5-11 (*continued*). **(E)** Axial T_2-weighted MRI (TR2500, TE90) obtained 4 days after the initial scan, demonstrating progression to central increased signal intensity consistent with extracellular methemoglobin (*arrow*). **(F)** CT scan demonstrating a focal area of abnormal increased density consistent with acute hemorrhage (*arrow*).

50 percent of patients who actually have shearing injury demonstrate findings of diffuse axonal injury on an initial CT study. However, MRI has been shown to have as much as 97 percent sensitivity for shearing injury as compared with 20 percent for early CT scanning (Gentry et al., 1988a; Orrison 1989; Orrison et al., 1994; Osborn, 1994). The appearance of shearing injury can vary over time, depending on the amount of hemorrhage present and the extent of surrounding edema. The MRI findings most often encountered in shearing injury include minimal or no changes on T_1-weighted sequences with focal areas of hyperintensity on T_2-weighted images. These lesions may appear similar to the white matter changes commonly encountered in the elderly, so these findings must be cautiously integrated in older patients (Fig. 5-13). When the initial shearing injury is hemorrhagic, or as hemorrhage develops over time, the MRI appearance will reflect the various stages of intraparenchymal hemorrhage discussed above. As with other forms of hemorrhage, evidence of shearing injury may only be evident on gradient-echo sequences when delayed-recall scans are performed. (Atlas et al., 1988; Osborn, 1994; Unger et al., 1989).

VENTRICULAR DILATION

Ventricular dilation may be observed in the acute post-traumatic phase or in conjunction with cerebral atrophy as one of the late sequelae that follow brain injury. In some cases post-traumatic ventricular dilation may be seen as a progressive form of obstructive hydrocephalus, presumably due to SAH, with a block at the level of the cerebral aqueduct or arachnoid granulations (Timming et al., 1982). Even relatively minor head injury may result in obstructive hydrocephalus when SAH is present. In these cases ventriculoperitoneal shunting may be effective. However, in other cases of early ventricular dilation, shunting is ineffective regardless of the timing of the procedure, and this appears to be an indicator of extremely severe head injury. In these cases the overall prognosis is poor (Timming et al., 1982). Prognosis is also poor when ventricular dilation is associated with loss of brain substance and atrophy. These forms of postventricular dilation do not represent obstructive hydrocephalus. Rather, they appear to reflect a loss of ventricular wall compliance from direct trauma or secondary to a loss of brain substance. Regardless of

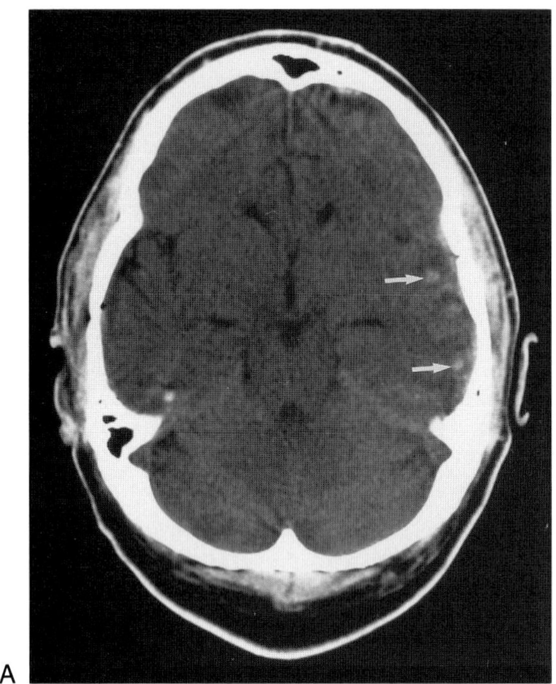

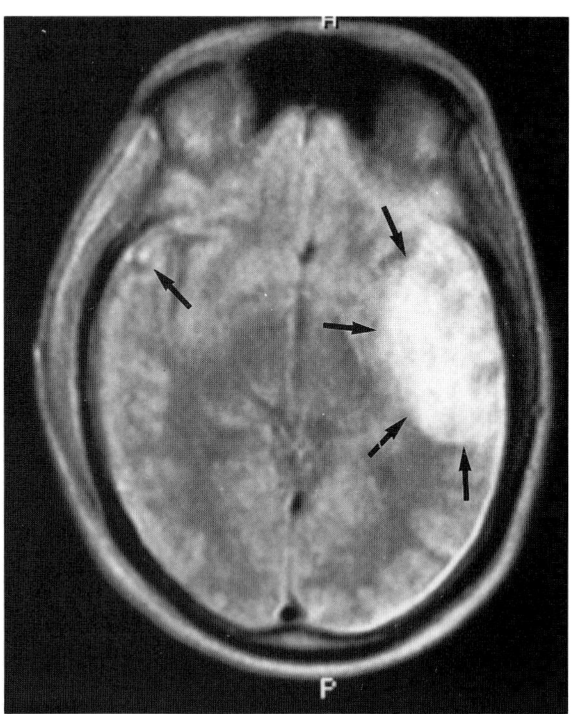

Fig. 5-12. **(A)** CT scan in a patient with acute head trauma. Note there are minimal focal areas of increased density in the left superficial temporal lobe (*arrows*). **(B)** Axial proton density-weighted MRI (TR2000, TE30) demonstrating a massive left temporal lobe contusion (*arrows*) and a smaller anterior right temporal lobe contusion (*arrow*). This scan was obtained at the same time as the CT scan in Fig. A.

the etiology, ventricular dilation is a predictor of extremely poor outcome following head trauma, especially when it is unresponsive to ventriculoperitoneal shunting.

PEDIATRIC HEAD INJURY

Nonaccidental trauma or child abuse is an extremely important condition for the clinician to recognize; neuroimaging studies are frequently the first examination to result in a suspicion of nonaccidental trauma. Cranial trauma is the leading cause of morbidity and mortality in nonaccidental trauma and is seen in approximately 50 percent of all cases (Ball, 1989; Osborn, 1994). There are several features of child abuse that can be revealed by neuroimaging techniques; the need for clinicians to be knowledgeable about these cannot be overemphasized, given the devastating results that may be seen from repeated abuse.

SDH is the most common finding on CT and/or MRI in nonaccidental trauma. As demonstrated above, CT may be adequate to exclude a surgical emergency, but MRI is far more sensitive for this abnormality, particularly in the subacute stage. Since blood has different characteristic appearances at varying ages on MRI, this study should be obtained in all cases of suspected child abuse. The presence of blood of various ages may be one of the strongest indicators of chronic nonaccidental trauma. In addition to the detection of SDH, both CT and MRI can demonstrate accompanying changes such as contusions, shearing injuries, and cerebral edema. The shaken baby syndrome tends to present with interhemispheric SDH, shearing injuries, SAH, and the clinical finding of retinal hemorrhages (Fig. 5-14). When smothering or strangling injuries are suspected, the neuroimaging methods may show evidence of watershed infarction, diffuse cerebral edema, or basal ganglia ischemia.

Multiple, bilateral, depressed, or complex fractures that are not readily explained by the clinical history should signal concern for the possibility of child abuse. When these findings are noted in com-

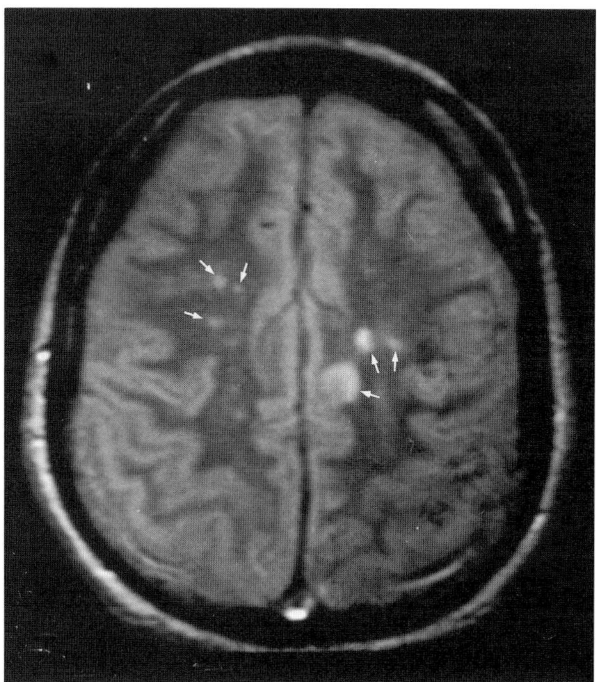

Fig. 5-13. Axial proton density-weighted MRI (TR2500, TE30) demonstrating multiple focal areas of abnormal increased signal intensity in the subcortical white matter representing shearing injuries from severe head trauma (*arrows*).

bination with healing or older fractures anywhere in the body, child abuse is the most likely diagnosis.

CONCLUSION

The primary goal of imaging procedures in head trauma is to facilitate acute patient care. Often the most expeditious procedure is required in order to maximize survival and to minimize morbidity. However, a correct and complete diagnosis will in general provide the optimum in patient care. Therefore, selection of the most appropriate imaging modality is critical, and this imaging must further be correlated with the management of an often critically injured patient. Such problems are frequently far from simple given the multiple organ systems that may be compromised following a major catastrophic insult. Unfortunately, the decisions regarding imaging in head trauma are often made in the middle of the night, under great duress, and after only a few minutes of patient evaluation. Nonetheless, these all-important studies form the basis for much of the research and teaching that is performed in the area of head trauma. In addition, these urgently obtained images are also an integral part of many medicolegal proceedings.

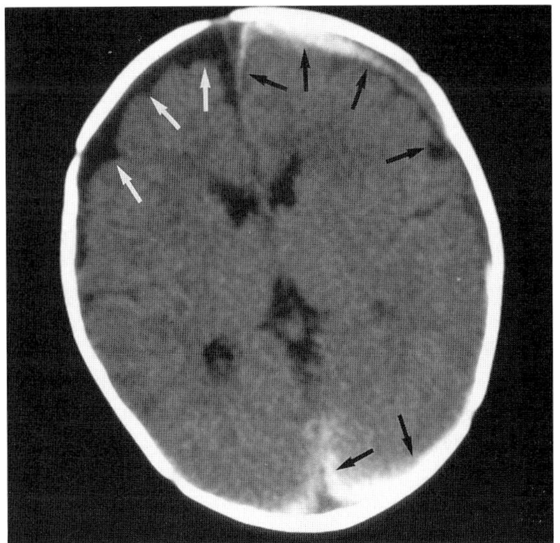

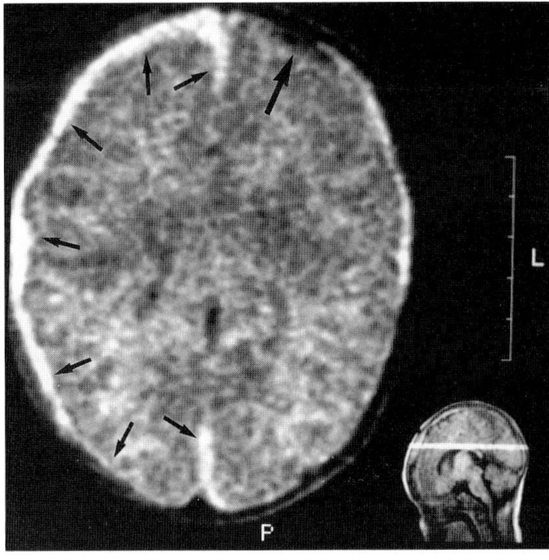

Fig. 5-14. **(A)** CT scan of patient with shaken baby syndrome, demonstrating a chronic subdural hematoma on the right (*white arrows*) and an acute subdural hematoma on the left (*black arrows*), which extends into the interhemispheric fissure both anteriorly and posteriorly. **(B)** Axial T_2-weighted MRI (TR2000, TE105) demonstrating decreased signal intensity (*large arrow*) in the region of more recent hemorrhage, with increased signal intensity (*arrows*) in the regions of chronic subdural hematoma.

Delayed images during the recovery phase of head trauma may also be important for documentation of either progression or resolution of injury. In addition, a negative imaging study may be an important part of the clinical management of many patients who continue to have difficulty following head trauma. There is no substitute for a thorough understanding of all the imaging modalities available when managing a head trauma victim. Appropriate timing and selection of these modalities can save lives and significantly reduce morbidity.

REFERENCES

Amendola MA, Ostrum BJ: Diagnosis of isodense subdural hematomas by computed tomography. AJR 129:693–697, 1977

Atlas SW, Grossman RI, Gomori JM et al: Hemorrhagic intracranial malignant neoplasms: spin-echo MR imaging. Radiology 164:71–77, 1987

Atlas SW, Mark AS, Grossman RI, Gomori JM: Intracranial hemorrhage: gradient-echo MR imaging at 1.5 T. Radiology 168:803–807, 1988

Ball WS Jr: Nonaccidental craniocerebral trauma (child abuse): MR imaging. Radiology 173:609–610, 1989

Barkovich AJ, Atlas SW: Magnetic resonance imaging of intracranial hemorrhage. Radiol Clin North Am 26:801–820, 1988

Boyko OB, Cooper DF, Grosseman CB: Contrast-enhanced CT of acute isodense subdural hematoma. AJNR 12:341–343, 1991

Brooks RA, DiChiro G, Petronas N: MR imaging of cerebral hematomas at different field strengths: theory and applications. J Comput Assist Tomogr 13:194–206, 1989

Bydder GM, Pennock JM, Porteous R et al: MRI of intracerebral hematoma at low field (0.15T) using T2 dependent partial saturation sequences. Neuroradiology 30:367–371, 1988

Chaney RK, Taber KH, Orrison WW Jr, Hayman LA: Magnetic resonance imaging of intracerebral hemorrhage at different field strengths: a review of reported intraparenchymal signal intensities. Neuroimaging Clin North Am 2:25–51, 1992

Clark RA, Wantanabe AT, Bradley WG, Roberts JD: Acute hematomas: effects of deoxygenation, hematocrit, and fibrin-clot formation and retraction on T2 shortening. Radiology 175:201–206, 1990

De La Paz RL, New PFJ, Buonanno FS et al: NMR imaging of intracranial hemorrhage. J Comput Assist Tomogr 8:599–607, 1984

DiChiro G, Brooks RA, Girton ME et al: Sequential MR studies of intracerebral hematomas in monkeys. AJNR 7:193–199, 1986

Dolinskas CA, Bilaniuk LT, Zimmerman RA: Computed tomography of intracerebral hematomas II. Transmission CT observations on hematoma resolution. AJR 129:681–688, 1977a

Dolinskas CA, Bilaniuk LT, Zimmerman RA: Computed tomography of intracerebral hematomas. II. Radionuclide and transmission CT studies of the perihematoma region. AJR 129:689–692, 1977b

Dooms AC, Uske A, Brant-Zawadzki M et al: Spin-echo MR imaging of intracranial hemorrhage. Neuroradiology 28:132–138, 1986

Edelman RR, Johnson K, Buxton R et al: MR of hemorrhage: a new approach. AJNR 7:751–756, 1986

Feuerman T, Wackym PA, Gade GF, Becker DP: Value of skull radiography, head computed tomographic scanning, and admission for observation in cases of minor head injury. Neurosurgery 22:449–453, 1988

Fong YT, Teal JS, Hieshima GB: Neuroradiology of Head Trauma. University Park Press, Baltimore, 1984

Gentry LR, Godersky JC, Thompson GH: MR imaging of head trauma: review of the distribution and radiopathologic features of traumatic lesions. AJNR 9:101–110, 1988a

Gentry LR, Godersky JC, Thompson B, Dunn VD: Prospective comparative study of intermediate-field MR and CT in the evaluation of closed head trauma. AJNR 9:91–100, 1988b

Gomori JM, Grossman RI: Mechanisms responsible for the MR appearance and evolution of intracranial hemorrhage. Radiographics 8:427–440, 1988

Gomori JM, Grossman RI, Goldberg HI et al: Intracranial hematomas: imaging by high-field MR. Radiology 157:87–93, 1985

Hackney DB: Skull radiography in the evaluation of acute head trauma: a survey of current practice. Radiology 181:711–714, 1991

Hamilton M, Wallace C: Nonoperative management of acute epidural hematoma diagnosed by CT: the neuroradiologist's role. AJNR 13:853–859, 1992

Hardy PA, Kucharczyk W, Henkelman RM: Cause of signal loss in MR images of old hemorrhagic lesions. Radiology 174:549–555, 1990

Hashimoto N, Sakakibara T, Yamamoto K et al: Two fluid-blood density levels in chronic subdural hematoma. J Neurosurg 77:310–311, 1992

Hayman LA, Taber KH, Ford JJ, Bryan RN: Mechanisms of MR signal alteration by acute intracerebral blood: old concepts and new theories. AJNR 12:899–907, 1991

Kishore PRS, Lipper MH, Becker DP: (1981). Significance of CT in head injury: correlation with intracranial pressure. AJR 137:829–833, 1981

Koo AH, LaRoque RL: Evaluation of head trauma by computed tomography. Radiology 123:345–350, 1977

Macpherson BCM, Macpherson P, Jennett B: CT incidence of intracranial contusion and hematoma in relation to the presence, site and type of skull fracture. Clin Radiol 42:321–326, 1990

Mills TC, Ortendahl DA, Hylton NM et al: Partial flip angle MR imaging. Radiology 162:531–539, 1987

Modesti LM, Binet EF: Value of computed tomography in the diagnosis and management of subarachnoid hemorrhage. Neurosurgery 3:151–156, 1978

Nelson AT, Kishore PRS, Lee SH: Development of delayed epidural hematoma. AJNR 3:583–585, 1982

Orrison WW Jr: Introduction to Neuroimaging. Little, Brown, Boston, 1989

Orrison WW Jr, Gentry LR, Stimac GK et al: Blinded comparison of cranial CT and MR in closed head injury evaluation. AJNR 15:351–356, 1994

Osborn A, Anderson RE, Wing SD: The false falx sign. Radiology 134:421–425, 1980

Osborn AG: Diagnostic Neuroradiology. Mosby-Year Book, St. Louis, 1994

Poon WS, Rehman SU, Poon CYF et al: Traumatic extradural hematoma of delayed onset is not a rarity. Neurosurgery 30:681–686, 1992

Reed D, Robertson WD, Graeb DA et al: Acute subdural hematomas: atypical CT findings. AJNR 12:341–343, 1991

Sipponen JT, Sipponen RE, Sivula A: Chronic subdural hematoma: demonstration by magnetic resonance. Radiology 150:79–85, 1984

Smith WP Jr, Batnitzky S, Rengachary SS: Acute isodense subdural hematomas: a problem in anemic patients. AJNR 2:37–40, 1981

Sweet RC, Miller JD, Lipper M: Significance of bilateral abnormalities on the CT scan in patients with severe head injury. Neurosurgery 3:16–21, 1978

Timming R, Orrison WW Jr, Mikula JA: Computerized tomography and rehabilitation outcome after severe head trauma. Arch Phys Med Rehabil 63:154–159, 1982

Tsai FY, Huprich JE, Gardner FC: Diagnostic and prognostic implications of computed tomography of head trauma. J Comput Assist Tomogr 2:323–331, 1978

Unger EC, Cohen MS, Brown TR: Gradient-echo imaging of hemorrhage at 1.5 tesla. Magn Reson Imaging 7:163–172, 1989

Weisberg LA: Computerized tomography in intracranial hemorrhage. Arch Neurol 36:422–426, 1979

Wilberger JE, Harris M, Diamond DL: Auto subdural hematoma: morbidity, mortality, and operative timings. J Neurosurg 74:212–218, 1991

Wilms G, Marchal G, Guesens E: Isodense subdural hematomas on CT: MR findings. Neuroradiology 34:497–499, 1992

Yeakley JW, Mayer JS, Patchell CC et al: The pseudodelta sign in acute head trauma. J Neurosurg 69:867–868, 1988

Zimmerman RA, Bilaniuk LT, Hackney DB: Head injury: early results of comparing CT and high-field MR. AJNR 7:757–764, 1986

Zimmerman RD, Heier LA, Snow RB et al: Acute intracranial hemorrhage: intensity changes on sequential MR scans at 0.5 T. AJR 150:651–661, 1988

Zimmerman RD, Leeds NE, Nadich TP: Ring blush associated with intracerebral hematoma. Radiology 122: 707–711, 1977

Functional Brain Imaging—Basic Principles and Application to Head Trauma*

6

Peter Herscovitch

Functional brain imaging refers to the use of techniques to obtain images of the brain that are related to physiology or biochemistry rather than to structural anatomy. Two approaches to functional brain imaging have been used to study patients with traumatic brain injury (TBI), namely positron emission tomography (PET) and single-photon emission computed tomography (SPECT). Both are reviewed in this chapter.

PET is a nuclear medicine technique for performing physiologic measurements in vivo. The PET scanner provides tomographic images of the distribution of positron-emitting radiopharmaceuticals in the body. From these images, measurements such as regional blood flow and glucose metabolism can be obtained. PET is still primarily a research tool, which has been used to study normal brain function and the pathophysiology of neurologic and psychiatric disease (Grafton and Mazziotta, 1992; Volkow and Fowler, 1992). Its role in the management of patients with brain disorders is at a much earlier stage (Powers et al., 1991). Conceptually, PET consists of three components: (1) tracer compounds labeled with radioactive atoms that emit positrons; (2) scanners, which provide tomographic images of the concentration of positron-emitting radioactivity in the body; and (3) mathematical models that describe the in vivo behavior of radiotracers, so that the physiologic process under study can be quantitated from PET images. The first tomographs for quantitative PET imaging were developed in the mid-1970s (Ter-Pogossian, 1992). Subsequently, instrument design has become more sophisticated, with improved spatial resolution and sensitivity. Radiotracer techniques have been developed to study regional cerebral blood flow (rCBF) and volume; glucose, oxygen, and protein metabolism; blood-brain barrier permeability; neuroreceptor-neurotransmitter systems; tissue pH; and the concentration of radiolabeled drugs in brain.

We also review SPECT, another nuclear medicine technique that provides tomographic images of radioactivity (Devous, 1989; George et al., 1991; Wyper, 1993). SPECT is simpler than PET because it uses radiopharmaceuticals labeled with conventional radionuclides such as technetium 99m (^{99m}Tc). However, its quantitative accuracy is inferior to that of PET and the variety of radiopharmaceuticals for studying the brain is relatively limited; it is used primarily to map cerebral perfusion. There is a strong interest in clinical SPECT brain studies, and improvements in instrumentation and radiopharmaceuticals are being actively pursued (Holman and Devous, 1992; Juni, 1994). There have been several reports of SPECT perfusion studies in acute and chronic TBI (Van Heertum et al., 1993; Wyper, 1993).

This chapter provides an overview of PET instrumentation, radiotracers, and mathematical modeling, emphasizing methods to measure cerebral hemodynamics and metabolism, the methods most relevant to TBI. In addition, SPECT instrumentation and radiopharmaceuticals are described. A discussion of the analysis and interpretation of functional brain images is followed by a review of the mechanisms by which head trauma causes abnormalities of CBF and metabolism. The published reports describing the use of PET or SPECT in head trauma are reviewed. Finally, the potential use of these methods in the diagnosis and management of individual patients rather than in the study of disease pathophysiology is discussed.

POSITRON EMISSION TOMOGRAPHY

PET Instrumentation

PET provides tomographic images of the distribution of positron-emitting radioactivity using rings of radiation detectors that are arrayed around the body. Because of the special nature of the positron and the techniques used for image reconstruction, it is possible to obtain *absolute* radioactivity measurements from these images.

Certain radioactive atoms, such as oxygen 15 (^{15}O) or fluorine 18 (^{18}F), decay by the emission of a positron from the nucleus. Positrons are "antimatter" particles to electrons; they have the same mass as electrons but are positively charged. After emission from the nucleus, positrons travel a variable distance in tissue, up to a few millimeters, losing kinetic energy. When almost at rest, they interact with orbital electrons of atoms, resulting in the "annihilation" of both particles. Their combined mass is converted into two high-energy photons, which travel in opposite directions from the annihilation site at the speed of light. Detection of these photon pairs is used to measure both the location and the amount of radioactivity in the field of view of the scanner. The two annihilation photons are detected by two opposing radiation detectors connected by an electronic coincidence circuit (Fig. 6-1). This circuit records a decay event when both detectors sense the almost simultaneous arrival of both photons. The site of the decay event is therefore localized to the volume of space between the two detectors. In practice, several rings of detectors are used. Opposing detector pairs in each ring are connected by coincidence circuits. With each decay event, the two resulting annihilation photons are detected as a coincidence line, so that the number of coincidence lines sensed by any detector pair is proportional to the amount of radioactivity between them. A computer records the coincidence events from each ring. Tomographic images of the underlying distribution of radioactivity are then reconstructed with the same mathematical technique that is used in conventional x-ray computed tomography (CT) (Hoffman and Phelps, 1986).

An important step in image reconstruction is a correction for the absorption or attenuation of annihilation photons that occurs owing to their interactions with tissue. This effect substantially decreases the number of coincidence counts detected. Although the amount of attenuation can be estimated by using an assumed value for the attenuating properties of tissue, actual measurements are more accurate. It is the ability to measure and correct for attenuation accurately that is one of the main features distinguishing PET from SPECT. Before the administration of radiotracer, a separate transmission scan is performed, with a source of positron-emitting radioactivity positioned between the subject's head and the detector rings. A similar measurement is made with nothing in the scanner field of view. The ratio of the

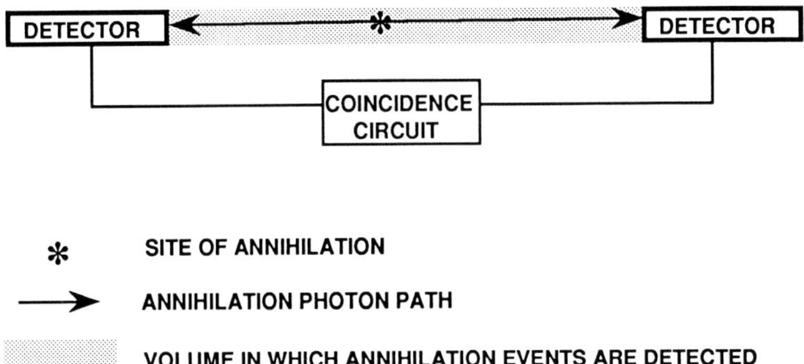

Fig. 6-1. The two high-energy photons resulting from a positron emission and annihilation are detected by two radiation detectors, which are connected by an electronic coincidence circuit. A decay event is recorded as a coincidence line between the detectors only when both photons are detected almost simultaneously. A very short time window for photon arrival, typically 5 to 20 ns, called the coincidence resolving time, is allowed for registration of a coincidence event. This coincidence requirement localizes the site of the annihilation to the volume of space between the detectors.

two measurements gives the amount of attenuation between each detector pair and is used to correct for attenuation.

The intensity of each point or pixel in the reconstructed PET image is proportional to the concentration of radioactivity at the corresponding location in the brain. To calibrate the scanner to obtain *absolute* radioactivity measurements, a cylinder containing a uniform solution of radioactivity is imaged. The radioactivity concentration of the solution is then measured with a calibrated well counter, and the scanner calibration factor is calculated to convert PET image counts to units of radioactivity concentration (e.g., $\mu Ci/cm^3$).

Many factors affect PET image quality and the ability to quantitate radioactivity accurately (Hoffman & Phelps, 1986; Karp et al., 1991). A critical issue in interpreting PET (and SPECT) images is the concept of image resolution. In PET, image resolution depends upon the accurate localization of positron-emitting nuclei. This is determined by the physics of positron annihilation and by detector design. Annihilation photons are produced only after the positron has traveled up to several millimeters from the nucleus; this limits the accuracy of locating the nucleus. In addition, the angle between the two annihilation photons deviates slightly from 180 degrees, causing a slight misplacement of the coincidence line. These effects result in a 1 to 3 mm resolution loss (Phelps and Hoffman, 1976). Detector size and shape determine how accurately the position of each coincidence line is recorded, smaller detectors providing better resolution. Resolution is measured by imaging a thin line-source of positron-emitting radioactivity (Fig. 6-2). Because of limited resolution, the radioactivity in the source appears blurred or spread out over a larger area; resolution is defined by the amount of spreading. The resolution of current scanners is about 4 to 5 mm in the image plane (DeGrado et al., 1994; Wienhard et al., 1994).

A PET system consists of many components (Council on Scientific Affairs, 1988; Hoffman and Phelps, 1986; Koeppe and Hutchins, 1992). Several rings of radiation detectors are mounted in a gantry. Each detector consists of a small scintillation crystal, which gives off light when the energy of an annihilation photon is deposited in it. The detector is coupled to a photomultiplier tube, which converts the light pulse to an electrical signal, which is fed into the coincidence circuitry. Current commercially available scanners have from 18 to 24 rings, each containing up to several hundred detectors (DeGrado et al., 1994; Wienhard et al., 1994). A tomographic slice is provided by each ring. In addition, "cross-slices" halfway between the detector rings are derived from coincidences between detectors in adjacent rings. Therefore, 47 contiguous slices can be obtained simultaneously by a 24-ring system. A dedicated computer is used to control the scanning process, collect the coincidence count information, and reconstruct and display the images.

A new approach to scanner design permits coincidence counts to be collected by opposing detectors, which do not have to be in the same or adjacent

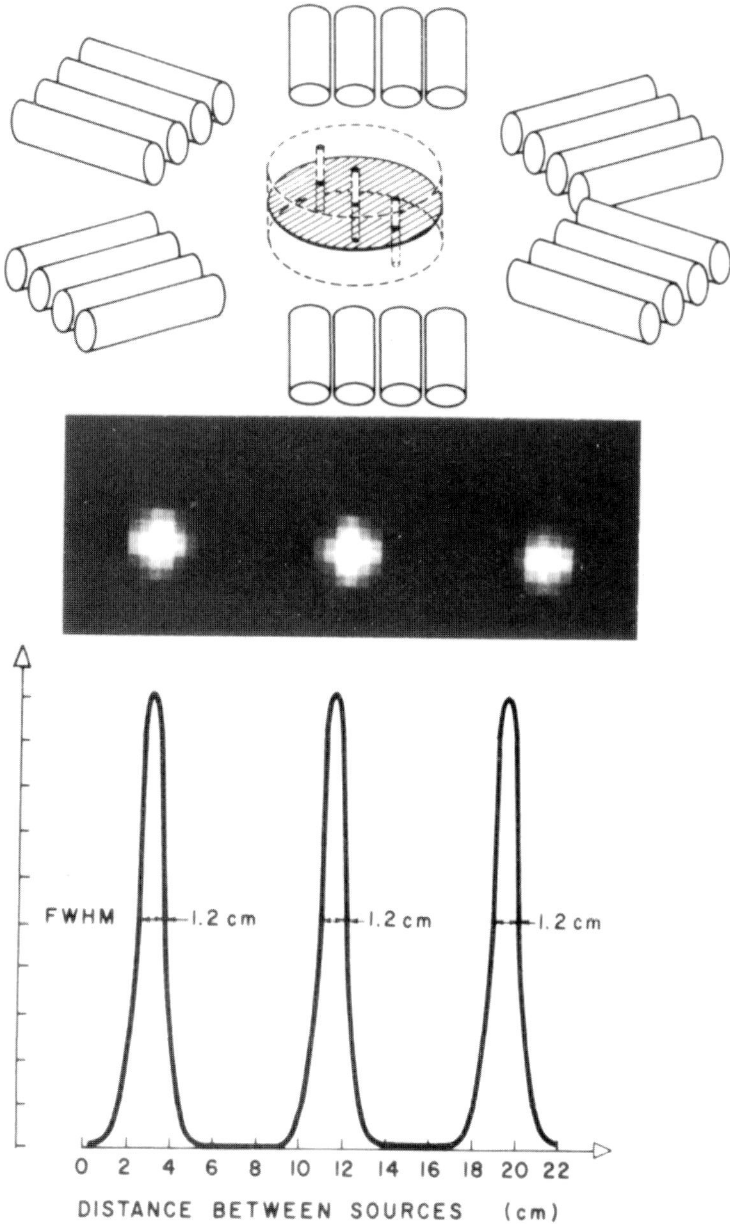

Fig. 6-2. The resolution of a PET scanner is defined and measured as shown here. Thin line sources of positron-emitting radioactivity perpendicular to the image plane are scanned (*upper panel*). Because of resolution limitations, the radioactivity in each source appears blurred or spread over a larger area (*middle panel*). Scanner resolution is defined by the amount of spreading that occurs. A plot of the image intensity along a line through the center of the images (*lower panel*) shows that this spreading approximates a bell-shaped or gaussian curve. The width of this curve at one-half of its maximum height, termed the full width at half maximum (FWHM), is the measure of resolution. Here the resolution is 1.2 cm. Another interpretation of the FWHM is that it is the minimum distance by which two points of radioactivity must be separated to be independently perceived in the reconstructed image. (From Ter-Pogossian et al., 1975, with permission.)

rings (Spinks et al., 1992). Because more coincidence lines are collected, scanner sensitivity is substantially increased. This improves image quality or alternatively permits the same number of image counts to be obtained with less administered radioactivity.

Positron-Emitting Radiotracers

The second requirement for PET is a radiotracer of physiologic interest that is labeled with a positron-emitting radionuclide. A radiotracer can be a naturally occurring compound in which one of the atoms is replaced with its radioactive counterpart, or it can be a labeled analogue which behaves in vivo similarly to the natural substance. Alternatively, it can be a synthetic substance, such as a radiolabeled drug, which interacts with a specific biologic system.

The positron-emitting nuclides most commonly used to label PET radiotracers (with their half-lives) are oxygen 15 (^{15}O, 2.05 minutes), nitrogen 13 (^{13}N, 10.0 minutes), carbon 11 (^{11}C, 20.3 minutes), and fluorine 18 (^{18}F, 109.8 minutes). (The half-life is the time required for radioactivity to decay to one-half of its original value.) The chemical nature of ^{15}O, ^{13}N, and ^{11}C is identical to that of their nonradioactive counterparts, which are basic constituents of living matter as well as of most drugs. Thus, they can be incorporated into radiotracers with the same in vivo behavior as the corresponding nonradioactive compound. ^{18}F is used to substitute for hydrogen or hydroxyl groups to synthesize analogues with characteristics similar to those of the unsubstituted compound. In addition, some drugs contain fluorine, so that ^{18}F-labeled forms can be synthesized. Because of their short half-lives (i.e., rapid decay), relatively large amounts of these radionuclides can be administered to provide good-quality images, but the radiation exposure is acceptable. The short half-lives, especially of ^{15}O, permit repeat studies in the same subject in one experimental session because of rapid physical decay after each administration.

The synthesis of PET radiotracers is demanding, however, because of these short half-lives. On-site production of radionuclides by means of a cyclotron is required (Wolf and Schlyer, 1993), and rapid techniques must be devised for radiotracer synthesis and quality control. These must yield products that are pure, sterile, and nontoxic. The tracer must have the appropriate properties to permit the desired physiologic measurement to be made (Dannals et al., 1993; Kilbourn, 1991). Important tracer characteristics include its permeability across the blood-brain barrier; the formation and fate of any radioactive metabolites; the ability to develop a mathematical model to describe the behavior of the tracer; and for neuroreceptor ligands, binding characteristics. Preclinical studies are typically performed, using tissue sampling or autoradiography in small animals and PET studies in large ones. A wide variety of positron-emitting radiopharmaceuticals have been synthesized (Fowler and Wolf, 1991) (Table 6-1).

Tracer Kinetic Modeling

A mathematical model is required to calculate the value of the physiologic variable of interest from measurements of radiotracer concentration in brain and blood. The model describes the in vivo behavior of the radiotracer (i.e., the relationship over time between the amount of tracer delivered to a brain region in its arterial input and the amount of tracer in the region). The use of models allows PET to be a quantitative physiologic technique rather than only an imaging modality (Carson, 1991; Huang and Phelps, 1986). Compartmental models are typically used, in which it is assumed that there are entities called compartments, which have uniform biologic properties and in which the tracer concentration is uniform at any instant in time. The compartments can be physical spaces such as the extravascular space or biochemical entities such as neuroreceptor binding sites. The model is described by one or more equations containing measurable terms, namely, the brain and blood radiotracer concentrations over time, and unknowns such as blood flow or receptor concentration that are of interest.

Several factors must be considered in developing a model. These include tracer transport across the blood-brain barrier, the behavior of the tracer in brain, the presence of labeled metabolites in blood, the potential for alterations in tracer behavior if there is pathology, and the ability to solve the model accurately for the unknown parameters. Error analysis and model validation are important. Error analysis consists of mathematical simulations to determine the sensitivity of the model to potential sources of measurement error. Validation experiments are usually performed to demonstrate that the method provides reproducible, accurate, and biologically meaningful measurements (Carson, 1991). This chapter describes the PET methods to measure regional cerebral blood flow (rCBF) and volume (rCBV), and

TABLE 6-1. Representative PET Radiotracers[a]

Physiologic Process or System	Radiotracer
Cerebral blood flow	$H_2{}^{15}O$ ^{15}O-butanol, ^{11}C-butanol, ^{11}C-fluoromethane, ^{18}F-fluoromethane
Cerebral blood volume	$C^{15}O$, ^{11}CO
Cerebral energy metabolism	
Oxygen metabolism	$^{15}O_2$
Glucose metabolism	^{18}F-fluorodeoxyglucose, ^{11}C-deoxyglucose, ^{11}C-glucose
Glucose transport	^{11}C-3-O-methylglucose
Neuroreceptor systems	
Dopaminergic	
Presynaptic dopamine pool	^{11}C-dopa, ^{18}F-fluorodopa
Dopamine reuptake sites	^{11}C-nomifensine, ^{11}C-cocaine, ^{18}F-GBR
Dopamine receptors	^{11}C-N-methylspiperone, ^{11}C-raclopride, ^{18}F-spiperone, ^{18}F-N-methylspiperone
Opiate	^{11}C-carfentanil, ^{11}C-diprenorphine, ^{18}F-cyclofoxy
Benzodiazepine	^{11}C-flumazenil
Serotonergic	
Presynaptic serotonin pool	^{11}C-α-methyltryptophan
Serotonin receptors	^{11}C-ketanserin, ^{18}F-setoperone
Protein synthesis	^{11}C-methionine, ^{11}C-methylmethionine, ^{11}C-leucine, ^{11}C-tyrosine
Tissue pH	$^{11}CO_2$, ^{11}C-DMO
Tissue drug kinetics	^{11}C-phenytoin, ^{11}C-valproate, ^{13}N-BCNU

[a] This table is a partial listing of the different radiotracers that have been used to study physiologic processes or systems in the brain with PET. The most commonly used radiotracer methods are those to measure regional cerebral blood flow and metabolism.

glucose and oxygen metabolism, the parameters potentially most relevant to studying patients with TBI. In addition, SPECT tracer methods for assessing cerebral perfusion are discussed.

PET Radiotracer Techniques

Cerebral Glucose Metabolism

The regional cerebral metabolic rate of glucose (rCMRGlu) is measured with ^{18}F-deoxyglucose (FDG). The approach is based on the technique to measure rCMRGlu in laboratory animals with ^{14}C-deoxyglucose and tissue autoradiography (Sokoloff et al., 1977). It was adapted for PET by using ^{18}F as the label (Huang et al., 1980; Phelps et al., 1979; Reivich et al., 1979). FDG is a glucose analogue in which a hydroxyl group has been replaced with an ^{18}F atom. FDG is transported across the blood-brain barrier and is phosphorylated in tissue, as is glucose, by hexokinase to form FDG-6-phosphate (FDG-6-P). Because of its anomalous structure, FDG-6-P cannot proceed further along the glucose metabolic pathway. Also, there is little dephosphorylation of FDG-6-P back to FDG. As a result of this "metabolic trapping," loss of FDG-6-P is negligible. This facilitates the calculation of rCMRGlu from measurements of local tissue radioactivity. Sokoloff's three-compartment model applied to FDG consists of plasma FDG in brain capillaries, free FDG in tissue, and FDG-6-P in tissue (Fig. 6-3A). Rate constants describe the movement of tracer between these compartments. An operational equation permits calculation of rCM RGlu from the tissue radioactivity concentration after FDG administration, of arterial plasma concentration of FDG over time, and of plasma glucose concentration (Fig. 6-3B). The equation also contains the rate constants and a factor termed the lumped constant, which corrects for the differences between glucose and FDG in blood-brain barrier transport and in phosphorylation. Neither the rate constants nor the lumped constant can be routinely determined for each experimental subject or condition. It has been found possible, however, to use standard values measured once in separate groups of normal subjects.

To implement the method, images are obtained starting 30 to 45 minutes after intravenous injection of 5 to 10 mCi of FDG. Blood is sampled to measure the concentrations of glucose and FDG in plasma

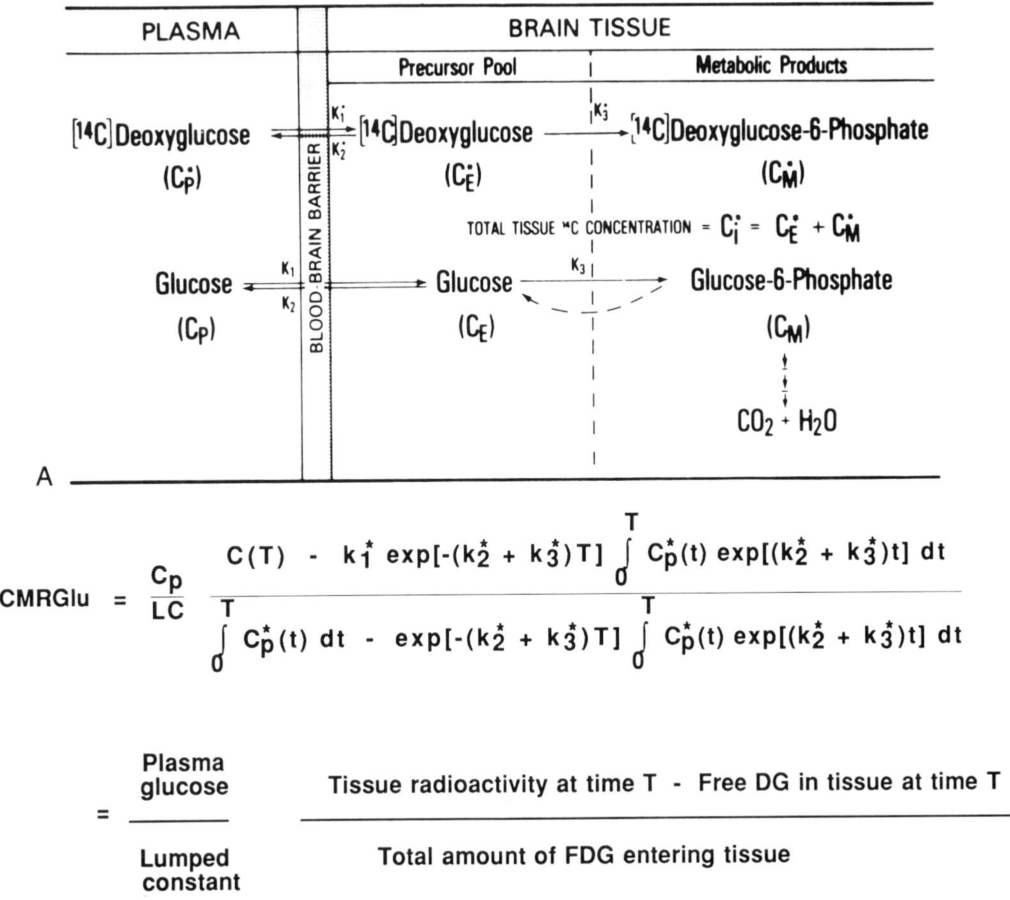

Fig. 6-3. **(A)** Diagrammatic representation of Sokoloff's three-compartment model used to measure rCMRGlu with deoxyglucose (DG). The compartments consist of DG in the plasma in brain capillaries, DG in brain tissue, and DG-6-P in tissue. Rate constants describe the movement of tracer between compartments, two for the bidirectional transport of DG across the blood-brain barrier between plasma and tissue (k_1^*, k_2^*), and one for the phosphorylation of DG to DG-6-P (k_3^*). In the adaptation of this model to PET, ^{18}F-labeled DG is used and a fourth rate constant, k_4^*, is added to account for the small amount of dephosphorylation of FDG-6-P back to FDG. The lower portion of the figure shows the metabolic fate of glucose. **(B)** Operational equation of the DG method. The word equation aids in understanding the model. The terms that are measured are C(T), the tissue radioactivity concentration at time T, typically 30 to 45 minutes after DG administration; $C_p^*(t)$, the plasma DG concentration over time; and (C_p), the plasma glucose concentration. The concentration of free DG in tissue at time T is calculated from [$C_p^*(t)$] and the rate constants. The difference between the two terms in the numerator is the concentration of DG-6-P that has been formed. The denominator equals the amount of DG delivered to tissue. Thus the ratio on the right-hand side is the fractional rate of phosphorylation of DG. Multiplying this ratio by C_p would give the rate of glucose phosphorylation if DG and glucose had the same behavior. Because this is not the case, the lumped constant is included to account for the difference. The adaptation of this equation to PET during FDG is more complex because of the inclusion of the fourth rate constant, k_4^*. (Fig. A from Sokoloff et al., 1977, with permission.)

over time. The operational equation with standard values for the rate constants and lumped constant is used to generate images of rCMRGlu (Fig. 6-4). Typical normal values of rCMRGlu are 6 to 7 mg/(min-100 g) in gray matter and 2.5 to 3 mg/(min-100 g) in white matter (Camargo et al., 1992; Hatazawa et al., 1988; Sasaki et al., 1986; Tyler et al., 1988).

The accuracy of using standard values for the rate constants and lumped constant has been the subject of considerable discussion (Baron et al., 1989; Cun-

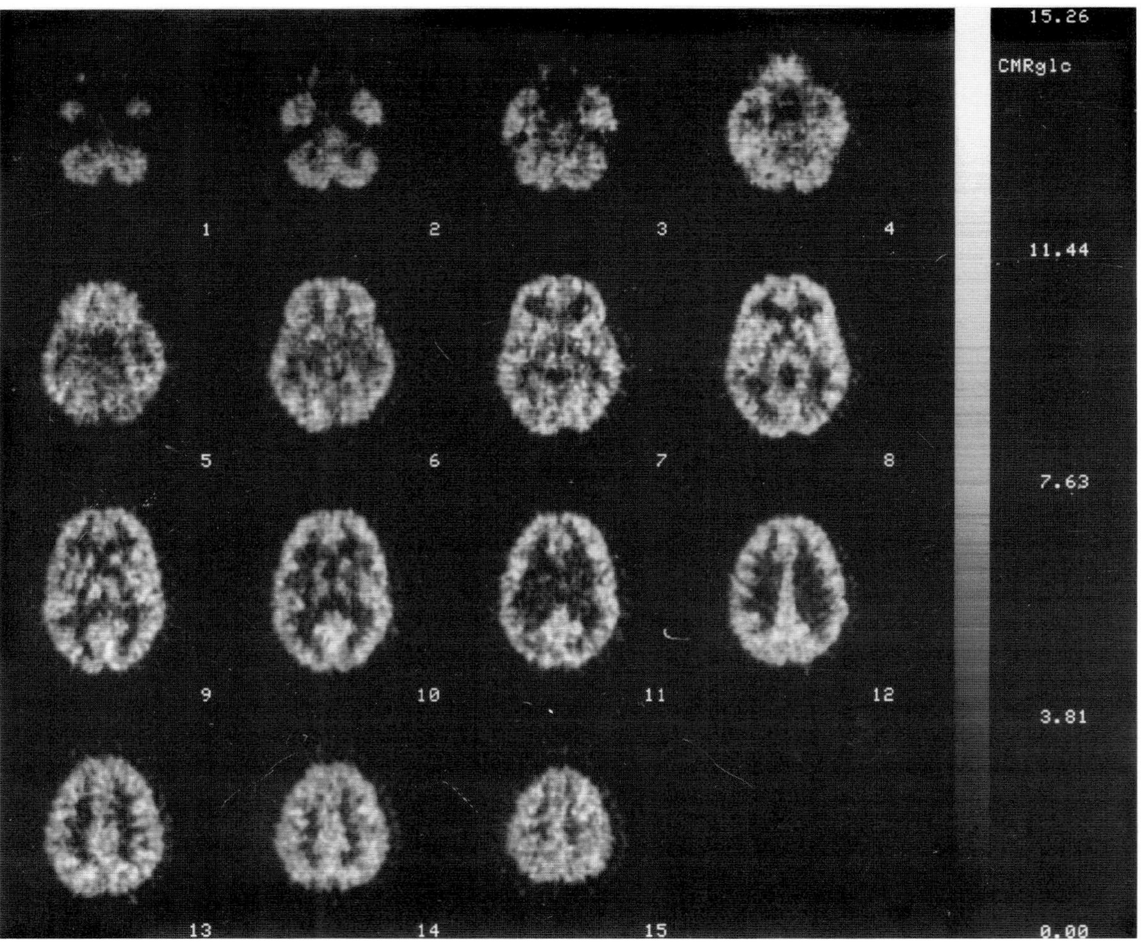

Fig. 6-4. Quantitative images of rCMRGlu obtained in a normal subject with FDG and application of Sokoloff's model. Anterior is up and left is to the reader's left. These images start at the level of the cerebellum (*upper left*) and proceed up through the brain. Note the bar scale at the right indicating the correspondence between glucose metabolic rates and gray levels in the image. (Figure courtesy of Cheryl Grady, Ph.D. Bethesda, MD)

ningham and Cremer, 1985). Their values may change in the presence of pathology, and the use of incorrect values results in inaccurate rCMRGlu calculations (Sokoloff, 1985; Sokoloff et al., 1977). Because the operational equation terms containing rate constants approach zero with increasing time (Fig. 6-3B), a 30- to 45-minute delay between FDG injection and PET imaging is used to minimize the error associated with using standard values. There can still be substantial error in cases of cerebral ischemia or tumor, however (Graham et al., 1989; Nakai et al., 1987; Wienhard et al., 1985). Several investigators have reformulated the operational equation to decrease its sensitivity to the rate constants and refined the methods to measure them (Brooks, 1982; Lammertsma et al., 1987). The lumped constant is uniform throughout brain and is constant under normal physiologic conditions. However, it does change in acute cerebral ischemia, recent cerebral infarction, and brain tumor (Gjedde et al., 1985; Greenberg et al., 1992; Nakai et al., 1987; Spence et al., 1990). Therefore, in pathologic conditions it is necessary to redetermine the lumped constant and rate constants to avoid errors in rCMRGlu calculation. This is difficult and has rarely been done in PET studies.

An alternative approach uses ^{11}C-glucose, which is transported and metabolized in the same way as glucose (Blomqvist et al., 1990). Therefore, a lumped constant correction factor is not required. A disadvantage is that the labeled metabolites of glucose, such as $^{11}CO_2$, are not all trapped in tissue, and therefore the tracer model must account for their egress. ^{11}C-Glucose may be more widely used in the future, especially in pathologic conditions.

Cerebral Blood Volume

Regional cerebral blood volume (rCBV) is measured by using trace amounts of ^{11}C- or ^{15}O-carbon monoxide administered by inhalation (Grubb et al., 1978; Martin et al., 1987). The tracer binds to hemoglobin and is confined to the intravascular space. Local radioactivity in brain is proportional to its red cell content, so that rCBV can be calculated from the ratio of the radioactivity in brain to that in peripheral blood. However, the hematocrit is less in brain than in peripheral large vessels owing to the behavior of blood in the brain microvasculature. Therefore the ratio of cerebral hematocrit to peripheral hematocrit (R) must be incorporated into the calculation (Grubb et al., 1978; Lammertsma et al., 1984; Martin et al., 1987). Equation (1) or a modification (Videen et al., 1987) is used to calculate rCBV in units of milliliters per 100 g from the radiotracer concentrations in tissue (C_t) and blood (C_{bl}):

$$\text{rCBV} = \frac{C_t}{C_{bl} \cdot R} \qquad (1)$$

The use of $C^{15}O$ has practical advantages over ^{11}CO (Martin et al., 1987). The 2-minute half-life of ^{15}O permits other PET studies to be performed with little delay and lowers radiation exposure, and the synthesis is more convenient. Normal values for rCBV are 4 to 6 ml/100 g in gray matter and 2 to 3 ml/100 g in white matter (Lammertsma et al., 1983; Perlmutter et al., 1987).

In cerebrovascular disease, rCBV reflects vasodilation in response to decreased cerebral perfusion pressure, as may occur with a narrowed internal carotid artery (Heiss and Podreka, 1993; Powers, 1991). Changes in rCBV can also be seen with elevated intracranial pressure (ICP) (Grubb et al., 1975). In addition, rCBV data may be required as part of other PET methods to correct for radiotracer located in the intravascular space in order to determine the amount of radiotracer that actually enters tissue.

Cerebral Blood Flow

Methods to measure rCBF with PET are based on a model developed by Kety to measure rCBF in laboratory animals (Kety, 1951; Landau et al., 1955). The model describes inert tracers that can diffuse freely across the blood-brain barrier. The technique involves infusing a radioactive tracer over a brief time period T (e.g., 1 minute); the animal is then killed. Frequent timed blood samples are obtained during the infusion to determine the arterial time versus radioactivity curve $C_a(t)$. Regional brain radioactivity at the end of the infusion, $C_t(T)$, is measured by quantitative tissue autoradiography. Tissue blood flow f (in units of ml/(min-100g)) is calculated from these measurements by Equation (2):

$$C_t(T) = f\int_0^t C_a(t)\exp[-f/\lambda(T - t)]\,dt \qquad (2)$$

where λ is the brain-blood partition coefficient for the tracer, defined as the ratio between the tissue and blood radiotracer concentrations when they are in equilibrium. Its value can be determined from independent experiments or can be calculated as the ratio of the solubilities of the tracer in brain and blood (Herscovitch and Raichle, 1985; Kety, 1951). Equation (2) is solved numerically for flow, using measured values for $C_t(T)$ and $C_a(t)$ and a specified value for λ.

Kety's method is the basis for methods to measure rCBF with PET. Although there are different approaches, they all involve administering a diffusible, positron-emitting radiotracer, blood sampling to determine the time-activity curve in arterial blood (typically from the radial artery), and the application of a modification of Equation (2) to generate images of rCBF from PET images of radioactivity. The tracer most commonly used is ^{15}O-water ($H_2{}^{15}O$) administered by intravenous injection. Because of the short half-life of ^{15}O, other PET measurements can be performed within 10 to 12 minutes.

The steady-state method was the earliest widely used PET method to measure rCBF (Frackowiak et al., 1980; Subramanyam et al., 1978). The subject inhales $C^{15}O_2$ delivered at a fixed rate. The action of carbonic anhydrase in red blood cells results in transfer of ^{15}O to water. $H_2{}^{15}O$ is constantly generated in the lungs and circulates throughout the body. A steady state is reached, at which the radioactivity delivered to brain tissue equals that leaving by decay and by venous washout. The brain distribution of radioactivity remains constant, and a simple equation can be used to calculate rCBF. This method was convenient with the early, single-ring tomographs, since multiple tomographic slices could be obtained by repositioning the patient during $C^{15}O_2$ inhalation. A limitation is the nonlinear relationship between rCBF and tissue radioactivity, which increases sensitivity to measurement errors (Baron et al., 1989; Herscovitch and Raichle, 1983; Lammertsma et al., 1981). Because of this, the long period required for CBF measurement, and the development of multislice scanners, the steady-state method has been largely supplanted.

Alternative approaches use bolus intravenous injections of $H_2{}^{15}O$ and an adaptation of Kety's equation. Equation (2) is not used directly because scanners cannot measure the instantaneous brain radiotracer concentration $C_t(T)$. It has been modified in different ways to account for the fact that scans are performed over many seconds, summing enough counts to obtain satisfactory images. With the PET/autoradiographic approach, $H_2{}^{15}O$ is administered by bolus intravenous injection, and a 40-second scan is obtained after the radiotracer arrives in the head (Herscovitch et al., 1983; Raichle et al., 1983). The relationship between tissue counts and rCBF is almost linear, so that errors in measurement of tissue radioactivity result in approximately equivalent errors in calculated rCBF. Because the PET image obtained with a brief scan (1 minute or less) closely reflects flow differences in different brain regions, useful information about relative CBF can be obtained without blood sampling. This approach is widely used in functional brain mapping experiments, in which $H_2{}^{15}O$ images are used to determine relative rCBF changes during neurobehavioral tasks (Frackowiak and Friston, 1994). Average values for rCBF in normal subjects obtained with either the steady-state method (Leenders et al., 1990) or the PET/autoradiographic method (Herscovitch et al., 1987; Perlmutter et al., 1987) are 40 to 60 ml/(min-100g) in gray matter and 20 to 30 ml/(min-100g) in white matter.

There are other methods for measuring rCBF based on the Kety model. One approach involves collecting several sequential, brief images after bolus intravenous administration of tracer (Koeppe et al., 1985). Parameter estimation techniques are used to estimate both rCBF and λ from the scan and blood radioactivity data. To simplify blood sampling for these $H_2{}^{15}O$ rCBF techniques, automated systems have been designed to continuously draw arterial blood past a radiation detector (Eriksson et al., 1988).

Methods using $H_2{}^{15}O$ assume that it is freely diffusible across the blood-brain barrier. However, there is a modest diffusion limitation, which results in an underestimation of rCBF at higher flows (Raichle et al., 1983). There are other tracers that do not have a diffusion limitation, such as ^{11}C- or ^{15}O-butanol (Berridge et al., 1991; Herscovitch et al., 1987). The diffusion limitation of $H_2{}^{15}O$ is accepted, however, because of the tracer's convenience. Also, in conditions with decreased rCBF, tracer diffusion limitation is less important.

Cerebral Oxygen Metabolism

The regional cerebral metabolic rate of oxygen ($rCMRO_2$) is measured using inhaled ^{15}O-oxygen ($^{15}O_2$). One method, developed in conjunction with the steady-state rCBF technique, uses continuous inhalation of $^{15}O_2$ (Frackowiak et al., 1980; Subramanyam et al., 1978). Another, a companion to the PET/autoradiographic rCBF method, uses a brief inhalation of $^{15}O_2$ (Mintun et al., 1984). The principles underlying these methods are similar. Approximately 35 to 40 percent of the oxygen delivered to brain is extracted and metabolized (Leenders et al., 1990; Perlmutter et al., 1987). Both methods measure this oxygen extraction fraction. There are essentially no stores of oxygen in brain, and all extracted oxygen is metabolized. Therefore, $rCMRO_2$ can be determined from the product of the oxygen extraction fraction and the rate of oxygen delivery to brain, which equals rCBF multiplied by arterial oxygen content. The tracer models describe the fate of the ^{15}O label following $^{15}O_2$ inhalation. Extracted $^{15}O_2$ is metabolized to $H_2{}^{15}O$, which is then washed out of brain. The $H_2{}^{15}O$ produced by brain as well as by the rest of the body recirculates to brain and diffuses into and out of brain tissue. Another component of the measured radioactivity is intravascular $^{15}O_2$ that is not extracted by brain. It is necessary to account for this component so that it is not attributed to radioactivity in tissue. Therefore, an independent measurement of rCBV is needed. Both PET methods require three scans to measure regional oxygen extraction fraction and $rCMRO_2$: an rCBF scan, an rCBV scan, and a scan obtained with $^{15}O_2$.

With the steady-state method, scanning is performed during continuous inhalation of $^{15}O_2$; rCBF is measured with continuous inhalation of $C^{15}O_2$ and rCBV with $C^{15}O$. The regional oxygen extraction fraction is computed from these scans and from measurements of blood radioactivity (Lammertsma et al., 1983). The alternative method for measuring regional oxygen extraction fraction and $rCMRO_2$ uses a brief inhalation of $^{15}O_2$ (Mintun et al., 1984; Videen et al., 1987). A 40-second scan is obtained following $^{15}O_2$ inhalation, and frequent arterial blood samples are collected for measurements of blood radioactivity. It also involves measurement of rCBF with $H_2{}^{15}O$ and the PET/autoradiographic method and measurement of rCBV with $C^{15}O$. The method was validated in baboons in a series of experiments that included very reduced $rCMRO_2$ (Altman et al., 1991; Mintun et al., 1984). This is relevant for PET studies of brain injury, in which reduced $rCMRO_2$ can occur. Average normal values for gray matter $rCMRO_2$ are 2.5 to 3.5 ml/(min-100g) (Leenders et al., 1990; Perlmutter et al., 1987).

SINGLE-PHOTON EMISSION COMPUTED TOMOGRAPHY

SPECT Instrumentation

The radionuclides used in SPECT decay by emitting a single photon or γ-ray from their nuclei. Detection of γ-rays is employed to image the radioactivity distribution. The most commonly used SPECT systems have one or more gamma camera "heads" (Devous, 1989; George et al., 1991; Holman and Devous, 1992; Masdeu et al., 1994). The gamma camera head has a large, relatively thin (e.g., ⅜ inch by 12 to 20 inches diameter) scintillation crystal of sodium iodide, which gives off a localized pulse of light when it absorbs a γ-ray. The front of the crystal is covered with a parallel-hole collimator, which is typically made up of lead perforated by an array of small hexagonal holes. The collimator limits the γ-rays that strike the crystal to those traveling along parallel lines perpendicular to the crystal face. An array of photomultiplier tubes and position logic circuits behind the crystal senses the light pulses and determine the location of each pulse in the crystal. This information is used to generate a planar image of the distribution of radioactivity in the body. In order to obtain tomographic images of the radioactivity distribution, the camera head is rotated around the body to obtain multiple views (Fig. 6-5), which are combined to reconstruct the tomographic images. To improve sensitivity, modern systems have two or three heads mounted in a gantry, which surround the body and rotate together. Alternative SPECT instrument designs, which are in limited use, employ either a circumferential array of small detectors or a single continuous cylindrical crystal that surrounds the patient (Holman et al., 1990).

SPECT devices have a spatial resolution of about 15 mm with single heads and 6 to 9 mm with multiple heads and different collimator designs. Sensitivity tends to be low, even with multiple head devices, because of the need for collimators, so that imaging time is typically 20 to 30 minutes. Therefore, radiotracers that provide a static, unchanging distribution are typically used. In contrast to PET, an accurate measured correction for attenuation is not convenient, and in some camera configurations is not possible at all. Currently, the most promising method requires a three-headed device in which one head acquires attenuation data while the other two acquire emission data. This approach is not widely used. Indeed, accurate correction for attenuation remains a major obstacle to quantitation in SPECT. Typically, radioactivity is not quantitated in absolute terms, but rather the tomographic images are used to obtain information about the relative amount of radioactivity in different regions. A major advantage is that single-headed cameras with SPECT capability are ubiquitous in nuclear medicine departments, and multiheaded systems are becoming more widespread.

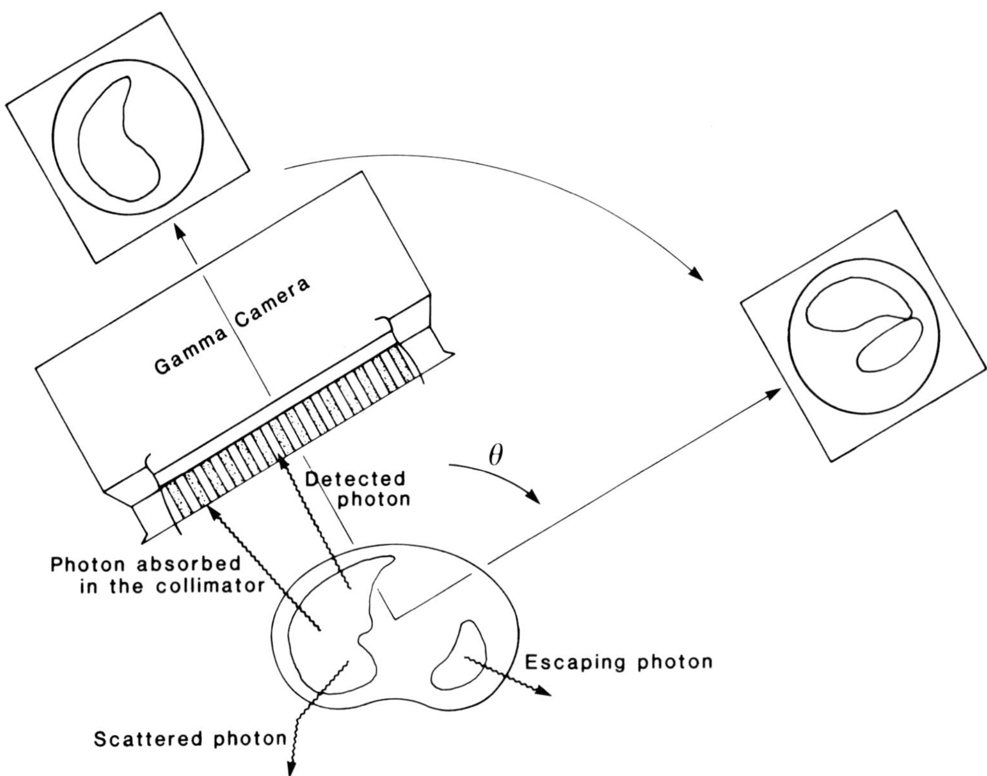

Fig. 6-5. SPECT data acquisition with a gamma camera. The collimator and the thin sodium iodide crystal detector behind the collimator are shown. γ-Rays or photons pass through the parallel holes in the collimator to the crystal and are registered by photomultipliers and electronic circuitry behind the crystal. Some photons strike the collimator septa at an angle and are absorbed, while others escape the body away from the view of the camera head and are not detected. As the head rotates around the patient, two-dimensional images are collected at each scanning angle. Scan profiles from these images are used as input for the SPECT reconstruction algorithm to obtain tomographic images of the distribution of radioactivity in the body. Some SPECT devices use two or three heads, which rotate around the body together in a gantry to increase scanner sensitivity. (From Sorenson and Phelps, 1987, with permission.)

In addition, a cyclotron is not required to obtain SPECT radiopharmaceuticals. The cost of SPECT instruments ranges from $250,000 to $1,000,000, primarily depending upon the number of heads, in contrast to the cost of PET scanners, which is about $2,500,000.

SPECT Radiotracer Methods

Most SPECT brain studies are performed with radiopharmaceuticals that map CBF. Several radiopharmaceuticals are available for this purpose (George et al., 1991; Holman and Devous, 1992; Van Heertum et al., 1993). The most commonly used radiotracer strategy is based on the microsphere method, a technique used to measure local flow in experimental animals (Warner et al., 1987). With that method, radioactive microspheres of a size appropriate to be trapped in capillaries are introduced into the left side of the animal's heart. They are distributed and trapped in tissue in proportion to flow, and then local radioactivity is measured in samples of tissue. SPECT uses lipophilic radiotracers with microsphere-like behavior, which are administered intravenously. Ideally they are freely diffusible across the blood-brain barrier and are completely extracted and retained by brain in a distribution that is proportional to local flow. The tracers have a stable distribution in the brain, facilitating imaging. Several SPECT perfusion agents are based on this principle, although their extraction or retention by brain is not complete (Gemmell et al., 1992).

The first widely-used SPECT CBF tracer was iodine 123 iodoamphetamine (^{123}I-IMP). It must be prelabeled by the commercial supplier, however, which is logistically difficult. Tracers using technetium 99m are preferable. ^{99m}Tc is more convenient to use since it is obtained from generators that are delivered regularly to nuclear medicine departments; thus on-site labeling is possible. In addition, its physical characteristics are more favorable for SPECT imaging. A widely-used ^{99m}Tc CBF agent is ^{99m}Tc-hexamethylpropylene amine oxime also called ^{99m}TC-exametazime (^{99m}Tc-HMPAO). Another compound, ^{99m}Tc-ethyl cysteinate dimer, or ^{99m}Tc-bicisate (^{99m}Tc-ECD), provides higher brain to background radioactivity ratios because of more rapid blood clearance and is more convenient to employ because of greater in vitro stability. It has recently been approved for clinical use in Europe and the United States. Although there are techniques to calculate absolute rCBF with these tracers, they are rarely used (Greenberg et al., 1990; Murase et al., 1992). Therefore, SPECT studies typically provide information only about relative rCBF, not absolute rCBF as does PET. Repeat SPECT studies cannot be performed rapidly because of the 6-hour half-life of ^{99m}Tc unless methods are used to subtract residual radioactivity. It is also possible to study rCBV with SPECT using ^{99m}Tc-labeled red cells (Kuhl et al., 1980); the approach is similar to that used for PET. However, there are no SPECT radiotracers to study cerebral metabolism.

An alternative approach for assessing cerebral perfusion uses inhaled xenon-133 gas, an inert tracer that freely diffuses into brain. A specialized SPECT device was designed for this purpose (Devous et al., 1986). The subject briefly inhales ^{133}Xe in air, and then a sequence of images is collected. rCBF is calculated with an algorithm based on the Kety flow model. The quality of the rCBF images is relatively poor and image resolution is low. Because of this and other factors, the rCBF values obtained are of somewhat limited accuracy (Rezai et al., 1988).

More recently there has been considerable progress in the development of receptor-binding ligands for SPECT, especially for dopamine and benzodiazepine receptors (Holman and Devous, 1992). Iodine 123 is typically used to radiolabel these ligands. The techniques of tracer kinetic modeling described above are applied to analyze image and blood radioactivity data (Laruelle et al., 1994a; Laruelle et al., 1994b).

DATA ANALYSIS

After a PET study has been completed, the relevant tracer model is applied to calculate the physiologic variable of interest. For the methods of measuring cerebral hemodynamics and metabolism described above, the model is applied on a point-by-point basis, and the intensity of the resultant image depends on the local value of the physiologic measurement (Fig. 6-4). Although visual inspection of PET images may reveal abnormalities, quantitative analysis is required for clinical research. Data reduction, analysis, and interpretation are very demanding. Newer scanners acquire up to 47 slices simultaneously, each containing data from many brain structures. Several different scan types may be obtained in one session (e.g., rCBF, rCBV, and rCMRO$_2$), and patients may have repeat studies on different days. The analysis of PET data is greatly facilitated by interactive computer programs. These permit regions of interest of arbitrary size and shape to be placed over different structures, for which the physiologic variable is then computed. Also, whole-brain measurements can be obtained by averaging over several PET slices.

PET measurements must be related to the underlying anatomy. Early approaches to data analysis used PET images obtained in standard planes (e.g., parallel to the canthomeatal line). The images are visually compared with corresponding anatomic sections in a brain atlas, and regions of interest are manually drawn. This method, however, is subjective and liable to observer bias. A refinement uses a template of standard regions to sample brain structures of interest, with visual adjustment to fit the template to the images. Alternative approaches have been developed, which relate PET images to anatomy more accurately and objectively. One method uses the principles of stereotactic localization to establish a correspondence between regions in a stereotactic brain atlas and specific regions of interest in the PET images (Fox et al., 1985). Other methods are required if there are structural abnormalities, as frequently occurs in head trauma. An approach widely used for both normal and abnormal brain is to obtain anatomic images with CT or MRI in the same planes as the PET slices. Methods to achieve this include head holders transferable between imaging modalities, fiducial markers affixed to the head, and most conveniently, automated computer techniques to register and reslice PET and MR or CT images (Evans et al.,

1991; Ge et al., 1994; Pelizzari et al., 1989; Wilson and Mountz, 1989; Woods et al., 1993). After coplanar anatomic and PET images have been obtained, regions of interest can be transferred between them. These automated techniques have also been used to register brain SPECT images with CT or MRI (Holman et al., 1991).

There is variability in regional and global PET measurements. The coefficient of variation (i.e., the ratio of the standard deviation to the mean value) for measurements of rCBF, rCMRGlu, and $rCMRO_2$ is 15 to 25 percent in groups of normal subjects (Camargo et al., 1992; Perlmutter et al., 1987; Tyler et al., 1988; Wang et al., 1994). This may reflect normal physiologic variation or methodologic inaccuracies. Approaches have been developed to facilitate detection of regional changes in spite of this variability. These techniques adjust for the effect of global variations by "normalizing" regional data, thereby decreasing their variance. This can be done by dividing regional values by the global average value or by the value in a structure presumed to be minimally involved in the disease being studied. Such techniques, however, can result in a loss of the information contained in the absolute values, especially if widespread changes occur. If the denominator as well as the numerator differs between groups, erroneous conclusions may be drawn. For example, in a study of Alzheimer's disease (Cutler et al., 1985), normalized rCMRGlu in thalamus was significantly *increased* because of a *decrease* in global metabolism. Therefore, normalized PET data must be carefully interpreted. In spite of the variability of PET measurements, it is possible to demonstrate meaningful physiologic abnormalities with absolute data (e.g., in cerebrovascular disease) (Powers, 1988).

SPECT perfusion studies typically do not permit quantitation of absolute rCBF, although the image intensity is proportional to flow. A normalization procedure is performed if regional tissue count data are to be averaged in a patient group or compared with data from normal subjects. This is accomplished by dividing the count data in individual regions of interest by the average count value (Goldenberg et al., 1992) or by the value in the cerebellum, assuming that it is not involved in the disease process. There are potential ambiguities with this approach. A region with the appearance of increased relative perfusion may actually have an elevated flow, but the finding may also reflect generally reduced flow in the other brain regions (Wilson and Wyper, 1992). Furthermore, any part of the brain may be involved in TBI, including the cerebellum, so that it is difficult to select an appropriate reference region (Gray et al., 1992).

Data from control subjects are required to analyze PET or SPECT measurements obtained in patients. Quantitative data obtained in appropriately selected normal subjects are used. Depending on the nature of the study, selection criteria must control for variables such as age, sex, handedness, and condition of general health. Average data from patients are statistically compared with the same regional measurements made in a group of normal control subjects. It is also possible to analyze regional data obtained in an individual patient (e.g., by determining whether the data are outside the range of normal). In comparing measurements obtained from many brain regions, it is possible that some regions will be found to be significantly different by chance because of the large number of multiple comparisons being made. One approach to avoid this error, which is rather conservative, is to adjust the study P value (typically .05) by dividing it by the number of measurements being made (the Bonferroni correction).

A rigorous approach is also required for the visual analysis of SPECT and PET images. SPECT images are frequently interpreted visually for abnormalities. The criteria for defining an abnormality are usually subjective, however, and further work must be done to define the sensitivity and specificity for detecting abnormalities (Juni, 1994; Stapleton et al., 1994). In some SPECT studies there is a clear definition of regional abnormality and scans are graded by agreement among two or more observers (Jacobs et al., 1994), whereas other studies use less rigorous approaches. This makes it difficult to compare different studies.

INTERPRETATION OF CHANGES IN CEREBRAL BLOOD FLOW AND METABOLISM

Physiologic Considerations

To interpret changes in PET and SPECT studies, it is necessary to understand the relationships among CBF, metabolism, and local neuronal activity as well as the mechanisms by which CBF and metabolism can become abnormal.

Normally, about 30 percent of the brain's energy metabolism supports synaptic transmission, 30 percent residual ion fluxes and transport, and 40 percent other processes such as axoplasmic transport and macromolecular synthesis (Astrup et al., 1981). In the resting state, the energy needs of the brain are met by the oxidative metabolism of glucose, and there is a proportional relationship, termed *coupling,* between rCBF and both $rCMRO_2$ and rCMRGlu (Baron et al., 1984; Fox and Raichle, 1986; Fox et al., 1988; Sokoloff, 1981). During increased local neuronal activity (e.g., with somatosensory or visual stimulation), there are increases in both rCBF and rCMRGlu in the brain regions involved (Fox and Raichle, 1984; Fox et al., 1988; Ginsberg et al., 1987; Leniger-Follert and Hossman, 1979; Toga and Collins, 1981; Yarowsky et al., 1983). Within physiologic limits, these increases parallel the stimulus rate and the rate of neuronal firing. Most of the brain's additional glucose consumption during increased neuronal activity is used to maintain ionic gradients across cell membranes, which must be restored after depolarization (Yarowsky and Ingvar, 1981). These observations form the basis for using measurements of rCBF and rCMRGlu as markers of local neuronal function (Raichle, 1987). PET studies in humans have shown, however, that there is only a slight increase in $rCMRO_2$ during functional activation (Fox and Raichle, 1986; Fox et al., 1988). This observation challenged the hypothesis that oxidative glucose metabolism or its products regulate the rCBF changes during neuronal activation. In fact, the processes responsible for coupling rCBF to rCMRGlu at rest and during activation remain to be elucidated (Edvinsson et al., 1993a; Lou et al., 1987; Raichle, 1991).

There are various mechanisms that can lead to abnormalities of CBF and metabolism that have relevance to studies of head trauma. Decreased neuronal activity in coma can decrease CBF and metabolism (Obrist et al., 1984), as can drugs and anesthetics that act on synapses or membranes to depress neuronal activity. Tissue damage or loss results in decreased flow and metabolism. In addition, coupled decreases in flow and metabolism can be seen in structures distant from a lesion. This phenomenon, called *diaschisis,* is attributed to a decrease in neuronal activity in a brain structure due to the loss of afferent projections from the damaged region (Feeney and Baron, 1986). For example, decreased flow and metabolism can be seen in the cerebellum contralateral to a cerebral infarct and in cerebral cortex ipsilateral to a small subcortical infarct or hemorrhage.

There are situations in which flow and metabolism are not coupled—for example, with changes in arterial blood gases (Edvinsson et al., 1993b) and in pathologic conditions such as cerebrovascular disease (Heiss and Podreka, 1993; Powers, 1988; Powers, 1991) or elevated intracranial pressure (Grubb et al., 1975). Hypercapnia causes vasodilation and increased CBF and hypocapnia causes the opposite effects, with little change in cerebral metabolism. Decreased arterial oxygen content, due to hypoxia or decreased hematocrit, leads to compensatory changes in cerebral vascular resistance and CBF so as to maintain oxygen delivery to brain (Brown et al., 1985). In both acute and chronic cerebrovascular disease, flow and metabolism may be uncoupled, and measurements of CBF alone are inadequate to characterize a given situation. In acute cerebral infarction, changes in CBF and $CMRO_2$ usually do not parallel each other, although after about 1 month there are relatively matched declines in both. Distal to a severely narrowed or occluded carotid artery, rCBF can be decreased but $rCMRO_2$ maintained by compensatory mechanisms such as local vasodilation and increased oxygen extraction. These mechanisms are also marshaled if cerebral perfusion pressure and CBF decrease owing to systemic hypotension. Thus, in these cases CBF does not reflect metabolism or neuronal function.

Effect of Limited Spatial Resolution

Artifactual abnormalities of CBF and metabolism can be observed with PET or SPECT because of the limited spatial resolution of the imaging devices. Limited resolution results in blurring of PET and SPECT images (Fig. 6-6). More important is its effect on the accuracy of radioactivity measurement (Hoffman et al., 1979; Mazziotta et al., 1981). Because the radioactivity appears spread out over a larger area, a brain region in the image contains only a portion of the radioactivity that was in the corresponding brain structure. In addition, some of the radioactivity in surrounding structures appears to be spread into the region. Because of this effect, called *partial volume averaging,* a regional measurement contains a contribution from both the structure of interest and surrounding structures. High radioactivity levels surrounded by lower values will be underestimated, while low radioactivity surrounded by high activity will be overestimated. These errors are less when the structure of interest

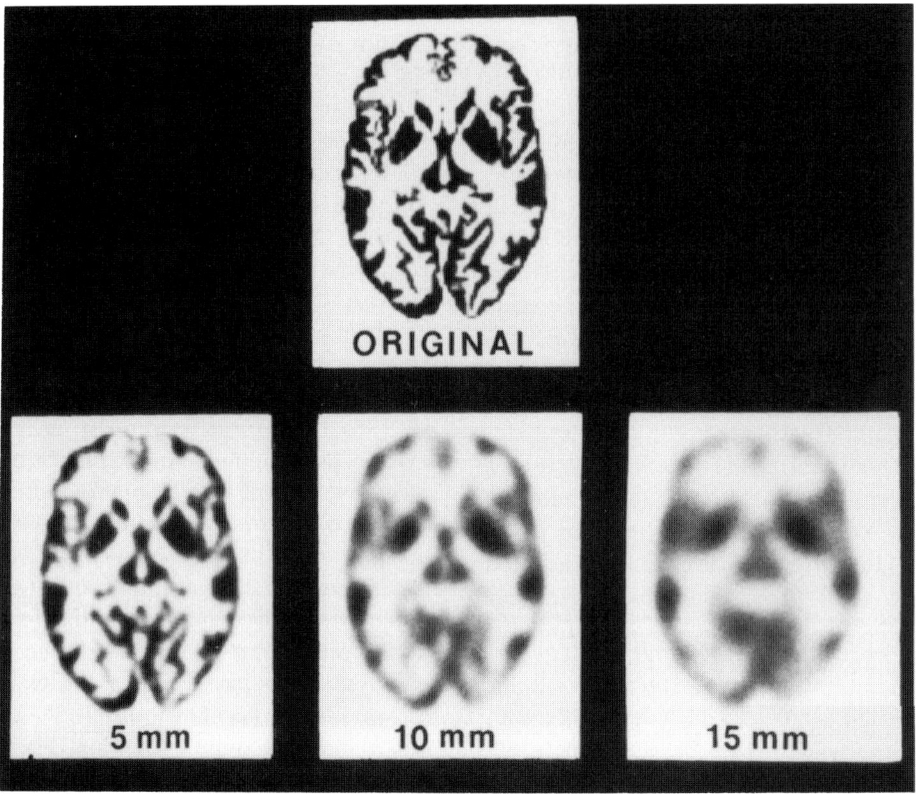

Fig. 6-6. This illustration simulates the effect of scanner resolution. At the upper center is a simulated "ideal" PET image of regional radioactivity, reflecting the higher metabolic activity in gray matter. Subsequent images simulate the effect of obtaining this image with tomographs of varying spatial resolution, from 5 to 15 mm FWHM. Note the blurring or spreading out of radioactivity, with gray matter structures appearing paler. As a result, radioactivity in cortical and subcortical gray matter regions is underestimated. Similar considerations hold for SPECT images. (From Mazziotta et al., 1981, with permission.)

is large with respect to scanner resolution. In a circular, uniform structure with a diameter twice the resolution, the radioactivity concentration will be accurately represented in the center. However, statistical considerations limit obtaining a measurement from such a small region. In general, it is not possible to measure pure gray matter radioactivity, especially in thin cortical regions.

Partial volume averaging with cerebrospinal fluid in sulci or ventricles can lead to an underestimation of tissue blood flow and metabolism. If there is cerebral atrophy, PET and SPECT measurements will be further reduced because of partial volume averaging with enlarged, metabolically inactive, cerebrospinal fluid spaces (Herscovitch et al., 1986; Videen et al., 1988). Beyond the border of a circumscribed region of decreased flow or metabolism, one would observe a gradual transition of the physiologic measurement to the value in surrounding normal tissue, also due to partial volume averaging (Powers, 1988). This gives rise to the false perception that the PET or SPECT "lesion" is larger than the actual abnormality.

FUNCTIONAL BRAIN IMAGING IN HEAD TRAUMA

With this background, it is possible to consider the abnormalities of CBF and metabolism that one might encounter in closed head injury. There have been several SPECT studies of patients with head trauma but relatively few PET studies. Some of the clinical situations to be discussed have been investigated with other techniques but are areas for future research with functional brain imaging. Because of the different mechanisms and issues involved, acute head trauma will be discussed separately from the postconcussive syndrome.

Acute Head Trauma

There are several mechanisms by which acute head trauma could produce SPECT or PET abnormalities. These include the effects of pathologic lesions as well as functional abnormalities such as elevated intracranial pressure and alterations in cerebrovascular regulation.

Functional Brain Imaging in Relation to Pathologic Abnormalities

Structural lesions include contusions, intracerebral hemorrhage, and diffuse axonal injury (Goodman, 1994; Richardson, 1990). A contusion is an area of hemorrhagic necrosis, usually on the crest of a convolution, which may involve the whole thickness of cortex and extend into white matter. One might expect decreased CBF and metabolism in a contusion. With small lesions, however, the decrease may be underestimated owing to partial volume averaging with surrounding uninvolved tissue. Brain tissue replaced by an intracerebral hematoma will appear as a region of absent flow and metabolism. Decreased CBF and metabolism may also be seen at a distance from an intracerebral hematoma (e.g., in contralateral cerebellum) because of the loss of afferent projections from or passing through the damaged region. Diffuse axonal injury occurring at the time of trauma due to shearing forces (Elson and Ward, 1994; Richardson, 1990) often underlies the severe impairment or coma of acute TBI. The mechanism is believed to be damage to the axolemma and cytoskeleton leading to loss of axonal continuity. Concussion and the sequelae of mild head injury may result from milder, reversible axonal dysfunction. Diffuse axonal injury results in deafferentation of the affected neurons, often in a scattered fashion (Povlishock and Valadka, 1994). This could cause coupled decreases in rCBF and metabolism.

There have been several reports of SPECT in acute head trauma, as well as at least two PET studies in the acute or subacute stages. SPECT with ^{99m}Tc-HMPAO has frequently shown hypoperfusion in areas of cerebral contusion or intracerebral hematoma demonstrated by CT or MRI (Abdel-Dayem et al., 1987; Bullock et al., 1992; Choksey et al., 1991; Nedd et al., 1993; Roper et al., 1991; Yamakami et al., 1993) (Fig. 6-7). PET studies have shown decreased rCBF, rCMRO$_2$, and rCMRGlu in cerebral contusion (Langfitt et al., 1986; Tenjin et al., 1990). Several authors have noted that the lesions visualized with SPECT are larger than those demonstrated by CT (Abdel-Dayem et al., 1987; Nedd et al., 1993; Tikofsky, 1994b). Although this may reflect functional disruption of flow and metabolism adjacent to the anatomically defined lesion, partial volume averaging of the lesion with surrounding normal brain would give the same appearance. Bullock et al. (1992) noted that although cerebral contusions or intracerebral hematomas had a surrounding zone of reduced perfusion, usually larger than the hemorrhagic lesion itself, such zones were not greater than the extent of the T$_2$-weighted MRI lesion corresponding to the surrounding edema.

It has frequently been reported that in acute head trauma there are more focal abnormalities on SPECT perfusion images than on CT (Abdel-Dayem et al., 1987; Nedd et al., 1993; Roper et al., 1991; Yamakami et al., 1993) (Figs. 6-7 and 6-8). Also, areas of decreased rCMRGlu have been observed on PET FDG scans without corresponding CT or MRI abnormalities (Langfitt et al., 1986). There are several potential explanations. In some cases the SPECT and CT studies were not done concurrently (Nedd et al., 1993). Some areas of cortical damage may not have been evident on CT but could have been demonstrated by MRI, which is more sensitive (Wilson and Wyper, 1992). It is possible that some functional imaging defects result from deafferentation of cerebral cortex due to axonal dysfunction. Also, the development of the SPECT or PET defect could precede the appearance of an anatomic lesion, so that sequential studies in these cases may be revealing. For example, Roper et al. (1991) performed repeat SPECT scans in four patients who initially had areas of hypoperfusion without a corresponding CT lesion. In two cases the SPECT changes normalized over time, while in the other two there was either no change or an increase in size of the perfusion defect in regions that demonstrated encephalomalacia on repeat CT.

In addition, there have been areas of contusion seen on CT without a corresponding SPECT abnormality (Roper et al., 1991). It has been hypothesized that these regions may have normal flow in spite of

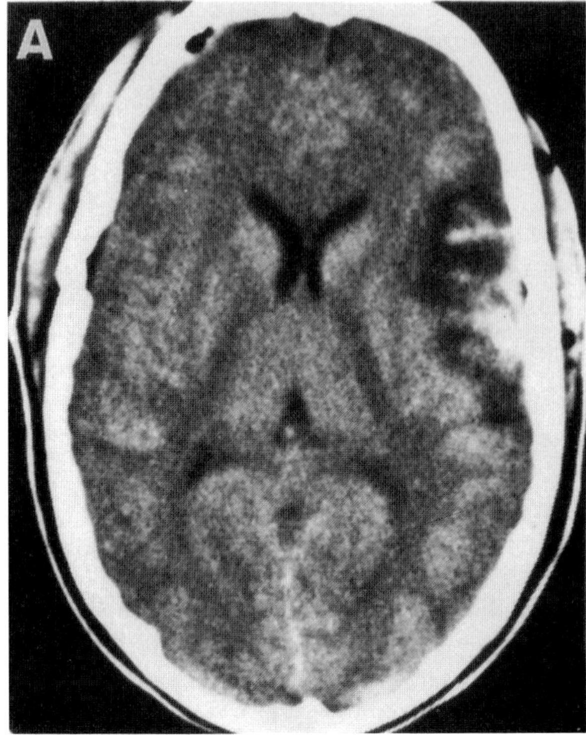

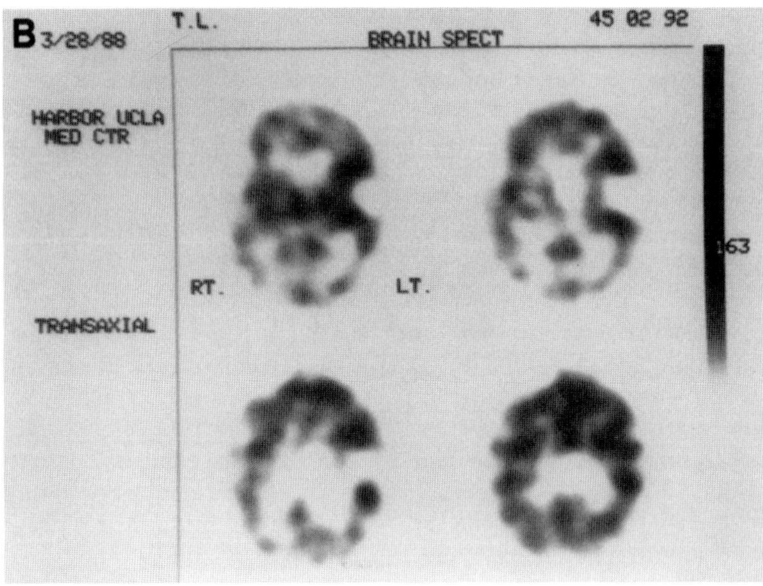

Fig. 6-7. CT and SPECT HMPAO images in a 19-year-old man obtained within 3 days of a nonpenetrating gunshot wound to the left temporal area. **(A)** X-ray CT shows a left frontotemporal contusion. **(B)** SPECT shows decreased perfusion in the area of the contusion, but also in the right frontal and right occipital areas, which were normal on CT. (From Roper et al., 1991, with permission.)

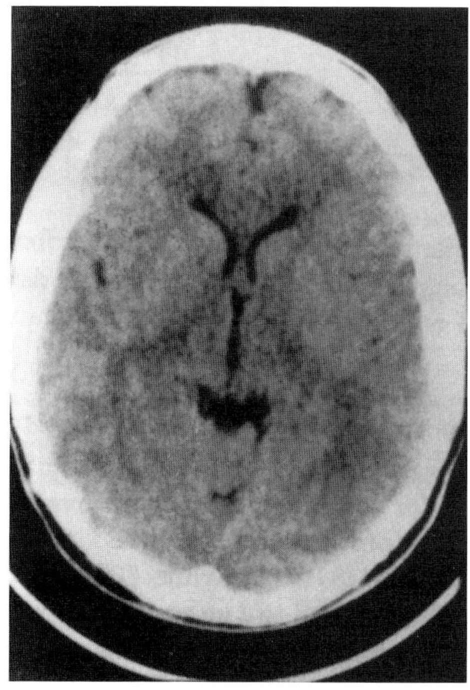
A

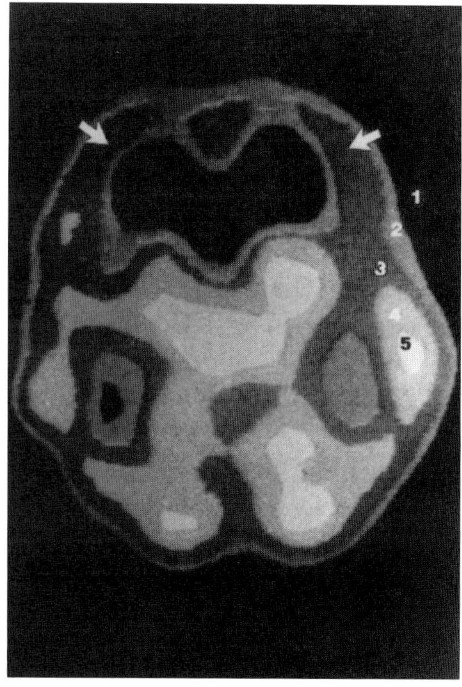

B

Fig. 6-8. **(A)** X-ray CT and **(B)** HMPAO SPECT images obtained in the acute phase of TBI. Although the CT scan was normal, SPECT showed decreased perfusion in both frontal lobes (*arrows*). (From Nedd et al., 1993, with permission.)

decreased metabolism (i.e., uncoupling of flow and metabolism), with flow in excess of the tissue's metabolic need. Bullock et al. (1992) observed zones of relative *hyperfusion* in several patients with contusion. The hyperemia occurred in tissue judged to be normal on the basis of both acute and late CT or MRI and typically resolved by the third week. Fumeya et al. (1990) noted in a preliminary report that rCBF assessed with ^{123}I-iodoamphetamine varied from hypoperfusion to hyperperfusion in contusions visualized on both CT and MRI. However, lesions showing only increased signal intensity on T_2-weighted MRI (believed to be edema) had normal or decreased flow. The PET study of Tenjin et al., (1990) using ^{15}O radiotracers and the steady-state method did not report values for the oxygen extraction fraction in contusion. However, on average, contusions showed a greater depression of $rCMRO_2$ than rCBF, suggesting that perfusion was in excess of the tissue's metabolic needs. To obtain a better understanding of the pathophysiology of contusions, serial PET measurements of both CBF and metabolism, with CT and MRI correlation, are required.

Functional Brain Imaging in Relation to Physiologic Abnormalities

In addition to contusion, hematoma, and diffuse axonal injury, several secondary physiologic abnormalities occur after head trauma, including elevated intracranial pressure, abnormal cerebrovascular regulation, depressed metabolism, and neurotransmitter abnormalities. These have been studied in experimental models or in patients by nontomographic techniques such as ^{133}Xe inhalation and are amenable to further investigation, especially with PET.

Cerebral perfusion pressure is the difference between systemic arterial and intracranial pressure. CBF is normally maintained over a wide range of perfusion pressure because of changes in the caliber of cerebral blood vessels, termed vascular autoregulation. Abnormalities in the regulation of CBF in response to changes in cerebral perfusion pressure as well as to changes in arterial carbon dioxide pressure occur in some patients with severe injury (Muizelaar and Obrist, 1992; Povlishock and Valadka, 1994). Changes in the cerebral circulation also occur as a result of elevated intracranial pressure, which decreases perfusion pressure. In the monkey, experimental elevation of intracranial pressure caused a rise in CBV, reflecting autoregulatory vasodilation to maintain CBF (Grubb et al., 1975). At very high intracranial pressure, CBF fell, but $CMRO_2$ do not significantly change, owing to increased oxygen extraction. Of interest, in the study by Kuhl et al. (1980) of CBV in acute TBI, the one patient with intracranial hypertension had increased CBV.

Abnormalities of global CBF and metabolism and of flow-metabolism coupling have been observed in severe TBI. There is a good correlation between global $CMRO_2$ and clinical state (i.e., as measured by the Glasgow Coma Scale [GCS] in acute head trauma); patients with GCS scores below 9 had $CMRO_2$ less than half normal (Obrist et al., 1984). Global CBF shows more variability. Early after injury (<12 hours), low CBF values have been observed that correlate with clinical status, but subsequently CBF tends to increase and the correlation is lost (Marion et al., 1991; Muizelaar and Obrist, 1992; Povlishock and Valadka, 1994). Obrist et al. (1984) identified two groups of patients with severe TBI on the basis of CBF findings. In about half, global CBF was reduced in proportion to $CMRO_2$ and the arteriovenous oxygen difference across the brain was normal, indicating that coupling between CBF and metabolism was maintained and that CBF reductions were secondary to depressed metabolic demand. In the remaining patients, CBF was normal or elevated in spite of decreased metabolism, indicating uncoupling. There was no consistent evidence of global cerebral ischemia (i.e., CBF insufficient to meet the tissue's metabolic needs). It should be noted, however, that in fatal head trauma ischemic tissue damage is often seen, including arterial border zone infarcts and diffuse ischemic damage (Goodman, 1994; Richardson, 1990). These may be due to episodes of hypotension or hypoxemia, which may occur even prior to hospitalization. Low global CBF is probably a reflection of tissue damage or decreased metabolic demand rather than a cause of ischemic lesions. The relationships among CBF, CBV, and metabolism, and clinical status and intracranial pressure in acute TBI are potential areas for investigation with PET. PET has the added ability to detect regional abnormalities that may be missed by global measurement techniques (Obrist et al., 1984). An important question is whether circumstances occur in TBI in which CBF is inadequate to meet the tissue's metabolic needs.

Finally, abnormal neurotransmitter release and receptor binding have been implicated in the pathogenesis of brain damage in experimental TBI. Excitatory amino acid neurotransmitters and endogenous opioids have received special interest (Hayes and Dixon, 1994). Thus, studies of receptor systems with SPECT or PET may be informative in acute head trauma. Wyper (1993) mentions the use of ^{123}I-MK801, a radiolabeled glutamate antagonist, to image N-methyl-D-aspartate (NMDA) receptors with SPECT in trauma. This research is of interest because of the potential role of excitatory amino acids in the pathogenesis of acute brain injury.

In summary, the primary and secondary anatomic and physiologic abnormalities that occur after acute TBI can lead to changes in cerebral hemodynamics and metabolism. The ability of PET to measure regional CBF, CBV, and metabolism make it a powerful approach to studying pathophysiology and effects of therapeutic interventions in acute head trauma. SPECT studies of cerebral perfusion, although more limited in scope, can also be informative. Because of the heterogeneity of patients with regard to structural brain damage and clinical status, such research requires careful design, with specific hypotheses applied to selected, well characterized patient groups. Anatomic information, obtained with CT or MRI, is needed to interpret PET and SPECT studies of head trauma because macroscopic lesions typically result in abnormalities of CBF and metabolism. It should be noted that there are logistical problems when imaging acutely ill, comatose, or unstable patients. It has been possible to examine such patients with PET or SPECT outside of an intensive care unit. However, the introduction of PET into the intensive care unit setting, which has been accomplished in at least one institution (personal communication from T. Videen, Washington University School of Medicine, St. Louis), will facilitate such studies.

Postconcussive Syndrome and Recovery from Head Injury

SPECT has been used to study patients beyond the acute phase of TBI (Gray et al., 1992; Newton et al., 1992; Prayer et al., 1993). There are perfusion deficits in areas of atrophy or encephalomalacia identified by CT or MRI. In addition, perfusion deficits have been observed without anatomically corresponding structural lesions, often in frontal and temporal regions. These may be due to interruption of white matter projections by diffuse axonal injury. However, not all CT or MRI abnormalities show corresponding SPECT changes. Attempts have been made to assess the prognostic value of SPECT imaging and to relate changes seen with functional brain imaging to neuropsychologic deficits.

Relation Among SPECT, CT, and MRI

Gray et al. (1992) performed ^{99m}Tc-HMPAO SPECT and x-ray CT in 53 patients at least 6 months after either minor (GCS score 13 to 15) or major (GCS score <9) TBI. Overall, 80 percent of patients showed perfusion deficits, while only 55 percent showed CT abnormalities (Fig. 6-9). There were more abnormalities with major TBI, but the difference between SPECT and CT was less in this group (90 versus 72 percent with CT abnormalities) than in the minor TBI group (60 versus 25 percent). Other investigators using MRI also observed discrepancies between structural and perfusion abnormalities. Newton et al. (1992) studied 19 patients 3 to 36 months after severe TBI by use of CT, MRI, and ^{99m}Tc-HMPAO SPECT and correlated these results with the Glasgow Outcome Scale (GOS). There were 43 perfusion defects on SPECT, 21 focal lesions on MRI, and 13 on CT; 31 of the 43 SPECT abnormalities were not seen on CT or MRI. However, several MRI or CT lesions were not apparent on SPECT. Although fewer lesions were detected with MRI than with SPECT, there was a similar inverse correlation between GOS and lesion number with either modality ($r = -0.84$ versus -0.82). Ichise et al. (1994), studying 29 patients, also found a discrepancy in lesion frequency with different modalities; 19 patients showed a total of 42 SPECT lesions, whereas 13 showed 29 MRI lesions and 10 showed 24 CT abnormalities. SPECT detected relatively more abnormalities than CT or MRI in the minor than in the major TBI group.

Prayer et al. (1993) performed MRI and ^{99m}Tc-HMPAO SPECT in 18 patients with normal CT scans 2 to 36 months after severe TBI (post-traumatic amnesia of at least 7 days). MRI scans were evaluated for evidence of diffuse axonal lesions of white matter, corpus callosum, or rostral brainstem and/or lateral ventricular enlargement. In contrast to other studies, both MRI and SPECT were abnormal in all patients, and the number of abnormalities was similar. However, 65 percent of the structural and functional abnormalities did not coincide topographically. MRI was superior for detecting white matter lesions while SPECT demonstrated more cortical changes. Evidence of diffuse axonal injury strongly correlated with poor outcome on the GOS. In the patients with diffuse axonal injury, SPECT showed reduced perfusion in large areas of frontal, temporal, and parietal cortex as well as in thalamus. The occurrence of cortical and thalamic hypoperfusion was attributed to multiple disconnections to these areas caused by diffuse axonal injury.

Prognostic Value of SPECT

Some studies have examined the potential of SPECT to provide prognostic information (Jacobs et al., 1994; Oder et al., 1991; Tikofsky, 1994b). Jacobs et al. (1994) scanned 67 patients within 4 weeks of TBI, 42 with moderate trauma (GCS score >10, retrograde amnesia for <24 hours, and/or abnormal CT) and 25 with minor trauma (no loss of consciousness, amnesia, or CT abnormalities, but with minor neurologic complaints). Patients received a neurologic examination, questioning about postconcussive symptoms, and memory and concentration tests (which were not otherwise described). After 3 months, patients received another clinical assessment and a repeat SPECT scan if the first one was abnormal. The moderate trauma group had more abnormalities on initial SPECT (60 percent) than the mild group (36 percent). The sensitivity of the initial SPECT scan for persistent sequelae was high, 95 percent of these patients having an abnormal scan. Specificity was lower, with only 70 percent of patients with no sequelae having a negative initial scan. A negative initial scan had a very high predictive value—97 percent of these patients had no clinical sequelae at 3 months. In contrast, the positive predictive value was poor, as only 59 percent of patients with positive scans had persistent sequelae. Although this study does suggest that a negative early scan predicts a favorable outcome in this patient group, it would have been strengthened if information about the patient's' clinical status had been provided, especially since many patients had very mild symptomatology.

Oder et al. (1991) compared long-term outcome with ^{99m}Tc-HMPAO SPECT scans performed 1 to 4 months after TBI in 12 patients with persistent vegetative state. Diffuse reduction of cortical perfusion with a frontal predominance occurred in four of six patients with poor outcome (GOS < 4), but in none of the six patients with a favorable outcome. Thus, in this small sample, the positive predictive value of

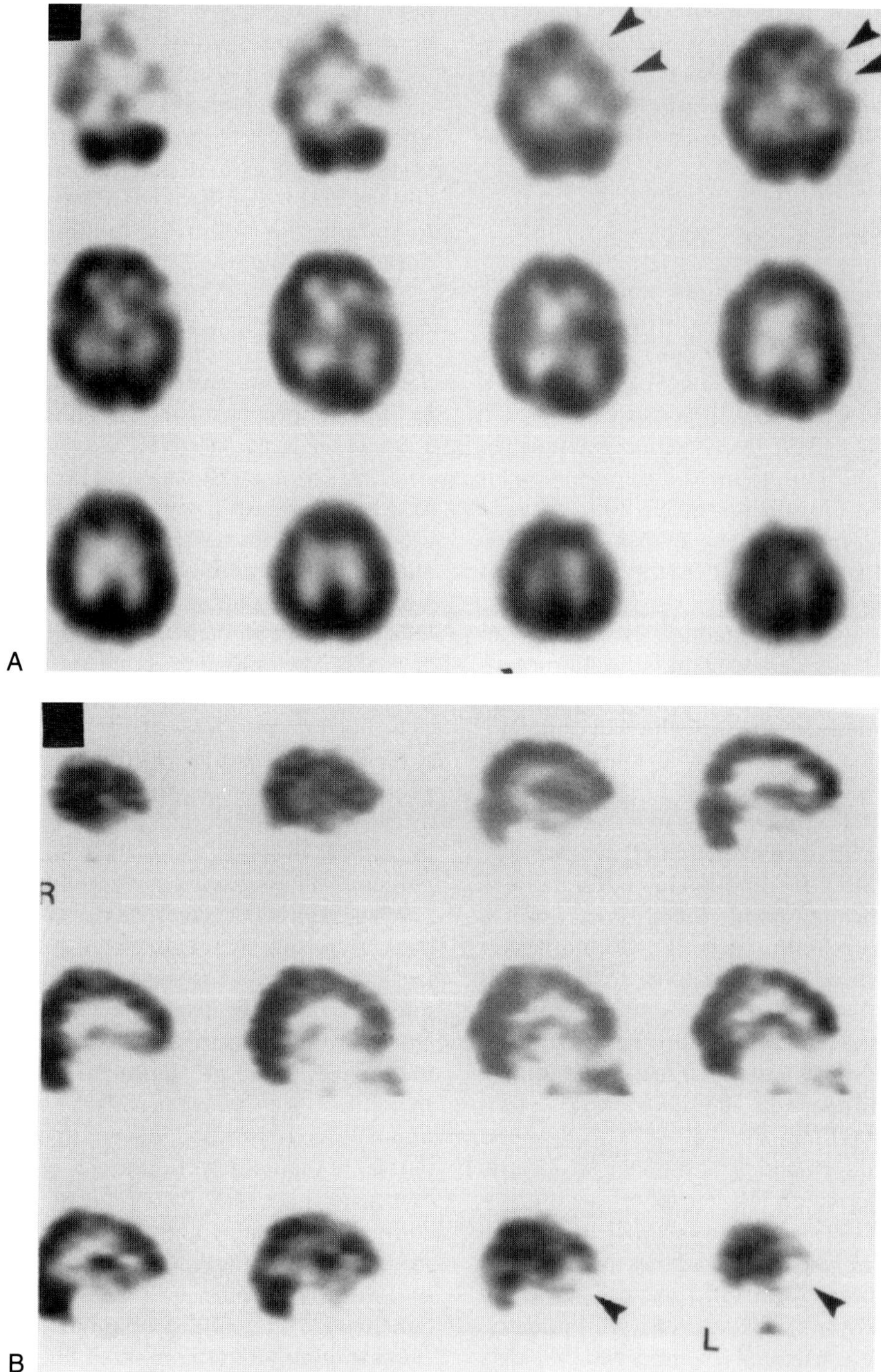

Fig. 6-9. SPECT HMPAO images obtained 53 months after mild TBI in a 50-year-old man with persistent decreased memory and concentration and emotional lability. CT and MRI scans were normal. There were focal perfusion deficits in the left inferior frontal and left anterior temporal lobes (*arrowheads*) seen in the **(A)** transaxial and **(B)** saggital images. (From Gray et al., 1992, with permission.)

global hypoperfusion for poor outcome was 100 percent, although the absence of this pattern did not reliably predict a good prognosis. MRI had even stronger predictive value; all of the patients with poor outcome, but none of those with good outcome, had evidence of diffuse axonal injury on MRI.

Relation Between Brain Imaging Abnormalities and Functional Deficits

Attempts to correlate SPECT or PET abnormalities with neuropsychological deficits have met with variable success. Goldenberg et al. (1992) studied 36 patients 7 to 66 months after severe TBI with SPECT. Regions of interest were drawn, and a quantitative perfusion index was calculated by dividing each region of interest count rate by the global average. Correlations were performed between regional SPECT data and test scores for executive function, memory, intelligence, and activities of daily living, with care taken to correct for multiple statistical comparisons. The hypothesized correlations between memory and regional perfusion and between temporal perfusion and test scores were not found. Correlations were observed, however, between right thalamic perfusion and vocabulary and executive function and between left thalamic perfusion and vocabulary, with weaker correlations found between right frontal perfusion and several tests. It was suggested that diffuse axonal injury could be responsible for the observed thalamic correlations by a diffuse effect on cognitive functions on the one hand and by interruption of connections to the thalamus on the other.

Wiedman et al. (1989) studied 16 patients with SPECT 5 to 12 months after diffuse or contusional TBI. Perfusion in 12 brain regions was visually assessed, and for each region cognitive test scores were compared between patients with and without a perfusion abnormality. Only 14 of 120 comparisons showed a relationship between perfusion defects and poor performance, but these favored anterior temporal and orbitofrontal regions. The most consistent relationships were found for nonverbal tasks in the right anterior temporal area and for visual memory tasks in the orbitofrontal areas.

Ichise et al. (1994) correlated SPECT with neuropsychological performance in 29 chronic TBI patients. They used count rates in cerebral cortex extending from frontal to occipital poles on midline saggital images to calculate an anteroposterior perfusion ratio. This index was based on the observation that TBI patients often have relative hypoperfusion anteriorly, which could be because contusions more often involve the anteroinferior aspects of the frontal and temporal lobes, or because diffuse axonal injury preferentially affects projections to these lobes. The ratio was lower in patients than in control subjects, and it correlated with 6 of 12 tests of memory, attention, or executive function. The correlations were weak however, with r^2 values of about 0.10 to 0.18, indicating that only a small amount of the variance in test performance is explained by differences in the SPECT perfusion ratio.

Further information on the relationship between SPECT and functional status can be obtained from the data of Jacobs et al. (1994). Within 4 weeks of mild to moderate TBI, abnormal scans were obtained in only 34 of 67 patients (51 percent) who had shown abnormalities on a clinical assessment consisting of neurologic examination, questioning about postconcussive symptoms, and memory and concentration tests. Furthermore, follow-up at 3 months showed 6 of 14 patients to have no sequelae but positive scans and 6 of 25 to have positive scans but no sequelae. Although the sensitivity of the follow-up SPECT study for sequelae was 95 percent, the specificity was only 57 percent and the positive predictive value 76 percent. Thus, the correlation between signs or symptoms and SPECT results was not particularly strong.

Ruff et al. (1989, 1994) studied chronic TBI patients with abnormalities on neuropsychological testing using PET and FDG. Regional PET data normalized to the whole slice average were defined as abnormal if they were two standard deviations below the values in controls. Abnormal rCMRGlu was frequently observed in the absence of CT abnormalities and often involved frontal and temporal brain regions. These were essentially case reports, however, and there was no systematic comparison of neuropsychological deficits to the PET data.

Use of Functional Brain Imaging to Study the Recovery Process

PET has been extensively used to map normal brain function. The rCBF changes that occur while subjects perform a sensorimotor or cognitive task in comparison with a control state reflect local neuronal function and are used to map the areas involved in the task (Frackowiak and Friston, 1994). The short (2-mintue) half-life of the flow tracer $H_2{}^{15}O$ permits multiple scans to be obtained during different tasks in a single experimental session. Such studies have been used to map the brain areas active during motor tasks in patients who have recovered from an ischemic motor stroke (Weiller et al., 1992) and could be used to study the recovery of sensorimotor and cognitive function after TBI. In addition, serial studies of resting CBF and metabolism during the recovery process in relation to the patient's improving clinical status could be of interest.

USE OF FUNCTIONAL BRAIN IMAGING IN PATIENT MANAGEMENT

A final area for consideration is the use of SPECT or PET in the management of individual patients with TBI. Although this has been suggested (Tikofsky, 1994a; Tikofsky, 1994b), in my view the current peer-reviewed literature does not support the use of either modality in the care of TBI patients. This may seem surprising, since SPECT and PET provide physiologic information about CBF and metabolism that is qualitatively different from the structural information provided by CT and MRI. However, physicians are experienced in dealing with anatomic and neuropathologic information (e.g., brain slices, surgical visualization) that CT and MRI provide noninvasively. There is no equivalent knowledge base for dealing with physiologic images, and there is little empirical support for using them in clinical decision making. Second, most studies using functional brain imaging were not specifically designed to examine its role in the diagnosis or management of the condition under investigation. Rather, they were performed to learn about disease pathophysiology, or more simply, to see what PET or SPECT would show. Thus, extrapolation of this information into the clinical arena is not justified. For example, many studies report the differences on functional brain imaging between a group of well characterized patients with a specific disease and normal control subjects. However, to establish diagnostic accuracy, one must compare patients with the full spectrum of the disease to control subjects with the full spectrum of conditions with which the disease may be confused in clinical practice (Powers et al., 1991).

The clinical value of a new diagnostic test can be assessed in a rigorous fashion in the same way that new treatments can be evaluated and compared with existing treatments in a randomized, controlled trial. Kent and Larson (1992) have listed the following criteria for assessing a diagnostic test: (1) Technical capacity (i.e., whether the test measures a phenomenon with precision); (2) diagnostic accuracy in the detection and classification of pathology, including information about disease detection (sensitivity) and exclusion (specificity); (3) diagnostic impact (i.e., a judgment of the test's accuracy and clinical value compared with existing alternatives); (4) therapeutic impact, which is the effect of the test on patient care (e.g., replacing a more costly, uncomfortable, or risky test or identifying patients who would not benefit from treatment); and (5) patient outcome (i.e., does the use of the test in a patient group prolong life, relieve suffering, or improve functional status?) More succinctly, the ultimate criterion is for a test to reduce morbidity and mortality or to save money (Powers et al., 1991). The utility of PET or SPECT in managing patients with TBI has not been demonstrated on the basis of these criteria. In fairness, it must be said that there is still controversy about the role of more widely used tests, such as MRI, in specific clinical situations (Kent et al., 1994). However, appropriate studies must be performed before functional brain imaging is routinely used in patients with TBI. This is a question not only of cost containment but also of ensuring that the decisions made using these tests will actually help rather than harm patients.

In head injury, the use of functional brain imaging is further complicated because its potential role is not necessarily to obtain a specific diagnosis. Rather, other uses have been suggested. Several authors have proposed using SPECT in both acute and chronic TBI because it may show more or larger lesions than CT or MRI. The clinical utility of this finding remains to be demonstrated, however. For example, in a patient with acute TBI and depressed consciousness, the presence or absence of an intracranial hematoma on CT has an obvious impact on patient management; the observation of several SPECT perfusion defects does not. It has been suggested that functional brain imaging has a role in determining patient prognosis (Tikofsky, 1994b). The study of Jacobs et al. (1994), discussed above, did find a very high negative predictive value of an initial normal SPECT scan in patients with TBI. However, detailed results of the initial clinical evaluation were not provided, and many of the patients had very mild symptoms, which might have also predicted prognosis. In a recent publication Worley, Hoffman, and Paine et al. (1995) concluded that although FDG PET in children and adolescents with traumatic brain injury correlated with outcome, it was no more useful than contemporaneous CT or MRI for prediction of outcome. Therefore, more work would be required before functional brain imaging is used to predict prognosis.

It has been proposed by Tikofsky (1994a) that SPECT "provides a useful tool for 'proving' the physiological basis for sustained cognitive impairment in patients with chronic TBI." Unfortunately, as noted above, the correlation between SPECT abnormalities and neuropsychological performance or clinical status is not particularly strong in large groups of patients, so that its use in individual patients is premature. Mayberg (1992), in discussing the use of functional brain imaging data in criminal trials, noted that it has "not reached the level of sophistication to predict any neurological or psychiatric deficit." Juni (1994), in a critical review of brain SPECT, noted that "while it may be possible in a given case to state that a particular scan defect is consistent with certain behavioral abnormalities, it is generally not possible to state with certainty that the two are causally related." Thus, the presence of SPECT or PET lesions does not prove that they are causing the patient's symptoms, nor does their absence prove that the patient's symptoms are not due to head trauma. It also follows that functional brain images cannot be used to prove or exclude malingering in a patient with post-traumatic complaints. Furthermore, abnormalities could be due to other conditions such as depression or substance abuse (Juni, 1994) or could even predate the trauma.

In conclusion, PET provides unique quantitative measurements of rCBF and metabolism. Although SPECT studies of cerebral perfusion are more limited in scope, they can also be informative. Both modalities could play an important role in clinical research studies designed to understand the pathophysiology of acute head trauma and its consequences. However, their role in the management of individual patients with TBI remains to be established.

REFERENCES

Abdel-Dayem HM, Sadek SA, Kouris K et al: Changes in cerebral perfusion after acute head injury: comparison of CT with Tc-99m HMPAO SPECT Radiology 165:221–226, 1987

Altman DI, Lich LL, Powers WJ: Brief inhalation method to measure cerebral oxygen extraction with PET: accuracy determination under pathologic conditions. J Nucl Med 32:1738–1741, 1991

Astrup J, Sorensen PM, Sorensen HR: Oxygen and glucose consumption related to Na^+-K^+ transport in canine brain. Stroke 12: 726–730, 1981

Baron JC, Frackowiak RSJ, Herholz K et al: Use of PET methods for measurement of cerebral energy metabolism and hemodynamics in cerebrovascular disease. J Cereb Blood Flow Metab 9:723–742, 1989

Baron JC, Rougemont D, Soussaline F et al: Local interrelationships of oxygen consumption and glucose utilization in normal subjects and in ischemic stroke patients: a positron emission tomographic study. J Cereb Blood Flow Metab 4:140–149, 1984

Berridge MS, Adler LP, Nelson AD et al: Measurement of human cerebral blood flow with [^{15}O]butanol and positron emission tomography. J Cereb Blood Flow Metab 11:707–715, 1991

Blomqvist G, Stone-Elander S, Halldin C et al: Positron emission tomographic measurements of cerebral glucose utilization using [1-^{11}C]D-glucose. J Cereb Blood Flow Metab 11:467–483, 1990

Brooks RA: Alternative formula for glucose utilization using labeled deoxyglucose. J Nucl Med 23:538–539, 1982

Brown MM, Wade JPH, Marshall J: Fundamental importance of arterial oxygen content in the regulation of cerebral blood flow in man. Brain 108:81–93, 1985

Bullock R, Sakas D, Patterson J et al: Early post-traumatic cerebral blood flow mapping: correlation with structural damage after focal injury. Acta Neurochir Suppl (Wien), 55:14–17, 1992

Camargo EE, Szabo Z, Links JM et al: The influence of biological and technical factors on the variability of global and regional brain metabolism of 2-[^{18}F]fluoro-2-deoxy-D-glucose. J Cereb Blood Flow Metab 12:281–290, 1992

Carson RE: Precision and accuracy considerations of physiological quantitation in PET. J Cereb Blood Flow Metab 11:A45–A50, 1991

Choksey MS, Costa DC, Iannotti F et al: ^{99m}T HMPAO SPECT studies in traumatic intracerebral hematoma. J Neurol Neurosurg Psychiatry 54:6–11, 1991

Council on Scientific Affairs: Instrumentation in positron emission tomography. JAMA 259:1351–1356, 1988

Cunningham V, Cremer JE: Current assumptions behind the use of PET scanning for measuring glucose utilization in brain. Trends Neurosci 8:96–99, 1985

Cutler NR, Haxby JV, Duara R et al: Clinical history, brain metabolism, and neuropsychological function in Alzheimer's disease. Ann Neurol 18:298–309, 1985

Dannals RF, Ravert HT, Wilson AA: Chemistry of tracers for positron emission tomography. pp. 55–74. Burns DH, Gibson RE, Dannals RF, Siegl PKS (eds): Nuclear Imaging in Drug Discovery, Development, and Approval. Birkhäuser, Boston, 1993

DeGrado TR, Turkington T, Williams JJ, Performance characteristics of a whole-body PET scanner. J Nucl Med 35:1398–1406, 1994

Devous MD Sr: Imaging brain function by single-photon emission computer tomography. pp. 147–234. In Andreasen NC (ed): Brain Imaging: Applications in Psychiatry. American Psychiatric Press, Washington, 1989

Devous MD Sr, Stokely EM, Chehabi HH, Bonte FJ: Normal distribution of regional cerebral blood flow measured by dynamic single-photon emission tomography. J Cereb Blood Flow Metab 6:95–104, 1986

Edvinsson L, MacKenzie ET, McCulloch J: Neurotransmitters: metabolic and vascular effects in vivo. pp. 159–180. In Cerebral Blood Flow and Metabolism. Raven Press, New York, 1993a.

Edvinsson L, MacKenzie ET, McCulloch J: Changes in arterial gas tensions. pp. 524–552. In Cerebral Blood Flow and Metabolism. Raven Press, New York, 1993b

Elson LM, Ward CC: Mechanisms and pathophysiology of mild head injury. Semin Neurol 14:8–18, 1994

Eriksson L, Holte S, Bohm C et al: Automated blood sampling systems for positron emission tomography. IEEE Trans Nucl Sci 35:703–707, 1988

Evans AC, Marrett S, Torrescorzo J et al: MRI-PET correlation in three dimensions using a volume-of-interest (VOI) atlas. J Cereb Blood Flow Metab 11:A69–A78, 1991

Feeney DM, Baron JC: Diaschisis. Stroke 17:817–830, 1986

Fowler JS, Wolf AP: Recent advances in radiotracers for PET studies of the brain. pp. 11–34. In M Diksic, RC Reba, (eds): Radiopharmaceuticals and Brain Pathology Studied with PET and SPECT. CRC Press, Boca Raton, 1991

Fox PT, Perlmutter JS, Raichle ME: A stereotactic method of anatomical localization for positron emission tomography. J Comput Assist Tomogr 9:141–153, 1985

Fox PT, Raichle ME: Stimulus rate dependence of regional cerebral blood flow in human striate cortex, demonstrated by positron emission tomography. J Neurophysiol 51:1109–1120, 1984

Fox PT, Raichle ME: Focal physiological uncoupling of cerebral blood flow and oxidative metabolism during somatosensory stimulation in human subjects. Proc Natl Acad Sci USA 83:1140–1144, 1986

Fox PT, Raichle ME, Mintun MA, Dence C: Nonoxidative glucose consumption during focal physiologic neural activity. Science 241:462–464, 1988

Frackowiak RS, Friston KJ: Functional neuroanatomy of the human brain: positron emission tomography—a new neuroanatomical technique. J Anat 211–225, 1994

Frackowiak RSJ, Lenzi G-L, Jones T, Heather JD: Quantitative measurement of regional cerebral blood flow and oxygen metabolism in man using ^{15}O and positron emission tomography: theory, procedure and normal values. J Comput Assist Tomogr 4:727–736, 1980

Fumeya H, Ito K, Yamagiwa O et al: Analysis of MRI and SPECT in patients with acute head trauma. Acta Neurochir Suppl (Wien) 51:283–285, 1990

Ge YR, Fitzpatrick JM, Votaw JR et al: Retrospective registration of PET and MR brain images—an algorithm and its stereotaxic validation. J Comput Assist Tomogr 18:800–810, 1994

Gemmell HG, Evans NTS, Besson JAO et al: Regional cerebral blood flow imaging: a quantitative comparison of technetium-99m-SPECT with $C^{15}O_2$ PET. J Nucl Med 31:1595–1600, 1992

George MS, Ring HA, Costa DC et al: Neuroactivation and Neuroimaging with SPECT. Springer-Verlag, London, 1991

Ginsberg MD, Dietrich WD, Busto R: Coupled forebrain increases of local cerebral glucose utilization and blood flow during physiologic stimulation of a somatosensory pathway in the rat: demonstration by double-label autoradiography. Neurology 37:11–19, 1987

Gjedde A, Wienhard K, Heiss WD et al: Comparative regional analysis of 2-fluorodeoxyglucose and methylglucose uptake in brain of four stroke patients. With special reference to the regional estimation of the lumped constant. J Cereb Blood Flow Metab 5:163–178, 1985

Goldenberg G, Oder W, Spatt J, Podreka I: Cerebral correlates of disturbed executive function and memory in survivors of severe closed head injury: a SPECT study. J Neurol Neurosurg Psychiatry 55:362–368, 1992

Goodman JC: Pathologic changes in mild head injury. Semin Neurol 14:19–31, 1994

Grafton ST, Mazziotta JC: Cerebral pathophysiology evaluated with positron emission tomography. pp. 1573–1588. In Asbury AK, McKhann GM, McDonald WI (eds): Diseases of the Nervous System: Clincial Neurobiology. WB Saunders, Philadelphia, 1992

Graham MM, Spence AM, Muzi M, Abbott GL: Deoxyglucose kinetics in a rat brain tumor. J Cereb Blood Flow Metab 9:315–322, 1989

Gray BG, Ichise M, Chung DG et al: Technetium-99m-HMPAO SPECT in the evaluation of patients with a remote history of traumatic brain injury: a comparison with x-ray computed tomography. J Nucl Med 33:52–58, 1992

Greenberg JH, Hamar J, Welsh FA et al: Effect of ischemia and reperfusion on λ of the lumped constant of the [^{14}C] deoxyglucose technique. J Cereb Blood Flow Metab 12:70–77, 1992

Greenberg JH, Kushner M, Rangno M et al: Validation studies of iodine-123-iodoamphetamine as a cerebral blood flow agent using emission tomography. J Nucl Med 31:1364–1369, 1990

Grubb RL Jr, Raichle ME, Higgins CS, Eichling JO: Measurement of regional cerebral blood volume by emission tomography. Ann Neurol 4:322–328, 1978

Grubb RL Jr, Raichle ME, Phelps ME, Ratcheson RA: Effects of increased intracranial pressure on cerebral blood volume, blood flow, and oxygen utilization in monkeys. J Neurosurg 43:385–398, 1975

Hatazawa J, Masatoshi I, Matsuzawa T et al: Measurement of the ratio of cerebral oxygen consumption to glucose utilization by positron emission tomography: its consistency with the values determined by the Kety-Schmidt method in normal volunteers. J Cereb Blood Flow Metab 8:426–432, 1988

Hayes RL, Dixon CE: Neurochemical changes in mild head injury. Semi Neurol 14:25–31, 1994

Heiss W-D, Podreka I: Role of PET and SPECT in the assessment of ischemic cerebrovascular disease. Cerebrovasc Brain Metab Rev 5:235–263, 1993

Herscovitch P, Auchus A, Gado M et al: Correction of positron emission tomography data for cerebral atrophy. J Cereb Blood Flow Metab 6:120–124, 1986

Herscovitch P, Markham J, Raichle ME: Brain blood flow measured with intravenous $H_2{}^{15}O$. I. Theory and error analysis. J Nucl Med 24:782–789, 1983

Herscovitch P, Raichel ME: Effect of tissue heterogeneity on the measurement of cerebral blood flow with the equilibrium $C^{15}O_2$ inhalation technique. J Cereb Blood Flow Metab 3:407–415, 1983

Herscovitch P, Raichle ME: What is the correct value for the brain-blood partition coefficient of water? J Cereb Blood Flow Metab 5:65–69, 1985

Herscovitch P, Raichle ME, Kilbourn MR, Welch MJ: Positron emission tomographic measurements of cerebral blood flow and permeability-surface area product of water using [^{15}O] water and [^{11}C]butanol. J Cereb Blood Flow Metab 7:527–542, 1987

Hoffman EJ, Huang S-C, Phelps ME: Quantitation in positron emission computed tomography: 1. Effect of object size. J Comput Assist Tomogr 3:299–308, 1979

Hoffman EJ, Phelps ME: Positron emission tomography: Principles and quantitation. pp. 237–286. In Phelps ME, Mazziotta JC, Schelbert HR (eds): Positron Emission Tomography and Autoradiography. Raven Press, New York, 1986

Holman BL, Carvalho PA, Zimmerman RE et al: Brain perfusion SPECT using an annular single crystal camera: initial clinical experience. J Nucl Med 31:1456–1461, 1990

Holman BL, Devous MS: Functional brain SPECT: the emergence of a powerful clinical method. J Nucl Med 33:1888–1904, 1992

Holman BL, Zimmerman RE, Johnson KA et al: Computer-assisted superimposition of magnetic resonance and high-resolution technetium-99m-HMPAO and thallium-201 SPECT images of the brain. J Nucl Med 32:1478–1484, 1991

Huang S-C, Phelps ME: Principles of tracer kinetic modeling in positron emission tomography and autoradiography. pp. 237–286. In ME Phelps, JC Mazziotta, HR Schelbert (eds): Positron Emission Tomography and Autoradiography. Raven Press, New York, 1986

Huang SC, Phelps ME, Hoffman EJ, Sideris K et al: Noninvasive determination of local cerebral metabolic rate of glucose in man. Am J Physiol 238:E69–E82, 1980

Ichise M, Chung DG, Wang P et al: Technetium-99m-HMPAO SPECT, CT and MRI in the evaluation of patients with chronic traumatic brain injury: a correlation with neuropsychological performance. J Nucl Med 35:217–226, 1994

Jacobs A, Put E, Ingels M, Bossuyt A: Prospective evaluation of technetium-99m-HMPAO SPECT in mild and moderate traumatic brain injury. J Nucl Med 35:942–947, 1994

Juni JE: Taking brain SPECT seriously: reflections on recent clinical reports in *The Journal of Nuclear Medicine.* J Nucl Med 35:1891–1895, 1994

Karp JS, Daube-Witherspoon ME, Hoffman EJ, Performance standards in positron emission tomography. J Nucl Med 32:2342–2350, 1991

Kent DL, Haynor DR, Longstreth WT Jr, Larsen EB: The clinical efficacy of magnetic resonance imaging in neuroimaging. Ann Intern Med 120:856–875, 1994

Kent DL, Larson EB: Disease, level of impact, and quality of research methods: three dimensions of clinical efficacy assessment applied to magnetic resonance imaging. Investig Radiol 27, 245–254.

Kety SS: The theory and applications of the exchange of inert gas at the lungs and tissues. Pharmacol Rev 3:1–41, 1951

Kilbourn M: Radiotracers for PET studies of neurotransmitter binding sites: design considerations. pp. 47–65. In Kuhl DE (ed): In Vivo Imaging of Neurotransmitter Functions in Brain, Heart and Tumors. American College of Nuclear Physicians, Washington, 1991

Koeppe RA, Holden JE, Ip WR: Performance comparison of parameter estimation techniques for the quantitation of local cerebral blood flow by dynamic positron computed tomography. J Cereb Blood Flow Metab 5: 224–234, 1985

Koeppe RA, Hutchins GD: Instrumentation for positron emission tomography: tomographs and data processing and display systems. Semin Nucl Med 22:162–181, 1992

Kuhl DE, Alavi A, Hoffman EJ et al: Local cerebral blood volume in head-injured patients: determination by emission computed tomography of ^{99m}Tc-labeled red cells. J Neurosurg 52:309–320, 1980

Lammertsma AA, Brooks DJ, Beaney Rp et al: In vivo measurement of regional cerebral haematocrit using positron emission tomography. J Cereb Blood Flow Metab 4:317–322, 1984

Lammertsma AA, Brooks DJ, Frackowiak, RSJ et al: Measurement of glucose utilization with [^{18}F]2-fluoro-2-deoxy-D-glucose: a comparison of different analytical methods. J Cereb Blood Flow Metab 7:161–172, 1987

Lammertsma AA, Jones T, Frackowiak, RSJ, Lenzi G-L: A theoretical study of the steady-state model for measuring regional cerebral blood flow and oxygen utilization using oxygen-15. J Comput Assist Tomogr 5:544–550, 1981

Lammertsma AA, Wise RJS, Heather JD et al: Correction for the presence of intravascular oxygen-15 in the steady-state technique for measuring regional oxygen extraction ratio in the brain: 2. Results in normal subjects and brain tumor and stroke patients. J Cereb Blood Flow Metab 3:425–431, 1983

Landau WM, Freygang WH Jr, Rowland LP et al: The local circulation of the living brain; values in the unanesthetized and anesthetized cat. Trans Am Neurol Assoc 80:125–129, 1955

Langfitt TW, Obrist WD, Alavi A et al: Computerized tomography, magnetic resonance imaging, and positron emission tomography in the study of brain trauma. J Neurosurg 64:760–767, 1986

Laruelle M, Baldwin RM, Rattner Z et al: SPECT quantification of [^{123}I]iomazenil binding to benzodiazepine receptors in nonhuman primates: I. Kinetic modeling of single bolus experiments. J Cereb Blood Flow Metab 14: 439–452, 1994a

Laruelle M, Van DC, Abi DA et al: Compartmental modeling of iodine-123-iodobenzofuran binding to dopamine D_2 receptors in healthy subjects. J Nucl Med 35:743–754, 1994b

Leenders KL, Perani D, Lammertsma AA et al: Cerebral blood flow, blood volume and oxygen utilization: normal values and effect of age. Brain 113:27–47, 1990

Leniger-Follert E, Hossman K-A: Simultaneous measurements of microflow and evoked potentials in the somatomotor cortex of rat brain during specific sensory activation. Pflügers Arch Eur J Physiol (Berlin), 380:85–89, 1979

Lou HC, Edvinsson L, MacKenzie ET: The concept of coupling blood flow to brain function: revision required? Ann Neurol 22:289–297, 1987

Marion DW, Darby J, Yonas H: Acute regional cerebral blood flow changes caused by severe head injuries. J Neurosurg 74:407–417, 1991

Martin WRW, Powers WJ, Raichle ME: Cerebral blood volume measured with inhaled $C^{15}O$ and positron emission tomography. J Cereb Blood Flow Metab 7:421–426, 1987

Masdeu JC, Brass LM, Holman BL, Kushner MJ: Brain single-photon emission computer tomography. Neurology 44:1970–1977, 1994

Mayberg HS: Functional brain scans as evidence in criminal court: an argument for caution. J Nucl Med 33: 18N–25N, 1992

Mazziotta JC, Phelps ME, Plummer D, Kuhl DE: Quantitation in positron computed tomography: 5. Physical-anatomical effects. J Comput Assist Tomogr 5:734–743, 1981

Mintun MA, Raichle ME, Martin WRW, Herscovitch P: Brain oxygen utilization measured with O-15 radiotracers and positron emission tomography. J Nucl Med 25:177–187, 1984

Muizelaar JP, Obrist WD: Cerebral blood flow and metabolism after severe head injury. pp. 47–79. In Stone JL (ed): Head Injury and Its Complications. PMA Publishing, Costa Mesa, CA, 1992

Murase K, Tanada S, Fujita H et al: Kinetic behavior of technetium-99m-HMPAO in human brain and quantification of cerebral blood flow using dynamic SPECT. J Nucl Med 33:135–143, 1992

Nakai H, Yamamoto YL, Diksic M et al: Time-dependent changes of lumped and rate constants in the deoxyglucose method in experimental cerebral ischemia. J Cerebr Blood Flow Metab 7:640–648, 1987

Nedd K, Sfakianakis G, Ganz W et al: ^{99m}Tc-HMPAO SPECT of the brain in mild to moderate traumatic brain injury patients: compared with CT—a prospective study. Brain Inj 7:469–479, 1993

Newton MR, Greenwood RJ, Britton KE et al: A study comparing SPECT with CT and MRI after closed head injury. J Neurol Neurosurg Psychiatry 55:92–94, 1992

Obrist WD, Langfitt TW, Jaggi J et al: Cerebral blood flow and metabolism in comatose patients with acute head injury. J Neurosurg 61:241–253, 1984

Oder W, Goldenberg G, Podreka I, Deecke L: HM-PAO-SPECT in persistent vegetative state after head injury: prognostic indicator of the likelihood of recovery. Intensive Care Med 17:149–153, 1991

Pelizzari CA, Chen GTY, Spelbring DR et al: Accurate three-dimensional registration of CT, PET, and/or MR images of the brain. J Comput Assist Tomogr 13:20–26, 1989

Perlmutter JW, Powers WJ, Herscovitch P et al: Regional asymmetries of cerebral blood flow, blood volume, oxygen utilization and extraction in normal subjects. J Cereb Blood Flow Metab 7:64–67, 1987

Phelps ME, Hoffman EJ: Resolution limit of positron cameras. J Nucl Med 17:757–758, 1976

Phclps ME, Huang SC, Hoffman EJ et al: Tomographic measurement of local cerebral glucose metabolic rate in humans with (F-18) 2-fluoro-2-deoxy-D-glucose: validation of method. Ann Neurol 6:371–388, 1979

Povlishock JT, Valadka AB: Pathobiology of traumatic brain injury. pp. 11–43. In Finlayson MAJ, Garner SH (eds): Brain Injury Rehabilitation: Clinical Considerations. Williams & Wilkins, Baltimore, 1994

Powers WJ: Positron emission tomography in the evaluation of cerebrovascular disease: clinical applications? In Theodore WH (ed): Clinical Neuroimaging. Alan R Liss, New York, 1988

Power WJ: Cerebral hemodynamics in ischemic cerebrovascular disease. Ann Neurol 29:231–240, 1991

Powers WJ, Berg L, Perlmutter JS, Raichle ME: Technology assessment revisited: does positron emission tomography have proven clinical efficacy? Neurology 41:1339–1340, 1991

Prayer L, Wimberger D, Oder W et al: Cranial MR imaging and cerebral ^{99m}Tc HM-PAO-SPECT in patients with subacute or chronic severe closed head injury and normal CT examinations. Acta Radiol 34:593–599, 1993

Raichle ME: Circulatory and metabolic correlates of brain function in normal humans. pp. 643–674. In Mountcastle VB, Plum F (eds): Handbook of Physiology. The Nervous System. American Physiological Society, Bethesda, MD, 1987

Raichle ME: The metabolic requirements of functional activity in human brain: a positron emission tomography study. pp. 1–4. In Vranic M, Efendic S, Hollenberg CH (eds): Fuel Homeostasis and the Nervous System. Plenum, New York, 1991

Raichle ME, Martin WRW, Herscovitch P et al: Brain blood flow measured with intravenous $H_2{}^{15}O$. II. Implementation and validation. J Nucl Med 24:790–798, 1983

Reivich M, Kuhl D, Wolf A et al: The [^{18}F]fluorodeoxyglucose method for the measurement of local cerebral glucose utilization in man. Circ Res 44:127–137, 1979

Rezai K, Kirchner PT, Armstrong C et al: Validation studies for brain blood flow assessment by radioxenon tomography. J Nucl Med 29:348–355, 1988

Richardson JTE: Clinical and Neuropsychological Effects of Closed Head Injury. Taylor & Francis, London, 1990

Roper SN, Mena I, King WA et al: An analysis of cerebral blood flow in acute closed-head injury using technetium-99m-HMPAO SPECT and computed tomography. J Nucl Med 32:1684–1687, 1991

Ruff RM, Buchsbaum MS, Tröster AI et al: Computerized tomography, neuropsychology, and positron emission tomography in the evaluation of head injury. Neuropsychiatry Neuropsychol Behav Neurol 2:103–123, 1989

Ruff RM, Crouch JA, Tröster AI et al: Selected cases of poor outcome following a minor brain trauma: comparing neuropsychological and positron emission tomography assessment. Brain Inj 8:297–308, 1994

Sasaki H, Kanno I, Murakami M et al: Tomographic mapping of kinetic rate constants in the fluorodeoxyglucose model using dynamic positron emission tomography. J Cereb Blood Flow Metab 6:447–454, 1986

Sokoloff L: Relationships among local functional activity, energy metabolism, and blood flow in the central nervous system. FASEB J 40:2311–2316, 1981

Sokoloff L: Basic principles in imaging of cerebral metabolic rates. pp. 21–49. In Sokoloff L (ed): Brain Imaging and Brain Function. Raven Press, New York

Sokoloff L, Reivich M, Kennedy C et al: The [^{14}C]deoxyglucose method for the measurement of local cerebral glucose utilization; theory, procedure, and normal values in the conscious and anesthetized albino rat. J Neurochem 28:897–916, 1977

Sorenson JA, Phelps ME: Physics in Nuclear Medicine. Grune & Stratton, Orlando, 1987

Spence AM, Graham MM, Muzi M et al: Deoxyglucose lumped constant estimated in a transplanted rat astrocytic glioma by the hexose utilization index. J Cereb Blood Flow Metab 10:190–198, 1990

Spinks TJ, Jones T, Bailey DL et al: Physical performance of a positron tomograph for brain imaging with retractable septa. Phys Med Biol 37:1637–1655, 1992

Stapleton SJ, Caldwell CB, Leonhardt CL et al: Determination of thresholds for detection of cerebellar blood flow deficits in brain SPECT images. J Nucl Med 35: 1547–1555, 1994

Subramanyam R, Alpert NM, Hoop B Jr et al: A model for regional cerebral oxygen distribution during continous inhalation of $^{15}O_2$, $C^{15}O$, and $C^{15}O_2$. J Nucl Med 19:13–53, 1978

Tenjin H, Ueda S, Mizukawa N et al: Positron emission tomographic studies on cerebral hemodynamics in patients with cerebral contusion. Neurosurgery 26: 971–979, 1990

Ter-Pogossian MM: The origins of positron emission tomography. Semin Nucl Med 22:140–149, 1992

Ter-Pogossian MM, Phelps ME, Hoffman EJ, Mullani NA: A positron-emission transaxial tomograph for nuclear imaging (PETT). Radiology 114:89–98, 1975

Tikofsky RS: Evaluating traumatic brain injury: correlating perfusion patterns and function. J Nucl Med 35:227, 1994a

Tikofsky RS: Predicting outcome in traumatic brain injury: what role for rCBF/SPECT? J Nucl Med 35:947–948, 1994b

Toga AW, Collins RC: Metabolic response of optic centers to visual stimuli in the albino rat: anatomical and physiological considerations. J Comp Neurol 199:443–464, 1981

Tyler JL, Strother SC, Zatorre RJ et al: Stability of regional cerebral glucose metabolism in the normal brain measured by positron emission tomography. J Nucl Med 29:631–642, 1988

Van Heertum, RL, Miller SH, Mosesson RE: SPECT brain imaging in neurologic disease. Radiol Clin North Am 31:881–907, 1993

Videen TO, Perlmutter JS, Herscovitch P, Raichle ME: Brain blood volume, flow, and oxygen utilization measured with ^{15}O radiotracers and positron emission tomography: revised metabolic computations. J Cereb Blood Flow Metab 7:513–516, 1987

Videen TO, Perlmutter JS, Mintun MA, Raichle ME: Regional correction of positron emission tomography data for the effects of cerebral atrophy. J Cereb Blood Flow Metab 8:662–670, 1988

Volkow N, Fowler JS: Neuropsychiatric disorders: investigation of schizophrenia and substance abuse. Semin Nucl Med 22:254–267, 1992

Wang G-J, Volkow ND, Wolf AP et al: Intersubject variability of brain glucose metabolic measurements in young normal males. J Nucl Med 35:1457–1466, 1994

Warner DS, Kassell NF, Boarini DJ: Microsphere cerebral blood flow determination. pp. 288–298. In Wood JH (ed): Cerebral Blood Flow: Physiologic and Clinical Aspects. McGraw-Hill, New York, 1987

Weiller C, Chollet F, Friston KJ et al: Functional reorganization of the brain in recovery from striatocapsular infarction in man. Ann Neurol 31:463–472, 1992

Wiedman KD, Wilson JTL, Wyper D et al: SPECT cerebral blood flow, MR imaging, and neuropsychological findings in traumatic head injury. Neuropsychology 3: 267–281, 1989

Wienhard K, Dahlbom M, Eriksson L et al: The ECAT EXACT HR: performance of a new high resolution positron scanner. J Comput Assist Tomogr 18:110–118, 1994

Wienhard K, Pawlik G, Herholz K et al: Estimation of local cerebral glucose utilization by positron emission tomography of [^{18}F]2-fluoro-2-deoxy-D-glucose: a critical appraisal of optimization procedures. J Cereb Blood Flow Metab 5:115–125, 1985

Wilson JTL, Wyper D: Neuroimaging and neuropsychological functioning following closed head injury: CT, MRI, and SPECT. J Head Trauma Rehab 7:29–39, 1992

Wilson MW, Mountz JM: A reference system for neuroanatomical localization on functional reconstructed cerebral images. J Comput Assist Tomogr 13:174–178, 1989

Wolf AP, Schlyer DJ: Accelerators for positron emission tomography. pp. 33–54. In Burns DH, Gibson RE, Dannals RF, Siegl PKS (eds): Nuclear Imaging in Drug Discovery Development and Approval. Birkhäuser, Boston, 1993

Woods RP, Mazziotta JC, Cherry SR: MRI-PET registration with automated algorithm. J Comput Assist Tomogr 17:536–546, 1993

Worley G, Hoffman JM, Paine SS et al: 18-Fluorodeoxyglucose positron emission tomography in children and adolescents with traumatic brain injury. Dev Med Child Neurol 37:213–220, 1995

Wyper DJ: Functional neuroimaging with single photon emission computed tomography (SPECT). Cerebrovasc Brain Metab Rev 5:199–217, 1993

Yamakami I, Yamaura A, Isobe K: Types of traumatic brain injury and regional cerebral blood flow assessed by ^{99m}Tc-HMPAO SPECT. Neurol Med Chir (Tokyo) 33:7–12, 1993

Yarowsky P, Kadekaro M, Sokoloff L: Frequency-dependent activation of glucose utilization in the superior cervical ganglion by electrical stimulation of cervical sympathetic trunk. Proc Nat Acad Sci USA 80:4179–4183, 1983

Yarowsky PJ, Ingvar DH: Neuronal activity and energy metabolism. FASEB J 40:2353–2362, 1981

The Electrophysiologic Evaluation of Head-Injured Patients: Value and Limitations

7

Jon Tippin
Thoru Yamada

Each year upward of 90,000 individuals will become chronically disabled because of head injuries (Goldstein, 1990). What is more, head injuries have become the leading cause of death in trauma centers around the country (Gennarelli et al., 1989). The impact of these injuries on the patients, their families, and society as a whole is particularly devastating because it is the young and potentially employable who are frequently affected (Dikmen et al., 1994). Depending on the severity of the injury, as many as 63 percent of surviving patients may be unable to return to work by 24 months after head trauma (Dikmen et al., 1994). To ensure that these patients are treated appropriately, an early and accurate assessment of cerebral function and prognosis for neurologic recovery is necessary.

The traditional means of assessing cerebral function in these patients include the clinical examination and neuropsychological batteries. Although the clinical evaluation is key, the Glasgow Coma Scale (GCS) may be an unreliable predictor of outcome in more severely affected patients because falsely pessimistic predictions occur commonly in this group (Karnaze et al., 1985; Gutling et al., 1995). Neuropsychological studies are frequently impossible to administer in the early postinjury period because of coma or other impairments that render the patient incapable of cooperating with the test. In an attempt to provide useful functional and prognostic information, the electroencephalogram (EEG) has also been used to study these patients. As early as 1940 Glaser and Sjaardema and Jasper et al. identified EEG abnormalities in traumatized patients, which commonly normalized as the patient recovered clinically. Later, studies using evoked potentials suggested that these techniques were useful in assessing the extent of cerebral injury, localizing areas of trauma, detecting complications (e.g., ischemia, metabolic derangements, and increased intracranial pressure) and establishing prognosis for neurologic recovery (Greenburg et al., 1977a; Greenberg et al., 1977b).

In this chapter we address the following questions:

1. What are the EEG and evoked potential patterns seen in head injury patients and how well do they assess the neurologic condition?
2. How effective are these procedures in predicting the long-term clinical outcome of these patients?
3. Do electrophysiologic studies confirm evidence of persistent neurologic dysfunction in patients with the postconcussive syndrome?
4. What additional information may be obtained by using sleep studies and quantitative EEG?
5. Perhaps most importantly, do these procedures provide information that cannot be obtained more reliably and accurately by other available means?

THE ROUTINE EEG

The EEG in the Setting of Acute Head Injury

Degree of EEG Abnormality in Relation to Severity of Head Trauma

Following an injury to the head, the EEG will show a large variety of patterns depending on the severity of injury, depth of coma, age of the patient, and time between trauma and recording of the EEG. Williams and Denny-Brown (1941) were the first to show experimentally that the initial EEG changes consist of immediate attenuation of cerebral activity, followed within seconds or minutes by generalized slow waves and eventually by return of normal electrical activity. In cases of mild head trauma, in which there has been little or no alteration of consciousness, the EEG is typically normal or shows subtle, nonspecific abnormalities; fewer than 20 percent of such patients have an abnormal record (Dow et al., 1944; Oshida et al., 1970; Yoshii et al., 1970). Hypersomnolence is common in this type of injury, and the EEG typically shows normal sleep patterns as these patients drift from wakefulness into drowsiness and sleep (Stockard et al., 1975). Children, however, tend to have a more abnormal EEG than would be anticipated by the relatively minor degree of trauma. In a study of 103 children with mild head injury, Liguori et al. (1989) found abnormal or borderline records in 52. The most common finding in this group was focal slow activity in the occipital regions followed by diffuse slowing. Karabudak et al (1992) compared the EEGs of 111 children with those of 21 adults with mild head injuries and linear skull fractures and found abnormalities in 61 percent of children but only 43 percent of adults. Again, abnormalities tended to consist of nonparoxysmal slow activity in the posterior quadrants. Similar results have been reported by Yoshii et al. (1970). Abnormalities such as these may persist for weeks or months following head injury despite normal consciousness (Stockard et al., 1975).

Older adults may also show a distinct EEG pattern in the acute setting following head trauma. In a study of 594 patients over the age of 50, Oshida et al. (1970) noted diffuse delta or alpha bursts in 50 percent and delta foci, primarily temporal, in 42.7 percent of abnormal records. These abnormalities tended to normalize rapidly; if not, an underlying structural lesion, such as intracerebral hemorrhage, was suspected. Yoshii et al. (1970) found abnormal records in 35.4% of patients over 50, findings that were intermediate between the findings in children (49.2 percent) and in young adults (23.8 percent). Again, older patients tended to have slow wave abnormalities that were either generalized or focal in the temporal regions. In any age group, the degree of abnormality tended to correlate with the duration of unconsciousness.

As the severity of head trauma increases, the EEG shows a greater degree of worsening and a more varied set of patterns. As a rule, there is good correlation between the EEG and depth of coma; progressive worsening of the EEG is associated with rostrocaudal deterioration (Rumpl et al., 1979). Table 7-1 shows the grading of these EEG abnormalities as proposed by Hockaday et al. (1965). In the mildest case, the

TABLE 7-1. EEG Grades

Grade	Description
Grade 1	Within normal limits Background activity consists of mostly alpha
Grade 2	Mildly abnormal Predominant theta activity with some alpha or delta
Grade 3	Moderately abnormal Predominant delta activity with minimal or no theta or alpha
Grade 4	Severely abnormal Burst suppression pattern
Grade 5	Extremely abnormal Nearly "flat" or electrocerebral silence

(Modified from Hockaday et al., 1965, with permission.)

EEG shows predominantly alpha activity with some intermixed theta. Patients in this stage are stuporous without abnormal motor activity. With increasing severity of head trauma, the EEG changes to primarily theta with some delta activity present (Fig. 7-1) and then to prominent high-voltage rhythmic and arrhythmic delta with less theta activity. Further clinical worsening is associated with diffuse, low-voltage delta activity. In the deepest stage of coma, in which the patient appears to be clinically brain dead, the EEG typically shows electrocerebral silence. This pattern of EEG deterioration has been described in head injury patients who have been studied serially as they progressed from higher midbrain syndromes to brain death (Rodin et al., 1965).

In addition to this relatively simple pattern of gradual slowing and amplitude reduction associated with progressive clinical worsening, a variety of other EEG patterns have been described in head injury patients. *Alpha coma,* as the name implies, is a pattern in which there is diffuse alpha activity that may be either reactive or unreactive to external stimuli (Westmoreland et al., 1975). The alpha activity tends to be maximal in the anterior regions and in some patients is seen superimposed on diffuse, small-amplitude delta. The *theta coma* pattern consists of intermittent rhythmic theta activity, maximal anteriorly, which is typically followed by periods of attenuation and may be superimposed upon diffuse delta activity. Like the alpha coma pattern, it may be either reactive or unreactive (Synek and Synek, 1984). A pattern with what appears to be typical stage II sleep elements has been referred to as *spindle coma* (Chatrain et al., 1963). Diffuse fast activity (8 to 15 Hz) has also been described (Loeb et al., 1959). Burst suppression, a pattern with prolonged intervals of markedly attenuated EEG activity interspersed with bursts of large amplitude, sharply contoured alpha, theta, and delta activity, is characteristically seen in deeply comatose, ventilator-dependent patients (Stockard et al., 1975). A variety of altered sleep patterns and epileptiform discharges may be seen in trauma; these are discussed below.

Focal EEG Abnormalities

Lateralizing signs on the EEG generally correlate well with the neurologic examination (Rumpl et al., 1979). These may consist of attenuated EEG activity, focal or hemispheric theta/delta activity, epileptiform discharges, and asymmetry of reactiivty (Courjon et al., 1971; Rumpl et al., 1979; Stockard et al., 1975). The presence of these lateralizing EEG patterns should alert the physician to the presence of a subdural, epidural, or intracerebral hematoma (Fig. 7-2). EEG attenuation and the presence of periodic lateralized epileptiform discharges (i.e., large-amplitude epileptiform discharges with a complex waveform lateralized to one hemisphere), have been attributed to subdural hematomas (Toyonaga et al., 1974). Usually, there is fairly good agreement between the EEG and the computed tomography (CT) scan (Synek, 1990b), but as noted earlier, children frequently have focal abnormalities that may not be associated with lesions visible on imaging studies. In the series reported by Liguori et al. (1989), asymmetric, diffuse slowing and focal slow-wave activity were seen in 39 of 103 children studied. CT showed extradural hematomas or cerebral contusions in only 10. Hence, especially in children, focal abnormalities on the EEG should be considered only suggestive of underlying structural pathology.

Role of Serial EEGs and EEG Monitoring

Serial EEG monitoring may provide clues to the presence of a variety of secondary complications. Metabolic derangements are more common in deeply comatose patients, in part owing to multiple organ trauma, and monitoring the EEG may alert the physican to the development of these (Courjon et al., 1971; Rumpl et al., 1979). Triphasic waves may be seen in coma from head trauma but are more frequently seen in metabolic encephalopathies (Bickford and Butt, 1955). The burst suppression pattern described earlier is probably seen only when there has been cerebral anoxia associated with the head injury (Stockard et al., 1975). Larson et al. (1973)

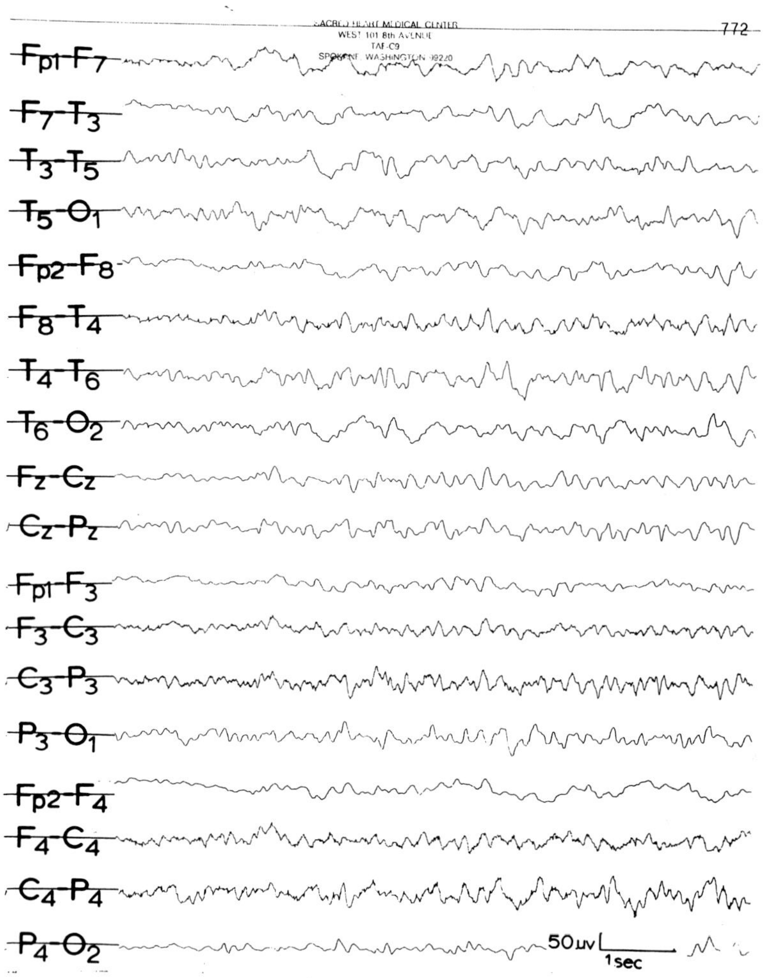

Fig. 7-1. EEG of a 45-year-old woman stuporous following head trauma. EEG shows slowing of background to 7 Ha with series of diffuse polymorphic delta activity.

have proposed continuous electrophysiologic monitoring as a means of identifying secondary ischemia due to increased intracranial pressure (ICP). However, it should be borne in mind that no specific EEG pattern has been consistently correlated with increased ICP (Munari and Calbucci, 1981). In a study of 73 patients admitted to an intensive care unit, five of whom had suffered a severe head injury, Jordan (1993) found continuous EEG monitoring to have a contributing impact on clinical management in four by identifying focal ischemia, diffuse hypoxia, and nonconvulsive seizures. EEG monitoring has been shown to be superior to following blood levels during pentobarbital coma for treatment of trauma-induced increased ICP (Winter et al., 1991). Serial EEGs may also be useful in following patients during therapeutic hyperventilation for increased ICP (Bricolo et al. 1972).

Epileptiform Activity

Isolated epileptiform activity (paraoxysmal bursts, sharps, spike and spike-wave discharges) are seen in a minority of patients (Courjon et al., 1971; Hutchinson et al., 1991; Rodin et al., 1965; Yoshii et al., 1970) and are poor predictors of subsequent epilepsy (Dusser et al., 1989). Such abnormalities are seen more frequently in children than in adults (Liguori et al., 1989; Yoshii et al., 1970). EEG seizure activity, consisting of runs of spikes and sharp waves, is seen early

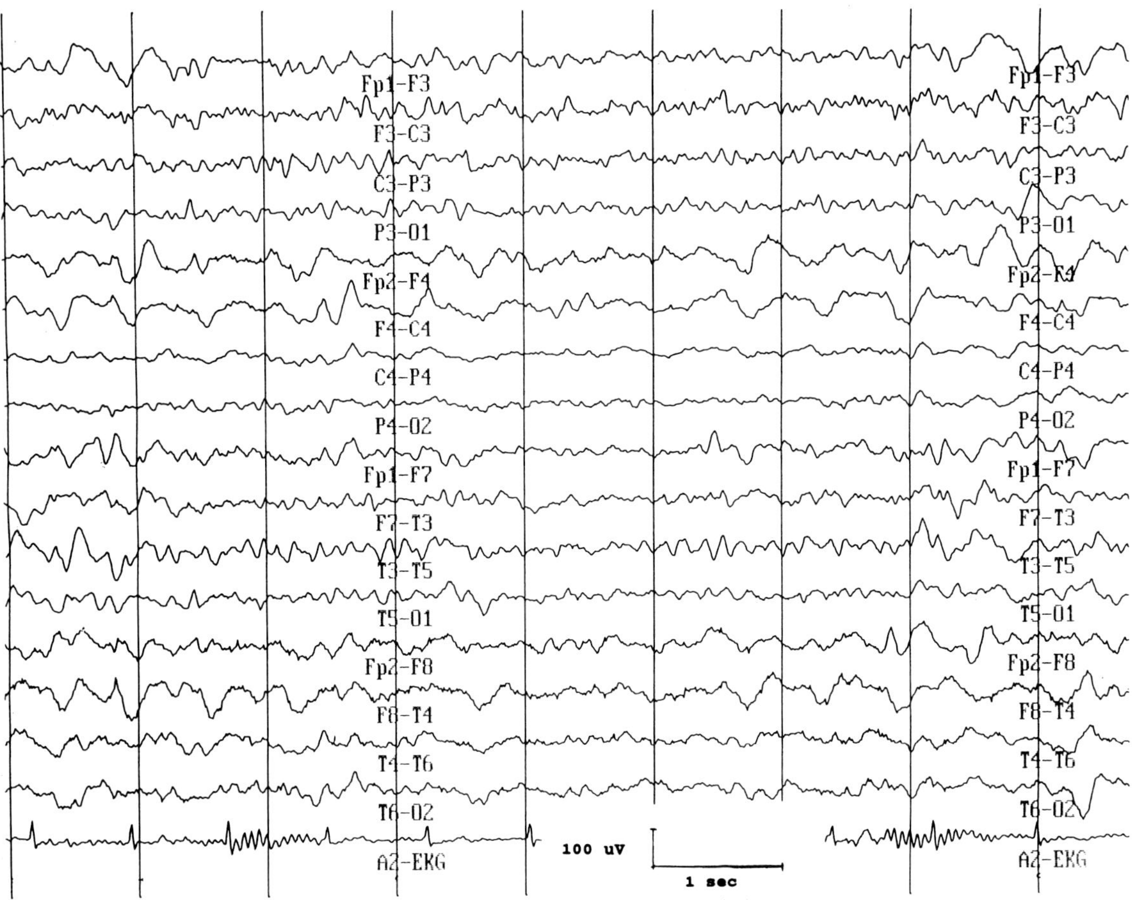

Fig. 7-2. EEG of a 32-year-old man with an acute right hemispheric subdural hematoma. Note attenuation of activity on the right associated with polymorphic delta activity most prominent in the right temporal area. In addition, there is diffuse theta-delta activity on both sides.

only in cases of severe trauma, and their presence may be of value in localizing a post-traumatic hematoma (Courjon and Scherzer, 1972). Also, the presence of focal seizure activity generally portends a worse outcome; mortality in such cases is three times that in cases without it (Stockard et al., 1975). A more involved discussion of post-traumatic epilepsy and associated EEG changes is found in Chapter 11.

Prognostic Value of EEG

One of the major uses proposed for EEG is in the prognostication of outcome of head-injured patients. In fact, EEG has been suggested by some authors to be superior to CT in determining outcome (Nau et al., 1979) and better than or equal to the clinical examination (Karnaze et al., 1982), although its usefulness has been questioned by others (De Bendedittis and Ettorre, 1974; Hutchinson et al., 1991). Unfortunately, there are as yet no data comparing EEG with magnetic resonance imaging (MRI) in this setting. Nau and Bock (1977) divided their patients into "survivors" and "nonsurvivors" based on the EEG. The surviving patients generally showed generalized polymorphic delta activity with some alpha and theta. After the third to fourth post-trauma day, the EEG showed an increase in background activity in these patients from 2 to 4 Hz, the appearance of faster activity (5 to 6 Hz), and some focal activity. Eventually, well organized alpha activity was seen. In those who did not survive, delta activity was persistent and there was a greater degree of disorganization. As the patient entered a terminal phase, there was progressive slowing and suppression of EEG activity. Prognosis was considered to be particularly poor if this pattern developed while the patient remained unchanged clinically. Dusser et al. (1989) found that if the EEG obtained after the third post-trauma day showed persistent, generalized delta ("slow monotonous" pattern), the duration of coma and period of awakening were longer and clinical outcome was poorer at 36 months after the inquiry. Also, a "prewakening" pattern on EEG (posterior hypersynchronous 2- to 3-Hz activity with anterior low voltage, fast activity) was always seen in those regaining consciousness. Both groups stressed the need for serial EEG recordings.

Attempts have also been made to predict outcome based upon a limited number of EEGs performed early in the patient's course. Synek (1990a, 1990b) devised an EEG rating scale based on that of Hockaday et al. (1965) (Table 7-1), which was expanded by including the presence or absence of reactivity, frontal rhythmic delta activity, epileptiform discharges, and alpha, theta, and spindle comas. Using survival and presence or absence of disability as end points, EEGs were divided into benign, malignant, and uncertain patterns as shown in Table 7-2. Benign patterns accurately predicted a good outcome; only 1 of 26 patients with this pattern was disabled at follow-up and none died. Most of the patients with uncertain patterns did well, but 20.2 percent of those with this pattern either died or were disabled at follow-up. All patients with a malignant pattern died. Reactivity (EEG desynchronization, attenuation, appearance of widespread delta or theta activity) was generally associated with a better outcome. Gutling et al. (1995) in fact found EEG reactivity to be highly predictive of outcome; 92 percent of their patients were correctly classified into good or bad outcome groups based on the presence or absence and type of reactivity. In contrast, Dusser et al. (1989) found no predictive value in EEG reactivity. Rae-Grant et al. (1991) devised a rating scale by using a variety of EEG patterns that have been ascribed prognostic significance by several authors, assigning them a weighted score based upon their perceived value, and placing them into a present or absent dichotomy. This scale was highly correlated with the patient's condition at discharge and showed good intra- and interobserver reproducibility.

Sleep-Wake Patterns

The notion that useful information can be obtained by observing sleep-wake patterns in the EEG of head-injury patients is supported by the fact that the mesencephalic-diencephalic region may be preferentially injured in these patients (Bergamasco et al., 1968). Hence, the preservation of normal-appearing sleep patterns would imply that functional integrity of these structures exists and that the degree of injury may be less severe than what is suggested clinically. The prognosis for recovery would be anticipated to be better if the severity of cerebral injury is less. By the same logic, sleep studies may be of value for localization; the presence of normal sleep elements in a comatose head-injury patient would suggest that the coma is primarily due to more rostral (i.e., telencephalic) injury (Bricolo et al., 1968).

The most commonly observed pattern in this setting consists of a predominance of stage II sleep,

TABLE 7-2. Interpretation of Benign, Uncertain, and Malignant Patterns Demonstrated on EEG

Frequency of Incidence	Benign	Uncertain	Malignant (if Persistent)
Frequent	Grade 1 Grade 2, (reactive)	Grade 2 (nonreactive) Grade 3, diffuse delta (reactive/nonreactive)	Low amplitude Grade 3 Burst suppression pattern (grade 4) Epileptiform discharges in grade 4 Low output EEG—grade 4 Isoelectric EEG—grade 5
Rare	Spindle pattern coma in grade 3 Frontal thythmic Delta grade 3 (reactive/ nonreactive)	Alpha Coma (reactive) Epileptiform discharges in grade 3	Alpha Pattern coma (nonreactive) Theta pattern coma

(From Synek, 1990b, with permission.)

with relatively less time spent in stages I, III, and IV (Bergamasco et al., 1968; Bricolo et al., 1968). Rapid eye movement (REM) time is typically decreased in these patients. In fact, REM is never seen except in the lightest level of coma (Bricolo et al., 1968). Ron et al. (1980) have also shown that a variety of other features may be seen: occasional large EEG and electromyographic (EMG) amplitudes in stage I; sporadic alpha bursts and an excessive amount of sleep spindles in stages II and III; abnormal EMG tremor in stage III; and fast waves, occasional spindles, and excessive EMG activity in stage IV. Fewer than normal eye movements may be seen in REM sleep, with excessive EMG activity and high-voltage, slow-wave bursts, which should not be present during that stage. In severely traumatized patients, it is common for there to be no discernible sleep stages; in these cases the night time EEG consists of either generalized slowing and hypersynchronization or diffusely attenuated activity with bursts of 4 to 6 Hz "sawtooth waves" in the frontocentral regions associated with REMs (Bergamasco et al., 1968).

As the coma resolves, there is a gradual, although frequently incomplete, normalization of these abnormalities (Bricolo et al., 1968; Ron et al., 1980). George and Landau-Ferey (1986) noted that even at 1 year after head injury, patients tend to have abnormally decreased amount of REM sleep and increased intrasleep arousals. These abnormalities persist regardless of the severity of the original trauma or the presence of residual neurologic deficits.

Whether or not the presence of sleep spindles provides any prognostic information is controversial. Spindles have been shown by several authors to be a frequent finding in early coma and their numbers have been found to steadily subside with subsequent recordings regardless of outcome (Chatrian et al., 1963; Courjon et al., 1971). However, Rumpl et al. (1983) have stressed that attention to the timing of the recording and noting of any atypical features may provide useful information. In their study, spindles were seen in the acute stage of coma in all patients who eventually made a good recovery. In later recordings, the proportion of spindles declined, but the waveforms remained typical and there was little asymmetry. Among patients who were left with moderate disability, spindles still occurred in 90 percent, but there were more atypical and asymmetric forms. Spindles that were fewer in number, asymmetric, and more atypical in appearance were seen in those who subsequently died or were severely disabled as follow-up.

Bergamasco et al. (1968) found that 13 of their 20 head-injured patients who had near-normal appearing sleep patterns on all-night polygraphic studies survived (no comment made about the quality of survival). However, the remaining seven patients who did not have sleep patterns eventually died. These authors considered that all-night recordings were superior to routine daytime EEGs. Bricolo et al. (1968), in contrast, could not demonstrate a consistent relationship between the degree of sleep pattern disorganization and outcome. However, it was noted that completely normal sleep patterns were never seen in those persisting in a severely comatose state. Ron et al. (1980) concluded that observing the sleep–wake cycle was not valuable for prognostication, but they did note that persisting REM abnormalities seen at follow-up correlated closely with cognitive deficits. The issue of post-traumatic sleep disturbances is further addressed in Chapter 12.

The EEG in the Late Post–Head Injury Stage

Recovery from Acute Head Injury

In those patients who recover from their head injury, the EEG typically shows a gradual increase in frequencies and the ultimate development of a reactive, posterior dominant alpha rhythm (Stockard et al., 1975). In adults this period of normalization may take days or a few weeks to occur, but in children the EEG may remain abnormal for many months or years (Kellaway, 1955). Focal abnormalities similarly show a pattern of improvement from delta to theta, and focal alpha activity may be replaced in time by a region of attenuated activity (Courjon and Scherzer, 1972). If persistent slowing is seen later in the patient's course, a fixed structural lesion, such as an intracerebral hematoma, may be present (Oshida et al., 1970). Nevertheless, focal abnormalities typically resolve more slowly than generalized ones even when no structural pathology exists (Courjon and Scherzer, 1972). Late in recovery there is less correlation between EEG abnormalities and the clinical examination than is seen in the acute period. Except in the most severely injured, abnormal EEGs tend to normalize regardless of clinical outcome (Courjon and Scherzer, 1972). This may reflect the relative insensitivity of the EEG in detecting pathology in subcortical structures, where trauma-induced diffuse axonal injury, a major cause of persisting disability, predominates (Gennarelli et al., 1982).

In those patients who make a poor recovery and are left in an apallic state, the EEG typically shows a monotonous pattern with a predominance of theta and delta activity, occasionally markedly attenuated records, and a loss of normal sleep patterns, especially spindles (Bricolo et al., 1968; Rumpl et al., 1983; Strnad and Strnadova, 1987). Prognostication based upon the EEG is characteristically problematic in this group, but those patients whose EEG shows an increase in frequency to faster rhythms and an alpha-like coma generally improve. Those with persistent delta activity or a rapid decrease in delta with apparent "normalization" unaccompanied by clinical improvement do poorly. In addition, those patients who show no improvement in their EEGs by 3 years typically show no further improvement in later recordings (Strnad and Strnadova, 1987). Focal EEG abnormalities have been reported in as many as 95 percent of patients with a prolonged post-traumatic amnestic syndrome lasting 1 week to 8 months (Koufen and Hagel, 1987). These abnormalities consist of intermittent temporal delta activity in most patients, while a persistent "delta focus" is seen in less than 10 percent. Normalization occurs within 3 months in 48 percent of these patients, while 22 percent still have focal abnormalities more than 2 years later. Generalized slowing is consistently seen during the period of amnesia, which tends to normalize as the amnesia clears. The majority of foci are bilateral; there is no support for the previously held notion that left-sided foci are more common in patients with post-traumatic amnesia.

Postconcussive Syndrome

In a number of patients who recover from the acute injury, symptoms of the postconcussive syndrome develop: headache, disequilibrium, sleep disturbances, depression, and complaints of cognitive impairment (Binder 1986; Jacome and Risko 1984). The EEG has been reported by some authors to show frequent abnormalities in these patients. Denker and Perry (1954) found that 50 percent of their patients who had their EEGs within 3 months of head trauma were abnormal. In those whose EEG was performed more than 3 months after trauma, 58 percent were abnormal, with 35 percent showing focal abnormalities while diffuse symmetrical abnormalities were seen in 17%, diffuse asymmetric changes in 3 percent, and amplitude asymmetries in another 3 percent. Torres and Shapiro (1961) studied 90 patients with either head trauma or whiplash injuries without head injury or loss of consciousness. The frequency of postconcussive symptoms was similar in the two groups. They found EEG abnormalities (either generalized or focal) in 44 percent of the head injury patients and in 46 percent of those with only whiplash. Rather difficult to explain are the findings that epileptiform discharges were seen more frequently in the whiplash group than in those who had suffered a direct blow to the head and that the follow-up EEGs were not uncommonly more abnormal than those performed initially. It should be noted that, like the report by Denker and Perry (1954), this study has several methodologic limitations; it was done before the era of CT and none of the patients had corroborating neuropsychological testing, and the results were not compared with those of a matched control group.

Using more rigidily defined criteria for abnormality than earlier investigators and recording both standard and 24-hour ambulatory EEGs, Jacome and Risko (1984) found no significant abnormalities in 54 patients with the postconcussive syndrome. They did note nonspecific paroxysmal abnormalities in three patients and specific focal or generalized epileptiform discharges in two. However, the EEG pattern in these patients appeared to be chronic in nature and probably predated the head injuries. Haglund and Persson (1990) studied 47 amateur boxers and compared the EEG findings in this cohort with a group of 50 soccer players and track-and-field athletes. Not only did they fail to find a significant difference in the frequency of EEG abnormalities in the two groups, but they were also unable to find a correlation between EEG abnormalities and such indirect measures of repetitive trauma as the numbers of lost fights and knockouts and the duration of boxing careers. Sulg and Dencker (1968) studied monozygotic twins discordant for head injury and found a high concordance rate in the twin pairs regardless of whether the EEG was abnormal or not. In addition, they were unable to find a correlation between EEG abnormalities and the twin who had suffered a blow to the head. Hence, it appears that the routine EEG is probably of little benefit in evaluating patients with remote mild head injuries or the postconcussive syndrome.

Reliability of EEG Interpretation

The degree to which an EEG may be clinically useful in the evaluation of head-injured patients is largely determined by the accuracy of its interpretation. This accuracy has been shown to be dependent upon the competency and experience of the electroencephalographer; those with board certification, more full-time EEG training, and more time spent in an active EEG laboratory interpret EEGs more accurately (Williams et al., 1985). In addition, EEG tracings typically include electrical activities of noncerebral origin that may mimic genuine cerebral activity and easily mislead the less experienced electroencephalographer. These artifacts can be of either physiologic or nonphysiologic origin (e.g., eye movements and electrode artifacts, respectively). Head and body movements occasionally create artifacts that resemble epileptiform activity or ictal discharges. Technical modifications, such as filter and sensitivity (amplifier gain) changes, can alter EEG patterns; for example, muscle twitch artifacts may be mistaken for spikes when a low-pass filter (high-frequency filter) of 15 Hz is used. Capable EEG technologists can contribute to better records and more accurate interpretations by identifying and minimizing these potentially confusing artifacts and technical factors. There are also EEG patterns that resemble epileptiform activity but are clinically insignificant. These include benign epileptiform transients of sleep ("small sharp spikes"), 6-Hz spike-waves ("phantom spike-waves"), 14- and 6-Hz positive spikes, and the rhythmic midtemporal theta of drowsiness. Experienced electroencephalographers distinguish these variables by visually characterizing a given EEG event by its waveform, potential field distribution, polarity, and timing in relation to the patient's level of consciousness. Even a computer cannot compete with the eyes of an experienced electroencephalographer and, as will be discussed later, may even confuse the interpretation further (Nuwer, 1990).

Conclusions

Whenever EEG clinical correlations are attempted, one must bear in mind that EEG changes in these patients can neither support nor exclude the presence of persisting nervous system dysfunction. This is particularly pertinent in those with milder degrees of trauma and those with the postconcussive syndrome. Prominent EEG abnormalities seen in these patients may have no relationship to head trauma, and a normal EEG does not rule out significant cerebral injury. In more severe injuries, serial EEGs are useful in the acute stage for determining the clinical course of brain recovery or deterioration and for predicting outcome. In contrast to what is seen in the acute setting, however, prognostication with the assistance of the EEG in later stages is fraught with considerable difficulties.

QUANTITATIVE EEG

Strictly speaking, the term *quantitative EEG* refers to a technique by which EEG activity is either displayed or analyzed following conversion of the raw EEG signal into a series of numerical values. The process is accomplished by feeding the amplified EEG analog signals to a digital converter, the output of which may be kept in its digital form for additional mathematical analysis or may be displayed graphically. The techniques discussed in this section are frequency spectral analysis by compressed spectral array (CSA) and topographic brain mapping. In the former process, the digitized EEG activity is displayed as a power spectrum showing the absolute or relative amplitudes of various frequencies of which the recorded EEG is composed. The mathematical process used to accomplish this is fast Fourier transformation. The displayed activity shows the distribution of frequencies in a prescribed period of time (e.g., 8 seconds), with each subsequent epoch stacked vertically to produce the CSA. The process by which brain mapping is produced is essentially the same, but an additional step is taken in which the amplitudes of the recorded EEG for a specific frequency band are displayed graphically as a topographic map. Blocks of amplitude ranges are displayed as different colors over a representation of the scalp. The purported benefits of these procedures include the ability to detect abnormalities not apparent with other techniques (particularly the routine EEG) and the improvement of long-term monitoring by eliminating seemingly unnecessary information, thus which makes the data of interest clearer by simplifying what is being seen and reduces the amount of data to be analyzed and stored (Nuwer, 1990).

Applications

Acute Head Injury

A number of authors have reported benefits of using the CSA to determine prognosis in patients with acute head injury. Bricolo et al. (1979) showed that if the CSA was characterized by a predominance of monotonous slow activity with a fixed frequency, mortality was 86 percent. If there was a fluctuating, changeable pattern or if a sleep-like pattern was recorded, death occurred in 41.3 and 13.3 percent respectively. Steudel and Kruger (1979) noted that the best indicator of survival was an increase in the amplitude of the parieto-occipital alpha and theta activities. They concluded that they could accurately predict outcome in 40 (80 percent) of the 50 severely head-injured patients they studied. Similar findings were noted by Strnad and Strnadova (1987), who also found that the predictive value of the alpha and theta spectra was often apparent by the second to third post-trauma day. Additional benefit may be realized by monitoring the EEG response to thiopental by CSA. Klein et al. (1988) noted that none of their survivors showed a general reduction in activity (especially alpha and beta) in response to the barbiturate, whereas the majority of nonsurvivors did. Conversely, all but 1 of 23 surviving patients showed an enhancement of beta activity. Of 17 patients who died, 3 showed this pattern, but they died of complications such as pneumonia rather than as a direct result of their head injury. Thus, these authors found a 100 percent correlation between lack of EEG response to thiopental and death, whereas accentuation correctly predicted a good outcome in 84 percent.

In terms of the predictive value of CSA in relation to the clinical examination, Hakkinen et al. (1988) showed a poor correlation between CSA and the GCS. They considered that CSA was better at predicting less severely injured patients, while GCS was more accurate in predicting those who died. Hence, a combination of the two techniques may be most useful. Karnaze et al. (1982) found that the GCS predicted outcome correctly in two patients in whom the CSA had been incorrect and that CSA identified three cases that were incorrectly predicted by GCS. Again, the suggestion was made that assessment of outcome by clinical examination and CSA are complementary. CSA has also been shown to be superior to the routine EEG in accurately predicting outcome in the acute setting by at least one group (Bricolo et al., 1979).

Chronic Stage After Head Injury

In patients with the postconcussive syndrome, CSA has been reported to show a shift of both alpha and beta activity to lower frequencies regardless of whether or not the patient actually suffered loss of consciousness (Tebano et al., 1988). The EEG was shown to be less able to detect these subtle frequency changes but was superior to CSA in identifying paroxysmal theta bursts. Using an analysis of coherence and phase, Thatcher et al. (1989) found an increase in coherence and a decrease in phase in the frontal and frontotemporal regions, a decrease in power differences between anterior and posterior regions, and a decrease in posterior alpha power. These abnormalities were noted within a few hours or days and showed very little decline over an extended period of observation. They speculated that these findings correlated with shear-strain and rotational white matter damage and localized gray matter contusions, although no imaging or pathologic information was reported. Thatcher et al. also believed that the 80 to 95 percent discriminant accuracy of these techniques compared favorably with the reported accuracy of neuropsychological studies.

Brain mapping has been reported by Jerrett and Corsak (1988) to be superior to routine EEG in head-injured patients,. In eight head injured patients, mapping was normal in four, all of whose EEGs were normal. However, abnormal brain maps were seen in four patients, only two of whom also showed abnormalities on routine EEG. The EEG most frequently missed low-amplitude slow activity. Another study of 135 patients who were evaluated by brain mapping several years after head injury showed abnormalities, mostly in the temporo-occipital regions, in 56 percent. In contrast, the routine EEG was abnormal in only 30 percent and consisted mostly of nonspecific, diffuse slowing (Hooshmand et al., 1989). However, Haglund and Persson (1990) found no additional benefit of CSA and brain mapping over routine EEG in boxers.

Conclusions

CSA appears to be of benefit in evaluating patients in the acute setting, especially if long-term monitoring is being used to assess prognosis. In later stages, CSA may also be helpful, particularly when more advanced techniques, such as analyses of coherence and phase, are used. Brain mapping is also suggested to be helpful in evaluating postconcussive syndrome cases. However, a word of caution is needed. Quantitative EEG recordings must be interpreted along with the routine EEG for accurate detection of common artifacts (electrocardiographic, electromyographic, eye blinks, and the like), which may not be obvious when looking at CSA or brain mapping alone. Also CSA is unable to recognize transient phenomena such as spikes or bursts. Therefore, rather than making analysis easier, there is an additional level of complexity inherent in the interpretation of these studies, and a firm understanding of routine EEG interpretation is still required of those reading them (Nuwer, 1990). As pointed out by Epstein (1994), the routine use of these techniques in head-injured patients should be discouraged. The medicolegal studies he reviewed were frequently flawed by poor technique, by misinterpretation of drowsiness, sleep, and medication effects as evidence of abnormality, and by misapplication of statistical analyses. The value of quantitative EEG in this setting has yet to be established.

EVOKED POTENTIALS

Evoked potentials (EPs) are generated in response to a repetitive sensory stimulus; with computer-assisted averaging, the desired signal is enhanced while unwanted background EEG signals and artifacts are suppressed. Visual, auditory, and somatosensory stimuli are the sensory modalities typically used. They are divided into short-, middle-, and long-latency responses, depending on the time period following the stimulus at which the potentials are recorded. For visual EP (VEP), responses within the first 200 ms are usually analyzed. Auditory EPs (AEPs) are divided into short-latency responses for those observed in the first 10 to 12 ms, middle for those seen between 12 and 50 ms, and long for those recorded more than 50 ms after the stimulus. Short-latency somatosensory EPs (SEPs) are those recorded in the first 25 to 30 ms after the stimulus, while long-latency responses occur later. VEP, middle- and long-latency AEP, and SEP peaks are usually named according to the polarity of the response (expressed as P for positive and N for negative), followed by the mean latency of that response (in milliseconds) recorded from normal controls (e.g., the P100 response of the VEP). The terminology used for the short-latency AEPs, which are commonly designated as brainstem auditory evoked potentials (BAEPs), is different; peaks are simply designated I through V.

Neural Generators of Short-Latency EPs

Although some controversy still remains, the neural generators for the short-latency EPs are known with a fair degree of certainty. The striate and peristriate occipital cortices appear to generate the P100 potential of the VEP when a pattern reversal stimulus is used. However, when a flash is used to stimulate the visual pathways, as is often the case in the acute postinjury phase, a more complex waveform is produced, which may be generated by a variety of cortical projection systems (Allison et al., 1977). Earlier BAEP studies proposed specific anatomic sites along the auditory pathway for the origins of waves I through V (I, auditory nerve; II, cochlear nucleus; III, superior olivary nucleus; IV, lateral lemniscus; V, inferior colliculus). More recently, the specificity of these anatomic origins has been questioned. At present, the consensus is that wave I correlates with the medulla, waves II and III with the lower pons, and waves IV and V with the upper pons and midbrain (Fig. 7-3). The origins of the various peaks of the SEP are dependent on the recording sites (Fig. 7-4, Table 7-3). The earliest potentials recorded following median nerve stimulation at the wrist originate in the brachial plexus (N9) and cervical spinal roots (N11). Later waves are produced in the cervical cord (N13), medial lemniscus (P13/14), and parietal cortex (N20). When recorded from ipsilateral central or from frontal electrodes, the subthalamic- or brainstem-originated N18 is recorded. The generators for the middle- and late-latency SEPs are more controversial but may include thalamocortical projections and primary and secondary cortical association areas (Yamada et al., 1984; Yamada et al., 1985; Mauguiere et al., 1983).

Long-Latency Responses

Short-latency responses are generally more stable and reliable, as they are less susceptible to the effects of sedatives or the patient's level of consciousness and show less inter- and intraindividual variability (Allison, 1965; Goff et al., 1966). However, as discussed below, several investigators have relied on these middle- and long-latency responses to evaluate head-injury patients. Latency and interpeak intervals have also been shown to be more reliable than an analysis of amplitude and waveform although the latter have been frequently used in the studies discussed below. However, computer-assisted analysis of these parameters has been suggested to be a more sensitive and reliable means of evaluating EP abnormalities in head-injured patients (Alter et al., 1990).

EP Studies in the Acute Postinjury Setting

Clinical Correlates

One of the values claimed for EPs is their ability to evaluate patients who are deeply comatose, under the influence of sedative and paralyzing medications,

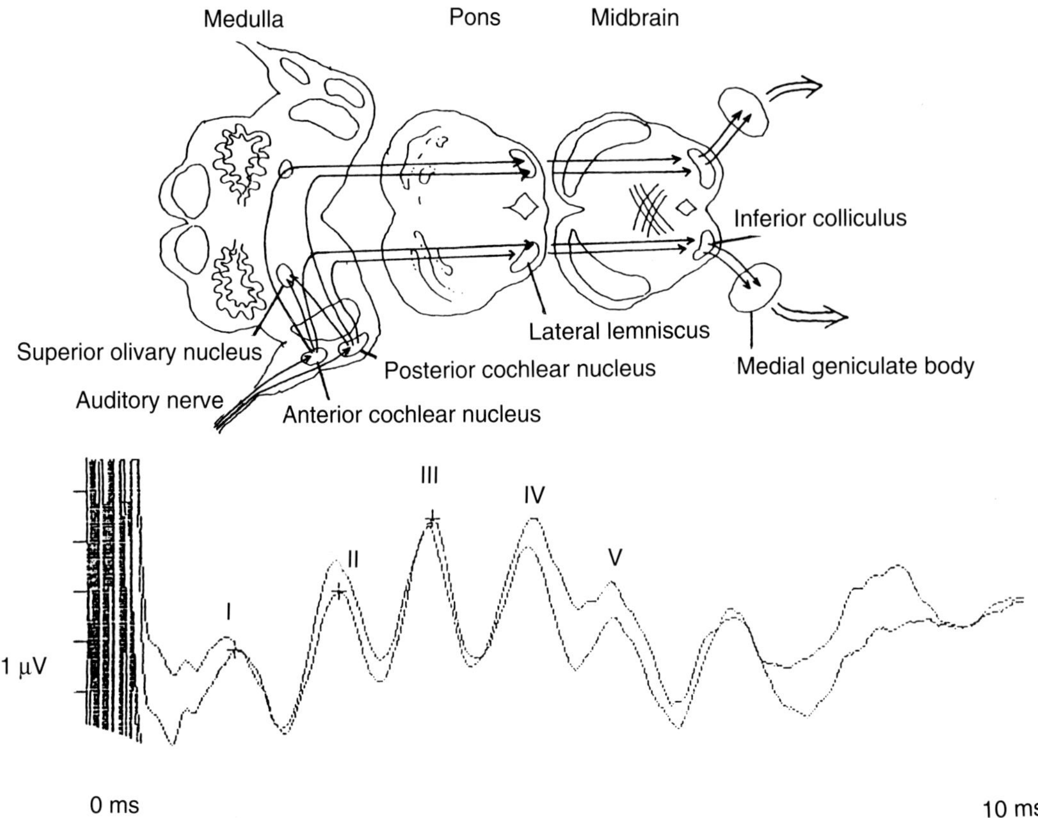

Fig. 7-3. Presumed generators of the short-latency BAEP. As discussed in the text, the specificity of these anatomic sites has been questioned.

or otherwise difficult to examine. Hence, EPs may provide a means of assessing the clinical status of such patients. BAEPs, and to a lesser degree SEPs, have been shown to correlate with the oculocephalic

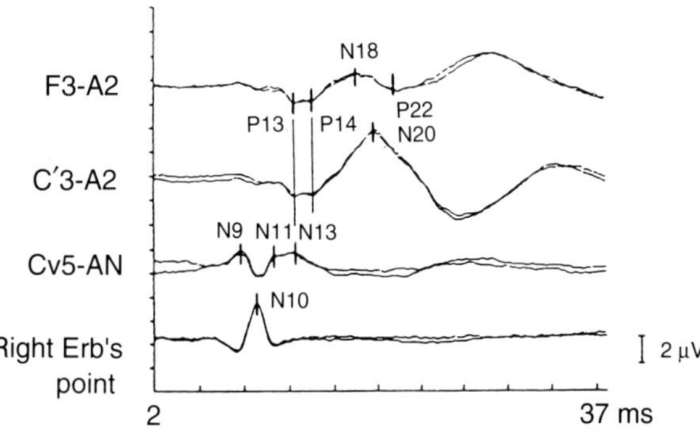

Fig. 7-4. Normal short-latency median SEP, right median nerve stimulation. Recording sites and presumed anatomic origins listed in Table 7-3.

reflex and pupillary light responses (Greenberg et al., 1977a; Karnaze et al., 1985). VEPs, SEPs, and middle- and long latency AEPs (but not BAEPs) have been correlated with the presence or absence of posturing (Greenberg et al., 1977a). The overall level of consciousness, as assessed by the GCS or similar measures, may also be reflected by EP abnormalities, especially the long-latency components (Greenberg et al., 1977b; Rappaport et al., 1981). However, it should be recalled that these components are susceptible to the sedative effects of medications, which makes it impossible to distinguish medication effects from those caused by the brain injury itself.

Localizing Value

Because EPs assess discrete sensory pathways, specific abnormal patterns may indicate focal cerebral lesions unsuspected by CT or the clinical examination (Cusumano et al., 1992). Using correlations with lesions confirmed pathologically, intraoperatively, or by CT

TABLE 7-3. Anatomic Origins of Short-Latency Median Nerve SEPs

	Recording Sites	Anatomic Origins
N9	Posterior neck (Cv5) to anterior neck	Distal brachial plexus
N10	Erb's point	Brachial plexus
N11	Posterior neck (Cv5) to anterior neck	Entry to cervical cord
N13	Posterior neck (Cv5) to anterior neck	Cervical cord
P13/P14	Scalp to noncephalic or ear	Brainstem/ medial lemniscus
N18	Frontal electrode to ear	Subthalamus, brainstem
P22	Frontal electrode to ear	Supplemental motor cortex
N20	Parietal (contralateral) to ear	Sensory cortex

and angiography, Greenberg et al. (1977a) found that SEPs were useful in localizing parietal lesions, while AEPs localized focal lesions in the temporal areas. VEPs could identify occipital lesions if the electroretinogram was used to exclude retinal pathology. When multiple scalp electrodes are used simultaneously to record SEP, a differential effect on the frontal N30 to P45 peaks from those recorded in the parietal areas may indicate predominant frontal lobe injury (Cusumano et al., 1992). Preferential brainstem injury may be suggested by preserved VEPs with abnormal BAEPs and by SEPs (N20 and later peaks). On the other hand, the cerebral hemisphere may be the primary site of injury when VEPs and cortical SEPs are abnormal while BAEPs and subcortical SEPs (P14, N18) are unaffected, although the issue remains unsettled (Ganes and Lundar, 1988; Greenberg et al., 1977a). It should be borne in mind, however, that because EPs assess discrete sensory pathways, considerable damage that will not be identified by these techniques may occur in areas through which EPs are not transmitted.

Prognostic Value

Perhaps the most useful role for EP studies in acute head injury is in predicting outcome. Although methods of assessing outcome have varied somewhat from one study to the next, a global assessment is typically used, patients with poor outcome being those who have died or been left severely disabled or in a persistent vegetative state. VEPs have generally been disappointing in this regard (Anderson et al., 1984; Firsching and Frowein, 1990; Greenberg et al., 1977a; Rappaport et al., 1981). This is in part due to technical difficulties in performing these studies in many head-injured patients and because they tend to be relatively insensitive to the patient's clinical status, showing abnormalities only in the most severely injured (Anderson et al., 1984). Their predictive value may be increased if considered along with other studies such as AEPs (Rappaport et al., 1981) or if the results are subjected to a computerized analysis of amplitude variability (Alter et al., 1990.)

The results from BAEP studies have been conflicting. Cant et al. (1986) found no correlation between BAEPs and outcome. Greenberg et al. (1977a) found no correlation with studies in the early postinjury period but did find BAEPs predictive if performed a mean of 14 days afterwards. Others have reported that as many as 40 percent of severely head-injured patients with normal or mildly abnormal BAEP studies will not survive (Anderson et al., 1984; Firsching and Frowein, 1990). On the other hand, Karnaze et al. (1985) reported BAEPs to be highly correlated with a favorable or unfavorable outcome, and these investigators found no falsely pessimistic predictions. Long-latency AEPs were also highly correlated with outcome but were falsely pessimistic in 7 of 39 patients. Rappaport et al. (1981) found that while BAEPs were not predictive of outcome, long-latency (not middle-latency) AEPs correctly predicted outcome, possibly because late components are sensitive to the level of consciousness. Alter et al. (1990) found that a computer-assisted analysis of AEPs was able to predict outcome and was particularly helpful in differentiating those patients who were left severely disabled from those who died or were left in a persistent vegetative state.

SEPs have been shown to be superior in predicting outcome to VEPs and AEPs, ICP monitoring, and CT by several investigators (Anderson et al., 1984; Cant et al. 1986; Cusumano et al., 1992; Firsching and Frowein, 1990; Greenberg et al., 1977a; Greenberg et al., 1982; Rappaport et al., 1981). Anderson et al. (1984) found that SEPs misjudged outcome in only 2 of 23 cases that they studied. These two patients had normal SEPs but poor outcome, one being left severely disabled while the other died. Firsching and Frowein (1990) found that 26 percent of patients with normal SEPs died, whereas the mortality was 45 percent for those with mild or moderate SEP abnormalities and 95 percent for those with completely absent responses. They noted that those patients with normal SEPs who died did so from delayed complications, such as gastrointestinal hemorrhage, septicemia, and cerebral infarction. Similar findings have been reported by others (Greenberg et al., 1981; Greenberg et al., 1982). Cusumano et al. (1992) recorded SEPs from frontal, central, and parietal electrodes and found the latency of the parietal P25 to be significantly correlated with outcome if recorded within the first 72 hours. Recordings made after the second week, however, demonstrated the superiority of the frontal N30–P45 amplitude in predicting outcome. They hypothesized that the superiority of the frontal recorded potentials lay in the predilection of this region of the brain to trauma (Fig. 7-5). The value of recording long-latency SEPs was stressed by Greenberg et al. (1982); long latencies correctly predicted outcome in 88 percent while short-latency responses were correct in only 58 percent of cases. Normal long-latency responses may also predict a good outcome in patients with intracranial hematomas who require surgery (Greenberg et al., 1981). In contrast to the ability of SEPs to predict global outcome, their value in predicting recovery of focal clinical deficits is unsettled (Cant et al., 1986; Greenberg et al, 1977a).

Multimodality Evoked Potentials

The evaluation of prognosis by multimodality evoked potentials (MEPs), in which a combined score is made for the three stimulus modalities, may provide additional information. Rappaport et al. (1981)

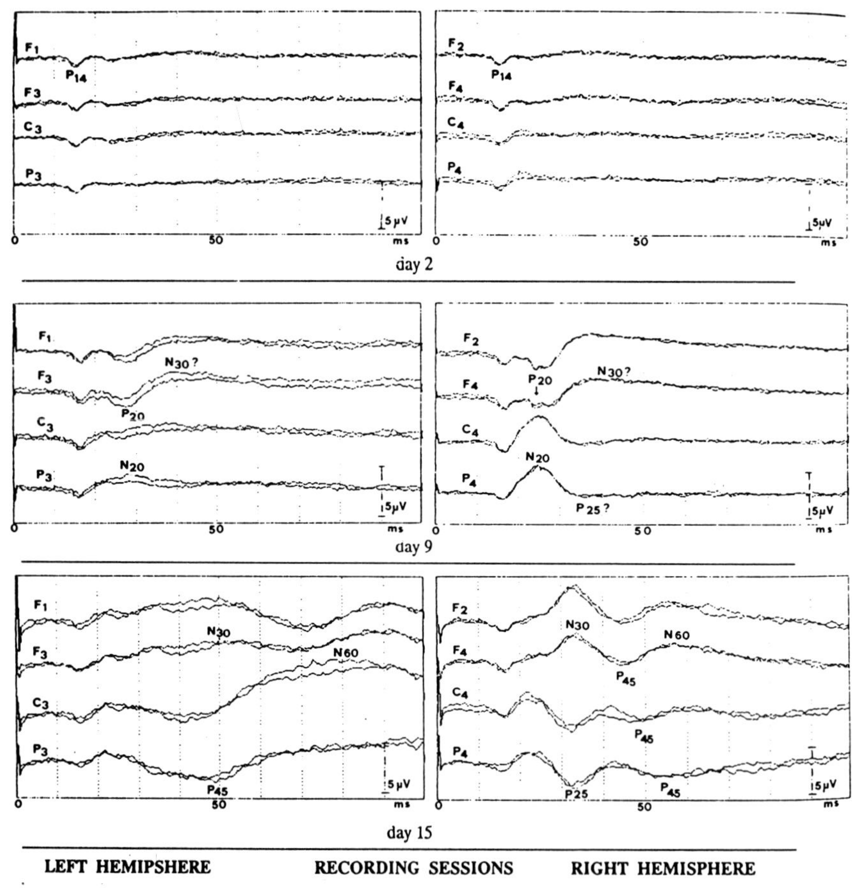

Fig. 7-5. SEP of a 22-year-old patient with bilateral orbital frontal contusions. Note diminished amplitude on the left, where single-photon emission tomography (SPECT) showed reduced regional uptakes unaccompanied by lateralized abnormalities on CT. On sequential recordings from the second to the fifteenth day, bilateral reappearance of frontal N30 predicted a favorable prognosis. (From Cusumano et al., 1992, with permission.)

found that the combined score of abnormalities for AEPs, VEPs, and SEPs was superior to the results of any one modality alone. Greenberg et al. (1981) found that 81 percent of patients with normal or mildly abnormal MEPs returned to normal functioning or were only moderately disabled at 1 year after injury. Likewise, 76 percent of the patients with severely abnormal MEPs had died or were left severely disabled. They also noted that those patients with normal MEPs were ''well on the way to ultimate recovery'' by 3 to 6 months. Those with more severe MEP abnormalities took longer to recover and required more intensive rehabilitation. However, in a later report by the same group (Greenberg et al., 1982) no difference was found between the predictive value of combined studies and SEPs alone.

EPs in Comparison with Clinical Assessments

One of the main questions to be answered is whether EPs provide any additional benefit relative to the clinical examination. As compared with the GCS, EPs (especially SEPs) have been shown to be superior in predicting outcome (Cusumano et al., 1992; Greenberg et al., 1982). Karnaze et al. (1985) found that BAEPs were better for prognostication than the GCS because only the former had no falsely pessimistic predictions. Cant et al. (1986) found the GCS to be predictive of outcome for patients at the extremes of the scale, but for those patients in the middle range SEPs were superior. EPs have also been shown to be superior to such variables as age, ICP, pupillary and oculocephalic reflexes, and motor responses (Anderson et al., 1984; Cant et al., 1986; Cusumano et al., 1992; Greenberg et al., 1982; Karnaze et al., 1985).

Prognostic Value in Comparison with EEG

Short-latency EPs also appear to be better for predicting outcome than the EEG, in large part owing to their stability in the face of sedative medications and other confounding variables (Hume et al., 1979; Hutchinson et al., 1991; Newlon et al., 1983). Hutchinson et al. (1991) compared SEPs with EEG using standardized grading systems and found not only that SEPs were better at distinguishing those patients who would have a favorable outcome from those who would not, but also that there was a direct relationship between the severity of SEP abnormalities and outcome. In another study (Ganes and Lundar, 1988), patients with electrocerebral silence on their EEG always had absent SEPs and VEPs but occasionally would have preservation of waves I to III of the BAEP. All patients with absent SEPs died within 2 days regardless of what the EEG showed at the time the SEPs were obtained. Hence, absence of SEPs alone was sufficient to predict an unfavorable outcome, and the EEG provided little additional prognostic information. However, Gutling et al. (1995) discovered that SEPs correctly predicted long-term outcome in 82 percent of their patients, while the presence or absence of reactivity was correct in 92 percent. By combining both SEPs and EEG reactivity, they were able to correctly classify 98 percent of their patients.

Value of Serial EP Testing

The use of intermittent, sequential EP monitoring has been suggested as a means of following a patient's clinical course and as a method by which complications that would require specific intervention may be identified (Jordan, 1993). EPs may identify cerebral ischemia, expanding hematomas (Larson et al., 1973), and a variety of toxic-metabolic aberrations (Hume et al., 1979). Attenuation of SEP amplitudes, including the subcortical P13/14, occurs in cases of increased ICP, primarily when central herniation is present (Cusumano et al., 1992; Ganes and Lundar, 1988). However, there appears to be no relationship between BAEPs and ICP (Karnaze et al., 1985); a not surprising fact given that these potentials only assess neural integrity up to the rostral brainstem. However, BAEPs become abnormal if there is sufficient distortion of the brainstem with central herniation (Nagao et al., 1983). It seems unlikely that EP monitoring would provide any additional benefit to traditional methods used to identify these complications. However, it is critical that these counfounding and potentially reversible factors be borne in mind by those interpreting EPs so that falsely pessimisitc predictions are avoided.

Evoked Potentials in the Chronic Setting

Clinical Outcome and EPs

EPs in the chronic phase of head injury have been suggested as being helpful in assessing the extent of cognitive impairment and predicting the potential for additional recovery. VEPs have been shown in one study (Gupta et al., 1986) to correlate with the extent of cognitive impairment. In this study, 50 percent of those with severe cognitive impairment had abnormal VEPs, while those with moderate or mild impairment had VEP abnormalities in 39 and 11 percent of cases, respectively. Prolongation of BAEP interpeak intervals may be seen in more than 25 percent of patients with the postconcussive syndrome (Benna et al., 1982). In a study using MEPs up to 1 year after head injury, those patients with persistently abnormal or deteriorating EPs had a poor outcome, while those with normal or improving EPs did well (Newlon et al., 1982). In this study EPs were found to correlate with outcome more accurately than the presence or absence of secondary complications. Of particular interest is the fact that an improvement in EP abnormalities was seen in some but not all patients before clinical improvement was apparent.

Not all studies have found EPs to be helpful in this setting, however. Rappaport et al. (1977) noted positive correlations with a disability rating scale only when long-latency VEPs and AEPs were recorded. Even with these responses, EPs were able to differentiate only those patients with very severe impairments from those with none; milder cases, in which the distinction is most critical, could not be differentiated from the more severely impaired. Shin et al. (1989) found no correlation between BAEPs and SEPs and a clinical evaluation of cognitive abilities. These EPs had only a 15 percent predictive power in assessing ultimate functional ability at the end of rehabilitation; the initial clinical evaluation and age of the patient were superior to EPs in this regard. EPs are particularly insensitive in comparison with such clinical features as age and duration of unconsciousness and amnesia in patients who have suffered mild head injuries (Werner and Vanderzant, 1991). The lack of predictive value in these later studies is probably reflected in the fact that EPs assess function indirectly; when the patient can be assessed directly, their value diminishes.

Event-Related Potentials and Cognitive Function

Another means of assessing patients in the later stage of their recovery is with event-related potentials. In contrast to the stimulus-specific EPs described above, event-related potentials are recorded independently of the type of sensory stimulus used and are considered to represent the electrophysiologic equivalent of the patient's psychological response to a novel stimulus (Oken, 1989). The precise nature of the psychologic processes being evaluated is not known with certainty but may include memory and attention (Olbrich et al., 1986; Papanicolaou et al., 1984). The two event-related potentials that have been studied most frequently in head-injured patients are the P300 response and contingent negative variation. The P300 is elicited by an anticipated stimulus (usually auditory) that occurs randomly in an "odd ball" pattern among frequent stimuli that the patient has been instructed to ignore. It is a large-amplitude positive potential with maximal distribution over the midline central and parietal regions. Contingent negative variation is a slow, negative potential, which is recorded between paired stimuli, of which the first acts as a warning and the second is an imperative stimulus to which the patient is instructed to make a response. The neural generators for these potentials is not known with certainty. Despite numerous studies in a variety of disease states, the sensitivity and specificity of these responses has not proved to be great (Oken, 1989).

In spite of the uncertainty of their value in assessing cognitive function, several investigators have attempted to use these event-related potentials to evalute head-injured patients. The P300 has been reported to be absent in patients who have suffered severe head injuries (Curry, 1980), while no significant abnormalities have been reported in milder cases (Werner and Vanderzant, 1991). Curry (1980) showed that P300 abnormalities correlated well with the severity of head injury and were able to differentiate severely injured patients from those with milder degrees of trauma. Olbrich et al. (1986) studied 18 severely head-injured patients acutely and 3 to 6 months later and found that the latency of P300 significantly correlated with impairments on initial neuropsychological testing. At follow-up, however, neuropsychological deficits had improved while the P300 remained abnormal in many patients. Hence, the event-related potentials of these patients were considered to be more sensitive in identifying residual congitive dysfunction than neurosychological testing. P300 abnormalities may represent the electrophysiologic correlate of post-traumatic amnesia (Papanicolaou et al., 1984) or impaired orientation and memory (Olbrich et al., 1986). Others have considered the P300 response simply a nonspecific alerting response in severely injured patients (Rappaport et al., 1991).

Contingent negative variation abnormalities in head-injured patients have included absence, attenuation, and asymmetry of responses, as well as an abnormal distribution with maximal negativity seen frontally (Curry, 1980; McCallum and Cummins, 1973). The latter finding has been seen in patients suffering diffuse frontal injury, which suggests that it represents a "release" phenomenon of normally suppressed processes originating in the frontal lobes (Curry, 1980). Despite the suggestion that contingent negative variation is able to identify specific areas of cerebral trauma, another study (Low, 1979) was unable to demonstrate any correlation between contingent negative variation abnormalities and proven brain lesions. Also, contingent negative variation was found to be even less reliable than the routine EEG in identifying cerebral pathology. As with quantitative EEG, there appears to be as yet no basis for the routine use of event-related potentials in head-injured patients (Epstein, 1994).

CONCLUSIONS

Returning to the questions raised at the beginning of this chapter, it appears that both EEG and EPs are able to assess the neurologic condition of patients following head injury. However, the correlation is time-dependent. The value of these studies is greatest early on when the patient is in coma or is difficult to evaluate clinically; when the patient's neurologic function is able to be studied directly, their value diminishes. Long-term EEG monitoring may identify a variety of complications, but the overall cost effectiveness of this labor-intensive procedure remains to be established. Neither routine EEGs nor EPs provide consistently useful and unique information in patients with the postconcussive syndrome. Although P300 studies and quantitative EEG may yet prove to be of some usefulness, their routine use in this setting should be discouraged. Prognostication is aided by electrophysiologic techniques when the course is unclear clinically. This is especially true for the EEG when a standardized rating scale with an assessment of reactivity or compressed spectral array is used and for EPs when attention is directed primarily to SEPs. In these specific situations it appears that the the EEG and EPs can provide unique, accurate, and reliable information in head-injured patients.

REFERENCES

Allison T: Cortical and subcortical evoked responses to central stimuli during wakefulness and sleep. Electroencephalogr Clin Neurophysiol 18:131–139, 1965

Allison T, Matsumiya Y, Goff GD, Goff WR: The scalp topography of human visual evoked potentials. Electroencephalogr Clin Neurophysiol 42:185–197, 1977

Alter I, John ER, Ransohoff J: Computer analysis of cortical evoked potentials following severe head injury. Brain Inj 4:19–26, 1990

Anderson DC, Bundlie S, Rockswold GL: Multimodality evoked potentials in closed head trauma. Arch Neurol 41:369–374, 1984

Benna P, Bergamasco B, Bianco C et al: Brainstem auditory evoked potentials in postconcussion syndrome. Ital J Neurol Sci 3:281–287, 1982

Bergamasco B, Bergamini L, Doriguzzi T: Clinical value of the sleep electroencephalographic patterns in post-traumatic coma. Acta Neurol Scand 44:495–511, 1968

Bickford RG, Butt, HR: Hepatic coma: the electroencephalographic pattern. J Clin Invest 34:790–799, 1955

Binder LM: Persisting symptoms after mild head injury: A review of the postconcussive syndrome. J Clin Exp Neuropsychol 8:323–346, 1986

Bricolo A, Formenton A, Turella G, Ore GD: Clinical and EEG effects of mechanical hyperventilation in acute traumatic coma. Eur Neurol 8:219–224, 1972

Bricolo A, Gentilomo A, Rosadini G, Rossi GF: Long-lasting post-traumatic unconsciousness. Acta Neurol Scand 44:512–532, 1968

Bricolo A, Turazzi S, Faccioli F: Combined clinical and EEG examinations for assessment of severity of acute head injuries. Acta Neurosurg suppl. 1, 28:35–39, 1979

Cant BR, Hume AL, Judson JA, Shaw NA: The assessment of severe head trauma by short-latency somatosensory and brain-stem auditory evoked potentials. Electroencephalogr Clin Neurophysiol 65:188–195, 1986

Chatrian GE, White LE, Daly D: Electroencephalographic patterns resembling those of sleep in certain comatose states after injuries to the head. Electroencephalogr Clin Neurophysiol 15:272–280, 1963

Courjon J, Naquet R, Baurand C et al: Valeur diagnostique et prognostique de l'EEG dans les suites immediates des traumatismes craniens [Value of the EEG in diagnosis and prognosis immediately after cranial trauma]. Rev Electroencephalogr Neurophysiol Clin 1:133–150, 1971

Courjon J, Scherzer E: Traumatic disorders. pp. 8–104. In Remond A, Magnus O, Courjon J, (eds.): Handbook of Electroencephalography and Clinical Neurophysiology. Vol. 14. Clinical EEG, IV. Part B. Elsevier, Amsterdam, 1972

Curry SH: Event-related potentials as indicants of structural and functional damage in closed head injury. Prog Brain Res 54:507–515, 1980

Cusumano S, Paolin A, Di Paolo F et al: Assessing brain function in post-traumatic coma by means of bit-mapped SEPs, BAEPs, CT, SPET and clinical scores. Prognostic implications. Electroencephalogr Clin Neurosphysiol 84:499–514, 1992

De Benedittis G, Ettore G: Focal EEG in post-traumatic mild coma. Follow-up study on unoperated patients. J Neurosurg Sci 18, 20–25, 1974

Denker PG, Perry GF: Postconcussion syndrome in compensation and litigation: analysis of 95 cases with electroencephalographic correlations. Neurology 4:912–918, 1954

Dikmen SS, Temkin NR, Machamber JE et al: Employment following traumatic head injury. Arch Neurol 51: 177–186, 1994

Dow RS, Ulett G, Raaf J: Electroencephalographic studies immediately following head injury. Am J Psychiatry 101:174–183, 1944

Dusser A, Navelet Y, Devictor D, Landrieu, P: Short- and long-term prognostic value of the electroencephalogram in children with severe head injury. Electroencephalogr Clin Neurophysiol 73:85–93, 1989

Epstein CM: Computerized EEG in the courtroom. Neurology 44:1566–1569, 1994

Firsching R, Frowein RA: Multimodality evoked potentials and early prognosis in comatose patients. Neurosurg Rev 13:141–146, 1990

Ganes T, Lundar T: EEG and evoked potentials in comatose patients with severe brain damage. Electroencephalogr Clin Neurophysiol 69:6–13, 1988

Gennarelli TA, Champion HR, Sacco WJ et al: Mortality of patients with head injury and extracranial injury treated in trauma centers. J Trauma 29:1193–1201, 1989

Gennarelli TA, Thibault LH, Adams JH et al: Diffuse axonal injury and traumatic coma in the primate. Ann Neurol 12:564–574, 1982

George B, Landau-Ferey J: Twelve months follow-up by night sleep EEG after recovery from severe head trauma. Neurochirurgia (Stuttg) 29:45–47, 1986

Glaser MA, Sjaardema H: The value of the electroencephalogram in craniocerebral injuries. West J Surg Obstet & Gynecol 48:689–695, 1940

Goff WR, Allison T, Shapiro A, Rosner BS: Cerebral somatosensory responses evoked during sleep in man. Electroencephalogr Clin Neurophysiol 21:1–19, 1966

Goldstein M: Traumatic brain injury: a silent epidemic. Ann Neurol 27:327, 1990

Greenberg RP, Becker DP, Miller JD, Mayer DJ: Evalaution of brain function in severe human head trauma with multimodality evoked potentials. Part 2: Localization of brain dysfunction and correlation with posttraumatic neurological conditions. J Neurosurg 46:163–177, 1977a

Greenberg RP, Mayer DJ, Becker DP, Miller JD: Evaluation of brain function in severe human head trauma with multimodality evoked potentials. Part 1: Evoked brain-injury potentials, methods and analysis. J Neurosurg 47:150–162, 1977b

Greenberg RP, Newlon PG, Becker DP: The somatosensory evoked potential in patients with severe head injury: outcome prediction and monitoring of brain function. Ann N Y Acad Sci 388:683–688, 1982

Greenberg RP, Newlon PG, Hyatt MS et al: Prognostic implications of early multimodality evoked potentials in severely head-injured patients. J Neurosurg 55: 227–236, 1981

Gupta NK, Verma NP, Guidice MA, Kooi KA: Visual evoked response in head trauma: pattern-shift stimulus. Neurology 36:578–581, 1986

Gutling E, Gosner A, Imnof H.-S, Landis T: EEG reactivity in the prognosis of severe head injury. Neurology 45:915–918, 1995

Haglund Y, Persson HE: Does Swedish amateur boxing lead to chronic brain damage? 3. A retrospective clinical neurophysiology study. Acta Neurol Scand 82: 353–360, 1990

Hakkinen VK, Kaukinen S, Heikkila H: The correlation of EEG compressed spectral array to Glasgow coma scale in traumatic coma patients. Int J Clin Monit Comput 5:97–101, 1988

Hockaday JM, Potts F, Bonazzi A, Schwab RS: Electroencephalographic changes in acute cerebral anoxia from cardiac or respiratory arrest. Electroencephalogr Clin Neurophysiol 18:575–586, 1965

Hooshmand H, Beckner E, Radfor F: Technical and clinical aspects of topographic brain mapping. Clin Electroencephalogr 20:235–247, 1989

Hume AL, Cant BR & Shaw NA: Central somatosensory conduction time in comatose patients. Ann Neurol 5:379–384, 1979

Hutchinson DO, Frith RW, Shaw NA et al: A comparison between electroencephalagraphy and somatosensory evoked potentials for outcome prediction following severe head injury. Electroencephalogr Clin Neurophysiol 78:228–233, 1991

Jacome DE, Risko M: EEG features in post-traumatic syndrome. Clin Electroencephalogr 15:214–221, 1984

Jasper HH, Kershman J & Elvidge A: Electroencephalographic studies of injury to the head. Arch Neurol 44:328–348, 1940

Jerrett SA, Corsak J: Clinical utility of topographic EEG brain mapping. Clin Electroencephalogr 19:134–143, 1988

Jordan KG: Continuous EEG and evoked potential monitoring in the neuroscience intensive care unit. J Clin Neurosphysiol 10:445–475, 1993

Karabudak R, Ciger A, Erturk I, Zileli T: EEG and the linear skull fractures. J Neurosurg Sci 36:47–49, 1992

Karnaze DS, Marshall LF, Bickford RG: EEG monitoring of clinical coma: the compressed spectral array. Neurology 32:289–292, 1982

Karnaze DS, Weiner JM, Marshall LF: Auditory evoked potentials in coma after closed head injury: a clinical-neurophysiologic coma scale for predicting outcome. Neurology 35:1122–1126, 1985

Kellaway P: Head injury in children. Electroencephalogr Clin Neurophysiol 7:497–502, 1955

Klein HJ, Rath SA, Goppel F: The use of EEG spectral analysis after thiopental bolus in the prognostic evaluation of comatose patients with brain injuries. Acta Neurochir Suppl (Wien) 42:31–34, 1988

Koufen H, Hagel KH: Systematic EEG follow-up study of traumatic psychosis. Eur Arch Psychiatry Neurol Sci 237:2–7, 1987

Larson SJ, Sances S, Ackmann JJ, Reigel DH: Noninvasive evaluation of head trauma patients. Surgery 74:34–40, 1973

Liguori G, Foggia L, Buonaguro A et al: EEG findings in minor head trauma as a clue for indication to CT scan. Childs Nerv Syst 5:160–162, 1989

Loeb C, Rosadini G, Poggio G: Electroencephalograms during coma. Neurology 9:610–618, 1959

Low MD: Event-related potentials and the electroencephalogram in patients with proven brain lesions. pp. 258–264. In Desmedt JE (ed): Progress in Clinical Neurophysiology: Cognitive components in cerebral event-related Potentials and Selective Attention. Vol. 6, Karger, Basel; 1979

Mauguiere F, Desmdet JE, Courgon J: Astreognosis and dissociated loss of frontal or parietal components of somatosensory evoked potentials in hemispheric lesion. Brain 106:271–311, 1983

McCallum WC, Cummings B: The effects of brain lesions on the contingent negative variation in neurosurgical patients. Electroencephalogr Clin Neurosphysiol 35:449–456, 1973

Munari C, Calbucci F: Correlations between intracranial pressure and EEG during coma and sleep. Electroencephalogr Clin Neurophysiol 51:170–176, 1981

Nagao S, Sunami N, Tsutsui T et al: Serial observations of brain stem function in acute intracranial hypertension by auditory brain stem responses—a clinical study. p. 474–479, In Ishii S, Nagai H, Bock M (eds); Intracranial Pressure Vol. 5. Springer-Verlag, Berlin, 1983

Nau HE, Bock WJ: Electroencephalographic investigations of traumatic apallic syndrome in childhood and adolescence. Acta Neurochir (Wien) 39:211–217, 1977

Nau HE, Bongartz EB, Bock WJ, Weichert C: Computerized tomography, electroencephalography, and clinical symptoms in severe cranio-cerebral injuries. Acta Neurochir (Wien) 45:209–216, 1979

Newlon PG, Greenberg RP, Enas GG, Becker DP: Effects of therapeutic pentobarbital coma on multimodality evoked potentials recorded from severely head-injured patients. Neurosurgery 12:613–619, 1983

Newlon, PG, Greenberg, RP, Hyatt MS et al: The dynamics of neuronal dysfunction and recovery following severe head injury assessed with serial multimodality evoked potentials. J Neurosurg 57:168–177, 1982

Nuwer MR: The development of EEG brain mapping. J Clin Neurophysiol 7:459–471, 1990

Oken BS: Endogenous event-related potentials. In Chiappa KH (ed): Evoked potentials in Clinical Medicine. 2nd Ed. Raven Press, New York, 1989

Olbrich HM, Nau HE, Lodemann E et al: Evoked potential assessment of mental function during recovery from severe head injury. Surg Neurol 26:112–118, 1986

Oshida K, Yoshii N, Mikami K et al: Electroencephalogram in the head injury of aged subjects. Keio J Med 19: 135–143, 1970

Papanicolaou AC, Levin HS, Eisenberg HM et al: Evoked potential correlates of posttraumatic amnesia after closed head injury. Neurosurgery 14:676–678, 1984

Rae-Grant AD, Barbour PJ, Reed J: Development of a novel EEG rating scale for head injury using dichotomous variables. Electroencephalogr Clin Neurophysiol 79: 349–357, 1991

Rappaport M, Hall K, Hopkins K et al: Evoked brain potentials and disability in brain-damaged patients. Arch Phys Med Rehabil 58:333–338, 1977

Rappaport M, Hopkins HK, Hall K, Belleza T: Evoked potentials and head injury. 2. Clinical applications. Clin Electroencephalogr 12:167–176, 1981

Rappaport M, McCandless KL, Pond W, Kraft MC: Passive P300 response in traumatic brain injury patients. J Neuropsychiatry Clin Neurosci 3:180–185, 1991

Rodin E, Whelan J, Taylor R et al: The electroencephalogram in acute fatal head injuries. J Neurosurg 23:329–337, 1965

Ron S, Algom D, Hary D, Cohen M: Time-related changes in the distribution of sleep stages in brain injured patients. Electroencephalogr Clin Neurophysiol 48:432–441, 1980

Rumpl E, Lorenzi E, Hackl JM et al: The EEG at different stages of acute secondary traumatic midbrain and bulbar brain syndromes. Electroencephalogr Clin Neurophysiol 46:487–497, 1979

Rumpl E, Prugger M, Bauer G et al: Incidence and prognostic value of spindles in post-traumatic coma. Electroencephalogr Clin Neurophysiol 56:420–429, 1983

Shin DY, Ehrenberg B, Whyte J et al: Evoked potential assessment: utility in prognosis of chronic head injury. Arch Phys Med Rehabil 70:189–193, 1989

Steudel WI, Kruger J: Using the spectral analysis of the EEG for prognosis of severe brain injuries in the first post-traumatic week. Acta Neurochir Suppl (Wien) 28:40–42, 1979

Stockard JJ, Bickford RG, Aung MH: The electroencephalogram in traumatic brain injury. pp. 317–367. In Vinken PJ, Bruyn GW, (eds): Handbook of Neurology. Vol. 23. Injuries of the Brain and Skull. Part 1. North-Holland, Amsterdam/Oxford, 1975

Strnad P, Strnadova V: Long-term follow-up EEG studies in patients with traumatic apallic syndrome. Eur Neurol 26:84–89, 1987

Sulg IA, Dencker SJ: Electroencephalographic findings in MZ twin pairs, discordant for closed head injury. Acta Genet Med Gemellol 17:389–401, 1968

Synek VM: Value of a revised EEG coma scale for prognosis after cerebral anoxia and diffuse head injury. Clin Electroencephalogr 21:25–30, 1990a

Synek VM: Revised EEG coma scale in diffuse acute head injuries in adults. Clin Exp Neurol 27:99–111, 1990b

Synek VM, Synek BJL: Theta pattern coma, a variant of alpha pattern coma. Clin Electroencephalogr 15: 116–121, 1984

Tebano MT, Cameroni M, Gallozzi G et al: EEG spectral analysis after minor head injury in man. Electroencephalogr Clin Neurophysiol 70:185–189, 1988

Thatcher RW, Walker RA, Gerson I, Geisler FH: EEG discriminant analyses of mild head trauma. Electroencephalogr Clin Neurophysiol 73:94–106, 1989

Torres F, Shapiro SK: Electroencephalograms in whiplash injury. Arch Neurol 5:28–35, 1961

Toyonaga K, Schlagenhauff RE, Smith BH: Periodic lateralized epileptiform discharges in subdural hematoma: case reports and review of Literature. Clin Electroencephalogr 5:113–118, 1974

Werner RA, Vanderzant CW: Multimodality evoked potential testing in acute mild closed head injury. Arch Phys Med Rehabil 72:31–34, 1991

Westmoreland BF, Klass DW, Sharbrough FW, Reagan TJ: Alpha coma: electroencephalographic, clinical, pathologic and etiologic correlations. Arch Neurol 32:713–718, 1975

Williams D, Denny-Brown D: Cerebral electrical changes in experimental concussion. Brain 64:223–238, 1941

Williams GW, Luders HO, Brickner A et al: Interobserver variability in EEG interpretation. Neurology 35: 1714–1719, 1985

Winer JW, Rosenwasser RH, Jimenez F: Electroencephalographic activity and serum and cerebrospinal fluid pentobarbital levels in determining the therapeutic end point during barbiturate coma. Neurosurger 29:739–742, 1991

Yamada T, Graff-Radford NR, Kimura J et al: Topographic analysis of somatosensory evoked potentials in patients with well-localized thalamic infarctions. J Neurol Sci 68:31–46, 1985

Yamada T, Kayamori R, Kimura J, Beck DO: Topography of somatosensory evoked potentials after stimulation of the median nerve. Electroencephalogr Clin Neurophysiol 59:29–43, 1984

Yoshii N, Matsumoto K, Oshida K et al: Clinicoelectroencephalographic study of 3200 head injury cases; a comparative work between aged, adults and children. Keio J Med 19:31–46, 1970

Post-Traumatic Headaches 8

Sue Barcellos
Matthew Rizzo

Headache is perhaps the most frequent complaint following trauma to the head or neck, especially from motor vehicle crashes. The reported incidence of these headaches varies quite broadly, and the pathologic underpinnings, natural course, and treatment remain ill-defined (Elkind, 1989a; Evans, 1992a; Goldstein, 1991; Haas, 1993a and b; Rasmussen and Olsen, 1992). Further confounding the attempts to understand the nature of post-traumatic headaches is the fact that they may occur as part of a postconcussive or post-traumatic syndrome that also includes dizziness, blurred vision, light and noise sensitivity, irritability, anxiety, fatigue, memory, insomnia and multiple cognitive complaints, including impaired concentration and attention (Evans, 1992a). That a headache may occur immediately after a severe head or neck injury is not surprising. In fact, in a Danish population study of all types of headache, 4 percent of individuals reported a new headache in association with trauma at some point in their lifetimes (Rasmussen and Olsen, 1993). The controversy exists in defining the association between head trauma and chronic headache (Olesen, 1988). Also, to be explained is the surprising claim that headaches following minor head trauma have a greater frequency and duration than those following major head trauma (Evans, 1992a; Yamaguchi, 1992).

It is also important to note that headache has a high base rate in the general population. Tension headache is ubiquitous, and most people have experienced such a headache in their lifetime. In fact, 70 to 90 percent of adults will have had a memorable headache in the past year (Rasmussen, 1993; Walters, 1974). Migraine headache is also common and is more prevalent in women than men (17.6 percent of women, 6 percent of men) (Lipton and Steward, 1993). Consequently, many patients with post-traumatic headache will have known pre-existing headaches. In a patient with significant previous headache it is sometime difficult to ascertain the role of trauma in the chronic headache.

When approaching the phenomena of post-traumatic headache, the main issues are (1) identifying the mechanisms by which the pain may be generated or maintained; (2) identifying psychological and social factors, including legal issues and secondary gain, that might sustain the complaint; and (3) establishing treatment approaches and coping styles that may resolve the condition rather than prolonging it. This chapter attempts to outline the terminology and proposed pathophysiology and to review current treatment approaches.

TERMINOLOGY

Numerous terms have been used to describe post-traumatic headaches according to the severity of trauma, location, or type of injury (Table 8-1). The introduction of the International Headache Society (IHS) Classification System was to have displaced these terms. In 1988 the IHS published Classification and Diagnostic Criteria for Headache Disorders, Cranial Neuralgia's and Facial Pain, which is an operational classification system attempting to group headaches by underlying mechanisms and response to therapy (Olesen, 1988) (Table 8-2). By a structured interview (example given in Table 8-3), it is possible to assign the headache complaints of most patients to a single classification category. In this system headaches such as migraine, tension-type, and cluster headaches that appear to occur independently of any other disease process are termed primary. Those headache conditions felt to have an identifiable medical cause factor are termed secondary. The term *post-traumatic headaches* is applied to secondary headaches that develop in close temporal association with head trauma.

TABLE 8-1. Post-Traumatic Headache Terminology

Post-traumatic headache (Goddard et al., 1994; Elkind 1989a, 1989b; Goldstein, 1991; Olesen, 1988)
Postconcussive headache (Goddard et al., 1994; Elkind, 1989a, 1989b; Evans, 1992a; Goldstein, 1991)
Post-head trauma syndrome (Elkind, 1989a, 1989b)
Mild head injury headache (Evans, 1992a)
Whiplash headache (Evans, 1992b; Radanov et al., 1993)
Post-traumatic migraine (Weiss et al., 1991; Haas 1993a, 1993b)
Post-traumatic cluster headache (Turkewitz et al., 1992)
Occipital neuralgia (Olesen, 1988; Ehni and Benner, 1984)
Cervicogenic headache (of Sjaastad) (Sjaastad et al., 1990)
Third occipital nerve headache (Bogduk and Marsland, 1986)
Minor intervertebral disorder (Bellavance et al., 1989)
Cervical migraine syndrome of Bartschi-Rochaix (Edmeads, 1988; Bartschi-Rochaix, 1968)
Posterior cervical sympathetic syndrome of Barre (Edmeads, 1988; Khurana and Niranhari, 1986)

By the IHS criteria (Table 8-4) (Olesen, 1988), the diagnosis of post-traumatic headache requires loss of consciousness, post-traumatic amnesia lasting more than 10 minutes, and relevant abnormalities in at least two of the following evaluations: (1) clinical neurologic examination, (2) radiography of the skull, (3) neuroimaging, (4) evoked potentials, (5) spinal fluid examination, (6) vestibular function test, and (7) neuropsychological testing. In addition, the headache must begin less than 14 days after the trauma (or after regaining consciousness). An acute post-traumatic headache becomes chronic if it continues beyond 8 weeks. A distinction is made for headaches after minor head trauma in which there was no loss of consciousness, no amnesia, and no confirming signs of injury. The compilers of the classification believed that a strong causal relationship exists between significant head trauma and acute or chronic headache and between mild head trauma or even whiplash (acceleration-deceleration injury) and acute headache. However, the development of chronic headache in mild head injury or whiplash is controversial. Indeed, chronic headache following trauma involves a "complex interrelationship between organic and psychosocial factors," which makes it "difficult to assess" (Olesen, 1988). This uncertainty has displaced the classification of *chronic post-traumatic headache from minor trauma* back into the descriptive terminology.

In the IHS scheme a secondary headache is named after the primary type it most resembles. The terms *post-traumatic migraine* (Haas, 1993a; Weiss et al., 1991) and *post-traumatic cluster* (Turkewitz et al. 1992) are examples. Cervical (cervicogenic) headache in the IHS system is a secondary headache associated with documented injury or disease of the cervical spine or contiguous neural structures (Olesen, 1988). Occipital neuralgia has a precise definition as a cranial neuralgia under the IHS system.

Despite the development of the IHS system, descriptive terminology abounds (see Table 8-1). The term *post-traumatic* is a catch-all (Goddard et al. 1994; Elkind, 1989b; Goldstein, 1991). The severity of trauma can further characterized on the basis of (1) degree of coma, (2) presence of absence of amnesia, and (3) observable injury on physical, radiologic, or cognitive evaluation (see Ch. 1). For example, in

TABLE 8-2. Classification of Headache Disorders, Cranial Neuralgias, and Facial Pain

1. Migraine
   - 1.1 Migraine without aura
   - 1.2 Migraine with aura
     - 1.2.1 Migraine with typical aura
     - 1.2.2 Migraine with prolonged aura
     - 1.2.3 Familial hemiplegic migraine
     - 1.2.4 Basilar migraine
     - 1.2.5 Migraine aura without headache
     - 1.2.6 Migraine with acute onset aura
   - 1.3 Ophthalmoplegic migraine
   - 1.4 Retinal migraine
   - 1.5 Childhood periodic syndromes that may be precursors to or associated with migraine
     - 1.5.1 Benign paroxysmal vertigo of childhood
     - 1.5.2 Alternating hemiplegia of childhood
   - 1.6 Complications of migraine
     - 1.6.1 Status migrainus
     - 1.6.2 Migrainous infarction
   - 1.7 Migrainous disorder not fulfilling above criteria
2. Tension-type headache
   - 2.1 Episodic tension-type headache
     - 2.1.1 Episodic tension-type headache unassociated with disorder of pericranial muscles
     - 2.1.2 Episodic tension-type headache associated with disorder of pericranial muscles
   - 2.2 Chronic tension-type headache
     - 2.2.1 Chronic tension-type headache associated with disorder of pericranial muscles
     - 2.2.2 Chronic tension-type headache associated with disorder of pericranial muscles
   - 2.3 Headache of the tension-type not fulfilling above criteria
3. Cluster headache and chronic paroxysmal hemicrania
   - 3.1 Cluster headache
     - 3.1.1 Cluster headache periodicity undetermined
     - 3.1.2 Episodic cluster headache
     - 3.1.3 Chronic cluster headache
       - 3.1.3.1 Unremitting from onset
       - 3.1.3.2 Evolved from episodic
   - 3.2 Chronic paroxysmal hemicrania
   - 3.3 Cluster headache-like disorder not fulfilling above criteria
4. Miscellaneous headache unassociated with structural lesion
   - 4.1 Idiopathic stabbing headache
   - 4.2 External compression headache
   - 4.3 Cold stimulus headache
     - 4.3.1 External application of a cold stimulus
     - 4.3.2 Ingestion of a cold stimulus
   - 4.4 Benign cough headache
   - 4.5 Benign exertional headache
   - 4.6 Headache associated with sexual activity
     - 4.6.1 Dull type
     - 4.6.2 Explosive type
     - 4.6.3 Postural type
5. Headache associated with head trauma
   - 5.1 Acute post-traumatic headache
     - 5.1.1 With significant head trauma and/or confirmatory signs
     - 5.1.2 With minor head trauma and no confirmatory signs
   - 5.2 Chronic post-traumatic headache
     - 5.2.1 With significant head trauma and/or confirmatory signs
     - 5.2.2 With minor head trauma and no confirmatory signs
6. Headache associated with vascular disorders
   - 6.1 Acute ischemic cerebrovascular disease
     - 6.1.1 Transient ischemic attack (TIA)
     - 6.1.2 Thromboembolic stroke
   - 6.2 Intracranial hematoma
     - 6.2.1 Intracerebral hematoma
     - 6.2.2 Subdural hematoma
     - 6.2.3 Epidural hematoma
   - 6.3 Subarachnoid hemorrhage
   - 6.4 Unruptured vascular malformation
     - 6.4.1 Arteriovenous malformation
     - 6.4.2 Saccular aneurysm
   - 6.5 Arteritis
     - 6.5.1 Giant cell arteritis
     - 6.5.2 Other systemic arteritides
     - 6.5.3 Primary intracranial arteritis
   - 6.6 Carotid or vertebral artery pain
     - 6.6.1 Carotid or vertebral dissection
     - 6.6.2 Carotidynia (idiopathic)
     - 6.6.3 Postendarterectomy headache
   - 6.7 Venous thrombosis
   - 6.8 Arterial hypertension
     - 6.8.1 Acute pressor response to exogenous agent
     - 6.8.2 Pheochromocytoma
     - 6.8.3 Malignant (accelerated hypertension)
     - 6.8.4 Preeclampsia and eclampsia
   - 6.9 Other vascular disorder
7. Headache associated with nonvascular intracranial disorder
   - 7.1 High cerebrospinal fluid pressure
     - 7.1.1 Benign intracranial hypertension
     - 7.1.2 High-pressure hydrocephalus
   - 7.2 Low cerebrospinal fluid pressure
     - 7.2.1 Postlumbar puncture headache
     - 7.2.2 Cerebrospinal fluid fistula headache
   - 7.3 Intracranial infection
   - 7.4 Intracranial sarcoidosis and other noninfectious inflammatory diseases
   - 7.5 Headache related to intrathecal injections
     - 7.5.1 Direct effect
     - 7.5.2 Due to chemical meningitis
   - 7.6 Intracranial neoplasm
   - 7.7 Headache associated with other intracranial disorders

(*Continued*)

TABLE 8-2. *(continued)* **Classification of Headache Disorders, Cranial Neuralgias, and Facial Pain**

8. Headache associated with substances or their withdrawal
   - 8.1 Headache induced by acute substance use or exposure
     - 8.1.1 Nitrate/nitrite-induced
     - 8.1.2 Monosodium glutamate-induced
     - 8.1.3 Carbon monoxide-induced
     - 8.1.4 Alcohol-induced
     - 8.1.5 Other substances
   - 8.2 Headache induced by chronic substance use or abuse
     - 8.2.1 Ergotamine-induced
     - 8.2.2 Analgesics abuse
     - 8.2.3 Other substances
   - 8.3 Headache from substance withdrawal (acute use)
     - 8.3.1 Alcohol withdrawal (hangover)
     - 8.3.2 Other substances
   - 8.4 Headache from substance withdrawal (chronic use)
     - 8.4.1 Ergotamine withdrawal
     - 8.4.2 Caffeine withdrawal
     - 8.4.3 Narcotics abstinence
     - 8.4.4 Other substances
   - 8.5 Headache associated with substances but with uncertain mechanism
     - 8.5.1 Birth control pills or estrogens
     - 8.5.2 Other substances
9. Headache associated with noncephalic infection
   - 9.1 Viral infection
     - 9.1.1 Focal noncephalic
     - 9.1.2 Systemic
   - 9.2 Baterial infection
     - 9.2.1 Focal noncephalic
     - 9.2.2 Systemic (septicemia)
   - 9.3 Other infection
10. Headache associated with mtetabolic disorders
    - 10.1 Hypoxia
      - 10.1.1 High-altitude headache
      - 10.1.2 Hypoxic headache (low-pressure environment, pulmonary disease causing hypoxia)
      - 10.1.3 Sleep apnea headache
    - 10.2 Hypercapnia
    - 10.3 Mixed hypoxia and hypercapnia
    - 10.4 Hypoglycemia
    - 10.5 Dialysis
    - 10.6 Other metabolic abnormalities
11. Headache or facial pain associated with disorders of cranium, neck, eyes, ears, nose, sinuses, teeth, mouth, or other facial or cranial structures
    - 11.1 Cranial bone
    - 11.2 Neck
      - 11.2.1 Cervical spine
      - 11.2.2 Retropharyngeal tendinitis
    - 11.3 Eyes
      - 11.3.1 Acute glaucoma
      - 11.3.2 Refractive errors
      - 11.3.3 Heterophoria or heterotropia
    - 11.4 Ears
    - 11.5 Nose and sinuses
      - 11.5.1 Acute sinus headache
      - 11.5.2 Other disease of nose or sinus
    - 11.6 Teeth, jaws, and related structures
    - 11.7 Temporomandibular joint disease (functional disorders are coded to group 2)
12. Cranial neuralgias, nerve trunk pain, and deafferentation pain
    - 12.1 Persistent (in contrast to tic-like) pain of cranial nerve origin
      - 12.1.1 Compression or distortion of cranial nerves and second and third cervical roots
      - 12.1.2 Demyelination of cranial nerves
        - 12.1.2.1 Optic neuritis (retrobulbar neuritis)
      - 12.1.3 Infarction of cranial nerves
        - 12.1.3.1 Diabetic neuritis
      - 12.1.4 Inflammation of cranial nerves
        - 12.1.4.1 Herpes zoster
        - 12.1.4.2 Chronic postherpetic neuralgia
      - 12.1.5 Tolosa-Hunt syndrome
      - 12.1.6 Neck-tongue syndrome
      - 12.1.7 Other causes of persistent pain of cranial nerve origin
    - 12.2 Trigeminal neuralgia
      - 12.2.1 Idiopathic trigeminal neuralgia
      - 12.2.2 Symptomatic trigeminal neuralgia
        - 12.2.2.1 Compression of trigeminal root or ganglion
        - 12.2.2.2 Central lesions
    - 12.3 Glossopharyngeal neuralgia
      - 12.3.1 Idiopathic
      - 12.3.2 Symptomatic
    - 12.4 Nervus intermedius neuralgia
    - 12.5 Superior laryngeal neuralgia
    - 12.6 Occipital neuralgia
    - 12.7 Central causes of head and facial pain other than tic douloureux
      - 12.7.1 Anesthesia dolorosa
      - 12.7.2 Thalamic pain
    - 12.8 Facial pain not fulfilling criteria in groups 11 and 12
13. Headache not classifiable

TABLE 8-3. Points Addressed in Structured Headache Interview

1. Frequency
2. Duration
3. Pain characteristics
   a. Location
   b. Quality (pulsatile, pressure, tic-like)
   c. Intensity (mild, moderate, severe)
   d. Aggravation by activity
4. Associated signs or symptoms
   a. Nausea and/or vomiting
   b. Photophobia and phonophobia
   c. Muscle tenderness
   d. Conjunctival injection
   e. Lacrimation
   f. Rhinorrhea
   g. Forehead and facial sweating
   h. Miosis
   i. Ptosis
   j. Eyelid edema
5. Accompanying neurologic deficits
   a. Preceding and resolving before the headache pain
   b. Occurring in association with the headache pain
6. Precipitating activities for headache
7. Response to medication
8. Complete general medical and neurologic interview

his review of post-traumatic headaches Evans (1992a) adopted criteria for mild head injury that require that the initial Glasgow Coma Scale score be 13 to 15 without subsequent deterioration, loss of consciousness less than 30 minutes, and the absence of any focal neurologic deficits, depressed skull fractures or intracranial hematomas. *Postconcussive* requires only that a period of unconsciousness occur at the time of trauma (Elkind, 1989a; Evans, 1992; Goddard et al., 1994; Goldstein, 1991). *Postcontusion* requires radiographic evidence of brain contusion. Applying *whiplash* to headache requires only onset or at the time of suspected whiplash (acceleration/deceleration) trauma (Evans, 1992b; Radanov et al., 1993).

The term *cervicogenic headache,* proposed by Sjaastad et al. (1990), describes a stereotypical headache and responses to therapy (Dieterich et al., 1993). It does not fulfill the secondary headache criteria put forth by the IHS because it does not require demonstrable pathology in cervical structures. The criteria of Sjaastad et al., 1990, for the diagnosis include tenderness to palpation of posterior and lateral neck structures and temporary pain relief following a local anesthetic nerve block. Thus it overlaps the IHS diagnostic criteria for *occipital neuralgia.* It also overlaps with other chronic cervical pain syndromes, including myofascial (Jaeger, 1989). Another type of cervicogenic headache is the "third occipital nerve headache," which (hypothetically) represents pain in the distribution of the third occipital nerve, due to trauma to the cervical spine, specifically to the C2-C3 zygapophysial joints (Bogduk and Marsland, 1986). Finally, *minor intervertebral disorder* headache has been attributed to trauma to any mobile segments of the cervical spine (invertebrate disks, auricular facets, and associated ligaments or muscles) (Bellavance et al., 1989). Additional labels describe pain thought to be due to injury to the vertebral artery or its associated sympathetic plexus. This includes the cervical migraine syndrome of Bartschi-Rochaix (Bartschi-Rochaix, 1968; Edmeads, 1988), and the posterior cervical sympathetic syndrome of Barré (Edmeads, 1988; Khurana and Niranhari, 1986; Winston, 1987).

MECHANISMS

Acute pain following head or neck trauma might arise from damage to the bones, blood vessels, or nerves and other tissues. Muscle trauma may result in the release of pain fiber-activating substances. How acute brain tissue injury might lead to acute headache is more puzzling. Brain tissue itself is insensitive to pain.

The proposed mechanisms whereby acute pain becomes chronic are extrapolated from studies in animals and remain speculative. Chronic pain is defined as pain continuing beyond the time of expected healing. Etiologic factors might include scarring of intracranial or extracranial tissue, neuroma formation, nerve entrapment in bony or muscular structures, or soft tissue injury. Chronic post-traumatic headache might be in the form of "neuropathic pain" in the distribution of the trigeminal, glossopharyngeal, or upper cervical nerves. Potential mechanisms invoke "disinhibition" from higher cortical centers (deafferent pain), or neural reprogramming, a dynamic change at the dorsal horn level as the result of altered peripheral or central nervous system inputs (Dubner and Ruda, 1992; see Fig. 8-3). This reprogramming alters the processing of nociceptive information, as in sunburn, where "touch" is perceived as pain.

Neural plasticity is the current mechanism to explain the chronic pain resulting from diverse conditions such as stroke, spinal cord injury, reflex sympa-

TABLE 8-4. International Headache Society Definition of Acute Post-traumatic Headache

5.1 Acute post-traumatic headache
- 5.1.1 With significant head trauma and/or confirmatory signs.
  Diagnostic criteria
  - A. Significance of head trauma documented by at least one of the following:
    1. Loss of consciousness
    2. Post-traumatic amnesia lasting more than 10 minutes
    3. At least two of the following exhibit relevant abnormality: clinical neurologic examination, skull radiograph, neuroimaging, evoked potentials, spinal fluid examination, vestibular function test, neuropsychological testing
  - B. Headache occurs less than 14 days after regaining consciousness (or after trauma if there has been no loss of consciousness)
  - C. Headache disappears within 8 weeks after regaining consciousness (or after trauma if there has been no loss of consciousness)
- 5.1.2 With minor head trauma and no confirmatory signs.
  Diagnostic criteria
  - A. Head trauma that does not satisfy 5.1.1A
  - B. Headache occurs less than 14 days after injury
  - C. Headache disappears within 8 weeks after injury

5.2 Chronic post-traumatic headache
- 5.2.1 With significant head trauma and/or confirmatory signs.
  Diagnostic criteria
  - A. Significance of head trauma documented by at least one of the following:
    1. Loss of consciousness
    2. Post-traumatic amnesia lasting more than 10 minutes
    3. At least two of the following exhibit relevant abnormality: clinical neurologic examination, skull radiograph, neuroimaging, evoked potentials, spinal fluid examination, vestibular function test, neuropsychological testing
  - B. Headache occurs less than 14 days after regaining consciousness (or after trauma if there has been no loss of consciousness)
  - C. Headache continues more than 8 weeks after regaining consciousness (or after trauma if there has been no loss of consciousness)
- 5.2.2 With minor head trauma and no confirmatory signs.
  Diagnostic criteria
  - A. Head trauma that does not satisfy 5.2.1A
  - B. Headache occurs less than 14 days after injury
  - C. Headache continues more than 8 weeks after injury

thetic dystrophy, fibromyalgia, myofascial pain, and post-traumatic headaches. Unfortunately, the evidence is lacking. In any case, it is reasonable (1) to treat the chronic post-traumatic headache pain in the same manner as the primary headache type it most closely resembles and (2) if this fails, to recruit the treatment approaches applied to other chronic neuropathic pain conditions.

HEADACHE TYPES

The syndrome of post-traumatic headache comprises multiple types. Currently the IHS classification is preferred, although there are other classification systems. Unfortunately, many of the published studies of post-traumatic migraine were made prior to the introduction of the IHS classification system, which complicates the interpretation of the literature.

Post-Traumatic Headaches Resembling Primary Headaches (IHS criteria)

Migraine

In the IHS scheme (Olesen, 1988) migraine is defined as a unilateral throbbing headache severe enough to inhibit or prohibit activity. The headache is made worse by exercise and is associated with the combination of photophobia, phonophobia, and nausea with or without vomiting (Table 8-5). It may have an associated aura, defined as a focal reversible neurologic deficit localizable to a specific cortical or brainstem area. The aura develops slowly, spreads

TABLE 8-5. International Headache Society Definition of Migraine Without Aura

1.1 Migraine without aura (previously used terms: common migraine, hemicrania simplex).
Diagnostic criteria
- A. At least five attacks fulfilling criteria B to D below
- B. Headache lasting 4 to 72 hours (untreated or unsuccessfully treated)
- C. Headache has at least two of the following characteristics:
  1. Unilateral location
  2. Pulsating quality
  3. Moderate or severe intensity (inhibits or prohibits daily activities)
  4. Aggravated by walking stairs or similar routine physical activity
- D. During headache, at least one of the following:
  1. Nausea and/or vomiting
  2. Photophobia and phonophobia
- E. At least one of the following:
  1. History, physical, and neurologic examinations do not suggest one of the disorders listed in groups 5 to 11 of Table 8-2
  2. History and/or physical and/or neurologic examinations do suggest such disorder, but it is ruled out by appropriate investigation
  3. Such disorder is present, but migraine attacks do not occur for the first time in close temporal relation to the disorder

over the cortex (similarly to a jacksonian seizure march), lasts less than 60 minutes, and resolves before the onset of a migrainous headache pain (Table 8-6). Three separate patterns of post-traumatic migraines have been described.

Acute post-traumatic migraines with aura have often been described following minor head injuries in children (Haas, 1993a) or injuries from contact sports such as football, soccer, wrestling, and rugby (Goldstein, 1991). In such cases hemiparesis, visual loss, scintillation, stupor, and convulsion may accompany headache. Vomiting may begin immediately or within a few hours of the trauma. The symptoms tend to clear in 24 hours (Haas, 1993a). In most cases there is a personal or strong family history of spontaneous migraines (Bennett et al., 1980). These pediatric headaches occur as a single event and without any neurologic sequelae. Caution is necessary to avoid missing conditions such as epidural hematomas, contusions, cerebral edema, or an ischemic or hemorrhagic process.

The pattern of recurrent migraines following trauma is usually without aura. A normal neurologic examination is expected during the headache. These headaches develop usually within hours, days, or weeks from the time of trauma (Haas, 1993a; Winston, 1987). Some persons reportedly develop a frequency greater than once a week (Weiss et al., 1991). Photophobia and phonophobia may be marked. Though not a part of the diagnostic criteria, dizziness without true vertigo is a frequent complaint. When not associated with other headache conditions or exacerbating factors, these headaches appear to have a favorable response to standard migraine management (Weiss et al., 1991; Winston, 1987).

The third type of migraine presentation is atypical and overlaps chronic tension-type headaches (Matthew, 1993a). These patients complain of a constant headache, often unilateral and usually mild in intensity. The headache generally does not inhibit activity. A moderate or severe unilateral headache associated with nausea, vomiting, photophobia, and/or phonophobia is superimposed. The non-IHS term *transformed migraine* has been applied to such a type. It is suspected to result from a "lowered headache threshold" due to muscular stressors, psychological stressors, or the pattern of acute analgesic use.

Tension-Type Headache

Tension-type headaches are perhaps the most common post-traumatic headaches. In the IHS system (Olesen, 1988) these headaches are characterized by bilateral pressure (nonthrobbing) pain. They may inhibit activity but usually do not prohibit it. Nausea, vomiting, photophobia, and phonophobia generally do not occur. Tension-type headaches are further defined as chronic or episodic. If the headache pain is present for more than 15 days out of a month or 180 days out of a year, the headache is termed chronic. The criteria for tension headache are listed in Table 8-7. The pathophysiology of chronic tension-type headaches is unknown, but a decreased pain threshold is suggested by demonstration of loss of inhibition of nociceptive reflexes (Langemark et al., 1993).

Episodic tension-type headaches usually respond to acute management and often do not create a hardship for the patient. Chronic tension-type headaches, however, are the most difficult to manage. The complaint so often occurs in patients who may give the appearance of being depressed or anxious that the National Institutes of Health Ad Hoc Classification System (1962) included the presence of anxiety and

TABLE 8-6. International Headache Society Definition of Migraine with Aura

1.2 Migraine with aura (previously used terms: classic migraine; classical migraine; ophthalmic, hemiparesthetic, hemiplegic, or aphasic migraine.
Diagnostic criteria
A. At least two attacks fulfilling criterion B below
B. At least three of the following four characteristics:
1. One or more fully reversible aura symptoms indicating focal cerebral cortical or brainstem dysfunction
2. At least one aura symptom develops gradually over more than 4 minutes, or two or more symptoms occur in succession
3. No aura symptom lasts more than 60 minutes. If more than one aura symptom is present, accepted duration is proportionally increased.
4. Headache follows aura with a free interval of less than 60 minutes. (It may also begin before or simultaneously with the aura.)
C. At least one of the following:
1. History, physical, and neurologic examinations do not suggest one of the disorders listed in groups 5 to 11 of Table 8-2.
2. History and/or physical and/or neurologic examinations do suggest such disorder, but it is ruled out by appropriate investigations.
3. Such disorder is present, but migraine attacks do not occur for the first time in close temporal relation to the disorder.

1.2.1 Migraine with typical aura.
Diagnostic criteria
A. Fulfills criteria for 1.2 migraine with aura, including all four criteria under B
B. One or more aura symptoms of the following types:
1. Homonymous visual disturbance
2. Unilateral paresthesias and/or numbness
3. Unilateral weakness
4. Aphasia or unclassifiable speech difficulty

depressed mood in the diagnosis, implying a role of psychological distress to produce the headache. In contrast, the IHS classified chronic tension-type headache as a primary headache (i.e., due to a physiologic process), although anxiety and/or depression play recognized roles. By the IHS criteria, any diagnosis of depression or anxiety disorder should meet DSM-IV (Diagnostic and Statistical Manual of Mental Disorders, 4th Edition) criteria. Other conditions that are believed to cause chronic daily headaches include oromandibular dysfunction, psychological stress, muscular stress, and the pattern of analgesics use. (Table 8-8).

By the IHS criteria, oromandibular dysfunction is defined by the presence of at least three of the following symptoms: temporomandibular joint noise on jaw movement, limited jaw movement, pain on jaw function, gnashing of teeth (bruxism), and related activity (e.g., tongue, lip, or cheek biting or pressing). The problem is limited to dysfunction of the mandible or temporomandibular joint and not related to muscular tenderness or stiffness. By this, a deliberate decision was made to exclude pericranial muscular tenderness that might represent a myofascial pain syndrome (Olesen, 1988). A discussion of the relationship of temporomandibular joint dysfunction to trauma is beyond the scope of this chapter (Burgess, 1991; Epstein, 1992; Heise et al., 1992). For the purpose of IHS headache classification, damage to the temporomandibular joint need not be demonstrated on radiographs.

With chronic tension-type headaches, psychological stressors are coded by the DSM-IV criteria (axis IV). It appears that multiple daily "hassles" have a stronger association than extreme or catastrophic stressors (DeBenedittis and Lorenzetti, 1992). They contribute to the maintenance of headache by the degree to which they generate a feeling of being unable to control the headache pain and its interruption of life activities. Psychogenic headaches are considered only as part of a "delusion or idea" or if they fulfill the DSM-IV criteria for somatoform or conversion disorders (Olesen, 1988).

Muscular stress refers to the presence of "long lasting tonic muscular contraction," possibly due to a sustained "unphysiologic position," and lack of rest or sleep (Olesen , 1988). This suggests that the process involved in the generation of myofascial pain may also contribute to chronic headache (see Ch. 13).

TABLE 8-7. International Headache Society Definition of Tension-Type Headache

2.1 Episodic tension-type headache (previously used terms: tension headache, muscle contraction headache, psychmygenic headache, stress headache, ordinary headache, essential headache, idiopathic headache, and psychogenic headache.
Diagnostic criteria
- A. At least 10 previous headache episodes fulfilling criteria B to D listed below. Number of days with such headaches <180/yr (<15/mon)
- B. Headache lasting from 30 minutes to 7 days
- C. At least two of the following pain characteristics:
  1. Pressing/tightening (nonpulsating) quality
  2. Mild or moderate intensity (may inhibit but does not prohibit activities)
  3. Bilateral location
  4. No aggravation by walking stairs or similar routine physical activity
- D. Both of the following
  1. No nausea or vomiting (anorexia may occur)
  2. Photophobia and phonophobia are absent, or one but not the other is present
- E. At least one of the following
  1. History, physical, and neurologic examinations do not suggest one of the disorders listed in groups 5 to 11 of Table 8-2.
  2. History and/or physical and/or neurologic examinations do suggest such disorder, but it is ruled out by appropriate investigations.
  3. Such disorder is present, but tension-type headache does not occur for the first time in close temporal relation to the disorder.

2.1.1 Episodic tension-type headache associated with disorder of pericranial muscles (previously used term: muscle contraction headache).
Diagnostic criteria
- A. Fulfills criteria for 2.1
- B. At least one of the following
  1. Increased tenderness of pericranial muscles demonstrated by manual palpation or pressure algometer.
  2. Increased EMG level of pericranial muscles at rest or during physiologic tests

2.1.2 Episodic tension-type headache unassociated with disorder of pericranial muscles (previously used terms: idiopathic headache, essential headache, psychogenic headache).
Diagnostic criteria
- A. Fulfills criteria for 2.1
- B. No increased tenderness of pericranial muscles. If studied, EMG of pericranial muscles shows normal levels of activity

2.2 Chronic tension-type headache (previously used term: chronic daily headache).
Diagnostic criteria
- A. Average headache frequency >15 days/mo (180 days/yr) for >6 months fulfilling criteria C and D
- B. At least two of the following pain characteristics:
  1. Pressing/tightening quality
  2. Mild or moderate severity (may inhibit but does not prohibit activities)
  3. Bilateral location
  4. No aggravation by walking stairs or similar routine physical activity
- C. Both of the following
  1. No vomiting
  2. No more than one of the following: nausea, photophobia, or phonophobia
- D. At least one of the following
  1. History, physical and neurologic examinations do not suggest one of the disorders listed in groups 5 to 11 of Table 8-2.
  2. History and/or physical and/or neurologic examinations do suggest such disorder, but it is ruled out by appropriate investigations.
  3. Such disorder is present, but tension-type headache does not occur for the first time in close temporal relation to the disorder.

2.2.1 Chronic tension-type headache associated with disorder of pericranial muscles

2.2.2 Chronic tension-type headache unassociated with disorder of pericranial muscles

TABLE 8-8. Factors Associated with Chronic Headache (International Headache Society Criteria)

1. Oromandibular dysfunction
2. Psychosocial stress (DSM-IV, axis 4)
3. Anxiety (DSM-IV)
4. Depression (DSM-IV)
5. Delusional disorder, somatic type or somatiform disorder (DSM-IV)
6. Muscular stress
7. Drug overuse
8. Others (as listed in groups 5 to 11 of IHS criteria, Table 8-2)

Analgesic overuse is probably a major contributor to chronic headaches. The monthly use of 45 g (approximately four 325-mg tablets per day) of aspirin or a similar analgesic, morphine-like drugs twice a month, or diazepam use exceeding 300 mg each month can each create a diffuse daily bilateral headache presenting shortly after awakening. Drug withdrawal is the suspected cause. Other agents such as caffeine, barbiturates, and codeine also may potentiate such headaches. The importance of appreciating analgesic overuse as withdrawal is that only resuming the offending agent will provide relief, and under these conditions no prophylactic intervention can be expected to work. Thus, the patient may be perceived as having intractable headaches or to be drug-seeking.

Cluster Headache

Cluster headache differs from migraine and tension-type headache by its frequency, duration, and associated autonomic signs (Table 8-9). One type of cluster headache is more common in men. The pain is severe, with a gnawing quality, and is located unilaterally in the orbital, supraorbital, or temporal areas. The pain lasts 15 to 180 minutes in association with one of the following on the side of the pain: (1) conjunctival injection, (2) lacrimation, (3) nasal congestion, (4) rhinorrhea, (5) forehead and facial sweating, (6) miosis, (7) ptosis, or (8) eyelid edema. It may occur at frequencies from once every other day to eight times per day. The headache is considered episodic if pain-free periods last longer than 14 days and chronic if the pain-free interval is shorter (Olesen, 1988).

Chronic paroxysmal hemicrania may be more common in women (Table 8-10). This form of cluster headache has a duration of 2 to 45 minutes and occurs more than five times per day. Most importantly, chronic paroxysmal hemicrania is completely responsive to indomethacin (Olesen, 1988).

The mechanism of cluster is not known, but one theory is a vasoregulary abnormality in the vessels of the cavernous sinus. There is no established association between cluster and trauma (Turkewitz et al., 1992). If such headache patterns developing after trauma the possibility of a lesion should be explored.

Other Post-Traumatic Headache Syndromes

It is important to consider all the secondary factors that may be contributing to headaches following trauma. These factors are listed in Table 8-2 (groups 5 to 11). Most commonly recognized in post-trauma cases are occipital neuralgia, cervicogenic headaches, and migraine-like headaches attributed to sympathetic damage.

Occipital Neuralgia

The term *occipital neuralgia* implies pain in the distribution of the greater and lesser occipital nerves, although it has also been loosely applied to any radiating pain triggered by palpation of occipital structures. Since its description in 1821 by Beruto y Lentijo and Ramas (Perelson, 1947) and again by many others (Ehni and Benner, 1984), it has been attributed to fibrosis or other organic processes that cause compression or irritation of the occipital nerve or nearby structures. Wolf (1963) proposed excessive muscle contraction and scarring of scalp tissue causing nerve entrapment. The International Association for the Study of Pain (Mersky, 1986) defines occipital neuralgia as "continuous aching, throbbing pain in the suboccipital region with radiation over the posterior and lateral scalp." Retro-orbital pain is common in severe attacks. Trigger zones are generally not present, although pressure on the occipital nerve can aggravate pain, adding "neuralgia consequent to injury associated with mild sensory changes—hyperalgesia, hyperesthesia, or hypoalgesia and hypoesthesia" (Bonica, 1990). The IHS classifies occipital neuralgia as a secondary headache. The criteria (Table 8-11) include pain of intermittent stabbing quality in the distribution of the greater or lesser occipital nerves, which may persist between the paroxysms; tenderness to palpation of the occipital nerve(s); and temporary easing of the pain condition by local anesthetic nerve blocks (Olesen, 1988).

TABLE 8-9. International Headache Society Definition of Cluster Headache

3.1 Cluster headache (previously used terms: erythroprosopalgia of Bing, ciliary or migrainous neuralgia (Harris), erythromelalgia of the head, Horton's headache, histaminic cephalgia, petrosal neuralgia (Gardner), spenopalatine, Vidian and Sluder's neuralgia, hemicrania periodica neuralgiformis).
Diagnostic criteria
- A. At least five attacks fulfilling criteria B to D
- B. Severe unilateral orbital, supraorbital, and/or temporal pain lasting 15 to 180 minutes untreated
- C. Headache associated with at least one of the following signs, which have to be present on the pain side:
  1. Conjunctival injection
  2. Lacrimation
  3. Nasal congestion
  4. Rhinorrhea
  5. Forehead and facial sweating
  6. Miosis
  7. Ptosis
  8. Eyelid edema
- D. Frequency of attacks: from one every other day to eight per day
- E. At least one of the following:
  1. History, physical, and neurologic examinations do not suggest one of the disorders listed in groups 5 to 11 of Table 8-2.
  2. History and/or physical and/or neurologic examinations do suggest such disorder, but it is ruled out by appropriate investigations.
  3. Such disorder is present, but cluster headaches do not occur for the first time in close temporal relation to the disorder.

3.1.1 Cluster headache periodicity undetermined
- A. Criteria for 3.1 fulfilled
- B. Too early to classify as 3.1.2 or 3.1.3

3.1.2 Episodic cluster headache (occurs in periods lasting 7 days to 1 year separated by pain-free periods lasting 14 days or more)
Diagnostic criteria
- A. All letter headings of 3.1
- B. At least two periods of headaches (cluster periods) lasting (in untreated patients) from 7 days to 1 year, separated by remissions of at least 14 days

Comment: cluster periods usually last between 2 weeks and 3 months

3.1.3 Chronic cluster headache (attacks occur for more than 1 year without remission or with remissions lasting less than 14 days).
Diagnostic criteria
- A. All letter headings of 3.1
- B. Absence of remission phases for 1 year or more with remissions lasting less than 14 days

3.1.3.1 Chronic cluster headache unremitting from onset (previously used term: primary chronic).
Diagnostic criteria
- A. All letter heading of 3.1.3
- B. Absence of remission periods lasting 14 days or more from onset

3.1.3.2 Chronic cluster headache evolved from episodic (previously used term: secondary chronic).
Diagnostic criteria
- A. All letter headings of 3.1.3
- B. At least one interim remission period lasting 14 days or more within 1 year after onset, followed by unremitting course for at least 1 year

Diagnostic difficulties arise because a similar clinical presentation, including a favorable response to local anesthetic occipital nerve blocks, may be seen in association with diverse etiologies, including abnormalities of the occipital musculature and C1, C2, and C3 cervical spine structures (Wilson, 1991), myofascial pain, migraine and chronic tension-type headache (Loeser, 1990), and cluster headaches (Anthony, 1985). Some of these points are discussed in more detail below in connection with cervicogenic headaches.

Myofascial pain syndromes involving the posterior cervical musculature may present a picture resembling occipital neuralgia (Graff-Radford et al., 1986).

TABLE 8-10. International Headache Society Definition of Chronic Paroxysmal Hemicrania

3.2 Chronic paroxysmal hemicrania (previously used term: Sjaastad's syndrome)
Diagnostic criteria:
A. At least 50 attacks fulfilling criteria B to E
B. Attacks of severe unilateral orbital, supraorbital, and/or temporal pain always on the same side lasting 2 to 45 minutes
C. Attack frequency above five per day for more than half of the time (periods with lower frequency may occur)
D. Pain is associated with at least one of the following signs/symptoms on the pain side:
1. Conjunctival injection
2. Lacrimation
3. Nasal congestion
4. Rhinorrhea
5. Ptosis
6. Eyelid edema
E. Absolute effectiveness of indomethacin (150 mg/day or less)
F. At least one of the following:
1. History, physical, and neurologic examinations do not suggest one of the disorders listed in groups 5 to 11 of Table 8-2.
2. History and/or physical and/or neurologic examinations do suggest such disorder, but it is ruled out by appropriate investigations.
3. Such disorder is present, but chronic paroxysmal hemicrania does not occur for the first time in close temporal relation to the disorder.

3.3 Cluster headache-like disorder not fulfilling above criteria.
Diagnostic criterion
A. Fulfilling all but one of the criteria for 3.2

The validity of considering these syndromes as a single disease entity remains subject to debate (see also Ch. 13). Symptoms include diffuse muscle soreness, the presence of myofascial trigger points, and nonrestful sleep (McCain, 1994; Sola and Bonica, 1990). This constellation of symptoms is believed to represent a "disorganization" of central neural processing resulting in a diffuse hyperesthetic state. The term *hyperesthetic* means that all sensory input is exaggerated (to be distinguished from hyperalgesic, which refers to increased responsiveness of only the pain fibers) (Mersky, 1986). The hallmark of myofascial pain syndromes is the presence of "active" myofascial trigger points (firm, hyperirritable loci found within taut bands of skeletal muscles or fasciae), which on palpation produce a radiation of pain in a "characteristic and reproducible referred pain pattern" not explainable along neural, ligamentous, or muscular structures (Travell and Simons, 1983). Trigger points located in five cervical muscles—the splenius capitis, splenius cervicis, multifidus, semispinalis capitis, and semispinalis cervicis—all have local suboccipital pain with extension to the vertex, periorbital, temple, and occipital areas (Graff-Radford et al., 1986) (Fig. 8-1). Response to an occipital nerve block does not differentiate between myofascial pain syndromes and occipital neuralgia.

Muscular structures generally have increased pain receptors near their points of insertion. Even in normal, non-headache conditions it is not unusual to have areas of point tenderness. Such tenderness may be distinguished from myofascial trigger points by the absence of pain radiation. Myofascial trigger points may be differentiated from true occipital neu-

TABLE 8-11. International Headache Society Definition of Occipital Neuralgia

Diagnostic criteria
Pain is felt in the distribution of greater or lesser occipital nerves.
Pain is stabbing in quality although aching may persist between paroxysms.
The affected nerve is tender to palpation.
The condition is eased temporarily by local anesthetic block of the appropriate nerve.

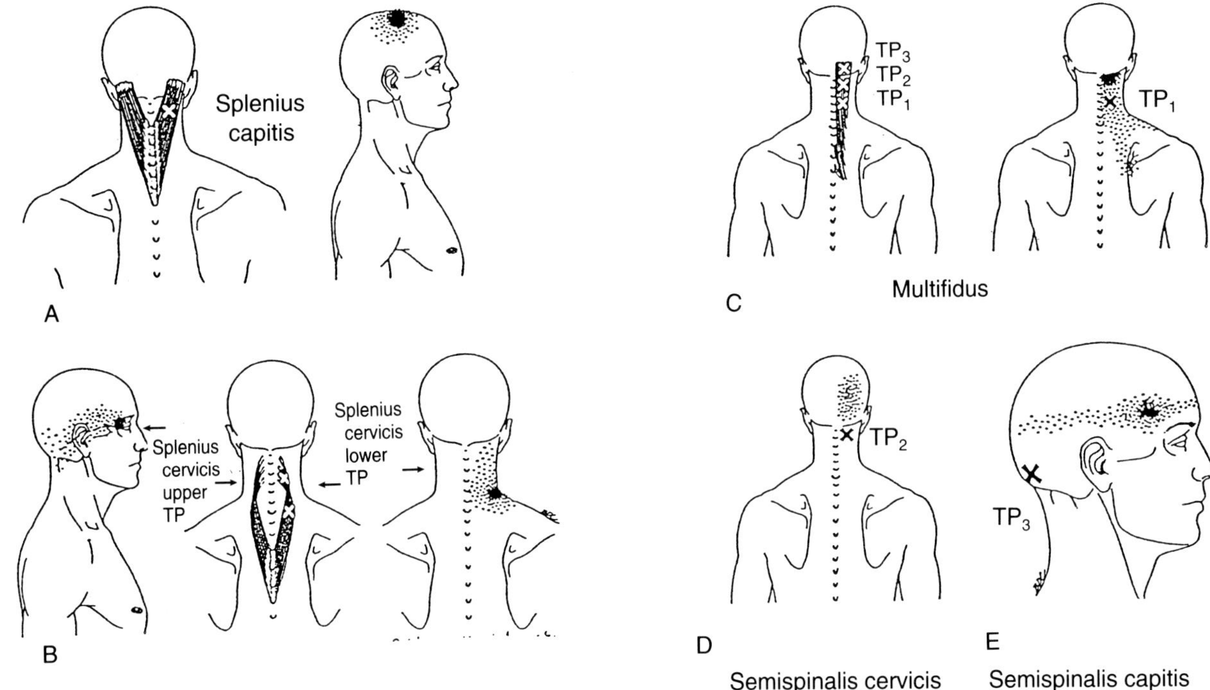

Fig. 8-1. Common cervical myofascial syndromes with pain radiation to the head. Trigger points (x) and referral pain pattern (dots) for posterior cervical muscles are depicted: (**A**) splenius capitis; (**B**) splenius cervicis; (**C**) multifidus; (**D**) Semispinalis cervicis; (**E**) semispinalis capititis. (From Travell and Simons, 1983, with permission.)

ralgia by identifying the location of the occipital artery (which lies adjacent to the occipital nerve), determining the proximity of tender points, and demonstrating evidence of altered sensory perception in occipital nerve distribution. The idea that occipital neuralgia may be due to nerve compression from spasm in the trapezius muscle must be questioned because the occipital nerve emerges through the aperture above the aponeurotic sling of the trapezius and the sternomastoid muscles, where it is not vulnerable to compression by the trapezius.

Cervicogenic Headaches

Certain congenital abnormalities (Arnold-Chiari malformations, basilar invagination, congenital atlantoaxial dislocation) (Khurana, 1991; Pascual et al., 1992; Stovner, 1993) are associated with head pain. So are acquired conditions, including tumors, infections, or fractures of the occiput or cervical spine (Edmeads, 1988; Wilson, 1991), and chronic conditions such as cervical spondylosis or degenerative arthritis (Edmeads, 1988; Wilson, 1991). Also, unilateral headaches have been reported to resolve following surgical correction of lower cervical root compressions (Michler et al., 1991). However, the role of cervical injury in the production and maintenance of post-traumatic headaches is unclear.

Cervicogenic headaches are a secondary headache type recognized by the IHS (Olesen, 1988). The criteria are listed in Table 8-12. The pain must be present in the neck and occipital region, with possible projection to the forehead, orbital region, temples, vertex, or ears, and must be precipitated or aggravated by neck movement or sustained neck position. A pathologic process must be identified; otherwise the headache is classified under the primary headache type it most closely resembles. There are, however, several headache syndromes described in the literature that are not accepted under IHS criteria.

Sjaastad et al. (1983) proposed a cervicogenic headache that is distinct from migraine or tension-type headaches and that could follow trauma to the neck or head. Criteria for the diagnosis of cervicogenic headache were later published by Sjaastad et

TABLE 8-12. Characteristics of Cervicogenic Headache

Major symptoms and signs
- I. Unilateral pain, without alternating sides
- II. Symptoms of neck involvement
  - A. Attacks provoked by
    - 1. Neck movement or sustained neck position
    - 2. Pressure over ipsilateral upper, posterior neck or occipital region
  - B. Ipsilateral neck, shoulder, and arm pain (vague, nonradicular)
  - C. Reduced range of motion

Pain characteristics
- III. Nonclustering episodes
- IV. Constant pain with fluctuations or discrete pain episodes of varying duration
- V. Moderate intensity, nonthrobbing
- VI. Pain initiates in neck with spread to oculofrontotemporal areas, maximal pain often in oculofrontotemporal area

Other important criteria
- VII. Anesthetic blocks of occipital nerve or C2 root on symptomatic side temporarily abolishes the pain at the site and in oculofrontotemporal areas
- VIII. Female sex
- IX. Head and/or neck trauma (whiplash) by history

Minor, more rarely occurring, nonobligatory symptoms and signs; various attack-related phenomena
- X. Autonomic symptoms and signs
  - A. Nausea
  - B. Vomiting
  - C. Ipsilateral edema; less frequently flushing in periocular area
- XI. Dizziness
- XII. Photophobia and phonophobia
- XIII. "Blurred vision" on eye ipsilateral to pain
- XIV. Difficulty swallowing

al. (1990) and are listed in Table 8-13. Unlike migraine, the unilateral headache pain does not alternate sides, and photophobia and phonophobia are not prominent complaints. The headaches are unresponsive to indomethacin unlike chronic paroxysmal hemicrania. The headache can be exacerbated by palpation of neck structures, and occipital nerve blocks offer relief (Bovim and Sand, 1992). The main distinction between the cervicogenic headache of Sjaastad and the IHS headache is that the latter requires specific radiologic evidence of a pathologic process.

Bogduk and his associates explored the mechanisms of cervicogenic headache by first mapping the structures innervated by the upper cervical nerves in cadavers (Bogduk, 1981; Bogduk, 1992; Bogduk et al., 1988) (see Table 8-14). There are several C2-innervated structures (C2 sinuvertebral nerve: dura matter of posterior cranial fossa, median atlantoaxial joint, cruciate ligament; C2 dorsal ramus: semispinus capitis, longissimus capitis, splenius capitis; C2 ventral ramus: lateral atlantoaxial joint, prevertebral muscle, trapezius, sternocleidomastoid). Bogduk (1981) also identified the relationship of the C2 spinal ganglion to the dorsal aspect of the atlantoaxial joint and established the radiologic landmarks to perform a selective C2 block. In those patients in whom selective C2 block relieved headache, he speculated that the nociceptive input from C2-innervated structures might establish or maintain the headaches. Direct injury to the C2 ganglion and nerve following whiplash has been speculated to occur by compression between the atlas and axis in the region of the lateral atlantoaxial joint when the force is generated "during rotation combined with extreme extension" (Keith, 1986).

Bogduk and Marsland (1986) proposed the existence of a "third occipital headache" due to traumatic arthropathy or degenerative arthritis of the C2-C3 zygapophysial joint. This joint is in the transition zone between cervical elements involved in rotation of the head and flexion and extension of the neck and may be prone to injury in whiplash-type trauma. The third occipital nerve also innervates the posterior

TABLE 8-13. International Headache Society Criteria for Cervicogenic Headache

A. Pain in the neck and occipital region with possible radiation to the forehead, orbit, temples, vertex or ears
B. Pain precipitated or aggravated by neck movement or sustained neck position
C. At least one of the following:
  1. Limitation of passive neck movements
  2. Changes in neck muscle contour, texture, tone, or response to stretching
  3. Abnormal tenderness of neck muscles
D. Radiologic evidence of at least one of the following:
  1. Movement abnormalities in flexion/extension
  2. Abnormal posture
  3. Fractures, congenital abnormalities, bone tumors, rheumatoid arthritis (not spondylosis or osteochondrosis)

(From Olesen, 1988, with permission.)

scalp, and a portion of the semispinalis capitis muscle provides the sole innervation of the C2-C3 zygapophysial joint. A third occipital nerve block may improve a posterior headache triggered by C2-C3 zygapophysial injury.

It appears that the trigeminal nociceptive system may also play a role in cervicogenic headaches. The terminations of trigeminal afferents within the spinal descending nucleus lie near the terminations of cervical afferents at the levels of C2, C3, and C4 (Fig. 8-2). In cats these cervical and trigeminal afferent nerve connections may merge on common second-order neurons (Kerr, 1960; 1972). The collection of cells in the upper cervical segments that receive nociceptive input from both the trigeminal and cervical nerves is called the *trigeminocervical nucleus*. According to Kerr (1960) any irritation to structures innervated by the cervical sensory nerves will activate the trigeminal nucleus and result in referred pain to the head.

A similar hypothesis of peripheral nociceptive drive has been proposed by Olesen (1991) (Fig. 8-3) to explain how cervical muscular tenderness or myofascial trigger points might act as generators for primary headaches. Patients with migraine may report neck pain and stiffness at some point during an attack. Injection of the tender muscles may relieve the migraine (Blau et al., 1994). Such injections may act at the level of the peripheral nerve or its more central connections. In the latter regard, palpation of cervical musculature, the occipital nerves, or the C2 spinous process may modulate head pain in the trigeminal distribution. Also, anesthetic occipital nerve or C2 nerve blocks may temporarily relieve pain in the frontal head areas not supplied by those nerves (Bogduk, 1981; Bovim et al., 1992a; Gawel and Rothbart, 1992).

Other proposed head pain triggers include arthrosis of the C1-C2 lateral articulation (Ehni and Benner, 1984), vascular compression of the cervical roots (Jansen et al., 1989a; Jansen et al., 1989b), injury to the second cervical ganglion (Keith, 1986), myofascial pain with trigger points (Jaeger, 1989), and stress (Muse, 1985).

Radiologic evaluation of patients with cervicogenic headaches (Pfaffenrath et al., 1987), including cerebral and cervical computed tomography (CT) and cervical spine films with flexion extension views, are generally unimpressive (Fredriksen et al., 1989). However, one radiologic study of post-traumatic headache patients suggested decreased extension-flexion at C2-C3, C5-C6, and C6-C7. The motion limitation was thought to represent muscular spasm (Jensen et al., 1990). The patients in this study also complained of "dizziness, visual disturbances, and ear symptoms."

TABLE 8-14. The Distribution of the C1 to C3 Spinal Nerves

C1 to C3 ventral rami
- Atlanto-occipital joint
- Lateral atlantoaxial joint
- Longus capitis
- Longus cervicis
- Rectus capitis anterior
- Rectus capitis lateralis
- Trapezius
- Sternocleidomastoid
- Dura mater of posterior fossa
- Vertebral artery

C1 to C3 sinuvertebral nerves
- Median atlantoaxial joint
- Transverse ligaments
- Alar ligaments
- Dura mater of spinal cord
- Dura mater of clivus
- C2-C3 intervertebral disc

C1 to C3 dorsal rami
- C2-C3, C3-C4 zygapophysial joints
- Suboccipital muscles
- Semispinalis capitis
- Semispinalis cervicis
- Multifidus
- Longissimus capitis
- Splenius capitis

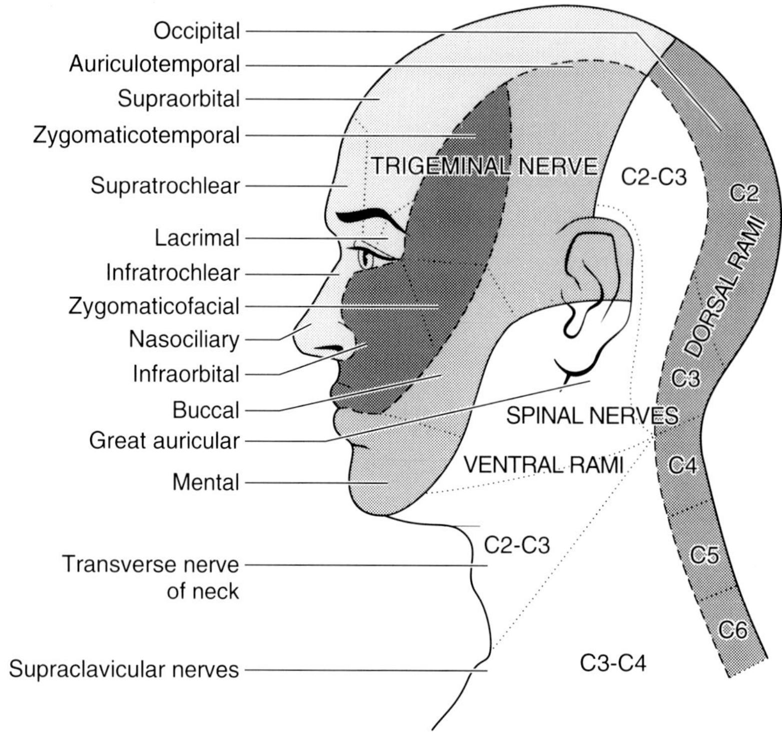

Fig. 8-2. Distribution of cutaneous nerves to head and neck. The ophthalmic, maxillary, and mandibular divisions of the trigeminal nerve are indicated by different shading. (Adapted from Romanes 1972, with permission.)

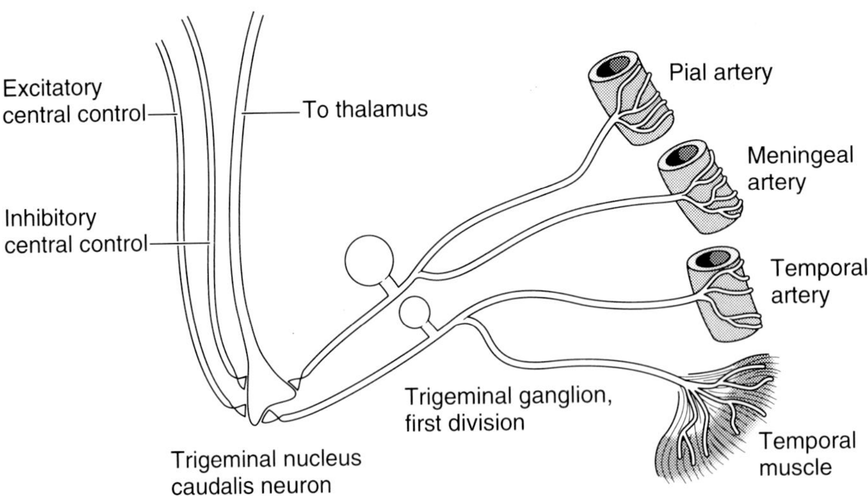

Fig. 8-3. Pain pathways relevant to headache. Schematic drawing of intracranial (vascular) and extracranial (vascular and myofascial) nociceptive nerve endings and their gradual convergence in the trigeminal ganglion and in the nucleus caudalis of the brainstem. The vascular-central-myogenic model predicts that convergence of supraspinal and peripheral inputs onto the same neuron may be crucial for migraine pain and perhaps for other headaches. (Adapted from Olesen, 1991, with permission.)

Indeed, the symptom of dizziness is commonly associated with post-traumatic headache (see also Ch. 9). One hypothesis is disruption of the neck afferents involved with spatial orientation and posture. However, electronystagmography and tests of spatial orientation were not found to be abnormal in patients with post-traumatic headaches and dizziness, nor was the dizziness influenced by C2 local anesthetic blocks (Dieterich et al., 1993).

In the final analysis, many questions remain about the relationship between cervical pathology or dysfunction and headache. Curiously, the severity of injury seems to be invisibly proportioned to headache. For example, it appears that migraine headaches are associated with new onset of back pain not due to trauma (Duckro et al., 1994). On the other hand, migraine does not seem to occur in some patients with extremely severe neck injuries, including spinal cord damage, with complete sensory levels between C2-C3 and C8 (Spierings et al., 1992).

Headaches Due to Sympathetic Injury

Bartschi-Rochaix (1986) described a series of patients with migraine-like headache as well as giddiness, blurred vision, scotoma, neck pain and dysesthesias, depression, and anxiety. Their symptoms were supposedly due to compression of vertebral arteries by trauma or osteophyte formation. In 1926 Barre described a similar collection of symptoms which he termed "posterior cervical sympathetic syndrome" and attributed to impingement on the sympathetic nerve plexus around vertebral arteries (Edmeads, 1988).

This pattern of symptoms in such cases differs from the pain of vertebral dissection. The latter pain has an acute onset in posterior head and neck areas and may remain severe over weeks, but range of motion is preserved and there is no cervical tenderness to palpation (Sturzenegger, 1994). Also, symptoms of ischemia of the brainstem or posterior circulation territory often accompany vertebral dissection. Of course, acute cerebrovascular ischemia itself may produce headache (Arboix et al., 1994; Olesen, 1988).

Vijayan (1977) described sympathetic symptoms with post-traumatic headaches without involving vertebral artery compression. His patients reported ipsilateral mydriasis, facial sweating, ptosis, and meiosis. Khurana and Niranhari (1986) reported similar cases. Currently, headache syndromes thought to be due to sympathetic injury are all grouped under the term *posterior migraine* (Edmeads, 1988). This is not an IHS classification.

PATIENT EVALUATION

A headache that immediately follows trauma raises the suspicion of cranial or cervical tissue injury. Emergent investigation aims to identify any process requiring immediate intervention. Conditions such as subarachnoid hemorrhage, major brain contusion with edema or ischemia, brainstem or spinal cord contusion, cervical fracture, or acute hydrocephalus are expected to be evident shortly after the trauma and to have associated neurologic abnormalities, which may progress if not treated. Description of the acute management of such conditions is beyond the scope of this chapter. Reassurance may be provided to the patient by close observation, by directed examination and studies, and by providing an expected time course for the headache. Post-traumatic headaches that arise as a consequence of these conditions usually resolve following their correction. Pain conditions that begin well after the trauma include post-stroke central pain, syrinx formation, neuroma formation, and disuse syndromes.

In the initial interview, several types of information should be obtained: (1) a description of the trauma, (2) the time elapsed since the trauma, (3) the characteristics of the headache, and (4) a general sense of the person's current functioning level. The type and severity of the trauma can be inferred from records of the physical examination, radiography, neuroimaging, or electrophysiologic data. Loss of consciousness and post-traumatic amnesia should be explored (Forrester et al., 1994). For the purpose of post-traumatic headache diagnosis, a retrospective assessment of when the patient "woke up" should be adequate for diagnostic classification.

By the IHS criteria, headache onset must occur within 2 weeks after the time of trauma or the time the patient regained consciousness to make a temporal association. If headache persists more than 8 weeks after trauma, it is considered chronic (Olesen, 1988). This cutoff does not directly apply to the legal definitions of chronic or permanent (Packard and Ham, 1993). The American Medical Association guidelines for the evaluation of permanent impairment (AMA, 1993) recommend estimating impairment due to chronic headache using the same approach as for other chronic pain.

Following establishment of the temporal association of the headache to the trauma, the severity of the head trauma, and the presence or absence of post-traumatic amnesia, it is necessary to establish if the headache pattern is consistent with any of the IHS primary headache types. This is best done systematically with a structured interview. The goal of establishing this association is to better predict successful treatment outcome.

Structured Interview

The main points addressed in the structured interview are outlined in Table 8-3.

Frequency

Migraine headaches occur as discrete episodes with headache-free intervals. Tension-type headaches are considered episodic if they occur less often than 15 days per month or 180 days per year; otherwise they are termed chronic. Cluster-type headaches are short periods of intense pain, which occur up to several times a day.

Duration

Simple migraine should last 4 to 72 hours. Tension-type headaches may have a duration of 30 minutes to 7 days. In the chronic form they may be daily or continuous. Cluster headaches occur either as short-duration (15-minute to 3-hour) gnawing severe pain in the male pattern or as repetitive brief jabs occurring over moments to 45 minutes in the female form (chronic paroxysmal hemicrania).

Pain Characteristics

Location

Is the headache unilateral or bilateral? Migraine and cluster-type headaches are usually unilateral while tension-type are bilateral. Migraine pain can occur in any area of the cranium, as can tension-type headache. Cluster headaches tend to localize to the orbital, frontal, or temporal area. Otherwise, constant head pain that consistently localizes in a discrete area (<5 cm diameter) suggests a focal pathologic process rather than a primary headache condition.

Quality

Each of the primary headache types has a characteristic pain quality: throbbing for migraine, pressure (tightness) for tension-type, and deep gnawing ache or "jab and jolts" for the cluster type. "Icepick-like pain may be associated with migraine. Pain descriptions associated with neuropathic pain includes "burning," "shooting," "electrical," "cold," "fullness," "numbness," and "pins and needles." Such qualities suggest possible nerve injury or neuroma formation.

Intensity

The IHS suggests a three-level verbal scale for reporting headache as mild, moderate, or severe. Mild does not influence daily activity, moderate does, and severe prohibits all activity. Tension-type headaches are usually mild to moderate, migraines are moderate to severe (in part owing to associated nausea and vomiting), and cluster headaches are usually severe.

Aggravation by Activity

Physical activity such as climbing stairs may worsen migraine headache pain but should have little influence on the pain of tension-type or cluster headaches. Neck movement or sustained neck posture is reported to worsen tension-type headaches. It may also distinguish cervicogenic headaches (of Sjaastad) from primary headaches.

Associated Signs or Symptoms

Nausea, with or without vomiting, photophobia, and phonophobia accompany migraine. Episodic tension-type headaches should not be accompanied by either nausea or vomiting. While light and sound may be irritating, photophobia or phonophobia should not accompany an episodic tension-type headache. If tension-type headache is chronic, nausea but not vomiting may be associated. Phonophobia or photophobia may also be present. With cluster or chronic paroxysmal hemicrania one or more of the following autonomic signs must be present during the attack: conjunctival injection, lacrimation, nasal congestion, rhinorrhea, forehead or facial sweating, miosis, ptosis, and eyelid edema.

Accompanying Neurologic Defects

A migrainous aura is a transient neurologic deficit of less than 60 minutes duration. As mentioned, it may represent dysfunction of a focal cortical or brainstem area, which precedes the pain of a migraine headache. To be classified as a simple aura the neurologic deficit must clear completely prior to the onset of pain. Any neurologic deficits at the time of headache pain may indicate a more sinister cause. One exception is the migraine headache with aura noted in children after head trauma, in which situation hemiplegia or other defects may accompany headache and not resolve until after a period of sleep.

Precipitating Activity

Precipitating activity is not required for diagnosis of primary headache type, but it does allow identification of factors that may be modified to better maximize treatment success. Precipitating activity becomes more valuable when considering those headache types that appear to fall between the classifications such as daily headaches with migrainous qualities or headache worsened with neck movement.

Response to Medications

A response to indomethacin (a poor acute migraine medication) may help differentiate between chronic paroxysmal hemicrania with subtle eye findings and an "icepick-type" migraine headache. Frequent use of medication may also trigger a headache that can replace or coexist with the original headache condition. Serotonin-selective medications such as sumatriptan are expected to be specific for migraine or cluster headaches, but one-third of tension-type headaches appear to respond. Only the response to indomethacin is considered diagnostic.

Contributing Factors

With the passage of time, it is important to establish if the character of the headache has changed since the time of trauma. Changes in the headache's character may reflect the influences of drug therapy or situational factors. Organic factors such as glaucoma, dental caries, sinus disease, hypertension, and infectious processes must not be overlooked. If the patient had a history of headaches prior to the trauma, it is valuable to determine if the current headache pattern reflects a new headache type or an exacerbation of a previous headache condition. Headache therapy may require adjustment.

In a patient who has deteriorated emotionally, cognitively, or physically following trauma, establishing the cause of this decline becomes important in individualizing headache treatment. Reactions to severe physical or cognitive injury or a major grief reaction to loss (such as loss of a spouse who may have been killed in the same traumatic event) qualify as severe or catastrophic stressors. Less severe physical or cognitive injury may alter a patient's usual pattern of activity and create "daily hassles" that are also associated with headache (DeBenedittis and Lorenzetti, 1992). Post-traumatic headaches are recognized to worsen around times of lawyer visits (Packard, 1992). Anxiety and depression after trauma are not unusual, and if they are severe enough to interfere with functioning, there exists a possible association with worsening headache (Olesen, 1988).

Certain medications first given during the acute headache phase might lead over time to a protracted course in susceptible people. Previously effective prophylactic and abortive therapies may become ineffective. When the medication is stopped, a withdrawl condition may develop, causing patients to seek the narcotic, sedative, or antianxiolytic they originally received. Furthermore, treatment with medications that "just take the edge off" may reinforce the pattern of frequent dosing. Such analgesic overuse headaches present daily, usually present upon awakening or shortly thereafter, and are associated with a sense of restlessness, memory difficulties, or anxiety. The headache may be relieved by the use of the causative medication, with the patient appearing tolerant to other acute medications. Such headaches are sometimes referred to as "rebound" headaches. Prophylactics are ineffective at the time the analgesic overuse is occurring.

Organized evaluation of muscles, especially in the cervical area, allows appreciation of possible muscular triggers or the presence of myofascial pain and/or post-traumatic fibromyalgia. The presence of these conditions would be expected to reduce the response to therapies directed at headache alone. Since these conditions are more refractory to treatment than headache, their coexistence suggests that treatment may be difficult. Myofascial pain is felt to be a consequence of inactivity. A patient fearful of increasing activity because of pain may become more prone to this condition. The patient may also have received advice from physicians and care providers that they must be careful and avoid activity. As a result of chronic disuse, the upper cervical flexors may become deconditioned and the head adopt a forward position (Watson and Trott, 1993).

TREATMENT

From the evaluation, a decision is made if the headache represents a treatable acute process or fulfills the criteria of a primary headache type. Identification is made of those factors that may influence the occurrence of headache and contribute to resistance to therapy. If the headache is chronic, past therapies should be reviewed, with careful attention to types of drug management and drug dosages as well as nondrug therapies.

Pharmacologic Management

Drug treatment for primary headache types includes both prophylactic and acute management approaches. The decision to treat prophylactically is based on a frequency of more than twice per month or the intolerability of the headache due to the severity or duration of the pain and associated symptoms (Baumel, 1994). The frequency of the headache also directs which medications may be effective. Another decision is what medication dosage schedules to adopt in order to avoid additional limitations due to intoxication, sedation, or "rebound" withdrawal symptoms associated with frequently dosed medications. Most headache drug trials have been applied to migraine headaches. The medications will be discussed under the head type for which they are most commonly used.

Migraine

Evidence has mounted against cranial vessel dilation as the cause of throbbing migraine pain, with the vascular involvement now appreciated as a component of the neuroinflammatory model (Moskowitz, 1993). In this model nerve activation results in the release of serotonin, substance P, and other vasodilators at the site of blood vessels and other nociceptive nerve endings. An inflammatory response occurs, further sensitizing nerve endings and causing nociceptive volleys into the central nervous system, which further sustain the nerve activation. Interruption of nerve-to-nerve and nerve-to-blood vessel interactions would be expected to halt the process. At this time the most successful agents for migraine management appear to work on inflammation or serotonin (5-hydroxytryptamine [5-HT]), receptors (Peroutka, 1993). 5-HT_1 receptor agonists are effective in acute management. Prophylaxis of migraine headache occurs as a result of 5-HT_2 antagonist activity. The similarity in the protein structure of α- and β-adrenergic, dopaminergic, and serotonergic receptors (Zemlan and Garver, 1990) and the effectiveness of medications working at these sites in controlling migraine suggest that our understanding remains incomplete.

Prophylaxis

β-adrenergic blocking agents are believed to function through their ability to moderate the discharge of serotonin neurons (Table 8-15). Propranolol is the agent of choice by which all the β-blockers and other medications are judged for effectiveness in migraine prophylaxis. That propranolol works through blocking β-adrenergic receptors was demonstrated by comparing active to inactive racemic forms (Tfelt-Hansen, 1986). Other β-adrenergic drugs, including metoprolol, nadolol, atenolol, and timolol, have been demonstrated to be effective in double-blind studies. Ineffectiveness of some drugs in this group is related to the presence of partial agonist activity (Tfelt-Hansen and Saxena 1993). Choice between the medications is based on dosing schedule, cost, and individual patient response.

Tricyclic antidepressants are believed to work through antagonism of 5-HT_2 receptors. Amitriptyline and imipramine have been the drugs of choice, with nortriptyline, desipramine, and doxepin also shown to be effective (Couch and Micieli, 1993; Mylechrane and Tfelt-Hansen, 1993) (Table 8-15). These medications appear to require approximately 2 weeks to take effect, which presumably is related to neurotransmitter shifts that occur during this period. There is a marked variability in the dose adequate to provide prophylaxis, ranging from 10 mg to more than 200 mg of amitriptyline. Limitation in the use of these drugs is primarily due to side effects, including sedation, dry mouth, cognitive difficulties, or effects related to orthostatic hypotension and urinary retention (Silberstein and Lipton, 1994).

Calcium channel-blocking drugs have been demonstrated to be effective in migraine headaches (Toda and Tfelt-Hansen, 1993) (Table 8-15). Flunarizime, a nonselective agent available in Europe but not in the United States, appears to be the most effective. However, it has major side effects of parkinsonism and depression limiting its usefulness. Of the approved agents available in the United States, verapamil and nicardipine appear to be the most effective. No standard dosing range has been determined for the calcium channel blocking agent. Their use is considered in patients who have contraindications for the use of β-blockers or tricyclic antidepressant drugs. The presence of Raynaud's phenomenon has

TABLE 8-15. Prophylactic Headache Management

Category	Drug	Headache Type	Receptor Activity	Daily Dose	Dosing Frequency	Contra-Indications	Treatment Considerations	Management Considerations	Side-Effects
β-Blockers			Partial agonist activity prevents effectiveness for migraine prophylaxis			Asthma, COPD, CHF, PUD, Raynaud's disease, insulin-dependent diabetes	Combined with amitriptyline may increase effectiveness. Combined with ergotamines may precipitate acute ergotism		Fatigue, exercise intolerance, depression, impotence
	Propranolol	MO, MA, TTH	Nonselective β-blocker, 5HT affinity	40–320 mg	Twice (long-acting: once)		Only FDA-approved migraine prophylactic medication	Beginning dose 20 mg bid	
	Metoprolol	MO, MA	β_1 selective	50–100 mg	Twice (long-acting, once)				
	Nadolol	MO, MA	Nonselective	40–240 mg	Once			May be administered without regard to meals	
	Atenolol	MO, MA	β_1 selective	50–200 mg	Once				
	Timolol	MO, MA	Nonselective	10–60 mg	Twice				
Ca channel blockers			Slow Ca channel block. Heterogeneous drug group			Bradycardia, conduction abnormalities, use of β-blockers	May inhibit cortical spreading depression; perhaps preferred for prolonged aura or vertebrobasilar migraine	May initially worsen headaches	Dizziness, headache, depression, tremor, gastric distress, peripheral edema, orthostatic hypotension, bradycardia
	Flunarizine	MO, MA		10 mg	Once	Pregnancy, parkinsonism, depression (including depression in first relative	Not available in United States		
	Verapamil	MO, MA, Cl		240–320 mg	tid, long-acting, once				
	Nicardipine	MO		40 mg	Once				
	Nifedipine	MA		30–90 mg	tid		Effective in patients with Raynaud's disease		

(Continued)

TABLE 8-15. *(continued)* **Prophylactic Headache Management**

Category	Drug	Headache Type	Receptor Activity	Daily Dose	Dosing Frequency	Contra-Indications	Treatment Considerations	Management Considerations	Side-Effects
Tricyclic anti-depressants			Norepinephrine, serotonin reuptake blocker, anticholinergic, antihistamine			Heart block, urinary retention, close-angle glaucoma	May reverse action of clonidine and similar antihypertensives. Choice of drug primarily based on side effects. Cimetidine inhibits clearance.	Begin with low dose. May increase as rapidly as every 3 days. Expect 2 weeks before observing effects.	Agitation, insomnia, sedation, tachycardia, tremor, sweating, blurred vision, constipation, urinary hesitation, orthostatic hypotension, weight gain, decreased libido, alopecia
	Amitriptyline	MO, MA, TTH		10–200 mg	Once				
	Nortriptyline			10–200 mg	Once				
	Imipramine			10–200 mg	Once				
	Disipramine			10–200 mg	Once				
	Doxepin			10–200 mg	Once				
Antiserotonin drugs									
	Metysergide	MO, MA, C1	Serotonin, antagonist, 5-HT, 5-HT2, 5-HT3	3–6 mg	tid	CVD, HTN, PUD, pregnancy, familial fibrotic disorders, renal or hepatic disease. H/O thrombophlebitis	May be more effective in migraine with aura	Vasomotor effects are additive to abortine ergotamine; drug holiday of 3–4 weeks every 6 months reduces risk of retroperitoneal fibrosis	1/5,000 incidence of retroperitoneal pulmonary or endocardial fibrosis; nausea, muscle cramps, claudication, hallucinations
	Cyproheptadine	MO, MA	5-HT_2 antagonist, antihistamine, anticholinergic	8–32 mg	tid-qid	Glaucoma, nursing mothers, asthma, hyperthyoridism, hypertension, cardiovascular disease, pyloroduodenal obstruction, prostatic hypertrophy, bladder neck obstruction	Efficacy not shown against placebo or by double-blind studies. May be more effective in children.	MAOI prolong and intensify anticholinergic effects	Sedation, weight gain, blurred vision, urinary retention, dry mouth, thickening of bronchial secretions

Anticonvulsants									
	Phenytoin	MO, MA	Na channels	300–800 mg	Once–tid		Efficacy not shown against placebo or by double-blind studies		
	Carbamazepine	MO, MA	Na channels	200–800 mg	bid–qid				
	Divalproex	MO, MA, TTH, C1	Na channels, serotonin, γ-amino-butyric acid	250–1,500 mg	bid–qid	1–2% risk of fetal abnorma-lities	May cause fatal hepatic failure. May cause thrombocytopenia, platelet inhibition. May decrease effectiveness of BCP	Monitor hepatic function. Measure platelets. Blood level range of 50 to 100 associated with good response	Sedation, nausea, diarrhea, tremor, ataxia, hair loss, acute paracreatinine
Selective serotonin reuptake inhibitors									
	Fluoxetine	MO, MA	Serotonin reuptake blocker	20–80 mg	qid	Pregnancy	Long half-life 2–3 days, may alter blood levels. May delay diazepam clearance. May inhibit renal clearance of TCAs	Anxiety may indicate potential mania. 25% of patients report headache as side effect	4% incident of rash. Anxiety, insomnia, weight loss, hypomania, seizures, impaired judgment
Other serotonin medications									
	Lithium	C1	Alters serotonin CNS receptor				May cause pseudotumor cerebri (idiopathic intracranial hypertension)		Tremor, nystagmus, dizziness, vertigo, incontinence, cardiac arrhythmia, hypotension, polyuria, thinning of hair, peripheral edema
Nonsteroidal anti-inflammatory drugs		MO, MA, MM				Pregnancy breast feedling, aspirin allergy, peptic ulcer disease	May be able to give just before menses to prevent headache	May inhibit diuretics, ↑ digoxin and metaclopramide levels, ↑ lithium levels	Gastric erosion, ulcer, renal compromise, platelet inactivation, mental changes
	Naproxen			550–1,100 mg	qid–bid–tid				
	Mechlofenamate			100–400 mg	tid				
	Flurbiprofen			50–200 mg	bid				
	Ibuprofen			300–1,200 mg	tid				

Abbreviations: MO, migraine without aura; MA, migraine with aura; TTH, tension type; MM, menstrual migraine; MAOI, monoamine oxide inhibitors; COPD, chronic obstructive pulmonary disease; CHF, congestive heart failure; CVD, cardiovascular disease.

been associated with a favorable response to nifedipine (Kahan, et al., 1983).

Antiserotonin drugs include methysergide and cyproheptadine. Because of the associated retroperineal fibrosis (in 1 in 5,000 cases), methysergide is not favored for migraine prophylaxis. Its common use is for cluster headache prophylaxis, and it will be discussed under that topic. Cyproheptadine has not been studied in a double-blind, randomized, placebo-controlled study, but it has been shown to be effective for migraine in open studies (Curran and Lance, 1964; Lance et al., 1970). It has 5-HT_2 antagonist, antihistamine H_1, and anticholinergic properties (Mylechrane, 1991). A consideration favoring the use of this drug is its relative safety except in those patients placed at risk by its anticholinergic properties (Tfelt-Hansen and Saxena, 1993).

The anticonvulsant medication valproic acid has been recently evaluated for effectiveness in migraine headache (Hering and Kuritsky, 1992; Jensen et al., 1994; Silberstein et al., 1993). One advantage of this medication was the demonstration that effectiveness did correlate with blood levels in the range believed to be therapeutic for seizures (Sianard-Gainko et al., 1993). Carbamazepine was shown to be effective in the management of migraine in one study. Phenytoin, considered to be effective in childhood migraine, has not demonstated effectiveness in the adult population, although Winston (1987) found good response in patients with whiplash-related migraine-type headaches (Table 8-15).

Acute Management

The most common limiting factor in treating posttraumatic headaches (Table 8-16) is their frequency. The migraine-specific ergotamines will induce headache if used too frequently, while the less specific analgesic medications such as aspirin, acetaminophen, or narcotics may cause rebound or dependence. Symptomatic treatments such as barbiturates or muscle relaxants also entail the risk of dependency. If a headache is found to respond to an acute nonaddicting medication but the headache is too frequent to allow its regular use, prophylaxis should be considered.

Ergotamines

Ergotamines have been the long-standing treatment for migraine headaches. The guidelines for their use have recently been outlined by the American Academy of Neurology. At the time of compilation of this chapter, only the oral and suppository forms of ergotamine were available in the United States. Ergotamine is a potent vasoconstrictor with 5-HT_1 and 5-HT_2, α-adrenergic agonist activity (responsible for peripheral arterial spasms) and dopaminergic activity (responsible for marked nausea and vomiting). (Tfelt-Hansen and Johnson, 1993). Ergotamines appear to stabilize the serotonin release from the dorsal raphe nucleus and to block neurogenic inflammation in the dura mater.

Ergotamine has poor bioavailability orally, although when used in combination with oral caffeine its bioavailability appears improved. Rectal bioavailability is better, but parenteral administration, usually in the form of dihydroergotamine, has the best bioavailability, as discussed below.

The major serious side effects of ergotamine are related to its vasoconstrictive properties. Mild symptoms of extremity paresthesias, leg cramps, and abdominal discomfort have occurred. In persons with coronary artery disease, myocardial infarction and cardiac arrest have followed. Cerebral vasospasm has been described, and caution is advised in the use of this drug for patients with migraine with aura. The constrictive effects of ergotamines last approximately 24 hours. For this reason their use should be separated from the use of sumatriptan or other potential vasoconstrictors by 24 hours (Panconesi et al., 1994). Ergotamine dose must be reduced when ergotamine is used in combination with methysergide prophylaxis because of the vasoconstrictive effects of methysergide. Half the usually effective dose of ergotamine is recommended.

Marked nausea and vomiting are due to the effect on the dopamine receptor, and this side effect is a major limiting factor in its use. Drug interactions include erythromycin and β-blockers. Erythromycin and other mycin antibiotics decrease the metabolism of ergotamine. β-Adrenergic blocking agents appear to potentiate acute ergotism.

Dihydroegotamine is a parenteral form of ergot alkaloid with agonist effects on 5-HT_1 and slightly less effect on 5-HT_2 receptors, noradrenoceptors, and dopamine receptors. Nausea is the most common side effect, which is lessened by co-treatment with parenteral antiemetics such as metoclopramide, prochlorperazine, or promethazine (Callahan and Raskin, 1986; Raskin, 1986). The severe side effects are related to vasoconstrictive properties and include paresthesias, abdominal cramps, leg cramps, and dizziness. There have been reports of severe peripheral arterial spasm or coronary spasm, believed to be due to idiosyncratic hypersensitivity. Dihydroergotamine IV combined with an antiemetic is the choice for migrainous status. In intractable headaches a dose of 0.5 to 1.0 mg in combination with an antiemetic may be given every 8 hours until relief (Raskin, 1990) Table 8-16). McBeath and Nanda (1994) reported that postconcussive syndrome patients had a favorable response to dihydroergotamine.

Nonsteroidal Anti-Inflammatory Drugs

Many migraine sufferers never come to the attention of the medical system because aspirin at doses below rebound potential are effective in aborting or significantly reducing headache pain. Of the other nonsteroidal anti-inflammatory drugs (NSAIDs) available, all the carboxylic acid forms but not the enolic forms (piroxicam) have some effectiveness. (Tfelt-Hansen and Johnson, 1993). Naproxen sodium is more rapidly absorbed than other NSAIDs, and in double-blind randomized trials it was shown to be better than placebo (Johnson et al., 1985) and better than or equal to ergotamine (Pradalier et al., 1985). Ibuprofen was also superior to placebo and acetaminophen (Kloster et al., 1992). Indomethacin is not considered to be effective in acute headache management. Dosing recomendations are aspirin 100 mg to be followed by a second dose of 1,000 mg in 1 to 2 hours, ibuprofen 1,200 mg followed by 400 mg in 1 to 2 hours, and Naprosyn 660 to 825 mg followed by 440 mg in 1 to 2 hours.

Limitations include the difficulty with oral administration if nausea and vomiting are pronounced. Aspirin in combination with metoclopramide has been suggested to have an effectiveness similar to that of sumatriptan (Oral Sumatriptan and Aspirin Plus Metoclopramide Comparative Study Group, 1992). Ketoralac is available parenterally in the United States and diclofenac is available parenterally in Europe, and both have been shown to be effective in relieving migraine. Caution is necessary in combining parenteral and oral NSAIDs, as renal compromise may be increased. Drug rebound and tachyphylaxis are common with all the NSAIDs.

Side effects include epigastric pain and risk of gastric ulcers, elevation of liver function tests, renal insufficiency or failure, somnolence, psychotic reactions, and worsening of asthma. Since NSAIDs have effects on bleeding time and platelet function, their use in individuals who may have increased bleeding risk should be avoided.

Acetaminophen has been marketed in combination with isometheptene, a sympathomimetic agent, and dichloralphenazone, a chloral hydrate derivative, for the acute management of migraine headache (Diamond, 1976). Isometheptene is a relatively mild sympathomimetic and is contraindicated only in patients with glaucoma, hypertension, severe renal disease, cardiac disease, or liver disease. Sedation agitation, and dizziness are side effects. An advantage to this medication is that its dosing regimen is two tablets at the onset of the headache, and one tablet each hour until relief, up to five tablets. A limitation of this medication is when the necessary dosage exceeds five tablets in 24 hours or 20 tablets in a week. As it contains acetaminophen, it carries a risk of rebound headache. Aspirin or acetaminophen is often combined with barbiturates with or without a caffeine component. This collection of medications was developed with the thought that mild sedation would relax and allow the patient to better tolerate the pain or to sleep until the headache resolved. The disadvantage of these medications is that a barbiturate increases the rebound potential and also carries a risk of addiction.

Steroids and Antihistamines

Dexamethasone (intramuscular or oral) and prednisone (oral) may be effective in aborting acute migraine headaches (Baumel, 1994). Although the mechanism is unclear, diphenhydramine is effective when used intramuscularly or intravenously fòr the acute abortion of headache. It may be more effective on those headaches that appear to have a histamine quality. Unfortunately its use is limited by station, dizziness, gastric distress, decreased coordination, thickening of bronchial secretions, hypertension, and excessive perspiration.

Serotonin Agonists

Serotonin-selective agents include sumatriptan, which is a 5-HT_1 agonist (Subcutaneous Sumatriptan International Study Group, 1991). It is the most serotonin-direct of all the antimigraine medications. It is available in Europe in an oral form and in the United States only in the subcutaneous form. The only apparent advantage of the subcutaneous instead of the oral form is a mild reduction in nausea. The medication may be taken at any time during

TABLE 8-16. Acute Headache Management

Category	Drug	Headache Type	Mechanism	Initial Dose	Route	Dosing Frequency	Treatment Consideration	Side Effects
Nonsteroidal anti-inflammatory drugs (NSAIDs)			Prostaglandin inhibition. Modified CNS serotonin release				Limit all NSAID use to <3 times per week. Tachyphylaxis may occur.	
	Aspirin	MO, MA, TTH		900–1,000 mg	Oral	900–1,000 mg in 1 h then q4 h	Risk of rebound (>50 mg/mo). Combining with metaclopramide increases effectiveness	Gastric erosion, ulcer, renal compromise, platelet inactivation, inhibit diuretics, ↑ digoxin and metaclopramide levels, ↑ lithium levels, mental status changes
	Acetominophen	MO, MA, TTH		1,000 mg	Oral	1,000 mg in 1 h then q4 h	If not effective, combine with aspirin or use in combination with isomethephene	Renal compromise
	Sodium naproxen	MO, MA, MM, TTH		600–825 mg	Oral	440–550 mg after 1–2 h	Limit 1,375 mg in 24 h	Gastric erosion, ulcer, renal compromise, platelet inactivation
	Ibuprofen	MO, MA, TTH		1,200 mg q4 h				Same as aspirin
	Flurbiprofen	MO, MA		100 mg	Oral	100 mg in 8 h	Limit 300 mg in 24 h	Same as aspirin
	Indomethacin	CPH		50 mg	Oral	50 mg in 8 h		
	Diclofenac	MO		50–75 mg	Oral	50–75 mg q12 hr	Parenteral form available in Europe	
	Ketoralac	MO, MA, TTH		60 mg	IM	60 mg q8 h	Parenteral form more bioavailable. Additive to other NSAIDs	
Combination								
	Isometheptene, dichloralphenazone, acetominophen	MO, MA, TTH	"Indirectly acting sympathomimetic, vasoconstriction and cardiac stimulation"	2 tablets at onset		MO, MA: 1 tablet q1 h until relief—up to 5 tablets q24 h. TTH: 2 tablets q4 h	Limit number of tablets to 10–20/week. Contains a sedative. Contraindications are glaucoma, HTN, severe renal disease, heart disease, hepatic disease	Sedation, agitation, dizziness

Steroids	Dexamethasone	MO, MA, Cl	Anti-inflammatory, anti-"vasculitis"	1.5 mg	Oral	1.5 mg q12 h for 48 h	Considered for refractory headache. Standard care for cluster headaches	Minimal with short course. Depression, acne, fluid retention
Antihistamines	Diphenhydramine	MO, MA, "vascular"	Antihistamine, anticholinergic	50 mg IV			Bilateral throbbing character to headache may predict response	Sedation, dizziness, poor coordination, epigastric distress, thickening bronchial secretions, hypotension, excessive perspiration
	Ergotamine	MO, MA, Cl	5-HT and 5-HT_2 agonist. Dopaminergic. Noradrenergic	2 mg	Oral	1 mg q30 h. Limit 6 mg. 1–2 mg at 1 h, limit 4 mg. Limit 10 mg/week	Preparations with combined caffeine may aid absorption. Vasoconstrictive. Action lasts 24 h	Nausea, vomiting, abdominal pain, acroparesthesia, leg cramps, diarrhea, intermittent claudication, pleural fibrosis
	Dihydroergotamine	MO, MA, Cl	5-HT_2 agonist. Dopaminergic agonist (alpha > beta). Noradrenergic	0.5–2 mg	IM/IV	0.5-2 mg q8 h. Limited to 72 h	Combined with antiemetic to lessen nausea (usually metoclopramide 10 mg)	
Serotonin-selective agonist		MO, MA, Cl	5H-T_1 agonist	6 mg	SQ	6 mg after 1 h. Limit 12 mg in 24 h	May have consistent pattern of headache return at 2–6 hours with total resolution after second dose	Flushing of neck. Jaw or chest tightening. Pain at injection site. Dizziness. Increased blood pressure
	Sumatriptan						Important not to use sumatriptan if diagnosis is not certain. Persons with sulfa allergies may be more prone to anaphylaxis. Vasoconstrictive additive to ergotamines	

(*Continued*)

TABLE 8-16. *(continued)* **Acute Headache Management**

Category	Drug	Headache Type	Mechanism	Initial Dose	Route	Dosing Frequency	Treatment Consideration	Side Effects
Antiemetics								
	Promethazine	MO, MA	Dopamine Antihistamine	25–50 mg 25 mg 25–50 mg	Oral Rectal Im	q6h q6h q6h Limit 100–200 mg/day	May lower seizure threshold. Used with caution in narrow-angle glaucoma, stenosis, peptic ulcer, urinary obstruction	Sedation, dizziness, dry mouth, extrapyramidal symptoms, akathesia, neuroleptic malignant syndrome, amenorrhea, hypotension, sun sensitivity, hyperpyrexia
	Prochlorperazine	MO, MA		10 mg 25 mg	IM suppl	None None	May diminish effect of oral anticoagulants	
	Chlorpromatine	MO, MA		25–50 mg 50–100 mg 25 mg	Oral Suppository IM	q4h (limit 100 mg) q8h none		
	Trimethobenzamide	MO, MA	Action on central chemoreceptor tirgger zone	250 mg 200 mg	Oral Suppository	q4h q4h	May precipitate Reye syndrome	Confusion, opisthotenos, parkinsonian-type symptoms
	Metaclopramide	MO, MA	Sensitizes tissue to action of acetylcholine. Dopamine	10–15 mg 10 mg 10 mg	Oral IM IV	q6h None q8h	*Often given with DHE. May be combined orally with aspirin	Sedation, parkinsonian-type tardive dyskinesia, galactorrhea, amenorrhea, hypotension
Other								
	Lidocaine	MO, MA, TTH	Action suspected at cord level	100 mg	IV	Once	For intratable headache. Patient not to drive after treatment. Used to abort cluster but also may assist prophylaxis	Seizure, cardiac arrhythmia, confusion
		Cl	Site: sphenopalative ganglia	4% 5% gel (3 swabs)	Intranasal	bid		
	Oxygen	Cl	Unknown	6–8 L for 5 min	By mask	Repeat immediately X2	Expected to be effective in uncomplicated cluster	None

Abbreviations: MO, migraine without aura; Cl, cluster; MA, migraine with aura; TTH, tension type; MM, menstrual migraine; DHE, dihydroergotamine.

the course of the headache but is limited to two doses within 24 hours, separated by 1 to 2 hours. The side effects of this medication include flushing of the skin, tightness of the neck, jaw, and/or chest, pain at the injection site, dizziness, and increased blood pressure. There has been a report of a possible cardiac collapse related to the use of this medication, although most of the cerebrovascular accidents and cardiac events have occurred either in combination with other vasoconstrictive agents or in individuals otherwise at risk for cerebrovascular accident or coronary artery ischemia. Imitrex appears to be effective in a subclass of tension-type headaches, which may suggest limitation of the diagnostic criteria (Brennum et al., 1992). In persons with sulfa drug allergies, there may be an increased risk of anaphylaxis. There does appear to be an increased vasoconstrictive effect when combined with ergotamine. When combined with monoamine oxidase inhibitors, the sumatriptan blood level is increased by 79 percent. As of the time of writing, dihydroergotamine 45 has not been commonly used subcutaneously owing to local irritative effects, but it may be available in the near future. It also may be available in a nasal delivery form in the near future. The introduction of dihydroergotamine by other than intramuscular or intravenous approaches will influence the choice between sumatriptan and DHE-45 in severe intractable headaches, especially those associated with nausea (Baumel, 1994).

Antiemetics

In an attempt to control the nausea component of migraine headaches, antiemetic drugs have been introduced (Lipton and Tfelt-Hansen, 1993). It appears that there may be a depoanergic component to migraine headaches, so that these agents are able to provide pain relief as well as antiemetic effects (Mathew, 1993b). The antiemetic drugs include promethazine, prochloperazine, and chlorpromatine. Metoclopramide, as mentioned previously, has been used also. Other agents that have been used in acute management of migraine headache include intravenous lidocaine, which is believed to exert its effect at a central spinal cord or brainstem level with direct suppression of trigeminal activity. Lidocaine is dosed at approximately 1 to 1.5 mg/kg IV, the potential risks being seizure, cardiac arrhythmias, and mental confusion (Maciewicz et al., 1988)

Tension-Type Headaches

β-Blockers and tricyclic antidepressants have been the primary prophylactic agents in the management of chronic tension-type headaches (Table 8-15). The effective agents in these groups overlap with those for migraine. Calcium channel blockers have not been shown to be particularly effective in the management of tension-type headaches. Of the anticonvulsive medications, valproic acid has been suggested to be effective in reducing the frequency of intensive chronic daily headaches (Mathew, 1991). Neither phenytoin nor carbamazepine has been shown to be effective. Of the serotonin-selective reuptake inhibitors, fluoxetine in doses of 10 to 80 mg daily has been suggested to have benefit in chronic tension-type headaches (Markley et al., 1991). Because of the long-term chronicity of the headaches, the use of the NSAIDs in prophylaxis has not been encouraged. In spite of this, especially during the period of drug removal for treatment of rebound headaches, long-acting NSAIDs such as naproxen have been found to be beneficial in covering the signs of withdrawal (Mathew, 1990).

Cluster-Type Headache

In the more classical (male-predominant) cluster-type headaches, cortical steroids, methysergide, periactin, calcium channel blockers, and lithium are the choices for prophylaxis (Ekborn and Sakai, 1993; Lance, 1993). Acute management involves attempting to break the cycle with the introduction of steroids, ergotamine agents, or methysergide and by treating acute attacks with sumatriptan, oxygen, or intranasal lidocaine. Cafergot has been suggested in a suppository form to be taken at bedtime if there is a frequent pattern of clusters awakening the patient during the night (Horton, 1952). Because of the short duration of cluster headaches, most acute medications, with the exception of sumatriptan or intranasal lidocaine, are ineffective. Oxygen may be abortive. In chronic paroxysmal hemicrania, by definition, the headaches are 100 percent responsive to indomethacin (Olesen, 1988). This is given at a dosing range of up to 50 mg tid for a minimum of 5 days. Piroxicam has been suggested to also be effective as a prophylaxis in chronic paroxysmal hemicrania.

Occipital Neuralgia

The clinical presentation of occipital neuralgia may occur independently or in combination with tension-type or migraine headaches. It may respond to treatment along with the primary headache type or may not respond until separately addressed. explain why the headaches have been refractory. Drug treatment specific to occipital neuralgia should be designed to address the neuropathic pain and possible focal inflammatory process, often beginning with the combination of NSAIDs and tricyclic antidepressants. The drug approach is combined with directed strengthening and increased flexibility exercises for the cervical area. Since it would be expected that conditions such as fibromyalgia or myofascial pain should be expected to also respond favorably to this treatment, improvement does not allow separation of these syndromes (McCain, 1994). While no controlled clinical trials have been made with a component muscle spasm or increased muscle tension present, muscle relaxants including methenesin-like agents (methocarbamol, carisoprodol, chlorzoxazone), baclofen, diazepam, and cyclobenzaprine have been suggested in the management (Mathew, 1993b). If there is strong clinical evidence of injury to the occipital nerve, neuropathic medications, including the anticonvulsants, may be considered. For those patients who have been completely refactory to medical management and conservative to nonpharmacologic management, the surgical approach has been suggested. Horowitz and Yonas (1993) have reviewed the literature recommending surgical treatment of occipital neuralgia (Table 8-17). It appears that the patients do better following surgery, although almost 100 percent will have return of their symptomatology to a degree that will still require another mode of therapy.

Cervicogenic Headaches

In cervicogenic headaches, it is unclear as to the best treatment approach. At this time exercise, NSAIDs, and centrally active pain control agents such as tricyclic antidepressants appear to be the accepted mode of therapy. Bovim and Sjaastad (1992) demonstrated a poor response to oxygen, ergotamine and morphine therapies. Those who support the concept of cervicogenic headaches as representing cervical pathology recommend trials of common headache approaches and if these fail, the surgical exploration for correctable conditions (Bovim et al., 1992b).

Post-Traumatic Headaches Due to Sympathetic Pain

As mentioned, post-traumatic sympathetic headaches have been grouped under migraine. They have been shown to respond to propranolol. If the migraine approach is ineffectual, consideration of medications for sympathetic pain conditions could include tricyclics, selective serotonin reuptake blockers, anticonvulsants, clonidine, nifedipine, and oral antiarrhythmics such as mexilitine. Stellate ganglion blocks to temporarily inhibit the sympathetic pathways to the head also might be considered in very refractory cases.

Summary of Pharmacologic Management

The drug therapy for major headache types is summarized in Tables 8-15 and 8-16. In all the choices of drug therapy for post-traumatic headaches, the most common determining factor is often coexisting disorders. In the presence of depression it may be more realistic to use selective serotonin reuptake agents developed for the treatment of depression such as fluoxetine, as this drug has been suggested to be effective against headache and the doses used will be closer to the antidepressant therapeutic ranges than they would be for the tricyclic antidepressants. With the tricyclic antidepressants, higher doses may be considered to address both the depression and the headache pain. Those tricyclics believed to be of value in axious depression may be considered in patients who present with components of anxiety. The use of antianxiolytics needs to be considered, not only for in relation management of the anxiety but also for their potential to produce rebound as well as addiction. Owing to the chronicity of the headache condition, it might be more reasonable to explore the possibility of treatment with imipramine or the β-blockers, as well as tegretol or valproic acid. Both tegretol and valproic acid should also be considered for use in patients with a possible post-traumatic seizure disorder. In patients who have significantly increased muscle tone, it was initially suggested to consider using muscle relaxants. As the majority of these also carry addictive potential, this recommendation has fallen into disfavor. A possible medication to consider is baclofen. In those conditions where disuse syndrome appears to occur, or with a frank reflex sympathetic dystrophy (RSD) or other evidence of sympathetic involvement, medications such

TABLE 8-17. Summary of 28 Articles on Occipital Neuralgia and Its Treatment

Author	No. of Patients	Etiology	Procedure	Outcome	Follow-up
Blume	114	Trauma 76 Anatomically abnormal 82 Nontraumatic 38 Normal anatomy 32	Radiofrequency	73.7%; complete relief (excellent) 4.4%; transitory pain (good) 4.4%; 50% reduction (fair) 17.5%; no relief (none) Traumatic etiology: 72%; excellent 6.6%; good 5.3%; fair 16%; none Nontraumatic etiology: 76%; excellent 24%; good Anatomically normal: 90%; excellent 3.5%; good 6.5%; fair 68%; excellent 6.1%; good 2.4%; fair 23%; none	6–24 mo
Chambers	35	?	Dorsal rhizotomy	10/22; complete relief 6/22; 75% improvement 6/22; <75% relief	3 mo–6.5 yr
Cox	490	Spasm (?#)	Scalenotomies; 395 Neurectomies; 95	Scalenotomies Excellent 30% Good 56% Poor 14% Neurectomies: Excellent 15% Good 71% Poor 9% (meaning of categories?)	?
Cusson	4	Nontraumatic 4/4	Dorsal rhizotomy	complete relief	5 weeks–1 yr
Dugan	10	Instability/miscellaneous	9; collar 1; no treatment	3; complete relief 7; partial relief/no relief	?
Ehni	7	C1-C2 arthrosis	5; fusion/decompression	Surgical; complete relief Conservative; partial relief	6 mo–10 yr
Gayral	3	Barré-Lieou osteoarthritis; 2 Fracture C_{3-4}; 1	Conservative therapy injections/traction	3/3; complete relief	1–4 yr
Graff-Radford	3	Myofascial pain; 2 Trauma; 1	Injection/traction	2/3; relief (myofascial patients) 1/3; residual pain (trauma patient)	1–2 yr

(*Continued*)

TABLE 8-17. *(continued)* **Summary of 28 Articles on Occipital Neuralgia and Its Treatment**

Author	No. of Patients	Etiology	Procedure	Outcome	Follow-up
Anthony	86		Injection	75/86; complete relief	Mean HA-free days, 31
	60		GON neurectomy	42/60; complete relief	Mean HA-free days, 244
Hammond	23	Trauma; 15 Spondylosis; 3 Rheum. arthritis; 2	Injection; 14 Neurectomy; 4 Collar; 5 Neurostimulation; 2 Medication; 9 External carotid ligation; 1	Poorly defined	<1 week–1 yr
Hunter	11	Trauma; 8	Avulsion GON Dorsal rhizotomy C2 Dorsal rhizotomy C2-C3	8 with trauma; relieved/benefited 3 without trauma; no relief	?
Jansen	12	Vasogenic; 9 Scar; 2 Disc; 1 Spondylosis; 1 Neuroma; 1	Decompression radiofrequency	14; complete relief 2; no relief	2–125 mo
Jundt	2	Temporal arteritis	Steroids	Complete relief	1–4 yr
Kelly	12	Fibrositis	Injection	11/12; complete relief	<1 yr
Knox	30	Whiplash; 1 Arthritis; 1 Miscellaneous; 16	Injection; 22	?	?
Martin	4	?	Peripheral section	4/4; complete relief	0–12 yr
Mayfield (includes Hunter study)	144	Whiplash	C_2 dorsal rhizotomy; 108 GON avulsion; 36	60/108; complete relief 18/36; temporary relief	?
Hilldebrandt	2	C2-C3 vascular compression	Vascular decompression	2/2; complete relief	12–26 mo
Koch	1		Alcohol rhizotomy	Complete relief	12 mo
Murphy	30	Trauma; 9 Arthritis; 9 Miscellaneous; 11 Trauma/arthritis; 1	Avulsion GON	Excellent; 18/30 Good; 7/30 Fair; 3/30	0–15 yr
Poletti	1	Foraminal stenosis	Decompression	Complete relief	2 yr
Poletti	2	Entrapment	Decompression	Complete relief	?
Schultz	92	?	Injection	52/92; complete relief 29/92; recurrence 11/92; no relief	2–14 mo
Scott	3	Chiari malformation	Decompression	3/3; complete relief	2–19 yr
Sharma	1	C2 vascular compression	Vascular decompression	Complete relief	1.5 yr

(*Continued*)

TABLE 8-17. *(continued)* **Summary of 28 Articles on Occipital Neuralgia and Its Treatment**

Author	No. of Patients	Etiology	Procedure	Outcome	Follow-up
Skillern	100	?	Injection	?	?
Smith	1	Syphilis	Antibiotics	Complete relief	3 mo
Star	9	Osteoarthritis	5/9; decompress/ fusion	4/5; no pain 1/5; some pain	22 mo
			4/9; medical management	1/4; no pain 3/4; some pain	18.5 mo

(From Horowitz and Yonas, 1993, with permission.)

as clonidine or nifedipine may be considered if agents such as the tricyclics or selective serotonin reuptake blockers and anticonvulsants more commonly used for neuropathic pain have proved ineffective. The presence of Raynaud's phenomenon suggests the increased possibility of a favorable response to nifedipine. New treatments such as tramadol are constantly evolving. Tramadol is a non-narcotic mu-opoid receptor agonist which also blocks monoamine receptors and is recommended for chronic pain (Lee et al., 1993).

Nonpharmacologic Management

The areas of non-drug-related therapy include exercise, transcutaneous electrical nerve stimulation (TENS) units, psychological and cognitive approaches to headache types associated with neck pain (Blau et al., 1994; Kidd and Nelsen, 1993), exercises that strengthen and tone the cervical muscles, and improved neck alignment, all of which may decrease post-traumatic headache severity or frequency (Watson and Trott, 1993). Ice packs have also been demonstrated to be effective in reducing the symptoms of migraine in post-traumatic headaches (Jensen et al., 1990b).

Patients with post-traumatic pain represent a subclass of chronic pain and would be expected to benefit from cognitive therapy directed at regaining a sense of control over their pain (Harkapaa et al., 1991). As demonstrated by the Minnesota Multiphasic Personality Inventory ($MMPPI_2$) profile, this headache group aligns with the highest elevation of pathologic scales. Relaxation therapy appears to have a benefit in the same range as the tricyclic antidepressants in migraine. However, it is unclear if it is equally effective in post-traumatic headaches. Recruitment of psychological support for evaluation and treatment may shorten the time until success of headache management.

CONCLUSION

Headaches following acute head or neck trauma are common. The hypothetical mechanisms are varied and draw from animal models and human anatomic and physiologic studies. The IHS classification system provides a framework for treatment by establishing similarities between the post-traumatic headache and primary headache types, with symptomatic treatment directed by these similarities. There is controversy surrounding the categorization of headache associated with cervical injury. The issue is clouded by an overlap with the syndromes of traumatic cervical pain. Psychological factors and litigation play a role in post-traumatic headache, especially in the setting of chronic complaints. The appropriate therapy includes medical treatment as well as encouraging increased activity and maximizing coping strategies. The aim is to limit the influence of headache on quality of life and to assist patients to establish a sense of control over their pain.

REFERENCES

Ad Hoc Committee on Classification of Headache, National Institutes of Health: Classification of Headache. JAMA 179:717–718, 1962

American Medical Association: Guides to the Evaluation of Permanent Impairment. 4th Ed. p. 312. American Medical Association, Chicago, 1993

American Psychiatric Association: Diagnostic and Statistical Manual of Mental Disorders [DSM-IV]; 4th ed. American Psychiatric Association, Washington, 1987

Anthony M: Arrest of attacks of cluster headache by local steroid injection of the occipital. pp 168–173. In Rose CF (ed), Karger, Basel, Switzerland, 1985

Arboix A, Massons J, Oliveres M, et al: Headache in acute cerebrovascular disease: a prospective clinical study in 240 patients. Cephalalgia 14:37–40, 1994

Bartschi-Rochaix W: Headaches of cervical origin. pp. 192–203. In Vinkey PJ, Bruyn GW (ed): Handbook of Clinical Neurology. Vol. 5. North-Holland, Amsterdam, 1968

Baumel B: Migraine: a pharmacologic review with newer options and delivery modalities. Neurology suppl. 3, 44:13–17, 1994

Bellavance A, Belzile G, Bergeron Y et al: Cervical spine and headaches. Neurology 39:1269, 1989

Bennett DR, Fuenning, SI, Sullivan G, Weber J: Migraine precipitated by head trauma in athletes. Am J Sport Med 8:202–205, 1980

Blau JN, Path FR, MacGregor EA: Migraine and the neck. Headache 34:88–90, 1994

Bogduk N: Local anesthetic blocks of second cervical ganglion: a technique with application in occipital headache. Cephalalgia 1:41–50, 1981

Bogduk N: The clinical anatomy of cervical dorsal rami. Spine 7:319–330, 1982

Bogduk N: The anatomical basis for cervicogenic headache. J Manipulative Physiol Ther 15:67–70, 1992

Bogduk N, Marsland A: On the concept of third occipital headache. J Neurol Neurosurg Psychiatry 49:775–780, 1986

Bogduk N, Windsor M, Inglis A: The innervation of the cervical intervertebral disks. Spine 13:2–8, 1988

Bonica JJ: General considerations of pain in the head. pp. 651–675. Bonica JJ, Loeser JD, Chapman CR, Fordyce WE (eds): The Management of Pain. Lea & Febiger, Philadelphia, 1990

Bovim G, Berg R, Dale LG: Cervicogenic headache: anesthetic blockades of cervical nerves (C2–C5) and facet joint (C2/C3). Pain 49:315–320, 1992

Bovim G, Fredriksen TA, Stott-Nielson A, Sjaastad O: Neurolysis of the greater occipital nerve in cervicogenic headaches: a follow-up study. Headache 32:175–179, 1992

Bovim G, Sand T: Cervicogenic headache, migraine without aura and tension-type headache. Diagnostic blockage of greater occipital and supra-orbital nerves. Pain 51:43–48, 1992

Bovim G, Sjaastad O: Cervicogenic headache: responses to nitroglycerin, oxygen, ergotamine and morphine. Headache 33:249–252, 1993

Brennum J, Kjeldsen M, Olesen J: The 5HT1-like agonist sumatriptan has significant effect in chronic tension type headache. Cephalalgia 12:375–379, 1992

Burgess J: Symptom characteristics in TMD patients reporting blunt trauma and/or whiplash injury. J Craniomandib Disorders: Fac Oral Pain 5:251–257, 1991

Callahan M, Raskin N: A controlled trial of acute migraine headache. Headache 26:168–171, 1986

Couch JR, Micieli G: Prophylactic pharmacotherapy. pp. 537–542. In Olesen J, Tfelt-Hansen P, Welch KMA (eds): The Headaches. Raven Press, New York, 1993

Curran DA, Lance JW: Clinical trial of methysergide and other preparations in the management of migraine. J Neurol Neurosurg Psychiatry 27:463–469, 1964

DeBenedittis G, Lorenzetti A: The role of stressful life events in the persistence of primary headaches: major events versus daily hassles. Pain 51:35, 1992

Diamond S: Treatment of migraine with isometheptene, acetaminophen, and dichloralphenazon combination: a double blind cross-over trial. Headache 16:282–287, 1976

Dieterich M, Pollmann W, Pfaffenrath V: Cervicogenic headache: electronystagmography, perception of verticality and postarography in patients before and after C2 blockade. Cephalalgia 13:285–288, 1993

Dubner R, Ruda MA: Activity-dependent neuronal plasticity following tissue injury and inflammation. Trends Neurosci 15:96–103, 1992

Duckro P, Schultz KT, Chibnell JT: Migraine as a sequela to chronic low back pain. Headache 34:279–281, 1994

Edmeads J: The cervical spine and headache. Neurology 38:1874–1878, 1988

Ehni G, Benner B: Occipital neuralgia and C1–2 arthrosis syndrome. J Neurosurg 61:961–965, 1984

Ekborn K, Sakai F: "Tension-type headache, cluster headache and miscellaneous headache" management. pp. 591–599. In Olesen J, Tfelt-Hansen P, Welch KMA (eds): The Headaches. Raven Press, New York, 1993

Elkind AH: Headache and head trauma. Clin J Pain 5:77–87, 1989a

Elkind AH: Headache and facial pain associated with head injury. Otolaryngol Clin North Am 22:1251–1271, 1989b

Epstein JB: Temporomandibular disorders, facial pain and headache following motor vehicle accidents. J Oral Maxillofac Surg 68:488–495, 1992

Evans RW: The postconcussive syndrome and sequelae of mild head injury. Neurol Clin North Am 10, 815–847, 1992a

Evans RW: Some observations on whiplash injuries. Neurol Clin North Am 10:975–997, 1992b

Evans RW, Evans RI, Sharp MJ: The physician survey on post-concussive and whiplash syndromes. Headache 34:268–274, 1994

Ferrari MD: Sumatriptan in treatment of migraine. Neurology, suppl. 3, 44:543–547, 1993

Forrester G, Encel J, Geffen G: Measuring post-traumatic amnesia (PTA): an historical review. Brain Inj 8:175–184, 1994

Fredriksen TA, Fougner R, Tangerud A, Sjaastad O: Cervicogenic headache: radiological investigations concerning head/neck. Cephalalgia 9:139–146, 1989

Gawel MI, Rothbart PJ: Occipital nerve block in the management of headache and cervical pain. Cephalalgia 12:9–13, 1992

Gawel MJ, Rothbart P, Jacobs H: Subcutaneous sumatriptan in the treatment of acute episodes of post-traumatic headache. Headache 33:96–97, 1993

Goddard MJ, Dean BZ, King JC: Pain rehabilitation. 1. Basic science, acute pain and neuropathic pain. Arch Phys Med Rehabil, suppl. 4, 75:4–8, 1994

Goldstein J: Posttraumatic headache and the postconcussion syndrome. Med Clin North Am 76:641–651, 1991

Graff-Radford SB, Jaegar, BJ, Reeves JL: Myofascial pain may present clinically as occipital neuralgia. Neurosurgery 19:610–613, 1986

Haas DC: Acute post traumatic headache. pp. 623–626. In Olesen J, Tfelt-Hansen P, Welch KMA (eds): The Headaches. Raven Press, New York, 1993a

Haas DC: Chronic post-traumatic headaches. pp. 629–637. In Olesen J, Tfelt-Hansen P, Welch KMA (eds): The Headaches. Raven Press, New York, 1993b

Harkapaa K, Jarvikoski A, Mellin G et al: Health locus of control beliefs and psychological distress as predictors for treatment outcome in low-back pain patients: results of a 3-month follow-up of a controlled intervention study. Pain 46:35–41, 1991

Heise AP, Laskin DM, Gervin AS: Incidence of temporomandibular joint symptoms following whiplash injury. J Oral Maxillofac Surg 50:825–828, 1992

Hering R, Kuritsky A: Sodium valporate in the treatment of migraine: a double-blind study with placebo. Cephalalgia 12:81–84, 1992

Horowitz MB, Yonas H: Occipital neuralgia treated by intradural dorsal nerve root sectioning. Cephalalgia 13:354–360, 1993

Horton BJ: Histamine cephalalgia. Lancet 2:92–98, 1952

Jaeger B: Are "cervicogenic" headaches due to myofascial pain and cervical spine dysfunction. Cephalalgia 9:157–164, 1989

Jansen J, Bardosi A, Hildebrandt J, Lücke A: Cervicogenic, hemicranial attacks associated with vascular irritation or compression of the cervical nerve root. C2 clinical manifestations and morphological findings. Pain 39:203–212, 1989a

Jansen J, Markakis E, Rama B, Hildebrandt J: Hemicranial attacks or permanent hemicrania—a sequel of upper cervical root compression. Cephalalgia 9:123–130, 1989b

Jensen OK, Justesen T, Nielsen FF, Brixen K: Functional radiographic examination of the cervical spine in patients with post-traumatic headache. Cephalalgia 10:295–303, 1990a

Jensen OK, Nielsen FF, Vosmar L: An open study comparing manual therapy with the use of cold packs in treatment of post-traumatic headaches. Cephalalgia 10:241–250, 1990b

Jensen R, Brinck T, Olesen J: Sodium valproate has prophylactic effects in migraine without aura: a triple-blind placebo controlled, cross over study. Neurology 44:647–651, 1994

Johnson ES, Ratcliffe DM, Wilkinson M: Naproxen sodium in treatment of migraine. Cephalalgia 5:5–10 1985

Kahan A, Weber S, Amor B et al: Nifedipine in the treatment of migraine in patients with Raynaud's phenomenon. N Engl J Med 308:110–113, 1983

Keith WS: "Whiplash"–injury of the 2nd cervical ganglion and nerve. Can J Neurol Sci 13:133–137, 1986

Kerr FWL: Central relationships of trigeminal and cervical primary afferents in the spinal cord and medulla. Brain Res 43:561–572, 1972

Kerr PWL: Mechanism to account for headache in cases of posterior fossa tumors. J Neurosurg 18:605–609, 1960

Khurana RK: Headache spectrum in Arnold-Chiari malformation. Headache 31:151–155, 1991

Khurana RK, Niranhari VS: Bilateral sympathetic dysfunction in post-traumatic headache. Headache 26:183–188, 1986

Kidd RF, Nelson R: Musculoskeletal dysfunction of neck in migraine and tension headache. Headache 33:566–569, 1993

Kloster R, Nestudd K, Vilmig ST: A double blind study of ibuprophen versus placebo in treatment of acute migraine attacks. Cephalalgia 12:169–171, 1992

Lance JW: Mechanism and Management of Headache. Butterworth-Heineman, Oxford, pp. 179–181

Lance JW, Anthony M, Sommerville B: Comparative trial of serotonin receptor antagonists in the management of migraine. Br Med J 2:327–329, 1970

Langemark M, Bach FW, Jensen TS, Olesen J: Decreased nociceptive flexion reflex threshold in chronic tension type headache. Arch Neurol, suppl. 10, 50:1061–1064, 1993

Lee CR, McTavish D, Sorlein EM: Tramadol: a preliminary review of its pharmacodynamic and pharmacokinetic properties and therapeutic potential in acute and chronic pain states. Drug 46:313–340, 1993

Lipton RB, Steward WF: Migraine in the United States: a review of epidemiology and health care use. Neurology, suppl. 3, 43:6–10, 1993

Lipton RB, Tfelt-Hansen P: Neuroleptic. pp. 349–352. In Olesen J, Tfelt-Hansen P, Welch KMA (eds): The Headaches. Raven Press, New York, 1993

Loeser JD: Cranial neuralgias. pp. 676–686. In Bonica JJ, Loeser JD, Chapman CR, Fordyce WE (eds): The Management of Pain. Lea & Febiger, Philadelphia, 1990

Maciewicz R, Borsook S, Strassman A: Intravenous lidocaine relieves acute vascular headache. Headache 28:309, 1988

Markley HG, Gasser PA, Markley ME, Pratt, SM: Fluoxetine in prophylaxis of headache: clinical experience. Cephalalgia, suppl. 11, 11:164–165, 1991

Mathew NT: Drug induced headaches. Neurol Clin 8:903–912, 1990

Mathew NT: Chronic refractory headache. Neurology, suppl. 3, 43:526, 1993a

Mathew NT: "Tension-type headache, cluster headache and miscellaneous headache" acute pharmacotherapy. pp. 531–542. In Olesen J, Tfelt-Hansen P, Welch KMA (eds): The Headaches. Raven Press, New York, 1993b

Mathew NT, Ali S: Valproate in treatment of persistent chronic daily headache. Headache 31:74–76, 1991

Mayou R, Bryant B, Duthie R: Psychiatric consequences of road traffic accidents. Br Med J 308:647–651, 1993

McBeath JG, Nanda A: Use of dihydroergotamine in patients with postconcussive syndrome. Headache 34:148–151, 1994

McCain GA: Fibromyalgia and myofacial pain syndromes. pp. 475–493. In Wall PD, Melzack R (eds): Textbook of Pain. Churchill Livingstone, Edinburgh, 1994

Mersky, H: Classification of chronic pain: description of chronic pain syndromes and definition of pain terms. Pain, suppl. 3, 51:1–225, 1986

Michler R-P, Bovim G, Sjaastad O: Disorders in the lower cervical spine: a cause of unilateral headaches? Headache 31:550–551, 1991

Moskowitz MA: Neurogenic inflammation in the pathophysiology and treatment of migraine. Neurology, suppl. 3, 43:16–20, 1993

Muse M: The stress-related post-traumatic chronic pain syndrome: criteria for diagnosis and preliminary report on prevalence. Pain 23:295, 1985

Mylechrane EJ: 5-Ht_2 receptor antagonists and migraine therapy. J Neurol 238:545–552, 1991

Mylechrane EJ, Tfelt-Hansen P: Miscellaneous drugs. pp. 379–402. In Olesen J, Tfelt-Hansen P, Welch KMA (eds): The Headaches. Raven Press, New York, 1993

Olesen J: Clinical and pathophysiological observations in migraine and tension-type headache explained by integration of vascular, supraspinal and myofascial inputs. Pain 46:125–132, 1991

Olesen J (and Headache Classification Committee of the International Headache Society): Classification and diagnostic criteria for headache disorders, cranial neuralgias, and facial pain. Cephalalgia 8:1–96, 1988

Oral Sumatriptan and Aspirin Plus Metoclopramide Comparative Study Group: A study to compare oral sumatriptan with oral aspirin plus metoclopamide in treatment of migraine. Eur J Neurol 32:177–184, 1992

Packard RC: Posttraumatic headache: permanency and relationship to legal settlement. Headache 32:496–500, 1992

Packard RC, Ham LP: Post-traumatic headache: determining chronicity. Headache 33:133–134, 1993

Panconesi A, Anselmi B, Curradi C. et al: Comparison between venoconstrictor effects of sumatriptan and ergotamine in migraine patients. Headache 34:194–197, 1994

Pascual J, Otorino A, Berciano J: Headache in type 1 Chiari malformation. Neurology 42:1519–1521, 1992

Perelson HN: Occipital nerve tenderness: a sign of headache. South Med J 40:653–656, 1947

Peroutka SJ: 5-Hydroxytryptamine receptor subtype, and the pharmacology of migraine. Neurology, suppl. 3, 43:34–38, 1993

Pfaffenrath V, Dandekar R, Pollmann W: Cervicogenic headache. The clinical picture, radiological findings and hypotheses on its pathophysiology. Headache 27:495–499, 1987

Pradalier A, Rancurel G, Dordain G et al: Acute migraine attack therapy: comparison of naproxen sodium and ergotamine tartrate compound. Cephalalgia 5:107–113, 1985

Radanov B, Sturzenegger M, DiStefano G et al: Factors influencing recovery from headache after common whiplash. Br Med J 307:652–655, 1993

Raskin NH: Repetitive intervenous dihydroergotamine as therapy for intractable migraine. Neurology 36:995–997, 1986

Raskin NH: Treatment of status migrainous; the American experience. Headache. suppl. 2 30:550–553, 1990

Rasmussen BK: Background to headache; epidemiology. pp. 15–20. Olesen J, Tfelt-Hansen P, Welch KMA (eds): The Headaches. Raven Press, New York, 1993

Rasmussen BK, Olesen J: Symptomatic and nonsymptomatic headache in a general population. Neurology 42:1225–1231, 1992

Rimel RW: Disability caused by minor head injury. Neurosurgery 9:221–228, 1981

Romanes GJ: The peripheral nervous system. p. 720. In Cunningham's Textbook of Anatomy. Oxford University Press, London, 1972.

Ruijs MBM, Gabreels FJM, Keyser A: The relationship between neurological trauma parameters and long-term outcome in children with closed head injury. Eur J Pediatr 152:844–847, 1993

Sianard-Gainko J, Lenaerts M, Basting E, Schoenen J: Sodium valproate in severe migraine and tension-type headache: clinical efficacy and correlations with blood levels. Cephalalgia 13:252, 1993

Silberstein SD, Lipton RB: Overview of diagnosis and treatment of migraine. Neurology, suppl. 7, 44:6–16, 1994

Silberstein SD, Saper J, Mathew N: The safety and efficacy of divalproex sodium in prophylaxis of migraine headache: a multicenter, double-blind, placebo controlled trial. Headache 33:264–265, 1993

Silberstein SD, Young W: For the Working Panel of the Headache and Facial Pain Section of the American Academy of Neurology: Safety and efficacy of ergotamine tartrate and dihydroergotamine in the treatment of migraine and status migrainosus. Neurology 45:577–584, 1995

Sjaastad O, Fredriksen TA, Pfaffenrath V: Cervicogenic headache: diagnostic criteria. Headache 30:725–726, 1990

Sjaastad O, Hovdahl H, Breivik H, Gronbael E: "Cervicogenic" headache, an hypothesis. Cephalalgia 3:249–256, 1983

Sola AE, Bonica JJ: Myofacial pain syndromes. pp. 352–367. In Bonica JJ, Loeser JD, Chapman CR, Fordyce WE (eds): The Management of Pain. Lea & Febiger, Philadelphia, 1990

Spierings ELH, Foo DK, Young RR: Headaches in patients with traumatic lesions of the cervical spinal cord. Headache 32:45–49, 1992

Stovner LJ: Headache associated with the Chiari type I malformation. Headache 33:175–181, 1993

Sturzenegger M: Headache and neck pain: the warning symptoms of vertebral artery dissection. Headache 34:187–193, 1994

Subcutaneous Sumatriptan International Study Group. Treatment of migraine attacks with sumatriptan. N Engl J Med 325:316–321, 1991

Tfelt-Hansen P: Efficacy of beta-blocking drugs in migraine: a critical review. Cephalalgia, suppl. 5, 6:15–24, 1986

Tfelt-Hansen P, Johnson ES: Antiemetics and prokinetic drugs. pp. 343–349. In Olesen J, Tfelt-Hansen P, Welch KMA (eds): The Headaches. Raven Press, New York, 1993

Tfelt-Hansen P, Lipton RB: Prioritizing acute pharmacotherapy. pp. 359–372. In Olesen J, Tfelt-Hansen P, Welch KMA (eds): The Headaches. Raven Press, New York, 1993

Tfelt-Hansen P, Saxena PR: Antiserotonin drugs. pp. 373–382. Olesen J, Tfelt-Hansen P, Welch KMA (eds): The Headaches. Raven Press, New York, 1993

Toda N, Tfelt-Hansen P: Calcium antagonists. pp. 383–389. In Olesen J, Tfelt-Hansen P, Welch KMA (eds): The Headaches. Raven Press, New York, 1993

Travell JG, Simons DG: Trigger Point Manual. Williams and Wilkins, Baltimore, 1984

Travell J, Simons DS; In: Myofacial Pain and Dysfunction, The Trigger Point Manual. Williams & Wilkins, Baltimore, 1983, pp. 296, 306

Turkewitz LJ, Wirth O, Dawson GA, Casaly JS: Cluster headache following head injury: a case report and review of the literature. Headache 32:504–506, 1992

Vijayan N: A new post-traumatic headache syndrome: clinical and therapeutic observations. Headache 17:19–22, 1977

Walters WE: The Pontypridd headache survey. Headache 14:81–90, 1974

Watson DH, Trott PH: Cervical headache: an investigation of natural head position and upper cervical flexor muscle performance. Cephalalgia 13:272–284, 1993

Weiss HD, Stern BJ Goldberg J: Post-traumatic migraine: chronic migraine precipitated by minor head or neck trauma. Headache 31:451–456, 1991

Wilson PR: Chronic neck pain and cervicogenic headache. Clin J Pain 7:5–11, 1991

Winston KR: Whiplash and its relationship to migraine. Headache 27:452–457, 1987

Wolf HG: Headache and Other Head Pain. Oxford University Press, New York, 1963, pp. 117–137

Yamaguchi M: Incidence of headache and severity of head injury. Headache 32:427–431, 1992

Zemlan FP, Garver DL: Depression and antidepressant therapy: receptor dynamics. Prog Neuropsychopharmacol Biolog Psychiatry 14:503–523, 1990

Neuro-Otologic Trauma and Dizziness

9

R. J. Tusa
S. B. Brown

Dizziness (vertigo, disequilibrium, lightheadedness) following head trauma occurs in 40 to 60 percent of patients (Friedman et al. 1945; Gannon et al. 1978). True vertigo is less frequent, with an incidence of 2 to 30 percent. The incidence of dizziness and vertigo is not closely related to the severity of the head trauma (Barber, 1969). Dizziness may occur from inner ear injury (benign paroxysmal positional vertigo [BPPV], endolymphatic hydrops, labyrinth concussion, perilymphatic fistula); brain injury (cerebellum, vestibular nuclei, temporal lobe); neck injury (vestibulospinal tract, cervical plexus, soft tissue); and psychological problems (Table 9-1). A clear delineation of the patient's symptoms and physical findings is critical to arriving at the correct diagnosis and treatment. In this chapter we describe the neuro-otologic disorders due to head trauma and offer an approach to assessing patients with dizziness.

ANATOMY AND PHYSIOLOGY

The external ear consists of the external acoustic meatus and tympanic membrane (Fig. 9-1). The middle ear consists of three small bones (auditory ossicles), which transmit sound vibrations to the oval

TABLE 9-1. Sites and Mechanisms of Trauma-Induced Dizziness

Site	Syndrome	Mechanism
Inner ear	Benign paroxysmal positional vertigo (BPPV)	Cupula or canal lithiasis
	Post-traumatic endolymphatic hydrops	Decreased endolymphatic absorption
	Perilymphatic fistula	Rupture in round or oval window or in membranous labyrinth
	Labyrinth concussion	Endolymphatic hemorrhage
	Temporal bone fracture	Disruption of bony or membranous labyrinth
Vestibular nerve	Temporal bone fracture	Disruption of 8th cranial nerve
Brainstem or vestibulocerebellum	Downbeat, upbeat, and torsional nystagmus, central positional vertigo, ocular tilt response, post-traumatic syndrome	Contusion or hemorrhage
Cerebral cortex	Tornado epilepsy	Post-traumatic seizures
Neck	Whiplash	Flexion-extension injury
Psychological	Panic disorder, chronic anxiety, depression, somatization, compensation neurosis	Psychogenic

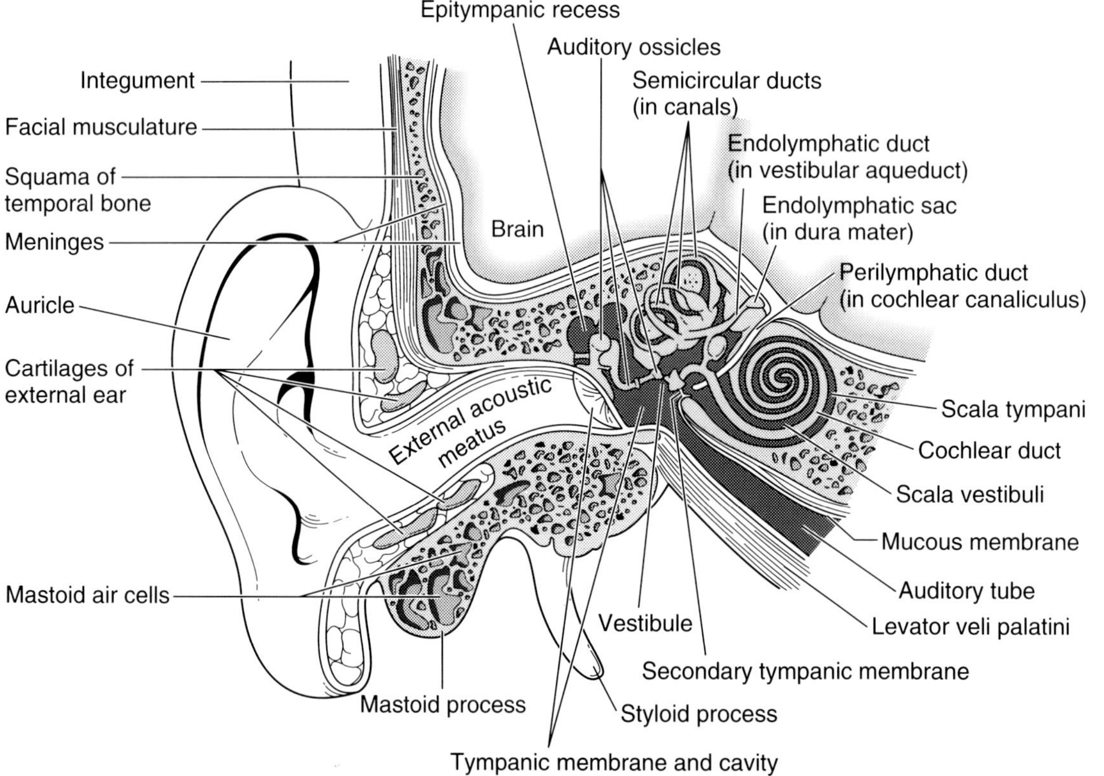

Fig. 9-1. Coronal section of the ear. (Adapted from Anson and Donaldson, 1973, with permission.)

window in the inner ear. Since the middle ear is a relatively closed cavity, its atmospheric pressure must be equalized to the environment, which is done via the auditory tube (eustachian tube). The inner ear lies in the petrous portion of the temporal bone and consists of two parts, the bony labyrinth (otic capsule) and the membranous labyrinth. The bony labyrinth is divided into three areas: the vestibule, bony semicircular canals, and bony cochlea. The membranous labyrinth is a continuous series of communicating sacs and ducts within the bony cavities. It consists of the utricle and saccule (otoliths) housed within the bony vestibule, the semicircular canals (or ducts) within the bony semicircular canals, the cochlear duct within the cochlea, and the endolymphatic duct and sac. The membranous labyrinth is filled with endolymph, which is actively secreted by structures in the labyrinth walls and reabsorbed by the endolymphatic sac. Between the membranous labyrinth and bony labyrinth is perilymph, which is cerebrospinal fluid (CSF) that communicates with the subarachnoid space via the cochlear aqueduct.

The semicircular canals repond to angular acceleration in three orthogonal planes. The neural receptors are hair cells embedded in a gelatinous material called the cupula. The otolith organs respond to linear acceleration and sustained head tilt relative to gravity. The neural receptors for both the canals and otoliths are responsible for stablizing the position of the eyes, head, and body in space and help to maintain an upright stance. This is mediated through three vestibular reflexes. The vestibulo-ocular reflex compensates for head movements and stabilizes eye movements with respect to the surroundings. The vestibulocollic reflex compensates for body movements and stabilizes the orientation of the head in space. The vestibulospinal reflex maintains the orientation of the body in space.

MIDDLE EAR DISORDERS

Injuries to the middle ear alone can cause conductive hearing loss and tinnitus but not dizziness. Trauma may cause hemorrhage or tear of the tympanic membrane, as well as ossicular chain dislocation or fracture (Brahe and Johansen, 1986). This is a frequent finding in longitudinal fractures of the temporal bone (Schuknecht and Davison, 1956; Tos, 1971) (see the section Temporal Bone Fractures below). Blast and explosive shock waves may also cause tympanic membrane perforation and ossicular chain fractures or dislocations (Kerr, 1980; Ziv et al., 1973) (see section Blast and Explosive Injury, below).

INNER EAR (LABYRINTH AND VESTIBULAR NERVE) DISORDERS

Benign Paroxysmal Positional Vertigo

Benign paroxysmal positional vertigo (BPPV) is one of the most common vestibular disorders following head trauma. It has been reported to occur in 15 to 33 percent of all patients with head trauma (Barber, 1964; Harrison 1956; Preber and Silferskiold, 1957; Proctor et al., 1956). The incidence increases with the age of the patient but not with the severity of the head trauma (Barber, 1964). Patients presenting with BPPV should be asked for a history of head trauma. Out of 500 patients with BPPV seen in two outpatient clinics, 17 percent had a history of recent head trauma (Baloh et al., 1987; Katsarkas and Kirkham, 1978). Patients with BPPV usually complain of vertigo lasting less than 1 minute in the morning when they get up or turn over in bed. Transient vertigo may also occur when they move their heads up or down. After a bad attack, they may complain of disequilibrium for several hours. The diagnosis is secured by eliciting torsional and upbeat nystagmus during the Hallpike-Dix maneuver when the affected ear is inferior (see the section Physical Examination below). This nystagmus has a 3- to 30-second latency, fatigues in 3 to 30 seconds, and habituates, unlike positional vertigo due to central causes. The mechanism is believed to involve calcium debris that has broken off from the utricle and within the endolymph of the posterior semicircular canal. The debris may be free-floating in the canal (canal lithiasis) or may be attached to the cupula (cupulolithiasis). We speculate that most cases of BPPV are due to canalithiasis based on the effectiveness of certain treatments and the fatiguability of the nystagmus (Herdman et al., 1993). In cupulolithiasis, we speculate that the nystagmus may not readily fatigue since the calcium will constantly pull down on the cupula. In a small number of patients, BPPV may also occur from calcium debris in the anterior canal, but the nystagmus will be torsional and downbeat. Finally, BPPV may involve the horizontal canal, but the nystagmus will be horizontal and directed toward whichever ear is inferior (Baloh et al., 1993). Although

BPPV usually occurs immediately after head trauma, it may also occur months to years later, but in those cases it can not be readily attributed to the trauma. It is possible that prior head trauma loosens otoconia in the utricle and increases susceptiblity to BPPV.

We design treatment according to the canal involved and whether we believe the vertigo is due to canal lithiasis or cupulo-lithiasis. For horizontal canal BPPV we use the repetitive movement of sitting and lying suggested by Brandt and Daroff (1980b). For anterior or posterior canalithiasis, we treat by a single slow maneuver of the head, which effectively moves the debris to an area in the labyrinth that does not cause symptoms Epley 1992; (Herdman et al., 1993) (Fig 9-2). For posterior cupulolithiasis we use Semont's maneuver (Herdman et al., 1993). The patient is seated on a table and the head is rotated 45 degrees toward the unaffected side. The patient is then moved quickly so as to lie on the side toward the affected ear (parallel to the plane of the affected posterior canal). After 4 minutes the patient is rapidly moved through the inital sitting position to the opposite side while the head is still positioned 45 degrees toward the unaffected side. The patient holds this position for 4 minutes and then moves slowly to a sitting position.

Post-traumatic Endolymphatic Hydrops

Post-traumatic endolymphatic hydrops can occur as a delayed complication of head injury from hemorrhage in the membranous labyrinth or trauma to the lining of the membranous labyrinth (Clark and Rees, 1977; Nadol et al., 1975; Paparella and Mancini, 1983). Hydrops may sometimes be delayed by 5 to 10 years after the insult (delayed endolymphatic hydrops). The mechanism is still unclear but is believed to involve decreased reabsorption of endolymph, which results in increased endolymphatic pressure and small leaks through the membranous labyrinth into the surrounding perilymph. Endolymphatic hydrops causes spells of roaring sound (tinnitus), ear fullness, and hearing loss often associated with vertigo lasting hours to a day. This disease entity may also present in nonclassical forms, with some symptom(s) absent. With repeat attacks, a sustained low-frequency sensorineural hearing loss and constant tinnitus usually develop. The diagnosis depends on documenting fluctuating hearing loss with audiograms, which may have to be done within 24 hours of a spell, as hearing may recover.

The treatment for endolymphatic hydrops is primarily prophylactic and includes elimination of alcohol and caffeinated products (including chocolate), restricting the diet to 2 g or less of sodium, and occasionally use of acetazolamide or another diuretic (Jackson et al., 1981). During acute attacks the patient is treated the same as for any other attack of acute vertigo (see the section *Acute Dizziness,* below), except that blood work and vestibular exercises are usually not necessary. When medical management fails, surgical ablation may be used if the disorder is unilateral (Shelton and Brackmann, 1989). Insertion of an endolymphatic shunt is the most benign surgical procedure; however, it is not always effective or it may stop working after a few years. Labyrinthectomy is appropriate in patients with disabling attacks of vertigo in whom there is a severe pre-existing hearing loss on the side of the defective labyrinth. Vestibular neurectomy is sometimes used in intractable cases in which hearing is preserved.

Labyrinthine Concussion and Semicircular Canal Paresis

Labyrinthine concussion and semicircular canal paresis may follow head trauma without bony fracture. Although the labyrinth is morphologically intact, it is rendered nonfunctional, possibly as a result of hair cell degeneration (Schuknecht, 1951). The disorder presents with acute vertigo, disequilibrium, nausea, hearing loss, and usually tinnitus. The vertigo is quite severe, and patients prefer to lie quietly with the affected ear up. Within a few days these symptoms begin to resolve, and the patient is left with a dynamic deficit (vertigo and disequilibrium induced by head movements), which can last for weeks to months until central compensation occurs. The diagnosis is based on sudden hearing and vestibular loss, which are usually profound and permanent. This condition should be treated in the same way as an acute vestibular defect (see the section*Acute Vertigo,* below). Physical therapy is useful after the acute vertigo subsides (Tangeman and Wheller, 1986). Episodic vertigo and ataxic gait may occur after recovery from labyrinthine concussion during ingestion of small amounts of alcohol, presumably from alcohol-induced impairment of central compensation (Thomke et al., 1990).

Perilymphatic Fistula

Perilymphatic fistula is an abnormal communication between the inner and middle ear with leakage of perilymph thought the defect. It is frequently due

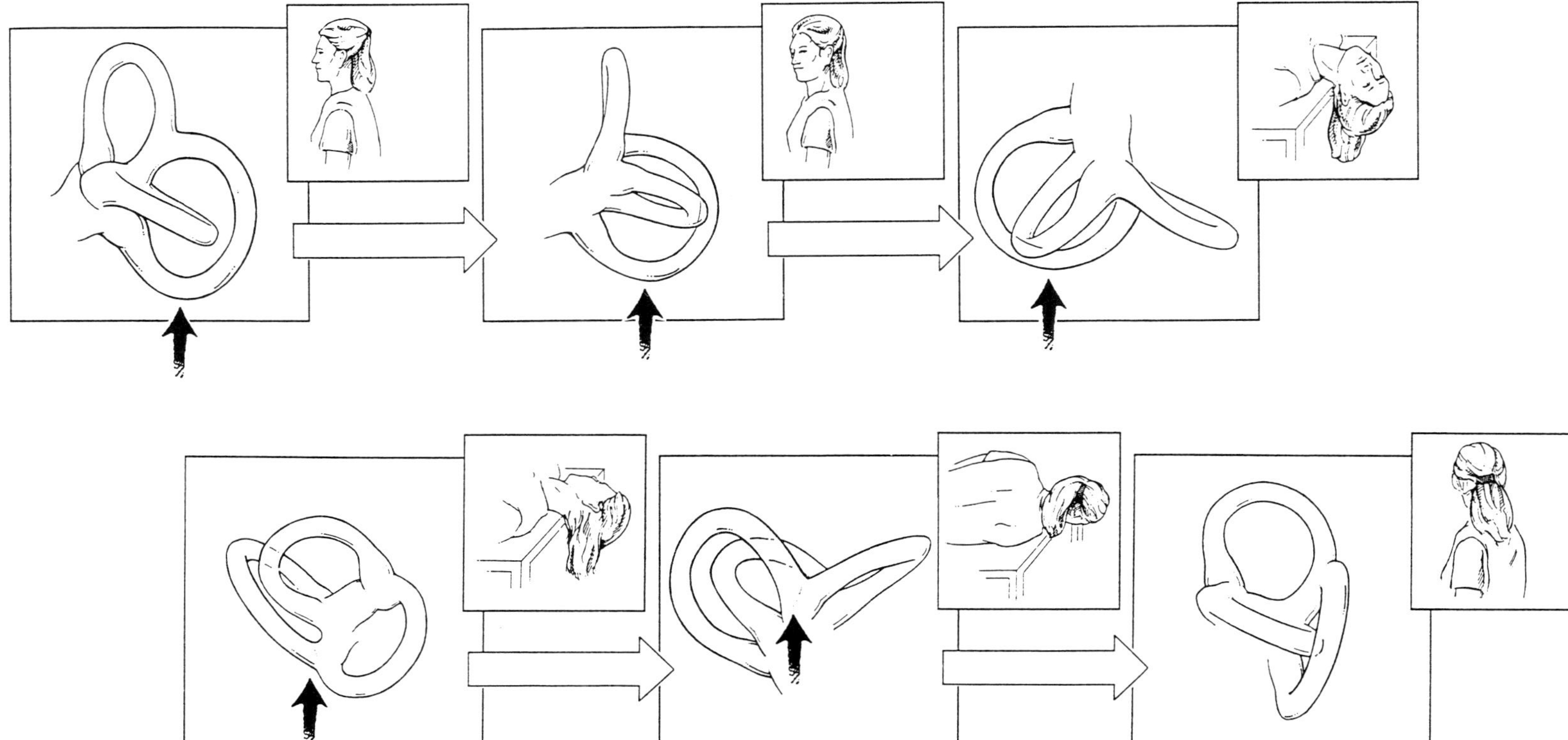

Fig. 9-2. Epley maneuver to treat BPPV. The arrows indicate the position of the free-floating debris in the left posterior semicircular canal during the different stages of the maneuver. The patient is quickly moved into the Hallpike-Dix position with the affected ear down (*top panels*). The patient is kept in that position for 4 minutes, and then the head is slowly rotated through extension until the opposite ear is down (*bottom left two panels*). The patient stays in that position for 4 minutes and then slowly sits up. (Adapted from Herdman et al., 1993, with permission.)

to head trauma including barotrauma, head injury, surgical trauma, violent coughing, and sneezing (Grimm et al., 1989). Barotrauma can cause oval or round window membrane rupture from an explosive route (sudden rise in CSF and perilymphatic pressure) or an implosive route (sudden increase in middle ear pressure relative to inner ear) (Goodhill, 1971). Perilymphatic fistula may also present at an early age spontaneously or from minor head trauma in children with congenital defects of the labyrinth, such as the Mondini defect and enlarged vestibular aqueduct syndrome (Jackler et al., 1987; Jackler and dela Cruz, 1989; Schuknecht, 1980). It presents with sudden, progressive, or fluctuating sensorineural hearing loss, tinnitus, and frequently vertigo and disequilibrium (Glasscock et al., 1992; Grimm et al., 1989). Common sites of perilymph leakage are the stapes footplate, the oval window membrane, and the round window membrane. Diagnosis of perilymphatic fistula is difficult but is facilitated by finding a positive Hennebert's sign, in which nystagmus or a drift of the eyes is induced by positive/negative pressure applied through the external auditory canal or by the Valsalva maneuver (Daspit et al., 1980). This sign may also be positive in 30 percent of the patients with hydrops (Nadol, 1977). Patients with perilymphatic fistula of the round or oval window or hypermobile stapes may experience vertigo from loud noises (the Tullio phenomenon) (Pyykko et al., 1992). Frequently the fistula will seal spontaneously, but some will remain open for several months following head trauma (Glasscock et al., 1992). A perilymphatic fistula may present with sudden hearing loss several years after a temporal bone fracture (Feldmann, 1987). Middle ear exploration is the only way to confirm the diagnosis, and common sites can be packed with soft tissue (Lehrer et al., 1984). Following surgical treatment, vertigo is the symptom most commonly improved, whereas improved hearing may be achieved only in 25 percent of patients (Glasscock et al., 1992).

Temporal Bone Fractures

Temporal bone fractures are divided into longitudinal (orthogonal to long axis of petrous pyramid) and transverse, with longitudinal fractures four times as common (Goodwin, 1983). Meningitis is a late complication of both types of fractures (Applebaum, 1960).

Longitudinal fractures result from temporal and parietal blows. They can extend through the clinoids to the mastoid air cells, and frequently lacerate the tympanic membrane and external auditory canal skin (Fig. 9-3A). They cause conductive hearing loss in 50 to 65 percent of cases (Tos, 1971), and also cause CSF and hemorrhagic otorrhea. Labyrinth concussion may occur, but the bony labyrinth is rarely fractured (Schuknecht and Davison, 1956). Damage to the vestibular and cochlear nerve is infrequent, and the facial nerve is involved in 10 to 20 percent of cases, usually in the labyrinthine segment or geniculate ganglion.

Transverse fractures usually result from frontal or occipital blows. In 80 to 95 percent of cases the fracture transects the inner ear, tears the membranous labyrinth, and lacerates the vestibular and cochlear nerve (Fig. 9-3B). This causes severe sensorineural hearing and vestibular loss. In 50 to 65 percent of cases the facial nerve is injured, usually in the labyrinthine segment. CSF often fills the middle ear and drains into the eustachian tube. The tympanic membrane usually remains intact, but hemotympanum is frequently seen. Both longitudinal and transverse fractures may occur simultaneously, as illustrated in Figure 9-4, which shows an axial CT scan of a 16-year-old girl who had severe right-sided hearing loss.

Among patients with temporal bone fractures, 50 percent will complain of dizziness, and positional nystagmus is the most common vestibular sign (Wennmo and Svensson, 1989). A review of 90 temporal bone fractures of both types revealed hemotympanum as the most common physical finding (46 ears), followed by bleeding from external ear canal (27 ears) and CSF otorrhea (13 patients) (Cannon and Jahrsdoerfer, 1983). Battle's sign from extravasation of blood along the path of the posterior auricular artery occurred in 8 patients, ossicular dislocation or fracture in 13, and facial paralysis in 14. Concussive injury sufficient to cause occipital fracture may also cause complete bilateral loss of cochlear and vestibular function, which is hypothesized to be due to axonal injury to the 8th cranial nerve and possibly the labyrinth (Feneley and Murthy, 1994).

Initial care of temporal bone fractures follows the A.B.C. preservation of airway, breathing, and circulation. Physical examination should include a sterile examination of the external auditory canal and tympanic membrane to evaluate for blood, CSF, and tympanic membrane tear. The cranial nerves 7th and 8th should be examined. Patients unable to respond can be electrically stimulated to evoke facial movement. If temporal bone injury is suspected, high-

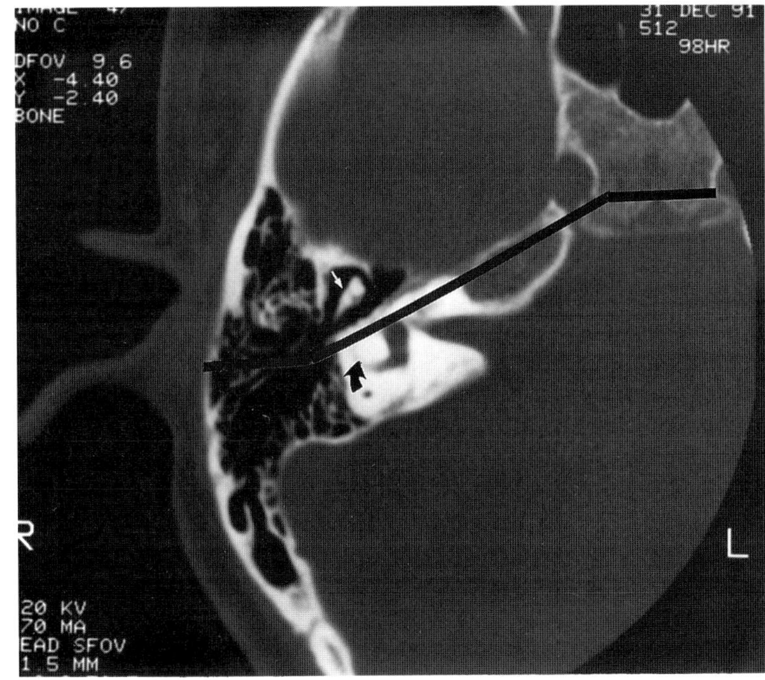

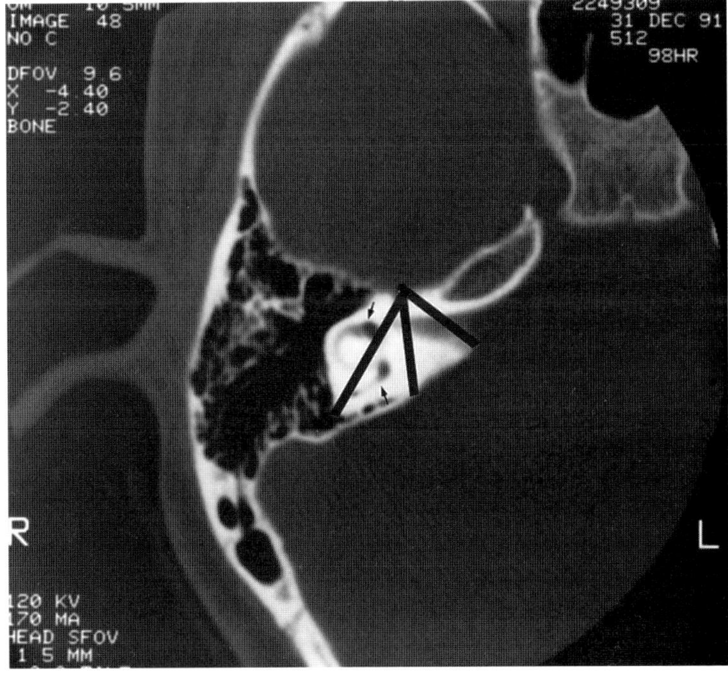

Fig. 9-3. CT scans of the skull base (axial view) showing sites of petrous bone fractures. (**A**) The broad line shows a common plane for longitudinal fractures. Notice that the fracture line can extend through the clinoids, even to the opposite side of the skull. The large arrow shows the vestibule and the smaller arrow the ossicular chain. Both the vestibule and ossicular chain can be disrupted from the fracture. (**B**) Three common planes for transverse fractures. The most lateral goes through the horizontal and posterior semicircular canals (*arrows*). The other two go through the internal auditory canal.

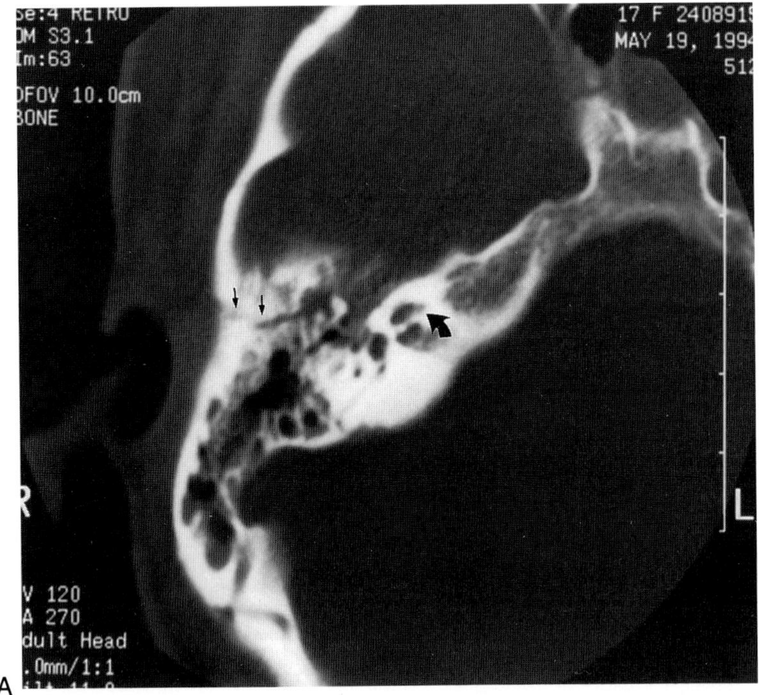

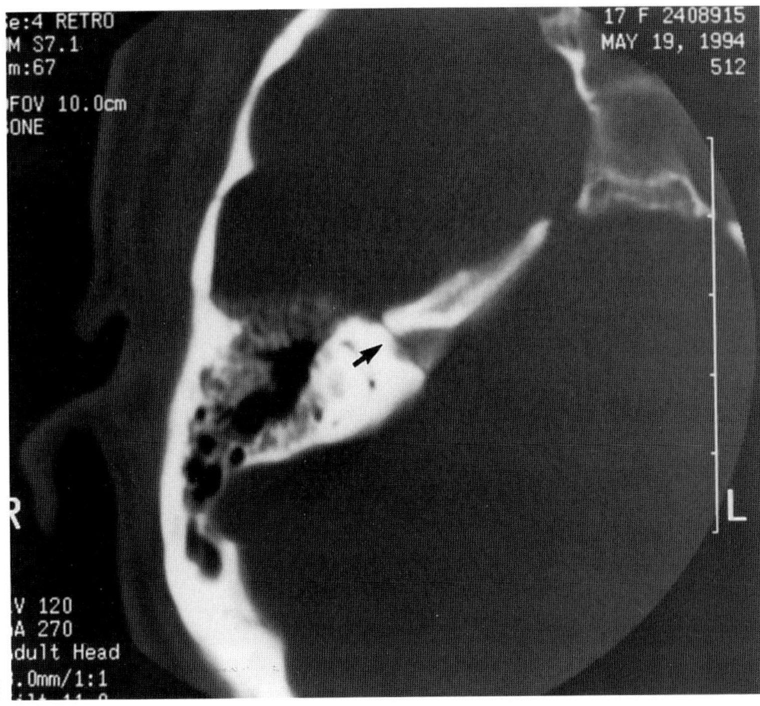

Fig. 9-4. CT scan of the skull base (axial view) of a 16-year-old girl who was involved in a car crash and suffered head injury. Her score on the Glasgow Coma Scale was 3 at the scene and 6 in the trauma center. Scans shows both longitudinal (**A**) and transverse fractures (**B**), which are indicated by arrows. Her examination demonstrated severe hearing loss in the right ear.

resolution computed tomography (CT) is the preferred method, with 1.5-mm cuts in coronal and axial planes (Avrahami and Epstein, 1991; Goligher and Lloyd, 1990; Liu-Shindo and Hawkins, 1988; Schubinger et al., 1986). When this is not available, lateral radiographic projections may reveal longitudinal fractures and Stenver projections may reveal transverse fractures.

Vestibular symptoms almost always fade by 1 year (Wennmo and Svensson, 1989) owing to central compensation, which can be facilitated by vestibular rehabilitation. If vertigo does not begin to resolve by several months, BPPV or perilymphatic fistula should be considered. If vertigo develops years after the trauma, delayed endolymphatic hydrops formation must be considered. Of patients with isolated low-frequency sensorineural hearing loss, 60 percent will have spontaneous partial recovery; 30 percent with isolated high-frequency sensorineural hearing loss will recover, but those with both low and high sensorineural hearing loss rarely experience significant recovery (Griffiths, 1979).

Blast and Explosive Injury

In an explosion, a shock wave spreads outward with an initial short, positive-pressure phase being followed by a longer, negative pressure phase. Damage caused by blast is correlated with peak pressure and duration of the positive-pressure phase. The middle and inner ear are the organs most sensitive to blast injury and frequently the only organs damaged (Kerr, 1980; Ziv et al., 1973). The most common injury is tympanic membrane perforation, which causes pain and conductive hearing loss. This has a spontaneous healing rate of up to 80 percent. Ossicular chain fractures or dislocations may also occur and cause conductive loss, which require surgical repair. Cochlear damage also occurs and causes tinnitus and sensorineural hearing loss which is usually severe. This hearing loss improves in a few days, but 25 to 45 percent of patients are left with some degree of permanent sensorineural hearing loss and tinnitus. Dizziness is less frequently reported, and the effect of blast injury on the vestibular system is less well known because it has been primarily observed on bedside examination (Cait et al., 1989; Kerr and Byrne, 1975). It mainly consists of BPPV, and it is unclear whether it is due to the blast itself or to subsequent head trauma from flying debris or a fall (Kerr and Byrne, 1975). On the basis of eye movement recordings, vestibular damage, including semicircular canal paresis, may be more common then previously believed (Shupak et al., 1993). These patients are usually not explored, and so it is unclear whether the vestibular defect is due to a perilymphatic fistula or to concussive injury to the labyrinth.

CENTRAL DISORDERS

Brainstem and Vestibulocerebellar Injury

Severe head trauma may produce axonal swelling and Wallerian degeneration in structures in the posterior fossa based on autopsy review (Oppenheimer, 1968; Peerless and Rewcastle, 1967; Pilz, 1983; Povlishock et al., 1983). To what extent focal damage to the brainstem can occur following head trauma is unclear. In animal models petechial hemorrhages and degenerative changes may occur in vestibular nuclei and the vestibulocerebellum with minor head trauma (Denny-Brown and Russell, 1941; Windle et al., 1944). These studies are difficult to extrapolate to humans since the animals were anesthetized during the head trauma. In careful serial sections of human brainstem in fatal blunt head injury, brainstem damage without damage to the rest of the brain was not found (i.e., brainstem injury is believed to occur as part of diffuse brain damage and not in isolation) (Makishima et al., 1976; Mitchell and Adams, 1973).

A variety of different types of central vestibular nystagmus, usually not associated with vertigo, may occur following head trauma. Downbeat nystagmus occurs from increased activity of central anterior semicircular canal pathways relative to the posterior semicircular canal (hemorrhage or contusion of cerebellar flocculus or of the medial longitudinal fasciculus in the floor of the fourth ventricle). Upbeat nystagmus occurs from increased activity of central posterior semicircular canal pathways relative to the anterior semicircular canal (hemorrhage or contusion of the brachium conjunctivum in the midbrain or the ventral tegmental tract in the dorsal pontomedullary junction). Gaze-position nystagmus occurs from decreased gain in the medial vestibular nucleus/nucleus prepositus hypoglossi in dorsal medulla or the flocculus. Positional-induced nystagmus from a peripheral vestibular basis (i.e., BPPV) is usually associated with vertigo. In contrast, positional-induced nystagmus from a central cause is rarely associated with vertigo, and when it occurs it is attributed to hemorrhage dorsolateral to the fourth ventricle (Brandt, 1990).

The ocular tilt reaction consists of head tilt, skew eye deviation (hypertropic eye contralteral to side of head tilt) and cyclodeviation of the eyes (excyclotropia of the hypotropic eye and incyclotropia of the hypertropic eye) (Brandt and Dieterich, 1987; Halmagyi et al., 1979). The patient primarily complains of verticle diplopia. This disorder is from a unilateral defect in the otolith and possibly in the posterior semicircular canal pahtways. Lesions of the labyrinth, 8th cranial nerve, and vestibular nuclei all cause an ipsilateral ocular tilt reaction (head tilt toward side of lesion), whereas lesions of the medial longitudinal fasciculus and interstitial nucleus of Cajal cause a contralateral ocular tilt reaction. Variations of the ocular tilt reaction include alternating skew deviation and seesaw nystagmus (Daroff, 1965; Keane, 1985).

Postconcussive Syndrome and Minor Head Trauma

Following minor head trauma with concussion and a brief period of amnesia, patients frequently complain of persistent headache (25 percent), anxiety (19 percent), insomnia (15 percent), dizziness (14 percent), and a host of other symptoms (Rutherford et al., 1977). To what extent these symptoms occur as a result of head trauma is unclear since these same symptoms are reported by patients without head trauma who are involved in litigation (Lees-Haley and Brown, 1993). The dizziness described by patients with postconcussive syndrome is usually nonspecific and often consists of a sense of swimming, lightheadedness, floating, rocking, and disorientation. Unfortunately, these terms are also used by patients with dizziness due to psychosomatic illness. One also needs to rule out peripheral vestibular defects and brainstem injury. Treatment of dizziness in this syndrome involves reassurance that there is no structural damage and that the symptoms are not unusual and usually resolve. Medication and pyschological intervention are useful when there is underlying anxiety and depression.

There have been two large neuro-otologic studies in patients with minor head injury. Tuohimaa (1978) studied 82 patients who were unconscious for 2 hours or less without evidence of skull fractures or intracerebral hemorrhage. Vestibular paresis from presumed labyrinth concussion was found in 17.1 percent of the patients within 4 days of the injury and persisted in 5.3 percent for up to 6 months. Their examination was not described beyond 6 months. Griffiths (1979) studied 84 patients within a few days of the traumatic incident who also had no skull fracture but did have direct injury to the skull with concussion (post-traumatic amnesia of less than 24 hours). Of these patients 56 percent had hearing loss based on audiogram, the majoirty of which were sensorineural loss, and 24 percent had vertigo of unknown etiology, 70 percent of which were associated with deafness. Vestibular studies were not done. Neither of these two studies described the initial neurologic exam during he first 24 hours, so the Glasgow Coma Scale (GCS) score could not be determined.

Seizures

The incidence of seizures following head trauma (post-traumatic seizures) is 7 to 10 percent, of which 20 to 36 percent are partial (Annegers et al., 1980; Hahn et al., 1988; Lee and Lui, 1992) (see also Ch. 12). Ninety-four percent of all seizures occur within 24 hours of the injury. The incidence increases as the GCS decreases, ranging from 5.9 percent for a GCS score higher than 13 to 35 percent for a GCS score below 8 (Hahn et al., 1988). Ictal vertigo with a true sense of rotation of self or environment (tornado epilepsy) is uncommon and primarily occurs in simple partial seizures, which usually evolve into complex partial seizures or generalize with loss of consciousness. In a series of 222 patients with partial seizures from traumatic and nontraumatic causes, 9 had ictal vertigo (Penfield and Kristiansen, 1951). Vertigo in some patients with partial siezures simulates endolymphatic hydrops without hearing loss (Nielsen, 1959). This is most likey due to stimulation of a vestibular cortical area in the superior temporal gyrus (Friberg et al., 1985). Seizures may also cause other neuro-otologic symptoms. Epileptic jerk nystagmus may occur in patients who remain conscious during the event, and is believed to be due to electrical activation of saccade eye fields and occasionally smooth pursuit and vestibular eye fields (Furman et al., 1990; Thurston et al., 1985; Tusa et al., 1990).

Cervical Trauma (Whiplash Syndrome)

Acute flexion-extension injuries of the neck often lead to symptoms referred to as the whiplash syndrome. Neck pain, headache, and limited range of motion of the neck are the most common symptoms, but dizziness usually described as lightheadedness, floating, and being off balance may follow. The acute injury is postulated to be mechanical strain with or without contusion or tears of the ligaments and muscles supporting the cervical spine (Macnab, 1971) (see also Ch. 13). Following significant neck trauma, disequilibrium may occur as a result of central cord syndrome. Vertigo can occur if there is associated vertebral artery thrombosis leading to a posterior inferior cerebellar artery syndrome. Often the physical examination is negative, leading the physician to be skeptical about these subjective complaints. Litigation is often involved, further confusing the etiology of the syndrome (see Ch. 27). There may be eye movement disorders in patients with whiplash, documented on electronystagmography (ENG) (Compere, 1968; Toglia, 1976; Rubin, 1973), but this is most likely the result of coincidental head trauma. In a population-based study by Sturzenegger et al. (1944) of 137 consecutive patients with whiplash (but no head trauma or neck fractures), complaints of tinnitus occured in 3.6 percent, vertigo in 4.4 percent, and unsteadiness in 16.8 percent at a mean delay of 7.2 days. These symptoms did not depend on the location of the person in the car or the presence of a seat belt or head restraint and were found to be more frequent in rear-end than in front or side collisions. The authors speculate that this is due to higher acceleration of the head caused by a larger physiologic movement posteriorly.

Cervical Vertigo

There is cervical input to the vestibular system that can enhance the vestibular-ocular reflex and contribute to self-motion. The cervico-ocular reflex functions synergistically with the vestibular-ocular reflex to generate slow-phase eye movements opposite to head movements to stabilize gaze during head movements. The cervico-ocular reflex can be demonstrated by measuring eye movements while moving the trunk with the head fixed. In normal subjects the response is extremely low, but it increases significantly in patients with bilateral vestibular deficits. This is possibly mediated by a multisynaptic pathway from the neck proprioceptors to the vestibular nuclei. Somatosensory receptors from neck muscles, tendons, and joints also contribute to self-motion during active locomotion. Arthrokinetic nystagmus can be evoked in the dark by human subjects and primates walking in place on a circular treadmill and also can be enhanced after bilateral labyrinth defects (Bles et al., 1983; Brandt et al., 1977).

Despite these findings, there is no evidence that injury to the neck causes significant vestibular deficits. Unilateral anesthesia of the posterolateral neck tissue rarely causes spontaneous nystagmus but can cause transient ipsilateral past-pointing, ataxia, and the sensation of numbness or floating (DeJong et al., 1977). These are the typical features of cervical vertigo, a controversial condition that has been proposed to explain somatic complaints of nonvertiginous dizziness in the absence of true peripheral or central vestibular dysfunction following whiplash injury. Numerous mechanisms have been proposed for cervical vertigo, including (1) vertebrobasilar insufficiency (Sandstrom, 1962); (2) cervical sympathetic irritation causing decreased blood flow to the labyrinth (Sandstrom, 1962); and (3) altered spinal proprioceptive fiber input (Hinoki, 1985).

Drug-induced Dizziness

Several hundred drugs may cause dizziness, especially in those over the age of 65 years (Ballantyne and Ajodhia, 1984; Wennmo and Wennmo, 1988). Table 9-2 lists the more common drugs along with their primary effects. Certain drugs cause vague complaints of dizziness including disequilibrium and lightheadedness. These include anticonvulsants, antidepressants, antihypertensives, antiinflammatories, hypnotics, muscle relaxants, and tranquilizers. Drugs used to treat dizziness and nausea (vestibular suppressants) are frequently also the cause of disequilibrium when used chronically. Sensitization to meclizine and scopolamine may occur after a few days of continuous use, and withdrawal symptoms will occur when the medication is stopped. This may be misinterpreted as recurrence of the problem, and so physicans should be cautious about restarting these medications. We try to restrict the use of these medications. We use meclizine, scopolamine, and other vestibular suppressants for a few days only during acute vestibular hypofunction such as labyrinth concussion or acute 8th cranial nerve transection. Then these drugs should be stopped; otherwise they can interfere with central compensation. Patients with brainstem medullary lesions may have nausea lasting for weeks and may require medication for a longer time. Certain drugs, including certain aminoglycosides and loop diuretics, may cause vestibular ototoxicity and spare hearing and lead to disequilibrium (Table 9-2). The other aminoglycosides affect hearing primarily.

TABLE 9-2. Drug-Induced Dizziness

Drug Type	Drugs That Can Cause Dizziness	Drugs That Interfere With Vestibular Compensation	Ototoxic (Vestibular) Drugs
Antiarrythmics			
Amiodarone, quinine			X (synergistic)
Anticonvulsants			
Barbiturates, carbamazepine	X		
Phenytoin, ethosuximide	X		
Antidepressants			
Amitriptyline, imipramine	X		
Antihypertensives			
Diuretics			
Hydrochlorthiazide	X		
Furosemide, ethaycrynic acid			X (synergistic)
α-Blockers			
Prazosine, terosine	X		
β-Blockers			
Atenolol, propranalol	X		
Calcium antagonists			
Nifedipine, verapamil	X		
Anti-inflammatory drugs			
Ibuprofen, indomethacin	X		
Aspirin			X (reversible)
Antibiotics			
Gentamicin, streptomycin			X
Tobramycin			X
Chemotherapeutics			
Cisplatin			X
Hypnotics			
Flurazepam, triazolam	X		
Muscle relaxants			
Cyclobenzaprine, orphenidrine	X		
Methocarbamol	X		
Tranquilizers			
Chlordiazepoxide	X		
Meprobamate	X		
Vestibular suppressants			
Meclizine, scopalamine	X	X	
Chloridazepoxide, diazepam	X	X	
Lorazepam	X	X	

Post-traumatic Migraine

Migraine can occur following trauma, including whiplash (Jacome, 1986; Winston, 1987) (see also Ch. 8), and certain types of migraine are a common cause of episodic vertigo and disequilibrium. To help standardize terminology and diagnostic criteria, we use the criteria of the International Headache Society (IHS) (1988). Below we briefly discuss the relevant types of migraine pertinent to neuro-otologic disorders. These types have not been specifically described following head trauma, although all can potentially occur.

Benign paroxysmal vertigo of childhood consists of spells of vertigo and disequilibrium without hearing loss or tinnitus (Basser, 1964; Parker, 1989). Headache is usually not a major feature of these spells initially. Spells occur mainly between 1 and 4 years of age but can occur at any time during the first decade. Vertigo and disequilibrium typically last for minutes but can last up to several hours. Patients may have visual disturbance, flushing, nausea, and vomiting. In the majority of cases the physical examination, audiogram, ENG, and electroencephalogram (EEG) are normal. Many of these patients eventually develop more typical migraine headaches, and there is frequently a positive family history for migraine. The incidence of migraine, however, is similar to that in the general population, and the age of onset is not described (Parker, 1989). Consequently, this is still a poorly understood entity even though it is listed as a type of migraine by the IHS. Since this entity is a diagnosis of exclusion, the diagnosis is aided by a positive response to treatment as discussed below.

Basilar migraine presents with symptoms in the distribution of the basilar artery, including vertigo, tinnitus, decreased hearing and ataxia (Bickerstaff, 1961; Harker and Rassekh, 1987). This disorder consists of two or more neurologic problems (vertigo, tinnitus, decreased hearing, ataxia, dysarthria, visual symptoms in both hemifields of both eyes, diplopia, bilateral paresthesia or paresis, decreased level of consciousness) followed by a throbbing headache. Vertigo typically lasts between 5 minutes and 1 hour. In the majority of cases audiograms are normal, but many patients have abnormal ENG studies (Eviatar, 1981; Olsson, 1991). There is frequently a positive family history for migraine.

Migraine management is based on the pathophysiology of this disorder and includes elimination of tyramine from the diet and the use of drugs that change vascular tone or block serotonin and prostaglandin receptors (Peroutka, 1990). In addition, migraine is triggered by a number of factors including stress, anxiety, hypoglycemia, estrogen, and nicotine, which should be removed if possible (Diamond, 1991; Silberstein and Merriam, 1991).

Psychogenic Dizziness

Panic attacks and hyperventilation causes spells that usually reach a crescendo within 10 minutes and consist of a variety of complaints, including a vague sense of dizziness, nausea, shortness of breath, palpitation, sweating, paresthesia, and fear. They may occur unexpectedly or be situational. These are anxiety disorders, and frequently there is a positive family history. Helpful diagnostic criteria can be found in the American Psychiatric Association Diagnostic and Statistical Manual Options Book (DSM-IV). Treatment includes patient education, behavioral modification, and if necessary supportive psychotherapy and medication, including antidepressants (imipramine).

Bouts of vertigo frequently results in chronic anxiety which often persists long after the organic vestibular deficit resolves. Patients may perceive prolonged disability and feel significantly handicapped out of proportion to any physical abnormality (Yardley et al., 1994). This may be more of a problem in patients with premorbid psychological disorders.

Psychogenic disorders of gait and stance have been well described (Keane, 1989; Lempert et al., 1991) and frequently occur following head trauma. Certain features help to identify a functional component, including knee buckling without fall, small-amplitude steps, uneconomical posture and movement, exaggerated sway during the Romberg test without fall, excessive slowness in gait, and fluctuations in level of impairment (Lempert et al., 1991).

PREFERRED APPROACH

History

The history is the most important part of the evaluation of the dizzy patient. Dizziness is an imprecise term used to describe a variety of problems, including vertigo, disequilibrium, presyncope, motion sickness and psychological problems, each of which has a different pathophysiologic mechanism (Table 9-3). It is sometimes helpful to ask patients to describe their symptoms without using the term dizziness. Frequently the cause of the dizziness is suggested by the temporal pattern of the symptoms and the conditions in which they occur (Table 9-4). For example, BPPV presents as spells of vertigo lasting for several seconds induced by a change in head position. Labyrinth concussion presents as a chronic problem. Initially, patients complain of spontaneous vertigo and poor balance. In time the vertigo primarily occurs only during head movements, but the poor balance persists.

Patient Presentations

Acute Vertigo

Acute vertigo is due to sudden imbalance of spontaneous neural activity in the vestibular nucleus due to disease in either the labyrinth, 8th cranial nerve, vestibular nucleus, vestibulocerebellum (nodulus and flocculus), or central otolith pathways (medial longitudinal fasciculus to interstitial nucleus of Cajal). Common etiologies of vertigo can be divided into those that impair and those that spare hearing

TABLE 9-3. Types of Dizziness

Type	Symptoms	Mechanism
Vertigo	Illusion of movement (rotation, tilt, or linear translation)	Imbalance of tonic vestibular signals
Disequilibrium	Imbalance or unsteadiness while standing or walking	Loss of vestibulospinal, visual, proprioception, or motor function
Presyncope	Lightheadedness	Decreased cerebral perfusion
Motion sickness	Dizziness, nausea, cold sweat, yawning	Visual-vestibular mismatch
Psychological	Floating, rocking, spinning inside of head	Chronic anxiety, panic attacks, depression, somatization

(Table 9-5). All patients with acute vertigo should have nystagmus on examination, at least during the day of the event. If nystagmus is not present, a vestibular defect is extremely unlikely. Table 9-6 lists guidelines for the management of acute vertigo. During the first few days, vestibular suppressants may be used (promethazine or phochlorperazine). Patients need hospitalization only if dehydrated or if a central lesion is suspected. After an acute insult, the imbalance of spontaneous neural activity in the vestibular nucleus usually corrects itself within several days. What remains is a dynamic deficit in vestibular function, in which patients perceive vertigo or unsteadiness during head movements. This dynamic deficit can only be repaired by vestibular adaptation. To facilitate vestibular adaptation, the patients are taught a series of vestibular exercises which encourages them to move their heads while viewing a stimulus (Tusa and Herdman, 1993). Preliminary results show that use of these exercises following acute unilateral vestibular loss does significantly improve balance and subjective complaints of vertigo (Herdman and Clendaniel, 1993). Vestibular suppressants delay vestibular adaptation. Consequently, these medications should be discontinued as soon as possible.

Chronic Dizziness

Chronic dizziness is primarily due to disequilibrium or a psychological problem. Normal balance depends on integration of sensory (visual, vestibular, and somatosensory) input and appropriate automatic postural responses involving the frontal lobe, basal ganglia, cerebellum, spinal cord, and peripheral nerves. More than 33 percent of survivors of severe closed head injury experience severe postural imbalance as measured by posturography, primarily anteroposterior sway (Wober et al., 1993). This may be more a function of cerebellar ataxia caused by lesion of the anterior cerebellar lobe. A low initial Glasgow Outcome Scale score is a valuable predictive parameter for later disturbances. Patients with vestibular and proprioceptive loss complain that their balance is worse in the dark (Baloh and Honrubia, 1990).

The clinical examination can be very helpful in the diagnosis of bilateral vestibular or static unilateral vestibular defects (see the section Physical Examination, below). These patients frequently have refixation saccadic eye movements following head thrust due to a decrease in the vestibular-ocular reflex gain. In addition, unilateral defects frequently cause nys-

TABLE 9-4. Temporal Pattern and Conditions of Dizziness

Tempo	Vertigo	Disequilibrium	Diagnosis
Spells (seconds to 1 min)	Positional-induced		BPPV
Spells (minutes to 1 hr)	Spontaneous	Spontaneous	Seizures
Spells (minutes to 1 hr)	Spontaneous or dynamic	Spontaneous	Post-traumatic migraine
Spells (hours to 1 day)	Spontaneous	Spontaneous	Endolymphatic hydrops
Chronic	Spontaneous, then dynamic	Spontaneous	Labyrinth concussion, canal paresis, temporal bone fracture
Chronic	Pressure or positional-induced	Pressure-induced	Perilymphatic fistula

TABLE 9-5. Hearing in Acute Vertigo

Hearing Usually Impaired	Hearing Usually Preserved
Endolymphatic hydrops	BPPV
Labyrinth concussion	Brainstem and vestibulocerebellar injury
Perilymphatic fistula	Postconcussive syndrome
Temporal bone fracture	Post-traumatic seizures
Blast and explosive injury	Cervical trauma
	Post-traumatic migraine
	Psychogenic

tagmus following horizontal head shaking, and bilateral lesions usually result in more than a four-line elevation in visual acuity during 2-Hz head oscillation and oscillopsia. The diagnosis should be secured by demonstrating a decreased vestibular-ocular response on the rotary chair test, and the peripheral nature of the defect should be identified by a decreased caloric test response.

Although vestibular neurectomy has been advocated for treatment of patients with post-traumatic unsteadiness with associated hearing impairment (Sanna and Ylikosky, 1983; Ylikoski et al., 1982), there have been no controlled trials comparing this form of treatment with vestibular rehabilitation. There is no physiologic basis for this type of treatment except for treatment-intractable spells of vertigo due to post-traumatic endolymphatic hydrops. In our opinion, there is no conclusive evidence that neurectomy facilitates vestibular compensation.

Treatment of bilateral vestibular defects should include avoidance of all ototoxins that may cause further permanent peripheral vestibular damage (gentamicin, streptomycin, tobramycin, ethacrynic acid, furosemide, quinine, cisplatin), avoidance of drugs that may transiently impair balance (sedatives, anti-anxiety drugs, antiepileptics, and antidepressants).

TABLE 9-6. Management of Acute Vertigo

Acute (Days 1–3)	Subacute
Bed rest	Begin vestibular exercises
Vestibular sedatives	Stop vestibular sedatives
Hospitalize if dehydrated or suspect central defect	Audiogram
CT/MRI of head if suspect central defect	Caloric and/or rotary chair tests to document vestibular loss

Vestibular rehabilitation may be very helpful for these patients.

Motion Sickness

Motion sickness consists of episodic dizziness, tiredness, pallor, diaphoresis, salivation, nausea, and occasionally vomiting induced by passive locomotion (e.g., riding in a car) or motion in the visual surround while standing still (e.g., viewing a rotating optokinetic stimulus). Motion sickness is believed to be due to a sensory mismatch between vision and vestibular cues (Brandt and Daroff, 1980a). Patients with migraine disorder are particularly prone to motion sickness, especially during childhood; 26 to 60 percent of patients with migraine have a history of severe motion sickness, compared with 8 to 24 percent in the normal population (Kayan and Hood, 1984; Kuritzky et al., 1981). The cause of this relation is not clear. Treatment consists of reassurance, reduction of circumstances that cause sensory mismatch, and medication if necessary (meclizine and scopolamine patch).

Hearing Loss

Sensorineural hearing loss is due to several causes, including labyrinthine concussion from blood or from loss of hair cells in the basal turn (an effect similar to that of high-intensity noise), disruption of the membranous labyrinth from transverse fracture of the temporal bone, disruption of the 8th cranial nerve and central pathways, and perilymphatic fistula in the stapes footplate when fractured and depressed into the vestibule (Healy, 1982; Proctor et al., 1956; Schuknecht, 1969; Ward, 1969). When skull fracture is not present, hearing loss is usually due to end organ abnormalities (Kochhar et al., 1990). Treatment is with use of a hearing aid.

Conductive hearing loss is usually due to longitudinal temporal bone fracture, which recovers spontaneously in 80 percent of patients (Tos, 1971). Another cause of hearing loss is ossicular chain disruption, which usually occurs at the incudostapedial joint and is usually amenable to surgical correction with excellent results (Hough, 1969). Hearing loss may also occur with tympanic membrane rupture, which usually heals spontaneously if no infection occurs.

Hearing loss is a common sequela of head trauma, and there have been a number of recent studies in children (Abd al-Hardy et al., 1990; Cockrell and Gregory, 1992; Dorman and Morton, 1982; Zimmerman et al., 1993). In a prospective study of 50 children admitted to a neurosurgery service following head trauma, 16 (32 percent) were found to have conductive hearing loss and 8 (16 percent) had sensorineural hearing loss (Zimmerman et al., 1993). All children with temporal bone fractures had conductive loss. Since hearing loss did not correlate with degree of head injury, close audiologic and otologic follow-up is strongly recommended in all children admitted with head injury. Hearing usually recovers in patients without skull fracture or ossicular chain damage (Dorman and Morton, 1982).

Facial Nerve Paresis

Facial nerve paresis has been reported in transverse fractures in 30 to 50 percent of cases and in longitudinal fractures in 10 to 15 percent of cases and is usually due to involvement of the geniculate ganglion and labyrinthine segment of the nerve (Fisch, 1974; Linderman, 1979). It may be due to transection or compression with edema. It should be treated with corticosteroids and followed with electromyography (EMG) of facial muscle (Crumley and Robinson, 1990). If denervation is found, then the nerve should be surgically explored through a combined middle cranial fossa and transmastoid approach to evaluate the entire length of the nerve. Exposure keratitis from incomplete eyelid closure must be prevented. Artificial tears should be used during the daytime, and Lacrilube ointment can be applied at night.

Tinnitus

Tinnitus is a common symptom which can be sustained or pulsatile, the latter being usually due to a vascular disturbance. It may occur for a few seconds or may be constant. Tinnitus occurs in 30 to 70 percent of all head injuries and is usually nonpulsatile and constant (Rouit and Murali, 1987). Tinnitus from head injury is described as more intense and bothersome than tinnitus from nontraumatic conditions but does not differ from that in nontraumatic conditions with respect to pitch, masking level, and general hearing level (Vernon and Press, 1994). The etiology of nonpulsatile and constant tinnitus is unclear but is speculated to be dysfunction of the cochlea, 8th cranial nerve, or central brainstem pathways and is usually associated with sensorineural hearing loss. An audiogram should be done. If there is significant hearing loss to speech discrimination, hearing aids may help. In addition, white noise at night may be useful. Tinnitus may be exacerbated by stress and anxiety, and antidepressant medication has been recommended (Marion, 1991).

Cerebrospinal Fluid Lead

The leakage of clear fluid from the ear or nose following head trauma (CSF otorrhea or rhinorrhea) is common with temporal bone fractures (Cannon and Jahrsdoefer, 1983). The majority of leaks will respond to bed rest, and those that fail may be surgically repaired. The location of the leak is best determined with a high-resolution CT scan of the temporal bone and paranasal sinuses following intrathecal injection of water-soluble contrast material (Hasso and Ledington, 1988). If the CSF leak is not patched, bacterial meningitis may occur.

PHYSICAL EXAMINATION

The elicitation of certain findings on clinical examination and laboratory testing helps confirm the correct diagnosis. ENG should be performed on any individual who demonstrates new-onset nystagmus or disequilibrium or complains of vertigo. If possible, computed dynamic posturography should be performed on patients with disequilibrium. The degree of impairment due to a vestibular abnormality can be quantified by using published guidelines (American Medical Association 1993), but this depends on obtaining objective clinic signs, diagnoses and test results. These guidelines have not been updated since 1972 but are expected to be revised in the next year by members in the American Academy of Otolaryngology. The guidelines as presently written are not meant to be used to determine degree of disability, since they do not take into account the patient's occupation, age, or ability to be retrained.

Eye Movements

Vestibular-Ocular Reflex

The vestibular-ocular reflex can be examined at the bedside by having the patient fixate on a target and oscillate the head vertically and horizontally at 2 Hz so that the tip of the nose moves 1 to 2 inches. This is above the frequency in which the patient can use pursuit eye movements to track the target. If the patient wears glasses for most of the day, the test should be done with the glasses on, since the vestibular

-ocular reflex adapts according to the refractive power of the lens. During this oscillation, the patient's eyes should move smoothly so that fixation is always maintained. Patients should read the lowest readable line on a Snellen chart during 2-Hz head oscillation. Patients whose lowest readable line is more than three lines above their static visual acuity probably have a vestibular defect. Finally, the examiner should have the patient fixate on a target and should examine the eyes after head thrusts horizontally and vertically. After the head thrust, a refixation saccade indicates decreased vestibular-ocular reflex (Halmagyi and Curthoys, 1988). Here, too, the patient needs to be tested with glasses on. With very young children and babies, the vestibular-ocular reflex can be assessed by picking them up and rotating them in outstretched arms while looking at thier eyes for nystagmus. Visual fixation should be blocked (e.g., with Frenzel lenses) to prevent the optokinetic response.

Smooth Pursuit, Vestibular-Ocular Reflex Cancellation, Saccades

The examiner should have the patient track a slowly moving target both horizontally and vertically with the head still (smooth pursuit) or with the head moving synchronously with the target (vestibular-ocular reflex cancellation). Lesions in the parieto-occipital cortex, pons, and cerebellum will all cause deficits in smooth pursuit (catch-up saccades) and cancellation or inappropriateness of the vestibular-ocular reflex for targets moving ipsilateral to side of the lesion. Impaired cancellation of the reflex has been reported after mild head and neck trauma (Herishanu, 1992). A review of oculomotor abnormalities from head and neck trauma has been recently published (Avrahami and Epstein, 1991; Hildingsson et al., 1989).

Nystagmus

The presence of spontaneous nystagmus should be checked with fixation blocked by Frenzel lenses or by ophthalmoscopy with the viewing eye covered (Zee, 1978) while the patient is seated and while the patient is supine with the head deviated to the left and right (position testing). Spontaneous nystagmus, with fixation blocked, of less than 5 degrees per second can be found in normal subjects and should not be used in isolation to diagnose a vestibular abnormality (Barber and Wright, 1973). Nystagmus due to an acute peripheral lesion is reduced with fixation and is usually horizontal or horizontal and torsional in direction (slow phases directed toward the defective side). Nystagmus present during fixation is always pathologic. Nystagmus should also be examined during the Hallpike-Dix maneuver for the presence of BPPV. In this maneuver the patient is seated on a flat examining table with the head rotated 45 degrees to one side. The patient is then quickly moved backward into a recumbent position with the head still deviated and hanging over the side of the table. Nystagmus from BPPV should begin within 30 seconds and last less than 30 seconds. If nystagmus persists in this position and is not present while the patient is sitting, it is likely due to a central problem (central positional vertigo). The presence of nystagmus following 20 horizontal head oscillations (head-shaking nystagmus) also indicates a vestibular imbalance (Hain et al., 1987). This sign may persist indefinitely after a peripheral or central unilateral vestibular lesion. Nystagmus or drift of the eyes should also be checked after positive and negative pressure directed to the external auditory canal (Hennebert sign), a Valsalva maneuver, or loud noises (Tullio's phenomenon) (Daspit et al., 1980; Pyykko et al., 1992). A positive sign is found in patients with perilymphatic fistula or hypermobile stapes and occasionally in those with post-traumatic endolymphatic hydrops.

Stance and Gait

Disorders in stance and gait are frequently found in patients following head trauma but are usually lumped under the nonspecific term of dizziness and so their frequency is not known (Friedman et al., 1945; Gannon et al., 1978). The Romberg and sharpened Romberg (tandem stance) tests, Fukuda stepping test, normal gait, and tandem gait all should be examined. In the Romberg tests the patient is asked to stand with feet closely approximated, first with eyes open and then with eyes closed. We ask patients to fold their arms across their chest and we time them for 30 seconds with eyes open and then 30 seconds with eyes closed. A positive Romberg test is one in which the patient can stand with eyes open but not with eyes closed. This result may be found in patients with acute vestibular defects or a proprioceptive defect. A positive sharpened Romberg test is also found in these circumstances as well as in patients with chronic vestibular defects and in some normal individuals over the age of 65 years. For the Fukuda stepping test, the subject should step in place for 50 steps with arms extended and eyes closed (Fukuda, 1959). Rotation of more than 30 degrees is abnormal. A positive Fukuda stepping test is frequently found in patients with a unilateral vestibular defect, but it is also found in patients with a leg-length discrepancy and other structural problems in the legs.

The Romberg test is also useful in identifying a functional component when patients rock backwards on their heels. Other features of stance and gait that help identify a functional component include knee buckling without fall, small-amplitude steps, uneconomical posture and movement, exaggerated sway during the Romberg test without fall, excessive slowness in gait, and fluctuations in level of impairment (Keane, 1989; Lempert et al., 1991). Some of these are features in astasia-abasia or Blocq's disease, in which the patient collapses or partially collapses when attempting to walk without an organic basis.

LABORATORY TESTS

Electronystagmography

ENG consists of eye movement recordings during visual tracking and during vestibular testing (by the rotary chair or caloric test, described below). It is difficult to interpret the findings of earlier papers recording ENG in patients complaining of post-traumatic vertigo, since slow-phase eye velocity of the spontaneous nystagmus and during the caloric test was not documented (Kirtane et al., 1982). Normal subjects have up to 5 degrees per second of spontaneous nystagmus. Despite that, these tests are objective and should be done in patients complaining of dizziness.

Rotary Chair Test

The rotary chair test is the most sensitive test to assess vestibular function. It can be performed in children of any age, although calibrations are usually only obtainable in infants 6 months or older (by using a happy face or similar stimulus). We usually have children under 4 years of age sit in the parent's lap. Eye movements are measured by electro-oculography. After calibration, peak slow-phase eye velocity is measured either during sinusoidal chair rotations or constant-velocity step rotations in the dark to assess vestibular-ocular reflex gain (eye velocity/chair velocity). This gain normally is near 1.0 at birth and decreases to about 0.7 in adults. Values less than 0.4 are abnormal and indicate vestibular hypofunction.

Caloric Test

As compared with the rotary chair technique, the caloric test is a less sensitive but more specific test of peripheral vestibular function. It is the best test for determining whether a vestibular defect is peripheral or central and on which side it is located. This test is usually not well tolerated by very young children, but a limited test can be done in children as young as 4 years of age and a complete test in children older than 8 years. Before the test is done, the internal auditory canal is checked with an otoscope and any wax or debris blocking the canal is removed. If there is a tympanic membrane performation, air at different temperatures instead of water should be used as the stimulus. The caloric test uses a nonphysiologic stimulus (usually water) to induce endolymphatic flow in the semicircular canals by creating a temperature gradient from one side of the canal to the other. Each ear is irrigated for usually 40 seconds with a constant flow rate of water at two temperatures (30° and 44°C). Eye movements are recorded at the start of irrigation and 2 minutes longer. At the end of this period, the ear is emptied of any remaining water and sufficient time (usually 5 minutes) is allowed for the nystagmus to stop before proceeding to the next irrigation. The order of irrigation can vary, but we usually use left cool, right cool, left warm, right warm. Figure 9-5 presents the summary of a caloric response indicating a vestibular deficit on the right side.

Posturography

One popular way to quantify postural sway is dynamic posturography, which measures sway in conditions in which visual and somatosensory cues are absent or altered and also measures automatic postural responses elicited by perturbations of the support surface. Deficits in a variety of different neural systems can be identified, including spinal cord (delayed onset of middle-latency EMG response), cerebral cortex (delayed onset of long-latency EMG response), and anterior cerebellum (3-Hz anteroposterior sway). Although the test is not specific for vestibular disorders, patients with uncompensated or severe vestibular deficits typically have difficulty maintaining their balance when both visual and somatosensory cues are altered. This test is also very useful in demonstrating objective signs

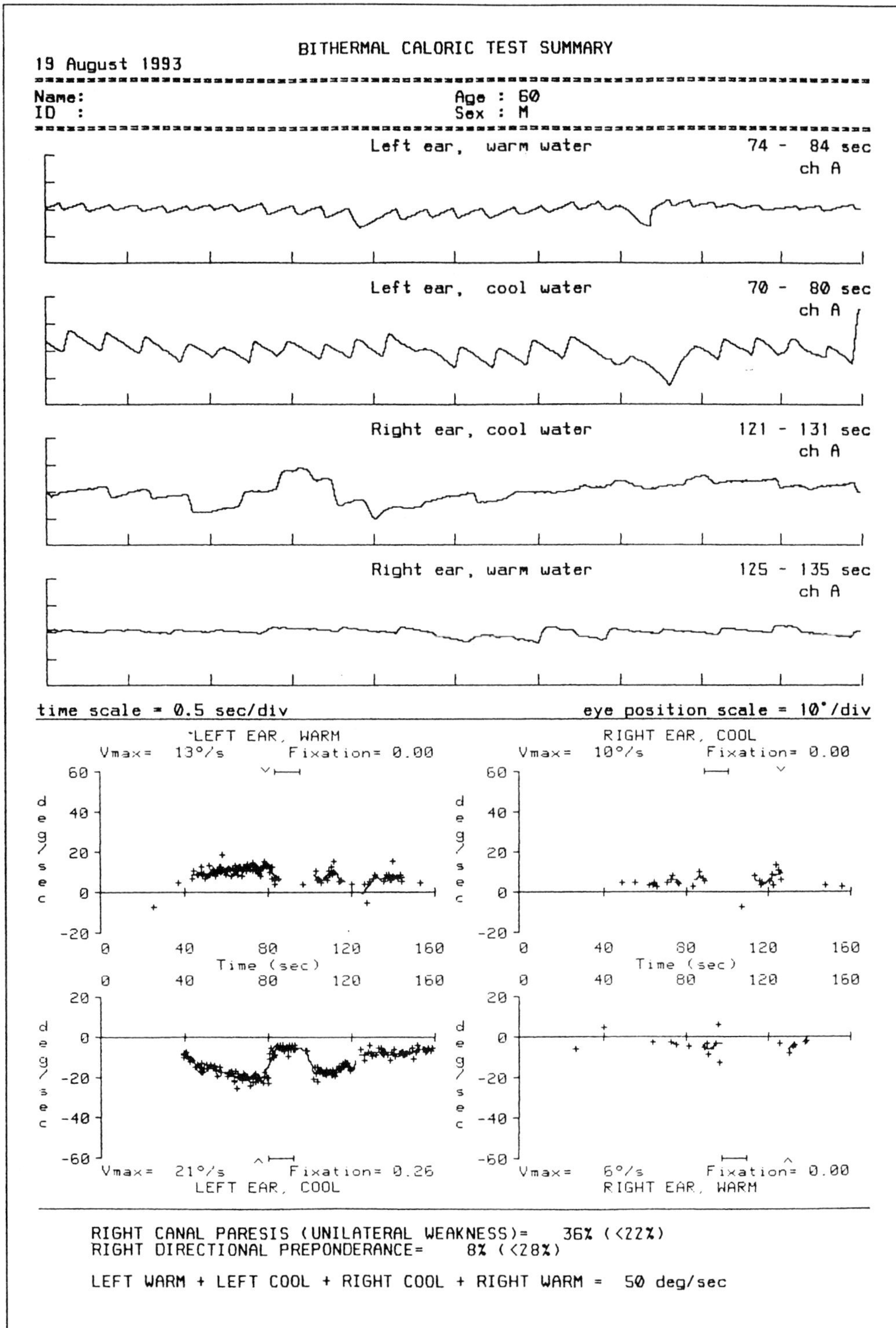

Fig. 9-5. Caloric test summary on a patient with right-sided vestibular paresis. The top half of the sheet shows a 10-second sample of the best response to each irrigation. The bottom half shows a plot of each slow-phase eye velocity against time. The degree of paresis is calculated by the formula:

$$\left[\frac{(R30 + R44) - (L30 + L44)}{(R30 + R44) + (L30 + L44)}\right] \times 100$$

In our laboratory, a significant vestibular paresis or directional preponderance is defined as greater than 22 percent.

for a functional component, including better performance on the more difficult portions of the test and a regular low-frequency sway (1 to 2 Hz). These findings raise the possibility of malingering.

Audiogram

An audiogram should be performed on all patients with head trauma-induced tinnitus and hearing loss. This should include both pure-tone and speech audiometry, acoustic reflexes, and middle ear function. Nonpulsatile and constant tinnitus without documented hearing loss is extremely rare. A nonorganic loss of hearing can be determined by the inconsistency of the audiogram (more than a 10-db change in threshold on successive trials), which may occur in up to 10 percent of head-injured patients (Berman and Fredrickson, 1978). The Stenger test is helpful in determining a nonorganic or exaggerated loss of hearing. In this test tones are presented simultaneously to both ears and the patient is asked to hold up a hand as long as the tone is on. As long as the tone is above the threshold in the good ear, the patient should respond regardless of the intensity in the suspect ear. A functional disorder is suspected when tones are presented simultaneously but the tone in the good ear is set below threshold and the tone in the suspect ear is set above the true threshold. In this case the patient's response is either inconsistent or absent.

Brainstem Auditory Evoked Responses

The brainstem auditory evoked response (BAER) is the averaged surface-recorded activity of the auditory neural generators of the auditory periphery and lower central auditory pathway. The BAER may be used to determine auditory threshold when standard audiograms cannot be obtained or give spurious results. It is also an excellent screening test for abnormalities involving 8th cranial nerve and central auditory brainstem pathways. The BAER has been reported to be abnormal in patients with postconcussive syndrome even when all other studies are normal (Noseworthy et al., 1981). The sensitivity of finding an abnormality in patients with head trauma by this test may increase when higher repetitive rates are used as the stimulus (Abd al-Hady et al., 1990).

Computed Tomography

High-resolution CT imaging of the temporal bone is best for evaluating petrous bone abnormalities, including labyrinthine defects, hearing loss, facial nerve paralysis, fractures, and other pathologies that are likely to entail bone erosion (Hasso and Ledington, 1988). The cause of conductive hearing loss and peripheral sensorineural hearing loss can usually be identified by the type of temporal bone fracture identified on CT (Momose et al., 1983). The location of CSF leaks is also best determined by high-resolution CT scan of the temporal bone following intrathecal injection of water-soluble contrast material.

Magnetic Resonance Imaging

Magnetic resonance imaging [MRI] with gadolinium enhancement with both coronal and horizontal sections through the 8th cranial nerve is the most sensitive test for evaluation of the internal auditory canal, cerebellopontine angle, and brainstem (Swartz and Harnsberger, 1990). Enhancement of the labyrinth has been reported in patients with inflammation of the labyrinth (Mark et al., 1992), but it is too early to determine the significance of these findings.

CONCLUSION

Dizziness occurs very frequently following head trauma and can be assessed in an organized way. There are many causes of dizziness, and it is imperative that the correct etiology be determined in order to offer the appropriate treatment. Meclizine and other vestibular suppressant drugs can be used excessively and inappropriately, usually without a good understanding of the cause of dizziness. These drugs delay vestibular compensation and frequently cause dizziness in their own right. In this chapter we have presented the key features of the history, physical examination, and laboratory data that allow one to ascertain the correct cause of dizziness. We have also described the most common causes of dizziness together with their treatment. Many causes of dizziness do respond to treatment. Peripheral causes respond much more readily than central causes. The most challenging problem in management is the frequently associated psychogenic component. This too can be managed with thoughtful discussion by the clinical provider and psychogenic intervention when appropriate.

REFERENCES

Abd al-Hady MR, Shehata O, el-Mously M, Sallam FS: Audiological findings following head trauma. J Laryngol Otol 104:927–936, 1990

American Medical Association: AMA Guides to the Evaluation of Permanent Impairment. 4th Ed. Chicago, 1993

Annegers JF, Grabow JD, Groover RV et al: Seizures after head trauma: a population study. Neurology: 30:683–689, 1980

Anson BJ, Donaldson JA: Surgical Anatomy of the Temporal Bone and Ear. WB Saunders, Philadelphia, 1973

Applebaum, E: Meningitis following trauma to the head and face. JAMA 173:1818–1822, 1960

Avrahami S, Epstein AD: Ocular motor abnormalities from head trauma. Surv Ophthalmol 35, 245–267, 1991

Ballantyne J, Ajodhia J: Iatrogenic dizziness pp. 217–247. In Dix MR, Hood JD (eds): Vertigo. John Wiley & Sons, Chichester, England, 1984

Baloh RW, Honrubia V: Clinical Neurophysiology of the Vestibular System. FA Davis, Philadelphia, 1990, p. 101

Baloh RW, Honrubia V, Jacobson K: Benign positional vertigo. Clinical and oculographic features in 240 cases. Neurology 37:371–378, 1987

Baloh RW, Jacobson K, Honrubia V: Horizontal semicircular canal variant of benign positional vertigo. Neurology 43:2542–2549, 1993

Barber HO: Positional nystagmus, especially after head injury. Laryngoscope 74:891–944, 1964

Barber HO: Head injury, audiological and vestibular findings. Ann Otolo Rhinol Laryngol 78:239–252, 1969

Barber HO, Wright G: Positional nystagmus in normals. Adv OtorhinoLarygol 19:276–284, 1973

Basser, LS: Benign paroxysmal vertigo of childhood. Brain 87:141–152, 1964

Berman JM, Fredrickson JM: Vertigo after head injury—a five year follow-up. J Otolaryngol 7:237–244, 1978

Bickerstaff ER: Basilar artery migraine. Lancet 1:15–17, 1961

Bles W, Klören T, Büchele W, Brandt T: Somatosensory nystagmus: physiological and clinical aspects. Adv Otorhinolaryngol 30:30–33, 1983

Brahe PC, Johansen L: Traumatic lesions of the middle ear: aetiology and results of treatment. Clin Otolaryngol 11:93–97, 1986

Brandt T: Positional and positioning vertigo and nystagmus. J Neurol Sci 95:3–25, 1990

Brandt T, Büchele W, Arnold F: Arthrokinetic nystagmus and ego-motion sensation. Exp Brain Res 30:331–338, 1977

Brandt T, Daroff RB: The multisensory physiological and pathological vertigo syndromes. Ann Neurol 7:195–203, 1980a

Brandt T, Daroff RB: Physical therapy for benign paroxysmal positional vertigo. Arch Otolaryngol Head Neck Surg 106:484–485, 1980b

Brandt T, Dieterich M: Pathological eye-head coordination in roll: tonic ocular tilt reaction in mesencephalic and medullary lesions. Brain 110:694–666, 1987

Cannon CR, Jahrsdoerfer RA: Temporal bone fractures. Review of 90 cases. Arch Otolaryngol Head Neck Surg 109:285–288, 1983

Chait RH, Casler J, Zajtchuk JT: Blast injury of the ear: historical perspective. Ann Otol Rhinol Laryngol Suppl 140:9–12, 1989

Cockrell JL, Gregory SA: Audiological deficits in brain-injured children and adolescents. Brain Inj 6:261–266, 1992

Clark K, Rees TS: Post-traumatic endolymphatic hydrops. Arch Otolaryngol Head Neck Surg 103:725–726, 1977

Compere, WE: Electronystagmographic findings in patients with "whiplash" injuries. Laryngoscope 78, 1226–1233, 1968

Crumley R, Robinson L: Traumatic facial nerve injury. pp. 97–101. In Gates GG (ed): Current Therapy: Otolaryngology Head and Neck Surgery. Vol. 4. B.C. Decker, Philadelphia, 1990

Daroff RB: See-saw nystagmus. Neurology 15:874–877, 1965

Daspit CP, Churchill D, Linthicum FH: Diagnosis of perilymph fistula using ENG and impedance. Laryngoscope 90:217–223, 1980

De Jong PTVM, de Jong JMBV, Dohen B, Jongkees LBW: Ataxia and nystagmus induced by injection of local anesthetics in the neck. Ann Neurol 1:240–246, 1977

Denny-Brown D, Russell WR: Experimental cerebral concussion. Brain 64:93–164, 1941

Diamond S: Dietary factors in vascular headache. Neurol Forum 2:2–11, 1991

Dorman EB, Morton RP: Hearing loss in minor head injury. N Z Med J 95:454–455, 1982

Epley, JM: The canalith repositioning procedure: for treatment of benign paroxysmal positional vertigo. Otolaryngol Head Neck Surg 107:399–404, 1992

Eviatar L: Vestibular testing in basilar artery migraine. Ann Neurol 9:126–130, 1981

Feldmann H: Late sequelae following laterobasal fractures, therapeutic and forensic viewpoints. Laryngol Rhinol Otol (Stuttg) 66:91–98, 1987

Feneley MR, Murthy P: Acute bilateral vestibulo-cochlear dysfunction following occipital fracture. J Laryngol Otol 108:54–56, 1994

Fisch V: Facial paralysis in fractures of the petrous bone. Laryngoscope 84:2141–2154, 1974

Friberg L, Olsen TS, Roland PE et al: Focal increase of blood flow in the cerebral cortex of man during vestibular stimulation. Brain 198:609–623, 1985

Friedman AP, Brenner C, Denny-Brown D: Post-traumatic vertigo and dizziness. J of Neurosurg 21:36–46, 1945

Fukuda T: The stepping test: two phases of the labyrinthine reflex. Acta Otolaryngol (Stockh) 50:95–108, 1959

Furman JMR, Crumrine PK, Reinmuth OM: Epileptic nystagmus. Ann Neurol 27:686–688, 1990

Gannon P, Wilson GN, Roberts ME, Pearse JH: Auditory and vestibular damage in head injuries at work. Arch Otolaryngol Head Neck Surg 104:404–408, 1978

Glasscock ME, Hart MJ, Rosdeutscher JD, Bhansali SA: Traumatic perilymphatic fistula: how long can symptoms persist? A follow-up report. Am J Ot 13:333–338, 1992

Goligher JE, Lloyd DM: View from within: radiology in focus. Fractures of the petrous temporal bone. J Laryngol Otol 104:438–439, 1990

Goodhill V: Sudden deafness and round window rupture. Larngoscope 81:1462–1472, 1971

Goodwin WJ: Temporal bone fractures. Otolaryngol Clin North Am 16:651–659, 1983

Griffiths, MV: The incidence of auditory and vestibular concussion following minor head injury. J Laryngol Otol 9:253–265, 1979

Grimm RJ, Hemenway WG, LeBray PR, Black FO: The perilymph fistula syndrome defined in mild head trauma. Acta Otolaryngol Suppl (Stockh) 464:1–40, 1989

Hahn YS, Fuchs S, Flannery AM et al: Factors influencing posttraumatic seizures in children. Neurosurgery 22:864–867, 1988

Hain TC, Fetter M, Zee DS: Head-shaking nystagmus in patients with unilateral peripheral lesions. Am J Otolaryngol 8:36–47, 1987

Halmagyi GM, Curthoys IS: A clinical sign of canal paresis. Arch Neurol 45:737–739, 1988

Halmagyi GM, Gresty MA, Gibson WPR: Ocular tilt reaction with peripheral vestibular lesions. Ann Neurol 6:80–83, 1979

Harker LA, Rassekh CH: Episodic vertigo in basilar artery migraine. Otolaryngol Head Neck Surg 96:239–250, 1987

Harrison MS: Notes on the clinical features and pathology of post-concussional vertigo with especial reference to positional nystagmus. Brain 79:474–482, 1956

Hasso AN, Ledington JA: Traumatic injuries of the temporal bone. Otolaryngol Clin North Am 21:295–316, 1988

Healy GB: Hearing loss and vertigo secondary to head injury. N Engl J Med 306:1029–1031, 1982

Herdman SJ, Clendaniel RA: Effect of early intervention on the recovery of function following resection of acoutic neuroma. Soc Neurosci Abstr 19:343, 1993

Herdman SJ, Tusa RJ, Zee DS et al: Single treatment approaches to benign paroxysmal positional vertigo. Arch Otolaryngol Head Neck Surg 119:459–454, 1993

Herishanu YO: Abnormal cancellation of the VOR after mild head and/or neck trauma. Neuro Ophthalmol 12:237–240, 1992

Hildingsson C, Wenngren BI, Bring G, Tooanen G: Oculomotor problems after cervical spine injury. Acta Orthop Scand 60:513–516, 1989

Hinoki M: Vertigo due to whiplash injury: a nuerological approach. Acta Otolaryngol Suppl (Stockh) 419:9–29, 1985

Hough JVD: Restoration of hearing loss after head trauma. Ann Otol Rhinol Laryngol 78:210–226, 1969

International Headache Society, Headache Classification Committee: Classification and diagnostic criteria for headache disorders, cranial neuralgias and facial pain. Cephalalgia, suppl 7, 8:1–96, 1988

Jackler RK, de la Cruz A: The large vestibular aqueduct syndrome. Laryngoscope 99:1238–1243, 1989

Jackler RK, Luxford WM, House WF: Congenital malformations of the inner ear: a classification based on embryogenesis. Laryngoscope, Suppl. 97:2–14, 1987

Jackson CG, Davis W, Glasscock ME III et al: Medical management of Meniere's disease. Ann Otol Rhinol Laryngolo 90:142–147, 1981

Jacome DF: Basilar artery migraine after uncomplicated whiplash injuries. Headache 26:515–516, 1986

Katsarkas A, Kirkham TH: Paroxysmal positional vertigo—a study of 255 cases. 7:320–330, 1978

Kayan A, Hood JD: Neuro-otological manifestations of migraine. Brain 107:1123–1142, 1984

Keane JR: Alternating skew deviation: analysis of 100 cases. Arch Neurol 32:185–190, 1985

Keane JR: Hysterical gait disorders: 60 cases. Neurology 39:586–589, 1989

Kerr AG: Trauma and the temporal bone. J Laryngol Otol 94:107–110, 1980

Kerr AB, Byrne JET: Concussive effects of bomb blast on the ear. J Laryngol Otol 89:131–143, 1975

Kirtane MV, Medikeri SB, Karnik PP: ENG after head injury. J Laryngol Otol 96:521–528, 1982

Kochhar LK, Deka RC, Kacker SK, Raman EV: Hearing loss after head injury. Ear Nose Throat 69:537–542, 1990

Kuritzky A, Ziegler DA, Hassanein R: Vertigo, motion sickness and migraine. Headache 21:227–231, 1981

Lee ST, Lui TN: Early seizures after mild closed head injury. J Neurosurg 76:435–439, 1992

Lees-Haley PR, Brown RS: Neuropsychological complaint base rates of 170 personal injury claimants. Arch Clin Neuropsychol 88:203–209, 1993

Lehrer JF, Rubin RC, Poole DC et al: Perilymphatic fistula—a definitive and curable cause of vertigo following head trauma. West J Med 141:57–60, 1984

Lempert T, Brant T, Dieterich M, Huppet D: How to identify psychogenic disorders of stance and gait. J Neurol 238:140–146, 1991

Linderman RC: Temporal bone trauma and facial paralysis. Otolaryngol Clin North Am 12:403–413, 1979

Liu-Shindo M, Hawkins DB: Traumatic injuries of the temporal bone. Otolaryngol Clin North Am 21:295–316, 1988

Macnab J: The "whiplash syndrome". Othop Clin North Am 2:389–403, 1971

Makishima K, Sobel SF, Snow JB: Histopathological correlates of otoneurological manifestations following head trauma. Laryngoscope 86, 1303–1314, 1976

Marion MS, Cevette MJ: Tinnitus. Mayo Clin Proc 66:614–620, 1991

Mark AS, Seltzer S, Nelson-Drake J et al: Labyrinthine enhancement on gadolinium-enhanced magnetic resonance imaging in sudden deafness and vertigo: correlation with audiologic and electronystagmographic studies. Ann Otol Rhinol Laryngol 101:459–464, 1992

Mitchell DE, Adams JH: Primary focal impact damage to the brain stem in blunt head injuries. Does it exist? Lancet 2:215–218, 1973

Momose KJ, Davis KR, Rhea JT: Hearing loss in skull fractures. Am J Neuroradiol 4:781–785, 1993

Nadol JB: Positive Hennebert's sign in Ménière's disease. Arch Otolaryngol Head Neck Surg 103:524–530, 1977

Nadol JB, Weiss AD, Parker SW: Vertigo of delayed onset after sudden deafness. Ann Otol Rhinol Laryngol 84:841–846, 1975

Neilsen JM: Tornado epilepsy simulating Ménière's syndrome. Neurology 9:794–796, 1959

Noseworthy JH, Miller J, Murray TJ, Regan D: Auditory brainstem responses in post concussive syndrome. Arch Neurol 38:275–278, 1981

Olsson JE: Neurotologic findings in basilar migraine. Laryngoscope suppl. 52, 101:1–41, 1991

Oppenheimer DR: Microscopic lesion in the brain following head injury. J Neurol Neurosurg Psychiatry 31:299–306, 1968

Paparella MM, Mancini F: Trauma and Meinere's syndrome. Laryngoscope 93:1004–1012, 1983

Parker W: Migraine and the vestibular system in childhood and adolescence. Am J Otol 10:364–371, 1989

Peerless S, Rewcastle N: Shear injuries of the brain. Can Med Assoc J 96:577–582, 1967

Penfield WG, Kristiansen K: Epileptic Seizure Patterns. Charles C Thomas, Springfield, IL, 1951

Peroutka SJ: The pharmacology of current anti-migraine drugs. Headache Suppl, 30:5–28, 1990

Pilz P: Axonal injury in head injury. Acta Neurochir Suppl (Wien) 32:119–123, 1983

Povlishock JT, Becker DP, Cheng CLY, Vaughan GW: Axonal changes in minor head injury. J Neuropathol Exp Neurol 42:225–242, 1983

Preber L, Silferskiold BP: Paroxysmal positional vertigo following head injury. Acta Otolaryngol (Stockh) 48:255–265, 1957

Proctor B, Gurdjain ES, Webster JE: The ear in head trauma. Laryngoscope 66:16–59, 1956

Pyykko I, Ishizaki H, Aalto H, Starck J: Relevance of the Tullio phenomenon in assessing perilymphatic leak in vertiginous patients. Am J Otol 13:339–342, 1992

Rouit RL, Murali R: Injuries of the cranial nerves pp. 141–158. In Cooper PR (ed): Head Injury. 2nd Ed. Williams & Wilkins, Baltimore

Rubin W: Whiplash with vestibular involvement. Arch Otolaryngol Head Neck Surg 97:85–87, 1973

Rutherford WH, Merrett JD, McDonald JR: Sequelae of concussion caused by minor head injuries. Lancet 1:1–4, 1977

Sandstrom J: Cervical syndrome with vestibular symptoms. Acta Otolaryngol (Stockh) 54:207–226, 1962

Sanna M, Ylikosky J: Vestibular neurectomy for dizziness after head trauma. A review of 28 patients. ORL J Otorhinolaryngol Relat Spec 45:216–225, 1983

Schubinger O, Valavanis A, Stuckman G, Antonucci F: Temporal bone fractures and their complications. Examination with high resolution CT. Neuroradiology 28:93–99, 1986

Schuknecht HF: An experimental study of auditory damage following blows to the head. Ann Otol Rhinol Laryngol 60:273–289, 1951

Schuknecht HF: Mechanism of inner ear injury from blows of the head. Ann Otol Rhinol Laryngol 78:253–262, 1969

Schuknecht HF: Mondini dysplasia. A clinical and pathological study. Ann Otol Rhinol Laryngol Supp 89:3–23, 1980

Schuknecht HF and Davison RC: Deafness and vertigo from head injury. Arch Otolaryngol Head Neck Surg 63:513–518, 1956

Shelton C, Brachmann DE: Current status of the surgical treatment of vertigo. Adv Otolaryngolo Head Neck Surg 3:125–151, 1989

Shupak A, Doweck I, Nachitgal D et al: Vestibular and audiometric consequences of blast injury to the ear. Arch Otololaryngol Head Neck Surg 119:1362–1367, 1993

Silberstein SD, Merriam GR: Estrogens, progestins, and headache. Neurology 41:786–793, 1991

Sturzenegger M, DiStefano G, Radanov BP, Schnidrig A: Presenting symptoms and signs after whiplash injury: the influence of accident mechanisms. Neurology 44:688–693, 1994

Swartz JD, Harnsberger HR: The temporal bone: magnetic resonance imaging. Top Magn Reson Imaging 2:1–16, 1990

Tangeman PT, Wheller J: Inner ear concussion syndrome: vestibular implications and physical therapy treatment. Top Acute Care Trauma Rehabil 1:72–83, 1986

Thomke F, Vogt T, Hopf HC: Alcohol-dependent unilateral vestibular impairment persisting after a closed head injury. J Neurol 237:326–327, 1990

Thurston SE, Leigh JR, Osorio I: Epileptic gaze deviation and nystagmus. Neurology 35:1518–1521, 1985

Toglia JU: Acute flexion-extension injury of the neck. Electronystagmographic study of 309 patients. Neurology, 26:808–814, 1976

Tos M: Prognosis of hearing loss in temporal bone fractures. J Laryngol Otol 85:1147–1159, 1971

Tuohimaa P: Vestibular disturbances after acute mild head injury. Acta Otolaryngol Suppl (Stockh) 359:1–67, 1978

Tusa RJ, Herdman SJ: Vertigo and dysequilibrium. pp. 8–14. Johnson RT, Griffin JW (eds): Current Therapy in Neurological Disease. Vol 4. Mosby-Year Book, St. Louis, 1993

Tusa RJ, Kaplan PW, Hain TC, Naidu S: Ipsiversive eye deviation and epileptic nystagmus. Neurology 40:662–665, 1990

Vernon JA, Press LS: Characteristics of tinnitus induced by

head injury. Arch Otolaryngol Head Neck Surg 120:547–551, 1994

Ward PH: The histopathology of auditory and vestibular disorders in head trauma. Ann Otolo Rhinol Laryngol 78:227–238, 1969

Wennmo C, Svensson C: Temporal bone fractures. Vestibular and other related ear sequelae. Acta Otolaryngol Suppl (Stockh) 468:379–383, 1989

Wennmo K, Wennmo C: Drug-related dizziness. Acta Otolaryngol Suppl (Stockh) 455:11–13, 1988

Windle WF, Groat RA, Fox CA: Experimental structural alterations in the brain during and after concussion. Surg Gynecol Obstet 79:561–572, 1944

Winston KR: Whiplash and its relationship to migraine. Headache 27:452–457, 1987

Wober C, Oder W, Kollegger H et al: Posturographic measurement of body sway in survivors of severe closed head injury. Arch Phys Med Rehabil 74:1151–1156, 1993

Yardley L, Luxon LM, Haacke NP: A longitudinal study of symptoms, anxiety and subjective well-being in patients with vertigo. Clin Otolaryngol 19:109–116, 1994

Ylikoski J, Palva T, Sanna M: Dizziness after head trauma: clinical and morphologic findings. Am J Otol 3:343–352, 1982

Zee DS: Ophthalmoscopy in examination of patients with vestibular disorders. Ann Neurol 3:373–374, 1978

Zimmerman WD, Ganzel TM, Windmill IM et al: Peripheral hearing loss following head trauma in children. Laryngoscope 103:87–91, 1993

Ziv M, Philipsohn BA, Leventon G, Man A: Blast injury of the ear: treatment and evaluation. Mil Med 138: 811–813, 1973

Neuro-Ophthalmologic Disturbances in Head Injury

10

Aditya V. Mishra
Kathleen B. Digre

Neuro-ophthalmic disturbances may account for a major source of morbidity in head-injured patients. Injuries to the anterior visual pathways are reported to occur in at least 5 percent of head-injured patients, and 13 percent suffer a cranial nerve injury (Baker and Epstein, 1991; Kline et al., 1984). Indeed, visual symptoms may actually be more frequent: a retrospective review of 188 consecutive closed head injuries revealed that 46 percent of patients had blurred or decreased vision and 30 percent had diplopia (Sabates, et al., 1991). Unfortunately, there are very few prospective studies outlining neuro-ophthalmic defects in head injury, and we are unaware of any that correlate the severity of head injury with the type of neuro-ophthalmic defect. Severely injured patients are a challenge to examine acutely since they often have a depressed level of consciousness. Behavioral and cognitive deficits also make their evaluation and treatment difficult. The clinical neuro-ophthalmologic examination is crucial to understanding the defects in such patients.

CLINICAL EVALUATION

History

In head trauma the history should be elicited in great detail because it can help indicate the mechanism of visual injury. For example, brow or frontal injury may lead to ipsilateral traumatic optic neuropathy, vertex injury to chiasmatic damage, and posterior head injury to occipital damage. If the patient is unconscious, the history will often be obtained from family members, witnesses to the injury, and emergency personnel. Important neuro-ophthalmic symptoms include blurred vision, scotomas, difficulty in reading, double vision, eye pain, drooping eyelids, and unequal pupils. Associated neurologic and systematic symptoms also need to be obtained, as well as past medical, surgical, and ocular history. Present medications and allergies should be listed. Blurred vision is a frequent complaint after head injury and even whiplash (Sturzenegger et al., 1994), and many causes are possible (see Table 10-1). A careful neuro-ophthalmologic examination is essential to delineate the etiology.

Neuro-Ophthalmic Examination

Visual Acuity

Examination begins with an assessment of best-corrected Snellen visual acuity at 20 feet. However, if the patient is bedridden, a hand-held near-vision card is an adequate substitute. If a refraction is not feasible, a pinhole acuity can be obtained. Eccentric fixation should be encouraged during the examination if a dense central scotoma exists. Visual acuity can be reduced in head injury patients because of either retinal or optic nerve injury. In the series of 21 patients with optic nerve trauma reported by Spoor et al. (1990), 20 had visual acuity of 20/200 or less. In Seiff's series (1990), NLP absence of light perception was more common in patients with optic canal fracture (63 percent) but even without a canal fracture 40 percent had no light perception. If letters on only one-half of the chart are seen, then a hemianopic defect is suspected. The causes may include a chiasmal or retrochiasmal lesion.

TABLE 10-1. Causes of Blurred Vision After Head Trauma

Refractive error
External injuries: cornea, lens, vitreal, or retinal abnormality
Traumatic maculopathy
Accommodation (loss or spasm)
Optic neuropathy
Chiasmal injury
Visual field defect
Convergence/divergence insufficiency
Diplopia from ocular motor palsy
Nystagmus
Poor vestibular-ocular reflex stabilization
Medication
Functional visual loss

Color Vision

Color vision can be assessed with standard plates (American Optical, Hardy-Rand-Ritter, or Ishihara plates). Abnormal performance suggests depressed color sensation usually due to optic nerve dysfunction. Central achromatopsia due to occipitotemporal damage is a rare complication of head trauma (Rizzo et al., 1993).

Confrontation Visual Fields

Confrontation visual fields are especially useful in the bedridden patient. Foveal defects can be detected by placing a red fixation target on the examiner's nose while simultaneously presenting a second test object in the patient's peripheral nasal field. With a central scotoma, the fixation target either is not seen or appears desaturated with a pink or orange color. Screening for hemianopic defects can be conducted by presenting one or more fingers in each peripheral quadrant while the patient fixates on the examiner's nose or by introducing simultaneous red targets in each hemifield and again looking for either absence of one target or color desaturation. Neglect can be assessed by simultaneously wiggling fingers in both hemifields. The patient may fail to report the presence of the finger in the neglected field.

Pupil Examination

The pupils may provide an index of visual function that can be assessed even in bedridden and obtunded patients. First, the pupils should be examined for anisocoria. A large, poorly reacting pupil may reflect direct damage to the iris sphincter. Another possibility is damage to the parasympathetic fibers of the third cranial nerve, which helps the iris to contract in bright light. This is accompanied by ptosis and eye muscle paralysis. The anisocoria increases in bright light owing to decreased contraction of the traumatized or denervated iris sphincter. Other signs of third cranial nerve dysfunction, such as upper lid ptosis or extraocular muscle paresis, are often associated with parasympathetic damage. However, if only the distal branches of the third cranial nerve are injured, perhaps as a result of an angle recession (diagnosed by gonioscopy), the only third nerve findings may be defective accommodation and a poorly reacting dilated pupil. If a pupil is dilated, dilute pilocarpine (<0.1 percent) should cause a denervated iris to contract. If it does not, iris injury or drug (e.g., scopolamine, atropine) effects should be suspected. When a pharmacologically dilated pupil is tested with 1 percent pilocarpine, minimal or no reaction is seen. Causes of mydriatic pupils after head trauma are listed in Table 10-2.

The other common pupil defect seen with closed head injury is a Horner's pupil. The smaller or miotic pupil is the abnormal pupil, and the anisocoria will increase in the dark as compared with bright light conditions; moreover a dilation lag is also seen. A mild ipsilateral upper lid ptosis and an upside-down ptosis of the lower lid suggest injury to the sympathetic fibers innervating Müller's muscle to the upper lid and the inferior tarsal muscle of the lower lid. The presence of a Horner's pupil can be confirmed with a cocaine drop test. A hydroxyamphetamine (Paredrine) drop test can be used to differentiate pre- and postganglionic lesions. Postganglionic lesions are frequently seen in cases of internal carotid artery dissection from trauma and often present with a painful Horner's pupil (Digre et al., 1991; Waltridge et al., 1989). Preganglionic lesions can occur after injuries to the spinal cord (C1 to C8, T1) nerve or brachial plexus (Lowenfeld, 1993).

TABLE 10-2. Causes of Post-Traumatic Mydriasis

Traumatic iris damage (gross; subtle)
Peripheral (orbital) 3rd cranial nerve damage
3rd cranial nerve palsy
Chemically induced mydriasis
Anxiety (Lowenfeld, 1993)
Post-traumatic tonic pupil

A relative afferent pupillary defect is sought by using the swinging flashlight test. A defect can be quantified by holding a series of progressively increasing neutral density filters, measured in logarithmic units, in front of the eye with the stronger pupillary reaction until the pupils react equally to an alternating light stimulus (Thompson, 1979). The presence of this pupillary defect suggests either an optic nerve abnormality or a large retinal injury. If retinal pathology (e.g., hemorrhage or detachment) is visible, no more than 0.6 logarithmic unit of afferent defect should be ascribed to any macular lesion and no more than 0.3 logarithmic unit to each quadrant of retinal detachment. (Thompson et al., 1982). If the defect appears out of proportion to the visible retinal lesions, an optic nerve injury should be suspected. An optic tract injury can also be associated with an afferent defect in the eye contralateral to the lesion. This is presumably because the optic tract receives more nerve fibers from the contralateral nasal retina than from the ipsilateral temporal retina.

Motility

The motility examination includes evaluation of ductions, versions, and vergences, as well as pursuit and saccade movements. The commonest cranial nerve palsy associated with closed head injury is a sixth nerve palsy, followed by third and fourth nerves. Sixth nerve dysfunction will manifest as an abduction deficit (Fig. 10-1) and an incomitant (not the same in all directions) esotropia. This defect is worse in the field of gaze of the paretic muscle and worse when measured with distant fixation as compared with near. The patient may adopt a head turn in the direction of the paretic nerve to force the eyes away from the field of gaze of the paretic muscle. Third nerve lesions may present with pupil dysfunction as described earlier, as well as with various degrees of dysfunction of ocular adduction, depression, elevation, and upper lid elevation. In time, signs of aberrant regeneration of the injured third nerve may be seen giving rise to confusing patterns of lid, pupil, and motility dysfunction patterns (e.g., signs of lid elevation, pupil constriction with attempted adduction, elevation, or depression or medial rotation of the eye with attempted elevation or depression) (see the section Third Nerve Injury).

Fourth nerve weakness presents with decreased depression in the adducted position (see Fig. 10-2) and an ipsilateral hypertropia on cover testing, which will

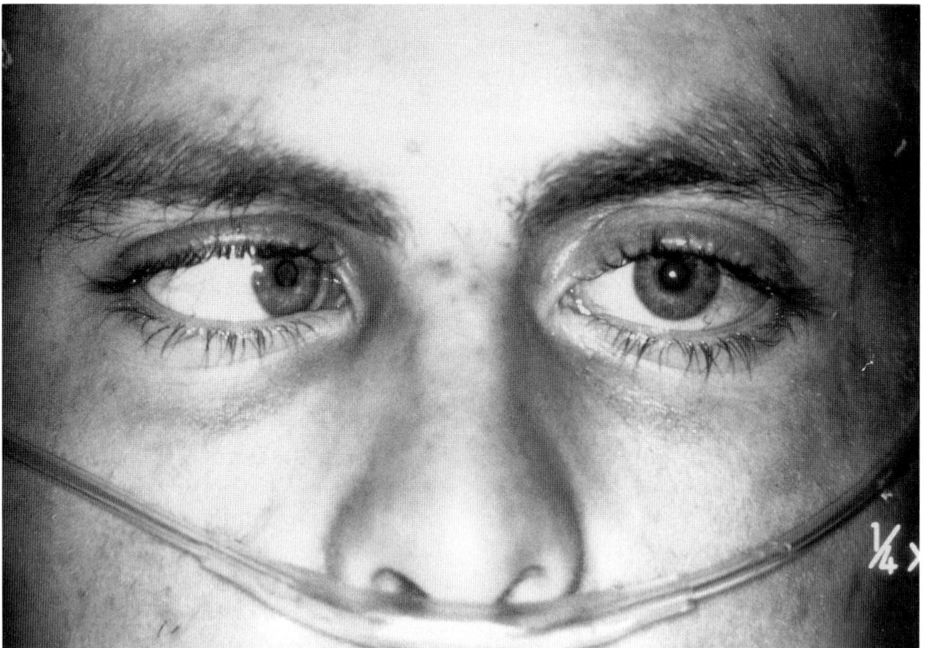

Fig. 10-1. Left abduction deficit secondary to post-traumatic sixth nerve palsy after closed head injuries.

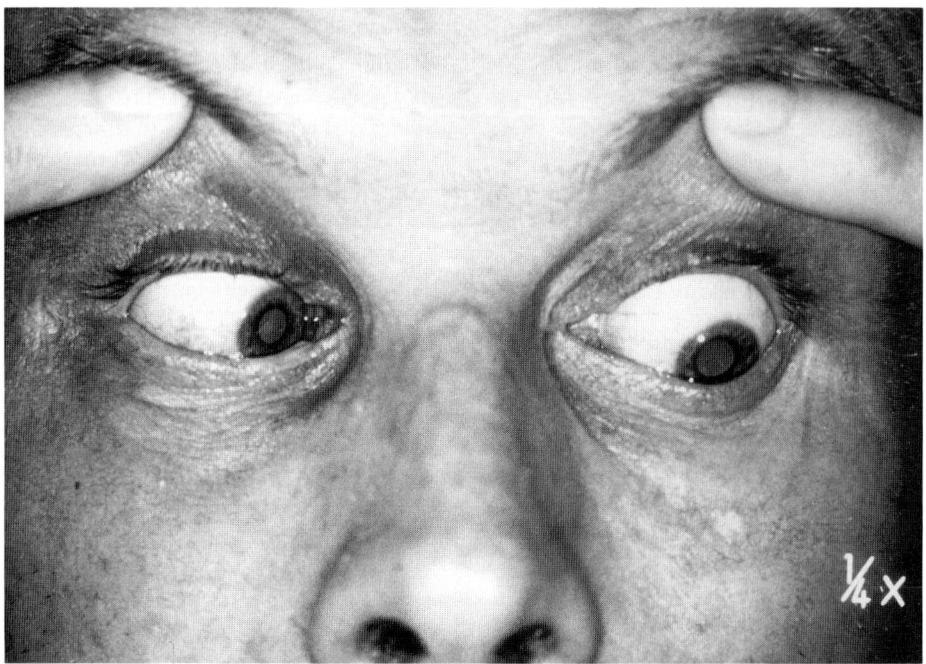

Fig. 10-2. Right fourth nerve palsy with limited depression in adduction of the right eye.

demonstrate a typical pattern on the diagnostic three-step test (Parks, 1958). The hypertropia becomes greater when measured in the gaze contralateral to the weakness and upon head tilt ipsilateral to the paretic muscle. The test must be performed with the patient in the upright position. The presence of torsion also supports the diagnosis of a fourth nerve palsy and can be measured with a double Maddox rod. (These rods consist of a set of parallel prism lenses in two colors, red and clear, over right and left eye which give a perpendicular line seen by each eye. The subject can align these lenses so that they appear straight, which provides the ability to measure torsional differences between the two eyes.) Excyclotorsion greater than 10 degrees suggests bilateral fourth nerve palsy (Sydnor et al., 1982). The presence of an alternating hypertropia in opposite gazes will also support this possibility.

An incomitant deviation that does not fit a cranial nerve palsy suggests the possibility of a restrictive lesion such as muscle entrapment related to an orbital blowout fracture. This can be confirmed by a forced duction test (see Baker and Epstein, 1991 for description of this test). If there is significant resistance, a muscle entrapment is likely.

Defective version movements are a sign of gaze palsy. A horizontal gaze palsy suggests a lesion at the level of the sixth nerve nucleus in the pons, which serves as the horizontal gaze center. Vertical gaze paresis is often more easily elicited with an optokinetic nystagmus drum rotated downward and is associated with convergence-retraction movements. Abnormal saccades can be detected by having the patient alternately fixate on two horizontally or vertically displaced targets while pursuit is examined by having the patient follow a slowly moving target.

The near point of accommodation is assessed with a Prince rule (a specialized ruler with an attached reading target, which measures in centimeters the reading distance, which is standardized for age) by having the patient fixate on a small accommodative target and moving it slowly closer to the patient. The distance at which the target blurs is recorded as the near point of accommodation. The point at which the target becomes diplopic or at which the patient's eyes are seen to diverge, indicating a loss of binocular fixation, is the near point of convergence. Normally it is 5 to 7 cm or less (Krohel et al., 1986). Fusional amplitudes are tested by placing a prism bar in front of the eyes and increasing the power until fusion is broken and diplopia elicited. Divergence is measured with the prism's base in, and convergence is measured with the prism's base out.

Slit-Lamp Examination

External and slit-lamp examination includes evaluation of any periorbital and conjunctival hemorrhages, lacerations, and foreign bodies. Slit-lamp examination can also evaluate for associated ocular injuries (i.e., corneal laceration, hyphema, cataract, and vitreous detachment or vitreous hemorrhage). Tonometry will rule out elevated intraocular pressure or hypotony.

If proptosis is suspected, Hertel exophthalmometry should be performed. The orbicularis function is tested by having the patient voluntarily and forcibly squeeze the eyes. Incomplete lid closure indicates abnormal seventh nerve function. Funduscopic examination will reveal most retinal and optic nerve lesions. A traumatic maculopathy can also be seen. However, in the early stages the funduscopic examination may be entirely normal in the presence of an indirect optic nerve injury. It is important not to dilate the pupil with pharmacologic agents until the patient is neurologically stable.

Ancillary Tests

Visual Field Testing

Formal visual field testing is not always possible in patients with acute head injury. When practical, it should be attempted. In the absence of retinal pathology, central scotomas and nerve fiber bundle defects suggest optic nerve damage. Owing to the anatomy of the optic canal, inferior visual field defects are more commonly seen with indirect optic nerve injury (Edmund and Godtfredsen, 1963; Turner, 1943). Serial visual fields can be important in documenting progressive field loss in patients with optic neuropathy who may be candidates for optic nerve decompression surgery. Uzzell et al (1988) found that patients with visual field defects also had a greater number of neuropsychological defects. In fact, visual field defects actually correlated with more severe head injury (Uzzell et al., 1988). After the patient has stabilized, characterization of the visual field defects (homonymous hemianopia, arcuate defects) may aid rehabilitative specialties with the patient's rehabilitative plan. In one study, 41 percent of the visual field defects were "tunnel-like." This defect was believed (after considerable testing) to be mainly functional (Sabates et al., 1991).

Visual Evoked Potentials

Visual evoked potentials (VEPs) are generally not practical in an emergency setting. However, their use has been advocated as a foveal function in coma and in cases of bilateral optic nerve injury in which signs of a relative afferent pupil defect may be lasting. A nonrecordable VEP often but not always indicates a poor prognosis for visual recovery (Striph et al., 1984). Importantly, the VEP may provide misleading results in uncooperative patients (Thompson, 1985), who are deliberately inattentive or who defocus their eyes. Medication effects constitute another confounding factor.

Imaging Studies

The modern imaging techniques of computed tomography (CT) and magnetic resonance imaging (MRI) have supplanted plain film radiography (see Ch. 5). High-resolution CT scanning with axial and coronal views and bone windows is the procedure of choice in orbital and facial injury patients, especially if optic nerve injury or orbital fracture is suspected (Manfredi et al., 1981; Nau et al., 1987) (Fig. 10-3). Coronal images are the most sensitive in detecting blowout fractures (Ball, 1987). Sphenoethmoid opacification also suggests optic nerve injury. In the series of Seiff et al. (1984) eight of nine patients with optic nerve injury had a fracture of either the optic canal or of bones adjacent to the canal. Axial and coronal CT at this time also gives exquisite detail of the optic nerve, as shown in Figure 10-4. MRI presently is not as good as CT in detecting bone injury but is much better in visualizing the posterior fossa and is often indicated as a supplement to CT in patients with suspected brainstem injury and also in evaluating patients with diplopia (Digre et al., 1994). In addition MRI may detect shear or contusion injuries in the occipital lobes.

Orbital echography is helpful in detecting dilated optic nerve sheaths (Fig. 10-5A) in patients with optic nerve injury with associated sheath hemorrhage and who may be candidates for optic nerve sheath decompression surgery. A-scan ultrasonography can detect extra fluid around the nerve (Fig. 10-5B & C). The neuro-ophthalmic examination identifies the areas of the visual system that are defective, thus aiding the neuroradiologist to perform the correct scan in the area of interest. Imaging recommendations for head trauma are listed in (Table 10-3).

TRAUMATIC OPTIC NEUROPATHY

Traumatic optic neuropathy can occur as a result of direct injury to the optic nerve from a penetrating missile or foreign body or as a result of indirect injury to either the anterior optic nerve (distal to the penetration of the central retinal vessels through the meningeal sheath of the nerve) or posterior optic nerve (proximal to the penetration of the central retinal vessels). This review deals with the indirect form of traumatic optic neuropathy.

Anterior indirect injury will often be identified by the presence of either disc edema or avulsion. Disc edema can occur as a result either of compression from a sheath hemorrhage or of anterior ischemic optic neuropathy by injury to the posterior ciliary vessels (Hedges and Gragoudas, 1981; Wyllie et al., 1972) (Fig. 10-6). Fluorescein angiography reveals normal retinal circulation but delayed filling of the vessels on the disc and peripapillary choroid, suggesting short posterior ciliary artery occlusion. Proposed mechanisms include compression of vessels and nerve from retrobulbar hematoma, avulsion of the vessels, thrombosis, elevated intraocular pressure, and vasospasm (Hedges and Gragoudas, 1981; Wyllie et al., 1972).

Optic nerve avulsion is a rare form of optic nerve injury and is often not recognized in the initial stages because of concurrent intraocular hemorrhage. If it is present, the disc is partially or totally absent, with a variable rim of surrounding retinal hemorrhage (Lowenstein, 1943) (Fig. 10-7). In cases with partial avulsion, serous retinal elevation is seen. Fluorescein angiography reveals transient initial slowing of the retinal circulation, but later angiograms will reveal normal filling. These findings suggest that the vessels are stretched rather than torn or that there is a preexisting communication between the retinal and choroidal circulations (Hillman et al., 1975; Park et al., 1971). If the medium is opaque, imaging with CT or echography may be helpful in showing a split between the nerve and globe.

Traumatic optic neuropathy as defined by Walsh and Hoyt (1969) refers to posterior nerve injury as a result of traumatic visual loss that occurs without external or initial ophthalmoscopic evidence of injury to the eye or optic nerve. Traumatic optic neu-

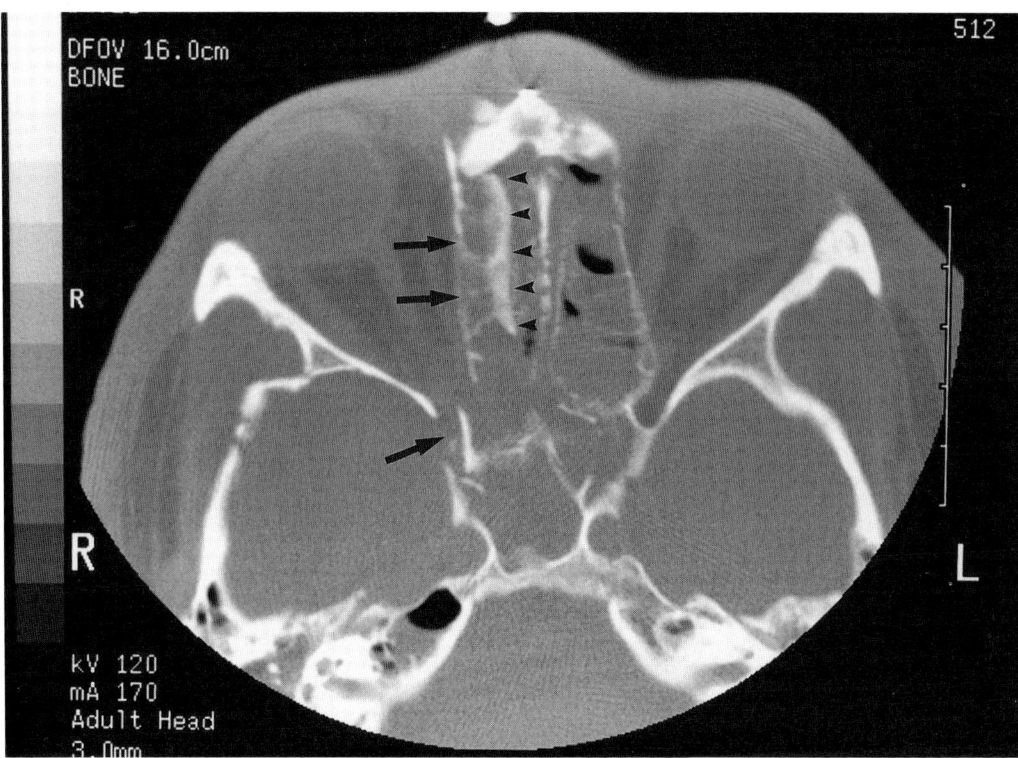

Fig. 10-3. Axial CT scan of the orbit in patient with traumatic optic neuropathy demonstrating blood in the ethmoid sinuses (*arrowheads*) and multiple fractures of right ethmoid bone and optic canal (*arrows*).

ropathy occurs in approximately 0.5 to 5 percent of closed head trauma cases (Gjerris, 1976; Kline et al., 1984; Steinsapir et al., 1994; Turner, 1943). A recent prospective study found an incidence of traumatic optic neuropathy in 2.5 percent of patients with midfacial fractures (Al-Qurainy et al., 1991). The commonest forms of injury occur from motor vehicle and bicycle accidents and falls (Steinsapir et al., 1994) and are related to ipsilateral frontal or midfacial trauma. The injury can result in partial or complete visual loss, with 43 to 56 percent of patients having a visual acuity of light perception or worse (Lessell, 1989; Mauriello et al., 1992; Spoor et al., 1990).

Anatomy

The optic nerve consists of approximately 1.2 million axons of the retinal ganglion cells as well as astrocytes and the central retinal vessels, is approximately 50 mm in length, and can be subdivided into five segments. The intraocular component is approximately 1 mm in length with a diameter of 1.75 mm vertically and 1.5 mm horizontally at the optic disc. It is typically unmyelinated and has a complex and controversial blood supply. According to Hayreh (1988), the surface nerve fiber layer is supplied by the retinal arterioles, the prelaminar region is supplied by centripetal branches of the peripapillary choroid artery, and the laminar region by centripetal branches of the short posterior ciliary arteries, which often anastomose to form the incomplete circle of Zinn-Haller. The intraorbital segment is S-shaped and mobile. The nerve acquires a myelin coat, which increases its diameter to 3 mm, and is also encased in meninges and surrounded by cerebrospinal fluid. The nerve and its meninges are surrounded by orbital fat and extraocular muscles, which originate from a tendinous ring at the orbital apex through which the optic nerve passes. The intraorbital nerve is approximately 25 mm long and can be subdivided into two portions. The anterior portion extends from the back of the globe to the point of entry of the central retinal vessels (approximately 10 mm). This region receives its blood supply from branches of the central retinal artery and branches of the pial system. The posterior

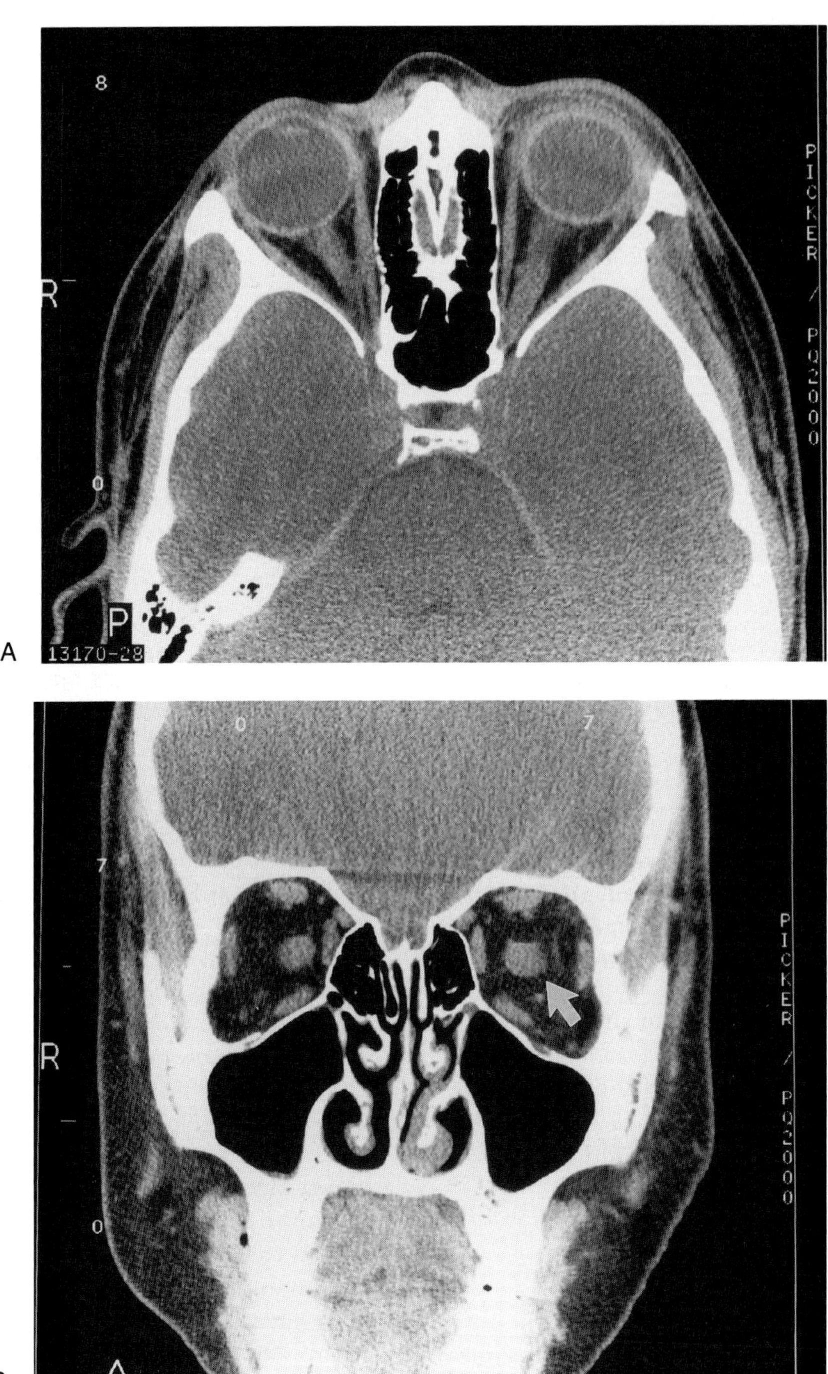

Fig. 10-4. Orbital (**A**) axial and (**B**) coronal CT scans demonstrate enlarged optic nerve on left of patient with traumatic optic neuropathy.

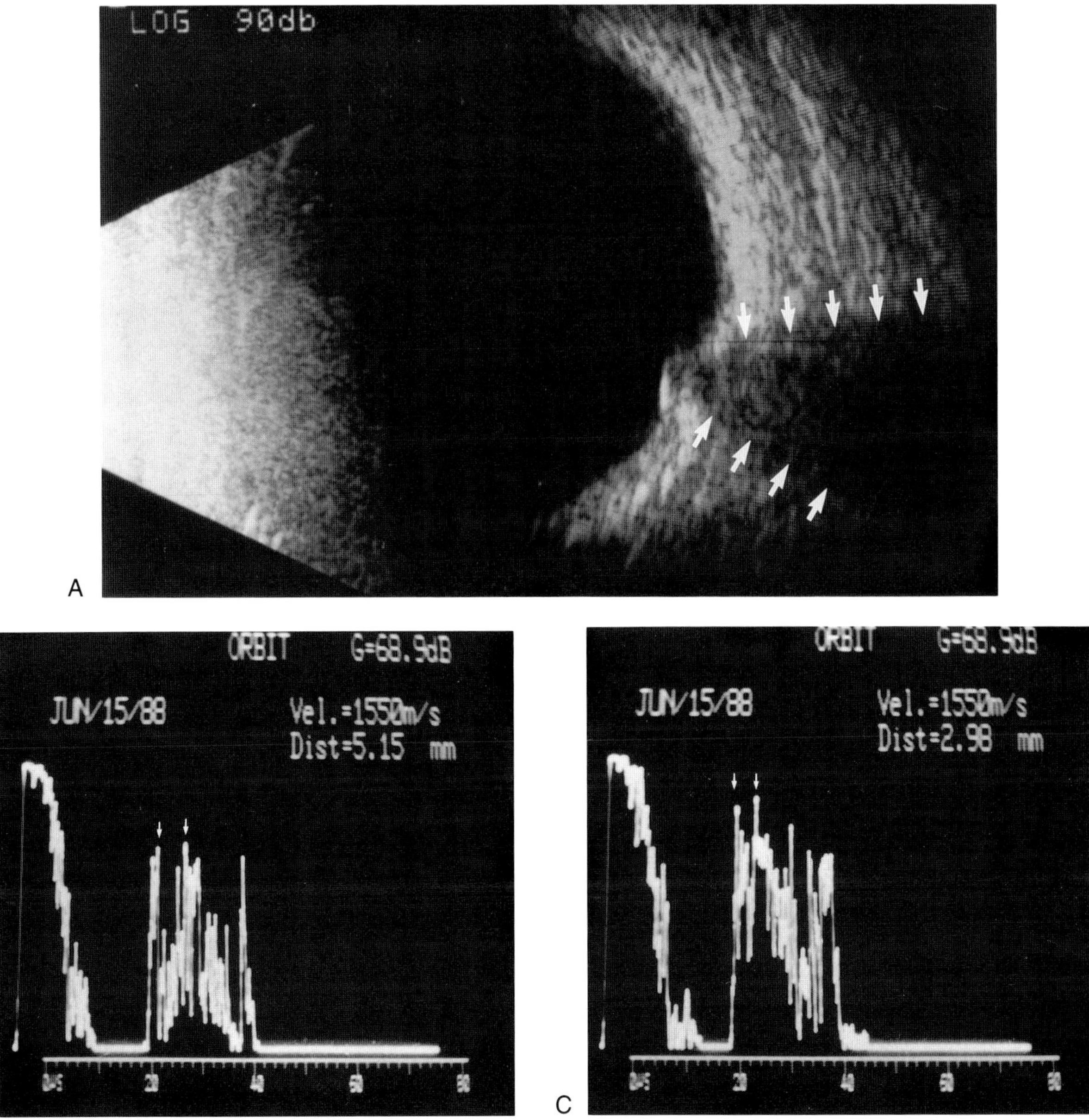

Fig. 10-5. (**A**) Echography: B-scan revealed dilated optic nerve sheaths. (**B & C**) Positive 30-degree test (same patient). (**C**) Notice the size of the optic nerve sheath complex decreases on 30 degrees. This means that there is excessive fluid around the optic nerve.

intraorbital portion extends from the point of entry of the central retinal vessels to the optic canal foramen at the orbital apex. This region receives its blood supply from the pial system, which is formed from branches of the ophthalmic artery. In rare cases, there may be a recurrent branch of the central retinal artery, giving the distal posterior orbital portion of the optic nerve a dual blood supply. The intracanalicular portion is approximately 10 mm in length and 4 mm in diameter. It is fixed within the optic canal

TABLE 10-3. Imaging Recommendations for Neuro-Ophthalmologic Problems after Head Injury

Injury or Symptom	Imaging Recommendation
Optic neuropathy	CT: Axial/coronal with bone windows of orbit with and without contrast. Ultrasound A and B scan
Chiasmal injury	MRI: Coronal, axial, sagittal views
Tract, occipital lobe injury	MRI: Axial, coronal
Diplopia with positive forced ductions (evidence of muscle entrapment)	CT—Orbital: axial, coronal views, possibly bone windows
Gaze palsies, INO, undiagnosed diplopia, nystagmus	MRI: Coronal, axial
Horner's syndrome	MRI: Pre- or postganglionic protocol

by the dura, which is tightly adherent to the bone of the canal, especially superiorly, which makes this portion of the nerve particularly susceptible to injury. The nerve receives its blood supply from a centripetal pial system fed from branches of the ophthalmic artery and internal carotid system.

The intracranial portion extends from the intracranial opening of the optic canal to the optic chiasm. Its length ranges from 3 to 16 mm depending on the fixation of the chiasm. The nerve rises to the chiasm at an angle of 45 degrees and is bounded laterally by the internal carotid artery, which gives rise to the ophthalmic artery just inferior to the nerve. The nerve is separated from the olfactory nerve by the anterior cerebral and anterior communicating arteries. The nerve receives its blood supply from branches of the internal carotid, anterior cerebral, and anterior communicating arteries.

Pathology

Crompton (1970) reported on 84 consecutive autopsies carried out soon after closed head injury. Blood was seen in the sheath spaces in 69 of the 84

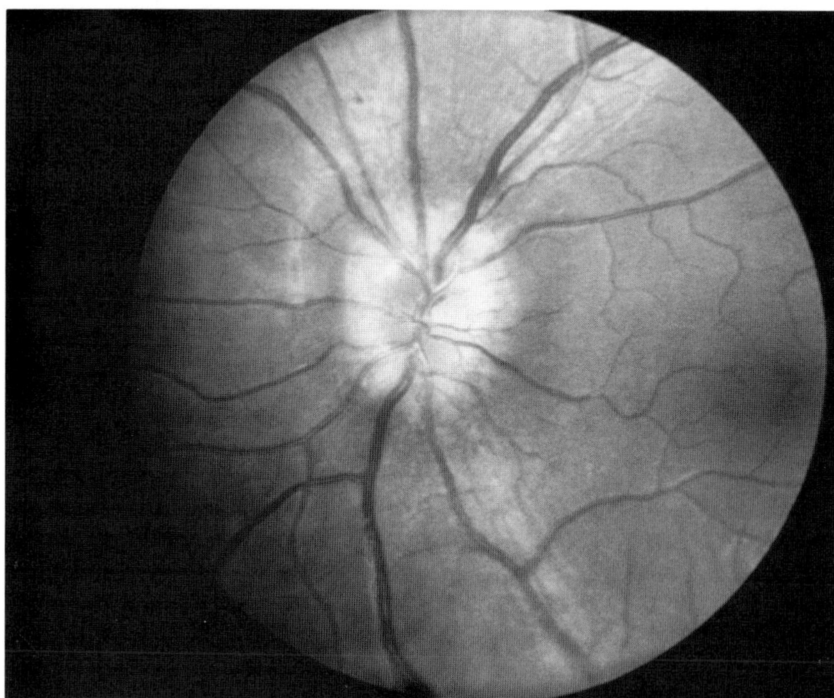

Fig. 10-6. Patient (whose images were seen in Figs. 10-4 and 10-5) with hand motion vision secondary to traumatic optic neuropathy with disc edema.

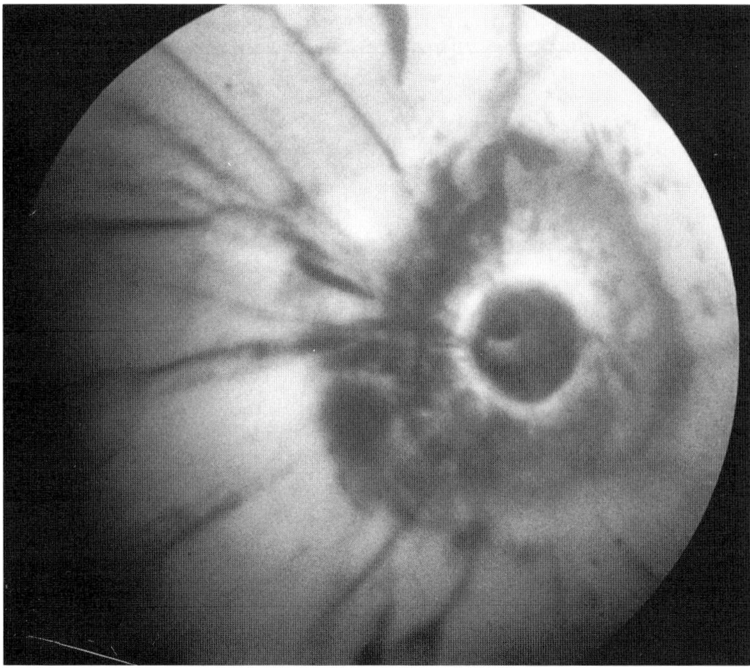

Fig. 10-7. Optic disc avulsion.

cases, and in 5 of these it was seen at the optic foramen. Hemorrhage within the nerve was present in 30 of the 84, and in 20 of these the canalicular portion was involved. Ischemic necrosis and shearing lesions were present in 37 cases, with the canalicular portion at the optic foramen involved in 30 and the intracranial segment in 20 of the 37. Crompton (1970) thought that sheath blood is an unlikely cause of visual impairment and noted that most of the hemorrhages occurred at sites where the optic nerve is tethered and immobile. He postulated that sudden movements of the orbital contents resulted in shearing of intradural veins at these sites. He noted the same sites for interstitial nerve hemorrhages. He believed that the major cause of visual loss was injury to the intracanalicular and intracranial optic nerve as a result of shearing of nerve fibers and blood vessels at the canalicular openings.

Other pathologic material from head injury patients revealed evidence of optic nerve sheath blood (Pringle, 1992), optic nerve laceration with nerve contusion (Hooper, 1951), collagenous fibrosis with infiltrate of lymphocytes, plasma cells, and iron pigment-containing phagocytes, degeneration in a triangular sector suggesting infarction, one case of intracanalicular discontinuity with necrosis (Hughes, 1962), and one case with total infarction and neutrophilic infiltrate associated with a canal fracture (Ramsay, 1979).

Walsh (1966) summarized clinicopathologic studies on 70 head-injured patients. He divided changes in the optic nerve into primary and secondary lesions. He defined primary lesions as those occurring at the moment of impact and consisting of (1) hemorrhages in the optic nerve, dura, and vaginal sheaths; (2) tears in the nerve; and (3) contusion necrosis. Secondary lesions occurred after the initial blow but could be rapid in onset. They included (1) edema; (2) necrosis of the nerve from generalized and localized circulatory disturbances and local compression of vessels; and (3) necrosis from vascular occlusion or spasm.

Management of Indirect Traumatic Optic Neuropathy

Management issues have been a source of controversy in dealing with traumatic optic neuropathy patients for several reasons (Kline et al., 1984; Miller, 1990). First the natural history has not been adequately defined. Furthermore there has not been a controlled prospective study carefully evaluating the various treatment options. Treatments have included observation, medical treatment with steroids, surgical decompression through several routes, and combined medical-surgical therapy.

Initial surgical results performed through a transcranial approach revealed little benefit. (Edmund and Godtfredsen, 1963; Hooper, 1951; Hughes, 1962; Lillie and Adson, 1934; Pringle, 1922). Subsequent reports in the Japanese literature (Fukado, 1975; Niho et al., 1970) using a transethmoidal approach suggested a much higher success rate in treating traumatic optic neuropathy with canal decompression than has been reported in the Western literature. In addition, these Japanese investigators report a much higher frequency of optic nerve injury with a higher percentage of optic canal fractures. Canal fracture was diagnosed on the basis of clinical findings, including loss or sluggishness of the pupillary reflex, a wound on the lateral aspect of the brow and nasal bleeding, and stereoscopic radiographs of the optic nerve. Surgery was performed up to 3 months after injury, and almost all patients had some improvement in vision. The results of these studies have not been universally accepted, as there appears to be a marked disparity in size between Fukado's study and others. Also, the increased incidence of canal fracture and exceptionally high success rate of surgical decompression in treating traumatic optic neuropathy has not been found in other reported studies. Nevertheless, these studies have shown that transethmoid-sphenoidectomy decompression is a relatively safe procedure.

Advocates for surgery alone have found some support from more recent reports (Kennerdell et al., 1976), including those of Girard et al. (1992), who noted improvement in 8 of 11 patients with traumatic optic nerve injury, and Fujitani et al. (1986), who noted improvement in 7 of 28 patients with no light perception treated with surgical decompression as compared with none of nine who were treated with oral prednisone therapy. However, the results in patients not entirely without light perception was similar between the two groups.

High-dose steroid therapy was believed to be beneficial in several series (Anderson et al., 1982; Lam and Weingeist, 1990; Matsuzaki et al., 1982; Mauriello et al., 1992; Seiff, 1990; Spoor et al., 1990). The rationale for the use of steroids is based on its anti-inflammatory effect in the treatment of brain edema and spinal cord injury data. It was felt that secondary optic nerve damage occurred as a result of nerve swelling within the optic canal causing nerve compression. However, recent studies involving "megadose" methylprednisolone in spinal cord injury reveals possible antioxidant effects separate from the glucocorticoid which protects the neural membrane from lipid peroxidation damage. (Bracken and Holford, 1993) In addition, better spinal cord blood flow which prevents ischemic damage has also been proposed. Treatment was found to be most effective if initiated within 8 hours of the time of injury (Bracken et al., 1990).

Although Walsh had believed that immediate total loss of vision at the moment of injury was a poor prognostic sign and that treatment would not be of much benefit, several reports indicate that vision can recover spontaneously (Wolin and Lavin, 1990), with steroid treatment (Wolin and Lavin, 1990; Spoor et al., 1990), with surgery (Fujitani et al., 1986), or with a combination treatment (Joseph et al., 1990; Mauriello et al., 1992). This would indicate that some of the initial damage is reversible and active treatment may help in maximizing recovery.

Anderson et al. (1982) reported some success with the use of high-dose steroids in some patients. They recommended initial treatment with high-dose dexamethasone and reserved surgical decompression for patients cases with delayed visual loss who failed to improve with steroids or those whose vision deteriorated after initial improvement with megadose steroids (Anderson et al., 1982).

Further, Lessell (1989) did not find any significant benefit from steroids alone as against observation, but the group that received steroids plus surgical decompression appeared to respond better. Subsequently, Joseph et al. (1990) reported improvement of 11 of 14 patients treated with combined steroid and transethmoid-sphenoidal decompression (Joseph et al., 1990).

If enlargement of the optic nerve sheath is noted on CT, MRI, or echography with or without the presence of disc edema, optic nerve sheath fenestration ought to be considered to evacuate any sheath hemorrhage and relieve pressure on the nerve. (Guy et al., 1989; Mauriello et al., 1992).

The management of indirect traumatic optic neuropathy will remain controversial until a well-designed controlled study is completed. Our approach is summarized in Table 10-4.

OPTIC CHIASM TRAUMA

Chiasmal injury is found infrequently (0.3 percent) incidence as compared with optic nerve trauma (Tang, 1993). It is usually related to a severe frontal

TABLE 10-4. Management of Traumatic Optic Neuropathy

1. Start intravenous methylprednisolone therapy (30 mg/kg loading dose followed by 5.4 mg/kg/h).
2. If orbital hemorrhage is present, perform canthotomy and cantholysis.
3. If subperiosteal hemorrhage is present, perform surgical drainage.
4. If nerve sheath is distended on CT, MRI, or ultrasound examination, consider optic nerve sheath fenestration.
5. If bone fragment is impinging on nerve, consider surgical decompression.
6. If no response occurs after 48 hours of methylprednisolone therapy, consider surgical decompression.
7. If vision is improving with methylprednisolone, continue high dose until maximum vision is achieved and then rapidly taper with oral prednisone.
8. If vision deteriorates with tapering dose, reinstitute high dose intravenous methylprednisolone and consider surgical decompression.

(Adapted from Steinsapir and Goldberg, 1994, with permission).

injury with associated change in mental status. Fracture of frontal, sella, or clinoid bones is commonly associated with chiasmal trauma along with other cranial nerve involvement (Tang, 1993). Patients often present with visual complaints, including blurred vision, visual scotomas, altered depth perception, and diplopia. On examination, visual field defects include bitemporal and junctional scotomas. Occasionally, seesaw nystagmus is seen in post-traumatic chiasmal damage. Endocrine abnormalities also occur if there is associated damage to the pituitary gland or stalk or the hypothalamus. Of patients with such abnormalities, 50 percent will have diabetes insipidus (Savino et al., 1980), characterized by increased thirst and unregulated urine output, which can be transient or permanent. Crompton (1971) found hypothalamic lesions in 40 percent of fatally injured head trauma patients. Other associated complications of injuries to the parasellar area include traumatic aneurysm, intrachiasmatic or suprasellar hematoma, carotid-cavernous fistula, meningitis, and cerebrospinal fluid leak.

Lindenberg et al. (1973) suggested that the chiasm may be damaged as a result of three mechanisms: (1) contusion hemorrhage, (2) contusion necrosis, and (3) contusion tears.

Surgical exploration has revealed a wide range of chiasmal appearances, including normal (Hughes, 1962); edematous and disintegrated (Anderson and Lloyd, 1964); containing a soft yellowish area probably resulting from infarction (Hughes, 1962); having a stretched appearance with an increased anterior chiasmatic angle (Obenchain et al., 1973); and complete sagittal transection (Rand, 1937).

The pathology found in autopsy cases includes sagittal tearing of the chiasm along with associated optic atrophy (Rand, 1937). Experimentally, Osterberg (1938) was able to produce macro- and microscopic tears by mechanically stretching the chiasm. Traquair et al. (1985) introduced a vascular mechanism whereby chiasmal injury can be caused by thrombosis of branches of the internal carotid artery supplying the chiasm. Hughes (1962) supported this hypothesis after examining 4 cases of chiasmal injury. He suggested that if the injury force is insufficient to cause sagittal tearing then it will also damage the vessels supplying the sagittal chiasm. Delayed visual loss can also accelerate as a result of intrachiasmal hemorrhage (Crowe et al., 1989).

Treatment of chiasmal injury includes management of associated endocrinologic abnormalities, surgical repair of any fractures compressing the chiasm, decompressment of hematomas, and steroid treatment already proposed (Tang, 1993).

OPTIC TRACT LESIONS

Optic tract injury was rarely reported before the advent of MRI. Walsh and Hoyt (1989) stated they had not seen any verifiable tract lesion on clinical examination but had seen random tract lesions on autopsy examination. Patients with tract lesions presented with incongruent homonymous hemianopic lesions, contralateral relative afferent pupillary defects, and subsequent bilateral optic atrophy. The atrophy was characterized by temporal disc pallor in the eye with nasal field loss and "bow-tie pallor" in the opposite eye (Walsh and Hoyt, 1989).

Pathogenesis is based on few pathologic autopsy reports. Crompton (1970) found only two cases of optic tract injury, with one case of interstitial nerve hemorrhage and one case of ischemic necrosis and shearing. Walsh and Hoyt (1989) suggest that injury occurs as a result of vascular compression secondary to increased pressure from intracranial hemorrhage or brain swelling rather than contusion. Often the injury and resultant field defect are masked by optic nerve and chiasmal defects.

OPTIC RADIATION AND OCCIPITAL CORTEX INJURY

Although optic radiation injury with closed head trauma has traditionally been thought to be uncommon (Gjerris, 1976), with newer radiologic techniques it may prove to be more frequent. Optic radiation injury occurs more frequently with penetrating trauma. Because of its long course, clinical features depend on the site of injury. Anterior lesions feature homonymous hemianopia associated with hemisensory loss, with or without hemiparesis. A "pie in the sky pattern" homonymous quadrantic defect is seen with anterior temporal lobe lesions. Parietal lobe lesions are associated with inferior homonymous quadrantanopsia and an absent or defective optokinetic nystagmus response when the drum is rotated in the direction of the lesion. Other features include hemisensory loss, aphasia, spatial orientation disturbance, and Gerstmann syndrome. Pursuit abnormalities also exist.

Occipital lobe injury typically presents with congruous homonymous hemianopia, with or without macular sparing. Bilateral defects portend a worse outcome than if no visual defect is present. These defects are more likely to be associated with secondary complications (e.g., herniation, edema, infarction).

A special syndrome of cortical blindness after frontal or occipital injury is seen in children (Griffith and Dodge, 1968). The onset of blindness is immediate or delayed and is associated with confusion or restlessness. The disorder usually lasts minutes to hours and has a good prognosis for visual recovery. The CT is usually normal in these patients. The cause is unknown, but Greenblatt (1973) proposed that these children may have underlying migranous or seizural predispositions based on the frequency of electroencephalographic (EEG) abnormalities detected over the occipital lobes in these patients. Others have hypothesized vasospasm or electrical depression as the underlying mechanism.

Occipital lesions related to closed head injury can be primary as a direct result of damage that occurs at the moment of impact or secondary as a result of the primary injury, including arterial occlusion from brain swelling. Cerebral contusion is the primary injury of head trauma. A contusion can be visualized macroscopically at the crest of the gray matter gyrus as small linear, triangular, perivascular hemorrhages in the cortex, with the apex facing the white matter and the base at the crest of the gyrus (Adams, 1984). Chronically they are seen as shrunken brown scars at the crest of the gyri. Primary occipital lobe injury can result from either coup lesons at site of impact or contrecoup contusions (Fig. 10-8). The latter occurs more often with deceleration injuries to a moving head than with a blow to a stationary head. Adams (1984) explains that contrecoup contusion is produced when the brain lags while the head is falling. At impact, acceleration and rotational forces stop; however, the brain continues to rotate, which subjects it to shearing stresses. Coup and contrecoup injury involving the occipital lobes may not spare the macular visual cortex since macular fibers terminate in the occipital poles. This is in contrast to occlusion of the posterior cerebral artery, which may spare the occipital pole as a result of its dual blood supply. Occlusion of the posterior cerebral artery occurs as a result of transtentorial herniation secondary to increased supratentorial hemorrhage resulting from brain swelling or hemorrhage. This leads to posterior cerebral artery compression at the tentorial edge, leading in turn to occipital lobe infarction. The injury often occurs as a result of a blow to the occipital region and is often associated with a skull fracture.

TRAUMATIC OCULAR MOTOR CRANIAL NEUROPATHY

Ocular motility damage occurs with closed head injury in up to one-third of patients (Sabates et al., 1991). The relative frequency of cranial nerve involvement varies with different practice patterns (Table 10-5). The sixth cranial nerve has been found to be the most frequently affected ocular motor nerve in both pediatric and adult populations (Harley, 1980; Rush and Younge, 1981; Kodsi and Young, 1992).

Ocular motility damage occurs as a result of several different mechanisms, including direct penetrating injury and indirect damage from acceleration injury,

A

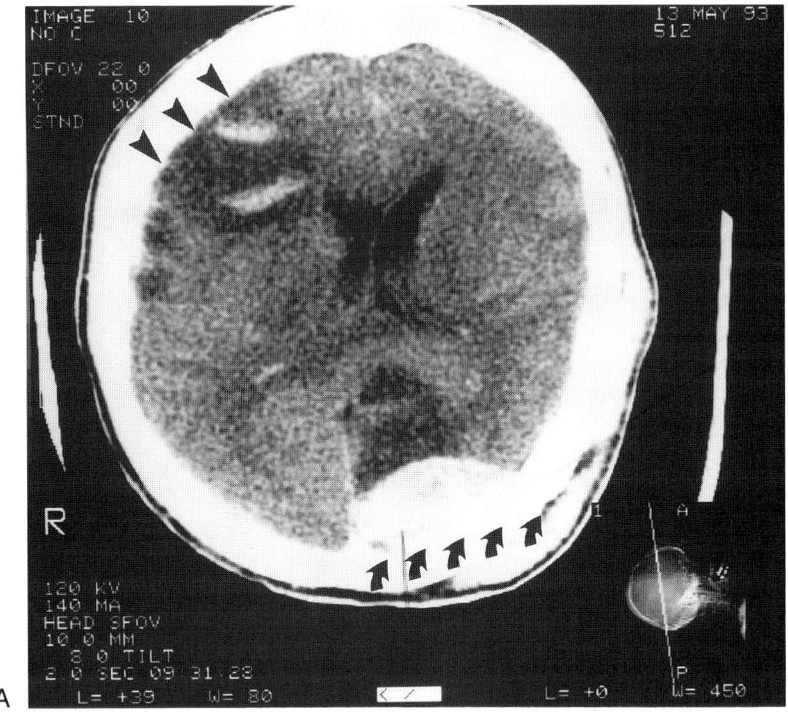

B

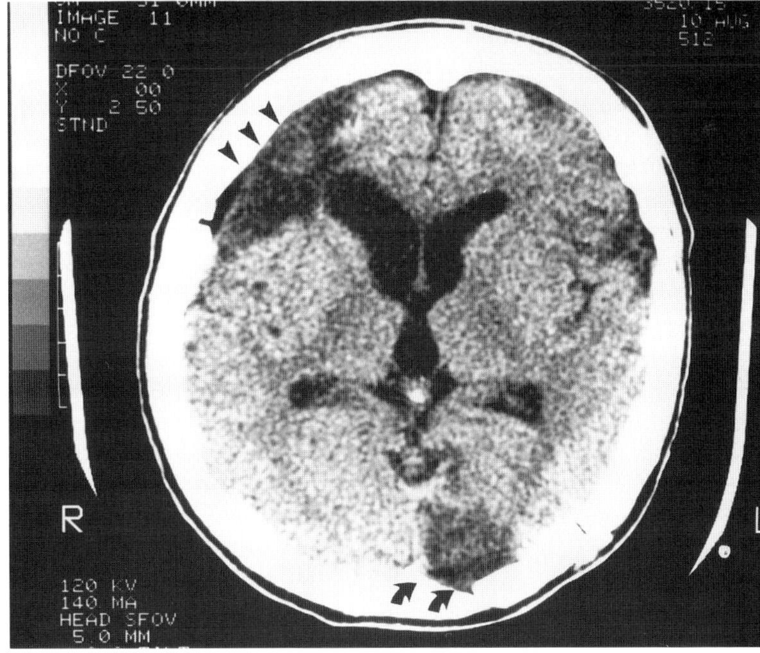

Fig. 10-8. (**A**) Acute: Head CT of patient with underlying hydrocephalus post-traumatic left occipital hematoma (arrows, coup lesion) and right frontal contusion (arrowheads, contrecoup). (**B**) Chronic: Same patient 1 year later.

TABLE 10-5. Recorded Cases of Traumatic Ocular Motor Palsies

Investigators, Year (No. with Multiple Palsies)	No. of Cases			
	Total	3rd Cranial Nerve	4th Cranial Nerve	6th Cranial Nerve
Rucker, 1966 (27)	112	34 (30%)	23 (21%)	55 (49%)
Rush & Young, 1981 (25)	172	47 (27%)	55 (32%)	70 (41%)
Richards et al., 1992 (64)	622	166 (27%)	169 (27%)	287 (46%)
Kodsi & Younge, 1992 (34)	246	61 (25%)	108 (44%)	77 (31%)
In pediatric population				
Harley, 1980	30	4 (13%)	5 (17%)	21 (70%)
Kodsi & Younge, 1992 (10)	58	14 (24%)	7 (12%)	37 (64%)

with propagation of shock waves from direct impact in closed head injury (Baker and Epstein, 1991). Shock waves distort the skull and cause skull fractures. The individual nerves are injured by either the shock waves or the fractures as the nerves enter the cavernous sinus. In one series skull fracture was present in over half of patients with a third, fourth, or sixth nerve palsy (Sabates et al., 1991). Nerves with a long intraosseous course are more likely to be injured by these mechanisms; hence, the great frequency of a sixth nerve palsy.

Acceleration injury causes both diffuse axonal injury, which can affect brainstem structures, and contusions, which can hemorrhage and affect cortex and brainstem (Adams et al., 1982; Lindenberg et al., 1973). The nerves can be stretched or torn as a result of gross brainstem displacement. The nerve is fixed to a nonmobile bone point at one end and moving brainstem at the other.

These primary mechanisms are further supported by the autopsy findings of Heinze (1969) in 21 cases of closed head injury. He found avulsion of the rootlets at the brainstem of the third, fourth, and sixth cranial nerves, as well as contusion necrosis and intraneural and perineural hemorrhage of the third nerve in the superior orbital fissure and sixth nerve disruption at the petrous bone (Heinze, 1969).

Secondary injury can occur with mass effect from supratentorial hemorrhage or edema leading to transtentorial herniation. The hippocampal gyrus descends and compresses the ipsilateral third nerve. As the supratentorial pressure increases the uncal herniation, the midbrain moves posteriorly and laterally, compressing the third nerve against the posterior clinoid (Lindenberg, 1966). Each third nerve is further stretched in the interpeduncular space because its origin is pulled down by the herniating midbrain. Also, the basilar artery, which is tethered to the pons by short pontine branches, moves downward with the brain, causing angulation and compression of the third nerves by the downwardly displaced posterior cerebral arteries (Sunderland and Hughes, 1946). Since pupil fibers are superficial, pupil dilation may be the first sign of herniation, along with impaired consciousness (Kerr and Hollowell, 1964; Sunderland and Hughes, 1946).

Herniation can also lead to occlusion and shearing of paramedian and short circumflex arteries, brainstem hemorrhage, and hemorrhagic necrosis (Adams, 1984; Gilbert and Deonna, 1972) (Table 10-6).

The oculomotor nucleus consists of several subnuclei at the level of the superior colliculus. The single midline caudate nucleus innervates the levator palpebrae superioris of each eye. The lateral paired nuclei supply the ipsilateral medial rectus, inferior rectus, inferior oblique, and the parasympathetic fibers to the sphincter pupillae and ciliary muscles, as well as the contralateral superior rectus. The nerve exits ventrally in the interpeduncular cistern and crosses the subarachnoid space to the cavernous sinus. The nerve passes medial and inferior to the ridge of the free edge of the tenorium and lateral to the posterior communicating artery. In the cavernous sinus the nerve is located in the lateral wall dorsal to the trochlear nerve. At the superior orbital fissure, the nerve divides into two trunks. The superior branch supplies the superior rectus and levator muscles while the inferior branch supplies the medial rectus, inferior rectus, inferior oblique, and sends parasympathetic branches to the ciliary ganglion (see Fig. 10-9).

TABLE 10-6. Neuro-Ophthalmic Findings in Brain Herniation

Site	Structure	Signs
Cingulate	Cingulate gyrus	N: leg weakness
	Anterior cerebral artery	N-O: gaze preference
Uncal	Third cranial nerve	N-O: ipsilateral 3rd nerve, ptosis, mydriasis, lateral deviation, occasional false 3rd nerve (contralateral)
	Cerebral peduncle	Hemiplegia (contralateral and/or ipsilateral)
	Posterior cerebral artery	Homonymous hemianopia
Tectal	Tectal plate	N-O: bilateral ptosis, upgaze paralysis
Central consciousness	Reticular formation	N: decreased consciousness
	Midbrain/pons	N-O: decreased eye movement
	Medulla	N: irregular breathing
	Corticospinal tracts	N: decerebrate rigidity
Tonsillar	Medulla	N: apnea

Abbreviations: N-O, neuro-ophthalmic finding; N, neurologic finding.
(Adapted in part from Miller and Becker, 1982, with permission.)

Third Nerve Injury

Brainstem injury to the third nerve nucleus and fascicle presents with bilateral ptosis. Also, the contralateral superior rectus will be weakened. Fascicular injury can be associated with contralateral hemiplegia (Weber syndrome) or hemidyskinesia (Benedikt syndrome). The nerve in the subarachnoid space is susceptible to avulsion and damage from transtentorial uncal herniation (Keefe et al., 1960). In late follow-up, signs of aberrant regeneration of the injured third nerve may be seen, giving rise to confusing patterns of lid, pupil, and motility dysfunction (Elston, 1984). Aberrant regeneration may manifest with signs of (1) lid elevation with attempted adduction or depression; (2) medial rotation of the eye with attempted elevation or depression; or (3) pupil constriction with attempted depression, elevation, or adduction. Because of the tonic innervation to the pupil from the misdirected fibers normally destined for the ocular muscles, the pupil will react poorly to light and dilate poorly to dark, creating a reversing anisocoria. In this situation the affected pupil can be the larger pupil in bright light, and the smaller pupil under dark room conditions.

Fourth Nerve Injury

The fourth nerve is less frequently identified as a cause of diplopia in head injury patients, which may reflect a greater difficulty in diagnosis. However, trauma is the most common cause of a fourth nerve palsy (Baker and Epstein, 1991; Burger et al., 1970; Keane, 1986, 1993; Khawam et al., 1967; Younge and Sutula, 1977). The trochlear nucleus is located ventral to the cerebral aqueduct and dorsomedial to the medial longitudinal fasciculus. It is the only cranial nerve to exit the brainstem dorsally and the only one to decussate completely. The nerve exits below the inferior colliculi, passes around the midbrain, and runs near the free edge of the tentorium toward the cavernous sinus. The nerve lies inferior to the third cranial nerve in the lateral wall of the sinus but passes over it prior to entering the superior orbital fissure outside the annulus of Zinn (the connective tissue band to which muscles are attached and through which the optic nerve and the 3rd and 6th cranial nerves pass to innervate muscles) (Fig. 10-9). The nerve is especially susceptible to trauma along the tentorial edge, and bilateral fourth nerve injury is likely to occur at the site of decussation in the anterior medullary velum, where the nerves are immediately adjacent to each other (Fig. 10-9).

Unilateral fourth nerve palsy is diagnosed by the presence of an ipsilateral hyperdeviation, which increases with opposite gaze and ipsilateral head tilt. In order to fuse the two images, patients will often tilt and turn their heads to the contralateral side. Occasionally some will tilt to the ipsilateral side, increasing the distance between the double images and thus making it easier to ignore the second image. Patients will also frequently complain of image tilt, which occurs secondary to excyclotorsion. The symptom of image tilt is believed to be present only in acquired fourth nerve palsy and not in the congenital

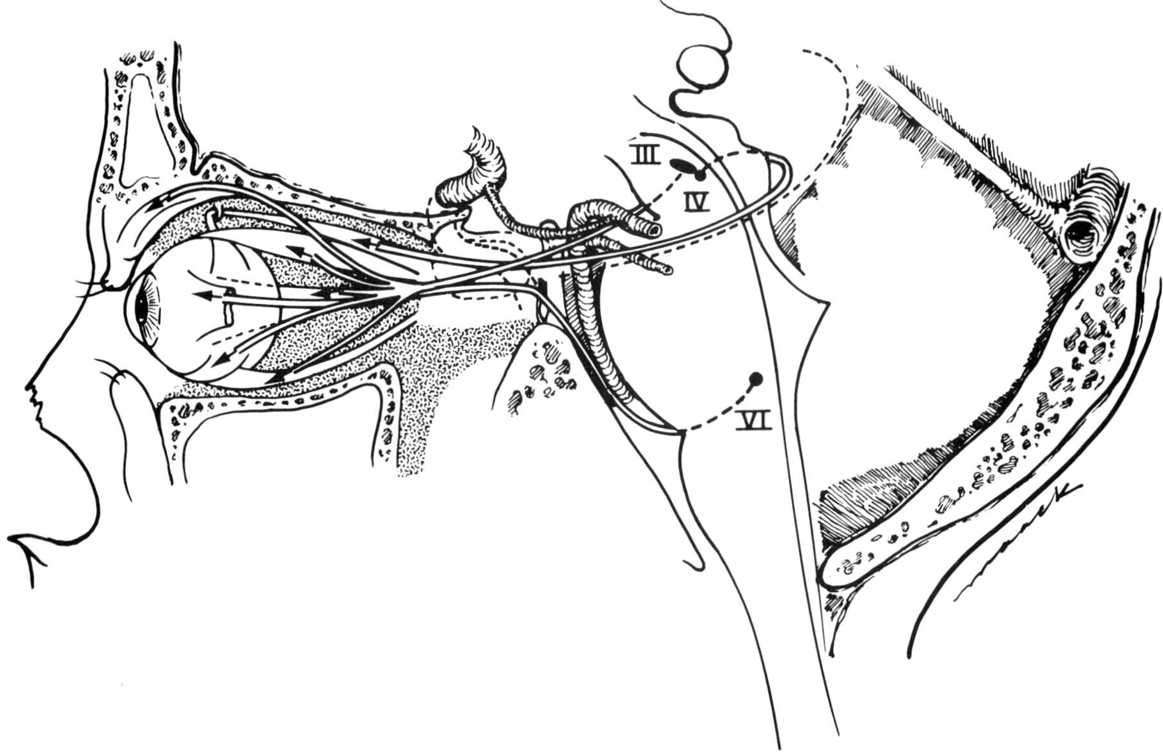

Fig. 10-9. Course of cranial nerves from brainstem to orbit. (From Digre et al., 1994, with permission.)

type (von Noorden et al., 1986). This can be measured with a double Maddox rod. Excyclotorsion greater than 10 degrees suggests bilateral involvement (Sydnor et al., 1982). A careful search for bilateral fourth nerve palsy should be undertaken prior to surgical treatment since the second palsy is frequently masked with only subtle findings (Hermann, 1981). CT can be helpful in demonstrating hemorrhage in the vicinity of the origin of the fourth nerve (Keane, 1986; Lavin and Troost, 1984). Occasionally, workup for cranial nerve palsy after head trauma will reveal an underlying, previously unsuspected structural disorder (Jacobson et al., 1988).

Sixth Nerve Injury

Sixth nerve palsy is frequently encountered in head trauma patients and is easily recognized by the presence of uni- or bilateral abduction defects (Fig. 10-1). Cover testing will reveal esotropia, which is worse in ipsilateral gaze into the field of action of the paretic muscle and worse with distant gaze as compared with near fixation. The nucleus is located at the pontomedullary junction near the midline beneath the facial colliculus. Injury in this area will present with a gaze palsy, since the nucleus is also the horizontal gaze center, with a population of interneurons that supply the contralateral medial rectus subnuclei via the medial longitudinal fasciculus, as well as with a seventh nerve palsy due to its proximity with the seventh nerve (Crouch and Urist, 1975). The fasciculus courses ventrally, exits at the pontomedullary junction, and ascends along the clivus before penetrating the dura 1 cm below the petrous bone. The nerve is vulnerable to blunt trauma at this point. The nerve may also be susceptible to raised intracranial pressure by stretching of the nerve in its subarachnoid course. It enters the cavernous sinus below the petroclinoid ligament, and unlike the other ocular motor nerves, it is located in the body of the cavernous sinus, adjacent to the internal carotid artery. The nerve is especially vulnerable to vascular lesions within the cavernous space because of this relationship. The nerve enters the orbit within the annulus of Zinn and innervates the lateral rectus muscle (Fig. 10-9). CT with bone window will occasionally demonstrate basal skull fracture involving the clivus (Fig.

10-10). Bilateral abducens nerve palsies can also occur with cervical fracture. The mechanism proposed is a stretching due to linear forces on the long course of the sixth nerve traveling through a canal (Arias, 1985).

Multiple Cranial Nerve Injury

Multiple cranial nerve injury with head injury usually occurs in the region of the cavernous sinus and orbital apex. The patient typically presents with complete ophthalmoplegia, a dilated pupil, ptosis, loss of accommodation, and loss of lid and ocular sensation. If the orbital apex is involved, decreased vision may also be present as a result of optic nerve damage. Signs of venous engorgement include lid edema, conjunctival chemosis, proptosis, and vein dilation. If a carotid-cavernous fistula is present, there are additional signs, including characteristic corkscrew conjunctival vessels, pulsating proptosis, and orbital bruit (Fig. 10-11A). CT or MRI imaging will reveal an enlarged cavernous sinus and dilation of the ophthalmic vein. The diagnosis is confirmed with angiography (Fig. 10-11B).

Treatment of diplopia due to third, fourth, and sixth nerve palsies is usually symptomatic (i.e., use of prisms for both horizontal and vertical diplopia). Fresnel plastic stick-on prisms are helpful since these can be changed periodically. If all else fails, opaque "magic-tape" over one lens of spectacles should be considered. Only about one-quarter of patients will eventually require surgical correction (Sabates et al., 1991). If the seventh nerve is also injured, tarsorrhaphy (surgical partial sealing of the upper and lower lids) may occasionally be necessary, especially if combined with fifth nerve injury, since lack of eyelid closure will lead to dry eyes, and when this is coupled with lack of sensation of irritation, corneal ulcers are likely to develop.

OTHER CAUSES OF DIPLOPIA AND BLURRED VISION

Orbital Fractures

Diplopia is a relatively frequent complaint in patients with blowout fractures. With orbital floor fractures, 36 to 86 percent of patients complained of diplopia (Baker and Epstein, 1991; Putterman et al., 1974). In most patients the diplopia gradually resolved over 4 to 6 months. It is believed that the

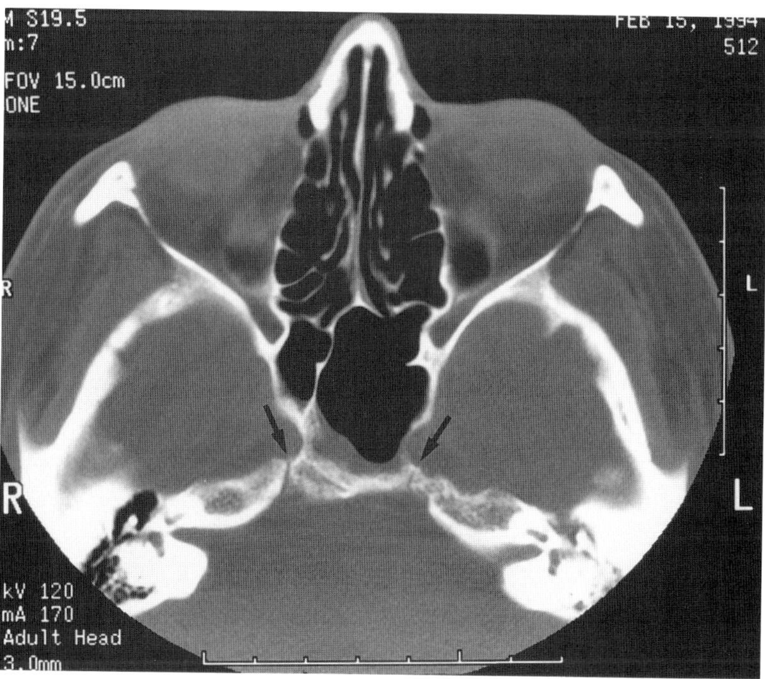

Fig. 10-10. Patient with sixth nerve palsy and basilar skull fracture (*arrows*).

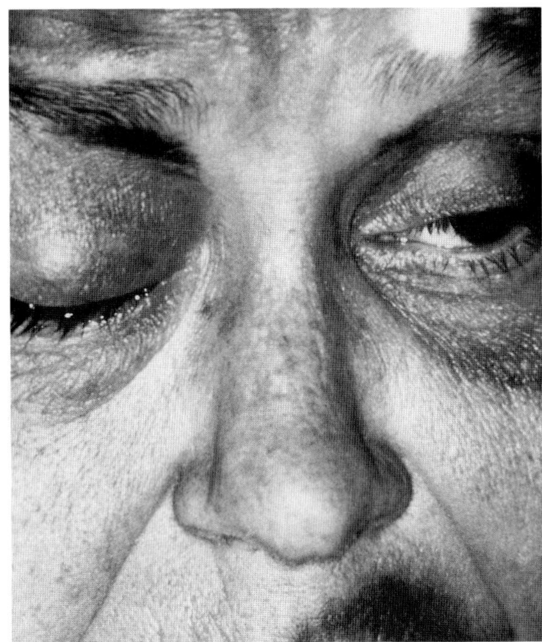

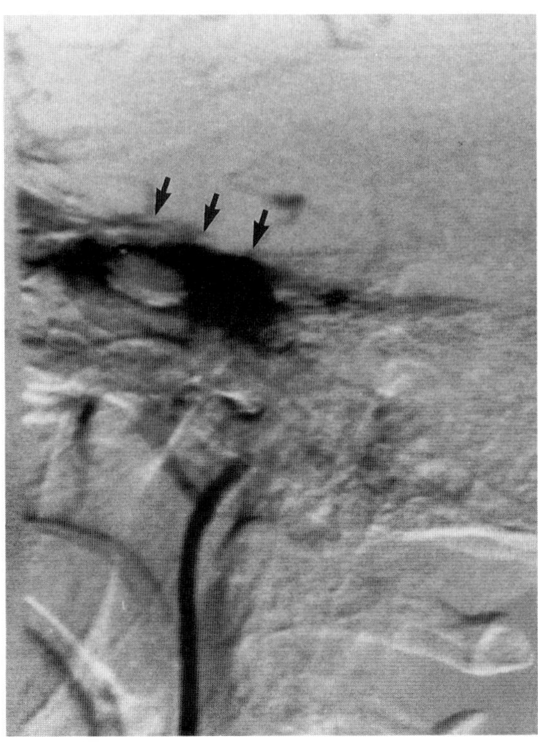

Fig. 10-11. (**A**) Patient with post-traumatic right proptosis and ptosis secondary to carotid-cavernous fistula. (**B**) Angiogram demonstrating patient's large fistula into the cavernous sinus.

initial diplopia in many cases is a result of edema and hemorrhage in the inferior orbit. More persistent diplopia occurs as a result of entrapment of muscle or perimuscular tissue in the fracture site, which can be diagnosed with a positive forced duction test (Baker and Epstein, 1991). The fracture and entrapment can be seen on coronal CT imaging, often with blood filling the associated sinus. These patients can also have either enophthalmos (eye sinking in) or proptosis (eye sticking out) in the acute phase and numbness in the distribution of the second maxillary nerve. Patients with persistent diplopia or significant enophthalmos can be treated with orbital surgery with or without strabismus surgery. Unless significant enophthalmos is present initially, surgery should be delayed for approximately 2 weeks (Emery et al., 1971).

Convergence Insufficiency

Patients with post-traumatic convergence insufficiency often complain of diplopia at near distance, difficulty in reading, eyestrain, headache, and blurred vision. They often use accommodative convergence to avoid diplopia and prefer to tolerate the blurred image (Carroll and Seaber, 1974). On examination, these patients will have a remote near point of convergence, decreased convergence fusional amplitudes, or both. In Kowals' series (1992), 14 percent of head injury patients had defective convergence. In the series of Burke et al. (1992), 15 percent of patients with whiplash had decreased convergence. Almost all cases resolved within 9 months. Treatment options include convergence exercises, prisms, and strabismus surgery in persistent symptomatic cases (Davies, 1956). The response to treatment is quite variable. The site of damage and the mechanism are unknown, but control centers have been postulated in the midbrain (Krohel et al., 1986).

Divergence Paralysis

Divergence paralysis is also seen in patients with severe head trauma, usually those with skull fracture and loss of consciousness but also in those with minor trauma without loss of consciousness. Patients complain of uncrossed diplopia at distance and have an esotropic deviation at distance, with full ductions and no evidence of a sixth nerve palsy. Many improve spontaneously without treatment, but prisms are helpful in alleviating diplopia in the acute stage (Rutkowski and Burian, 1972).

Disorders of Accommodation

Disorders of accommodation after head injury include accommodation paresis and accommodative spasm. In a series of 161 head injury patients, 19 percent had accommodative spasm and 16 percent had poor accommodation (Kowal, 1992). The diagnosis of accommodative spasm was made on the basis of blurred distant vision, which improved with myopic correction, and evidence of either emmetropia or hypertropia with cycloplegic refraction. Poor accommodation was diagnosed on the basis of blurred near vision in patients under age 35, which improved with extra plus lenses and a remote near point of accommodation. A large percentage had persistent symptoms 1 year later (Kowal, 1992). Poor accommodation can be seen with the use of some medications. Anticholinergics such as tricyclic antidepressants, frequently used in post-traumatic headache and depression, may inhibit the ciliary muscle and reduce accommodation. Narcotics and sedatives reduce conciousness level and may impair accommodation.

Skew Deviation

Skew deviation is a vertical misalignment of the eyes secondary to either brainstem or cerebellar lesions. Trauma is a relatively uncommon cause of skew, being responsible for only 5 among 100 patients with skew deviation (Keane, 1975). It is a disorder of supranuclear pathways and can be produced by disrupting the otolith pathways, which ascend via the medial longitudinal fasciculus from the medulla to the third and fourth nuclear complexes. Frequently the pons is the site of the lesion. The vertical deviation can be comitant or incomitant but does not step out to a cranial nerve palsy and is not associated with any cyclodeviation or torsion, a helpful feature in distinguishing skew from fourth nerve palsy (Trobe, 1984).

Gaze Paresis

Horizontal gaze paresis is a relatively infrequent finding in closed head injury patients. Keane (1986) found only one case among 96 patients involved in motorcycle accidents. Frontal lobe lesions will cause loss of voluntary gaze to the opposite side, which usually recovers with time. Pontine lesions involving the pontine paramedian reticular formation cause ipsilateral conjugate horizontal gaze paresis. These lesions are usually associated with loss of consciousness and have decreased response to the doll's head maneuver or caloric testing. There is a good prognosis for recovery.

Internuclear Ophthalmoplegia

Internuclear ophthalmoplegia is characterized by absent or slow-adducting saccades and dissociated nystagmus of the abducting eye. The lesion can be bilateral or unilateral, and it occurs as a result of demyelinating, ischemic, or shear injury to the medial longitudinal fasciculus. Although several cases have been reported (Baker, 1979; Beck and Meckler, 1981; Rich et al., 1974), it is relatively uncommon. Patients with bilateral lesions can also have impaired convergence, impaired vertical movements, and skew deviation.

Pursuit, Saccades, and Vestibular-Ocular Reflex

Eye movements such as pursuit (the ability to track smoothly an object moving slowly in space), which should depend on dorsolateral structures in a parieto-occipital pathway, and saccades (fast reflexive or volitional eye movements), which may depend on frontal eye fields in the frontal lobe) can be abnormal in patients with head trauma. Frequently, saccades are initially abnormal as compared with controls in latency, refixations, and accuracy (Williams et al., 1995). After 1 year, however, some of these parameters actually improve.

The vestibular-ocular reflex is a complex reflex representing vestibular input into ocular motor centers. The suppression of the reflex is required when movement of the head occurs during fixation. Trauma to the vestibular end organ and eighth cranial nerve may disrupt the reflex; suppression of the reflex can be disturbed by cerebral trauma. The patient complains of blurred vision with movement such as walking down a grocery aisle, driving a car, and walking in crowded malls. The problem is fairly common, being seen in about one-third of patients with head trauma (McLeish et al., 1991).

Finally, oscillopsia (a sense that the world is moving or jiggling) results from nystagmus. It may be interpreted by the patient as blurred or double vision. A search for damage to the brainstem or cerebellum is helpful. Downbeat, periodic alternating, and seesaw nystagmus have been reported (Leigh and Zee, 1991). Treatment with clonazepam (low-dose) may be helpful in decreasing symptoms on the basis of our experience.

FUNCTIONAL VISUAL LOSS

No discussion of neuro-ophthalmic findings after head injury would be complete without a discussion of the types of functional visual loss and suggestions for detecting them on examination. In order to appreciate the diversity of patients and subtleties of examination, clinicians should read the excellent review by Thompson (1985). He classifies functional patients as representing a continuum from those who are innocently suggestible to deliberate malingerers. Several clever tasks are outlined in this paper.

The first type of functional loss is feigned blindness of one eye. Wih the lack of a relative afferent pupillary defect and a completely normal examination, the examiner must surreptitiously fog the good eye by various means in order to demonstrate good vision. For example, a +2.00 cylinder can be raised in front of the supposed goodly eye, and the patient told to read with both eyes the 20/20 line. In this way, the patient will use the "bad" eye. Red/green glasses may be used in this way as well (Thompson, 1985). Testing visual stereopsis in patients with feigned monocular loss is helpful, since any patient who is able to do nine stereo dots in the Titmus test, must have at least 20/40 vision in both eyes or 40 seconds of stereo vision.

When both eyes are supposedly blind, an optokinetic nystagmus (OKN) drum moved in any direction will confirm sight, or a mirror moved in front of the patient's eyes will cause the sighted to follow with their eyes. Frequently, we distract patients with "Now I am going to check your neurologic examination" and with this ask them to touch their noses and then the examiner's finger. The obstacle course made up of furniture in the office from one end to the other is also helpful to show that such patients have vision.

Visual field changes after head trauma that can be functional include tunnel visual fields. A trip to the tangent screen with a field marked at 1 m and 3 m will frequently show the 3-m field *within* the 1-m isopter—obviously *not* physiologic visual field expansion.

Keane (1979) recognized a specific hysterical hemianopic visual field with part of a visual field missing in one eye, a normal visual field in the opposite eye. With both visual fields tested together, the hemianopic field defect remained—again an unphysiologic field.

Finally, cranial nerve and mild gaze palsies can be mimicked by patients with covergence spasms or spasm in the near (Cogen and Freece, 1955). While taking more history or distracting the patient with other tests, a full range of eye movement can be seen.

Approaching the patient with functional visual loss takes an understanding of the patient type. The innocently suggestible will be reassured and happy that there is really nothing wrong while the deliberate malingerer may be angry and seek many other opinions. Frequently telling the patient that the problem will certainly improve and not cause long-term problems is successful.

ACKNOWLEDGMENTS

Supported in part by a grant from Research to Prevent Blindness, Inc., New York, NY to the Department of Ophthalmology, University of Utah.

We thank Tiffany Parkin for typing assistance.

REFERENCES

Adams JH: Head injury. pp. 85–124. Adams JH, Corsellis JAN, Duchen LW (eds): Greenfield's Neuropathology. John Wiley & Sons, New York, 1984

Adams JH, Graham DI, Murray LS et al: Diffuse axonal injury due to non-missile head injury in humans: an analysis of 45 cases. Ann Neurol 12:557–563, 1982

Al-Qurainy A, Stassen LFA, Dutton GN et al: The characteristics of midfacial fractures and the association with ocular injury: a prospective study. Br J Oral Maxillofacial Sur 29:291–301, 1991

Anderson DL, Lloyd LA: Traumatic lesion of the optic chiasm: a report for four cases. Can Med Assoc J 90:110–115, 1964

Anderson RL, Panje WR, Gross CE: Optic nerve blindness following blunt forehead trauma. Ophthalmology (Rochester) 89:445–455, 1982

Arias MJ: Bilateral traumatic abducens nerve palsy without skull fracture and with cervical spine fracture. Neurosurgery 16:232–234, 1985

Baker RS: Internuclear ophthalmoplegia following head injury. J Neurosurg 51:552–555, 1979

Baker RS, Epstein AD: Ocular motor abnormalities from head trauma. Surv Ophthalmol 35:245–267, 1991

Ball JD Jr: Direct oblique sagittal CT of orbital wall fractures. AJR 148:601–608, 1987

Beck RW: Ocular deviations after head injury. Am Orthoptic J 35:103–107, 1985

Beck RW, Meckler RJ: Internuclear ophthalmoplegia after head trauma. Ann Ophthalmol 13:671–675, 1981

Bracken MB, Holford TR: Effects of timing of methylprednisolone or naloxone administration on recovery of segmental and long-tract neurologic function in NASCIS. 2. J Neurosurg 79:500–507, 1993

Bracken MB, Shepard MJ, Collins WF et al: A randomized, controlled trial of methylprednisolone or naloxone in the treatment of acute spinal-cord injury. Results of the Second National Acute Spinal Cord Injury Study. N Engl J Med 322:1405–1411, 1990

Burger LJ, Kalvin NH, Smith JL: Acquired lesions of the fourth nerve. Brain 93:567–574, 1970

Burke JP, Orton HP, West J et al: Whiplash and its effect on the visual system. Graefes Arch Clin Exp Ophthalmol 230:335, 1992

Carroll RP, Seaber JH: Acute loss of fusional convergence following head trauma. Am Orthopt J 24:57–59, 1974

Cogan DG, Freese CG: Spasm of the near reflex. Arch Ophthalmol 54:752–759, 1955

Crompton MR: Visual lesions in closed head injury. Brain 93:785–792, 1970

Crompton MR: Hypothalamic lesions following closed head injury. Brain 94:165–172, 1971

Crouch ER Jr, Urist MJ: Lateral rectus muscle paralysis associated with closed head trauma. Am J Ophthalmol 79:990–996, 1975

Crowe NW, Nickles TP, Troost T, Elster AD: Intrachiasmal hemorrhage: a cause of delayed post-traumatic blindness. Neurology 39:863–865, 1989

Davies CE: Etiology and management of convergence insufficiency. Am Orthopt J 6:124–127, 1956

Digre KB: Trauma to the brain with attention to the occipital lobe. North American Neuroophthalmic Society Mtg., Big Sky, MT, 1993

Digre KB, Osborne AO, Subbaratum H: Neuro-radiologic evaluation of supranuclear and intranuclear disorders of gaze. Ophthalmol Clin North Am 7:459–486, 1994

Digre KB, Smoker WRK, Johnston P et al: Selective MR imaging approach for the evaluation of Horner's syndrome. AJNR 13:223–227, 1992

Edmund J, Gotdfredsen E: Unilateral optic atrophy following head injury. Acta Ophthalmol (Copenh) 41:693–697, 1963

Elston JS: Traumatic third nerve palsy. Br J Ophthalmol 68:538–543, 1984

Emery JM, von Noorden GK, Schlernitzauer DA: Orbital floor fractures: long-term follow-up of cases with and without surgical repair. Trans Pa Acad Ophthalmol Otolaryngol 75:802–812, 1971

Fujitani T, Inoue K, Takahashi T et al: Indirect traumatic optic nerve neuropathy—visual outcome of operative and nonoperative cases. Jpn J Ophthalmol 30: 125–134, 1986

Fukado Y: Results in 400 cases of surgical decompression of the optic nerve. Mod Prob Ophthalmol 14:474–481, 1975

Gilbert JJ, Deonna T: Unusual brainstem finding following closed head injury. J Pediatr 81:343–345, 1972

Girard BC, Bouzas EA, Lamas G et al: Visual improvement after transethmoid decompression in optic nerve injuries. J Clin Neuro Ophthalmol 12:142–148, 1992

Gjerris F: Traumatic lesions of the visual pathways. pp. 27–57. In Vinken PJ, Bruyn CW (eds): Handbook of Clinical Neurology. Vol. 24. North Holland, Amsterdam

Greenblatt SH: Post-traumatic cerebral blindness. JAMA 225:1073–1076, 1973

Griffith JF, Dodge PR: Transient blindness following head injury in children. N Engl J Med 278:648–651, 1968

Guy J, Sherwood M, Day AL: Surgical treatment of progressive visual loss in traumatic optic neuropathy. Report of two cases. J Neurosurg 70:799–801, 1989

Harley RD: Paralytic strabismus in children: etiologic incidence and management of the third, fourth, and sixth nerve palsies. Ophthalmology 86:24–43, 1980

Hayreh SS: Arterial blood supply of the eye. pp. 1–23. In Bernstein EF: Amaurosis Fugax. Springer-Verlag, New York, 1988

Hedges TR, Gragoudas ES: Traumatic anterior ischemic optic neuropathy. Ann Ophthalmol 13:625–628, 1981

Heinze J: Cranial nerve avulsion and other neural injuries in road accidents. Med J Aust 2:1246–1249, 1969

Hermann JS: Masked bilateral superior oblique paresis. J Pediatr Ophthalmol Strabismus 18:43–48, 1981

Hillman JS, Myska V, Nissim S: Complete avulsion of the optic nerve. Br J Ophthalmol 59:503–509, 1975

Hooper RS: Orbital complications of head injury. Br J Surg 39:126–138, 1951

Hughes B: Indirect injury of the optic nerves and chiasm. Johns Hopkins Med J 1:98–126, 1962

Jacobson DM, Warner JJ, Choucair AK et al: Trochlear nerve palsy following minor head trauma. J Clin Neuro Ophthalmol 8:263–268, 1988

Joseph MP, Lessell S, Rizzo J, Momose KJ: Extracranial optic nerve decompression for traumatic optic neuropathy. Arch Ophthalmol 108:1091–1093, 1990

Keane JR: Ocular skew deviation. Analysis of 100 cases. Arch Neurol 32:185–190, 1975

Keane JR: Hysterical hemianopsia. Arch Ophthalmol 97:865–866, 1979

Keane JR: Trochlear nerve pareses with brainstem lesions. J Clin Neuro Ophthalmol 6:242–246, 1986

Keane JR: Fourth nerve palsy: historical review and study of 215 inpatients. Neurology 43:2439–2443, 1993

Keefe WP, Rucker CW, Kernohan JW: Pathogenesis of paralysis of the third cranial nerve. Arch Ophthalmol 63:585–592, 1960

Kennerdell JS, Amsbaugh GA, Myers EN: Transantral-ethmoidal decompression of optic cranial fracture. Arch Opthalmol 94:1040–1043, 1976

Kerr FWL, Hollowell OW: Location of pupillomotor and accommodation fibers in the oculomotor nerve: experimental observation on paralytic mydriasis. J Neurol Neurosurg Psychiatry 27:473–481, 1964

Khawam E, Scott AB, Jampolsky A: Acquired superior oblique palsy: diagnosis and management. Arch Ophthalmol 77:761–768, 1967

Kline LB, Morawetz RB, Swaid SN: Indirect injury of the optic nerve. Neurosurgery 14:756–764, 1984

Kodsi SR, Young BR: Acquired oculomotor, trochlea and abducent cranial nerve palsies in pediatric patients. Am J Ophthalmol 4:568–574, 1992

Kowal L: Ophthalmic manifestations of head injury. Aust N Z J Ophthalmol 20:35–40, 1992

Krohel GB, Kristan RW, Simon JW, Barrows NA: Posttraumatic convergence insufficiency. Ann Ophthalmol 18:101–104, 1986

Lam BL, Wingeist TA: Corticosteroid-responsive traumatic optic neuropathy. Am J Opthalmol 109:99–101, 1990

Lavin PJM, Troost BT: Traumatic fourth nerve palsy: clinicoanatomic correlations with computed tomographic scan. Arch Neurol 41:679–680, 1984

Leigh RJ, Zee DS: The Neurology of Eye Movements. FA Davis, Philadelphia, 1991, pp. 386, 391, 392, 415–421, 432

Lessell S: Indirect optic nerve trauma. Arch Ophthalmol 107:382–386, 1989

Lillie WI, Adson AW: Unilateral central and annular scotoma produced by callus from fracture extending into optic canal. Arch Ophthalmol 12:500–508, 1934

Lindenberg R: Significance of the tentorium in head injuries from blunt sources. Clin Neurosurg 12:129–142, 1966

Lindenberg R, Walsh FB, Sacks JJ: Neuropathology of Vision: an Atlas. Lea & Febiger, Philadelphia, 1973, pp. 220–223

Lowenfeld I: The Pupil. Iowa State University Press, Ames IA, 1993, pp. 1477–1568

Lowenstein A: Marginal haemorrhage on the disc. Partial cross-tearing of the optic nerve. Br J Ophthalmol 27:208, 1943

Manfredi SJ, Mohammad RR, Sprinkle PS et al: Computerized tomographic scan findings in facial fractures associated with blindness. Plast Reconstr Surg 68:479–490, 1981

Matsuzaki H, Kunita M, Kawai K: Optic nerve damage in head trauma: clinical and experimental studies. Jpn J Ophthalmol 26:447–461, 1982

Mauriello JA, Deluca J, Krieger A et al: Management of traumatic optic neuropathy a study of 23 patients. Br J Ophthalmol 76:349–352, 1992

McLeish M, Digre KB, Keane JR et al: Investigation of visual changes following closed head injury. North American Neuroophthalmology Society Mtg, Park City, UT, 1991

Miller JD, Becker DP: General principles and pathophysiology of head injury. pp. 1896–1937. In Youmans JR (ed): Neurological Surgery. WB Saunders, Philadelphia, 1982

Miller NR: The management of traumatic optic neuropathy, editorial. Arch Ophthalmol 108:1086–1087, 1990

Nau HE, Gerhard L, Foerster M et al: Optic nerve trauma: clinical, electrophysiolgical and histological remarks. Acta Neurochir (Wien) 89:16–27, 1987

Niho S, Niho M, Niho K: Decompression of the optic canal by the transethmoidal route and decompression of the superior orbital fissure. Can J Ophthalmol 5:22–40, 1970

Obenchain TG, Killeffer FA, Stern WE: Indirect injury of the optic nerve chiasm with closed head injury: report of three cases. Bull Los Angeles Neurol Soc 38:13–20, 1973

Osterberg G: Traumatic bitemporal hemianopia (sagittal tearing of the optic chiasma). Acta Ophthalmol (Copenh) 16:466–474, 1938

Park JH, Frenkel M, Dobbie JG, Choromokos: Avulsion of the optic nerve. Am J Ophthalmol 72:969–971, 1971

Parks NM: Isolated cyclovertical muscle palsy. Arch Ophthalmol 60:1027–1035, 1958

Pringle JH: Atrophy of the optic nerve following diffuse violence to the skull. Br Med J 2:56–57, 1922

Putterman AM, Stevens T, Urist MJ: Nonsurgical management of blowout fractures of the orbital floor. Am J Ophthalmol 77:232–239, 1974

Ramsay JH: Optic nerve injury in fracture of the canal. Br J Ophthalmol 63:607–610, 1979

Rand CW: Chiasmal injury complicating fracture of the skull. Bull Los Angeles Neurol Soc 2:91–94, 1937

Rich JR, Gregorius FK, Hepler RS: Bilateral internuclear ophthalmoplegia after trauma. Arch Ophthalmol 92:66–68, 1974

Richards BW, Jones FR, Younger BP: Causes and prognosis in 4,278 cases of paralysis of the oculomotor, trochlear and abducens cranial nerves. Am J Ophthalmol 3:489–496, 1992

Rizzo M, Smith V, Pokorny J, Damcesis AR: Color perception profiles in central achromatopsia. Neurology 43:995–1001, 1993

Rucker CW: The causes of paralysis of the third, fourth, and sixth cranial nerves. Am J Ophthalmol 61:1293–1298, 1966

Rush JA, Younge BR: Paralysis of cranial nerves III, IV, and VI: cause and prognosis in 1000 cases. Arch Ophthalmol 99:76–79, 1981

Rutkowski PC, Burian HM: Divergence paralysis following head trauma. Am J Ophthalmol 73:660–662, 1972

Sabates NR, Gonce MA, Farris BK: Neuro-ophthalmological findings in closed head trauma. J Clin Neuro Ophthalmol 11:273–277, 1991

Savino PJ, Glaser JS, Schatz NJ: Traumatic chiasmal syndrome. Neurology 30:963–970, 1980

Seiff SR: High dose corticosteroids for treatment of vision loss due to indirect injury to the optic nerve. Ophthalmic Surg 21:389–395, 1990

Seiff SR, Berger MS, Guyon J, Pitts LH: Computed tomographic evaluation of the optic canal in sudden traumatic blindness. Am J Ophthalmol 98:751–755, 1984

Spoor TC, Hartel WC, Lensink DB, Wilkinson MJ: Treatment of traumatic optic neuropathy with corticosteroids. Am J Ophthalmol 110:665–669, 1990

Steinsapir KD, Goldberg RA: Traumatic optic neuropathy. Surv Ophthalmol 38:487–518, 1994

Striph GG, Slamovits TL, Burde RM: Visual recovery following prolonged amaurosis due to compressive optic neuropathy. J Clin Neuro Ophthalmol 4:189–195, 1984

Sturzenegger M, Distefans G, Radamor BP et al: Presenting symptoms and signs after whiplash injury: the influence of accident mechanism. Neurology 44:688–693, 1994

Sunderland S, Hughes ESR: The pupillo-constrictor pathway and the nerves to the ocular muscles in man. Brain 69:301–309, 1946

Sydnor CF, Seabor JH, Buckley EG: Traumatic superior oblique palsies. Ophthalmology 89:134–138, 1982

Tang R: Chiasm trauma. North American Neuroophthalmology Society Mtg, Big Sky, MT, 1993

Thompson HS: Putting a number on the relative afferent pupillary defect. pp. 157–158. In Thompson HS, Daroff R, Frisen L et al (eds): Topics in Neuro-Ophthalmology, Baltimore, Williams & Wilkins, 1979

Thompson HS: Functional visual loss. Am J Ophthalmol 100:209–213, 1985

Thompson HS, Montague P, Cox TA et al: The relationship between visual acuity, pupillary defect, and visual field loss. Am J Ophthalmol 93:681–688, 1982

Traquair HM, Dott NM, Russell WR: Traumatic lesions of the optic chiasma. Brain 58:398–404, 1935

Trobe JD: Cyclodeviation in acquired vertical strabismus. Arch Ophthalmol 102:717–720, 1984

Turner JWA: Indirect injury of the optic nerves. Brain 66:140–151, 1943

Uzzell DP, Dolinkas CA, Langefelt TW: Visual field defects in relation to head injury severity. Arch Neurol 45:420–424, 1988

Von Noorden GK, Murray E, Wong SY: Superior oblique paralysis: a review of 270 cases. Arch Ophthalmol 104:1771–1776, 1986

Walsh FB: Pathological-clinical correlations. I. Indirect trauma to the optic nerves and chiasm. II. Certain cerebral involvements associated with defective blood supply. Invest Ophthalmol Vis Sci 5:443–449, 1966

Walsh FB, Hoyt WF: Clinical Neuro-Ophthalmology. 3rd Ed. Williams & Wilkins, Baltimore, 1969, pp. 2331–2518

Waltridge CB, Muhlbauer MS, Lowery RD: Traumatic carotid artery dissection: diagnosis and treatment. J Neurosurgy 71:854–857, 1989

Williams IM, Ponsford JL, Gibson K, et al: Cerebral control of saccades and neuropsychological test results after head injury. J Clin Neurosci (in press)

Wolin MJ, Lavin PJM: Spontaneous visual recovery from traumatic optic neuropathy after blunt head injury. Am J Ophthalmol 109:430–435, 1990

Wyllie AM, Mcleod D, Cullen JF: Traumatic ischaemic optic neuropathy. Br J Ophthalmol 56:851–853, 1972

Younge BR, Sutula F: Analysis of trochlear nerve palsies: diagnosis, etiology, and treatment. Mayo Clin Proc 52:11–18, 1977

Post-Traumatic Epilepsy 11

Mark A. Granner

Epilepsy is a relatively rare consequence of head injury, but the sheer number of annual head injuries leads to a sizable population of people with post-traumatic epilepsy. This is especially true in teenagers and young adults, in whom trauma is the leading cause of symptomatic (noninherited) epilepsy (Annegers, 1993). The magnitude of the public health problem is compounded by the costs of epilepsy, including clinic and emergency department visits, medications, and lost job productivity.

The relationship between head trauma and epilepsy was noted as early as 400 B.C., when Hippocrates observed that left-sided cranial trauma was associated with right body motor seizures (Temkin, 1971). Global conflicts of the past century have provided abundant material for the study of head injury, and have greatly enhanced our understanding of post-traumatic epilepsy and its pathology, natural course, and possible treatment.

DEFINING THE DISORDER

Seizure

For the purposes of this discussion, a seizure will be defined as a paroxysmal hyperexcitability of a population of cortical neurons, which is associated with a corresponding behavioral change. Depending on its location and extent, this electrophysiologic event may or may not be visible on routine scalp electroencephalography (EEG). The behavioral change may be subjective (e.g., a visual sensation or limb tingling) or objective (e.g., limb jerking), and may or may not be discernable to an observer. Epileptic seizures tend to be self-limited, with clear-cut beginnings and endings, except in the case of status epilepticus, which is defined as "a seizure that persists for a sufficient length of time or is repeated frequently enough that recovery between attacks does not occur" (Commission on Classification and Terminology of the International League Against Epilepsy, 1981).

To facilitate discussion and help with rational therapy decisions, the Commission on Classification and Terminology of the International League Against Epilepsy published a classification scheme of seizures, which was updated in 1981 (Table 11-1). The classification is based on commonly observed clinical features of the various types of seizures and is supported by reproducible patterns in electrophysiology as demonstrated on the EEG. The main distinction is between generalized seizures (involving all neocortex at onset) and partial seizures (involving a focal area or region of neocortex at onset). Generalized sei-

TABLE 11-1. Classification of Epileptic Seizures

Classification	Subclassification
Partial seizures	Simple partial seizures (consciousness not impaired)
	With motor signs
	With somatosensory or special sensory symptoms
	With autonomic symptoms or signs
	With psychic symptoms
	Complex partial seizures (with impairment of consciousness)
	Simple partial onset followed by impairment of consciousness
	With impairment of consciousness at onset
	Partial seizures evolving to secondarily generalized seizures
Generalized seizures	Absence seizures
	Myoclonic seizures
	Clonic seizures
	Tonic seizures
	Tonic-clonic seizures
	Atonic seizures
Unclassified seizures	

(Modified from Commission on Classification and Terminology of the International League Against Epilepsy, 1981, with permission.)

zures are further subclassified as tonic (sustained increased muscle tone), clonic (repetitive limb jerking), tonic-clonic (a tonic phase followed by a clonic phase), myoclonic (a sudden, single jerk), atonic (sudden loss of muscle tone), and absence (cessation of activity, with staring and unresponsiveness, followed by prompt resumption of activities). As both cerebral hemispheres are involved in generalized seizures, they all involve some alteration in consciousness, although myoclonic seizures are usually too brief to tell. The major subclassification of partial seizures is into simple and complex partial seizures, with the former involving no alteration in consciousness and the latter involving some (or complete) alteration in consciousness. A partial seizure may start with simple symptomatology, then progress to a complex partial seizure (related to spread of the seizure beyond its originating focus). A partial seizure may likewise spread to involve both cerebral hemispheres, producing a partial seizure with secondary generalization. Finally, if a seizure can not be placed into one of the generalized or partial categories, it is called unclassified. Vague terms such as "epileptiform disorder," "epilepsy spectrum disorder," and "seizure-like syndrome" are nonstandard, misleading, and have no prognostic value. Their use is to be discouraged.

Epilepsy

The terms epilepsy and seizure are not synonymous. A seizure is a single event. Epilepsy is a syndrome, with a multitude of possible causes, manifestations, and courses. An epileptic syndrome is defined by its seizure type(s), age of onset, genetics (if any), etiology, course, EEG pattern, examination findings, and response to therapy. In simple terms, epilepsy is the tendency to have recurrent unprovoked seizures (which distinguishes it from seizures occurring in the setting of severe illness, fever, or metabolic disturbance).

A classification scheme analogous to that for seizures exists for epileptic syndromes (Table 11-2), which is based on whether the syndrome is primarily focal (or "localization-related"), generalized, or of undetermined nature. Within each group syndromes are subclassified as idiopathic (usually with a genetic basis), symptomatic (due to some known or suspected underlying brain disease), or cryptogenic (due to presumed but as yet undisclosed brain disease). Specific epilepsy syndromes are described elsewhere (Committee on Classification and Terminology of the International League Against Epilepsy, 1989).

An estimated 10 percent of all people will have at least one seizure during their lifetimes. The majority are single, isolated seizures (usually in the setting of an acute illness) and therefore do not constitute epilepsy. The prevalence of epilepsy in America is estimated to be 0.6 percent of the population, or around 2 million people (Scheuer and Pedley, 1990).

Post-Traumatic Epilepsy

Post-traumatic epilepsy is an epileptic syndrome caused by head trauma. As will be discussed, its seizure type is usually partial (simple or complex), with

TABLE 11-2. Classification of the Epilepsies and Epileptic Syndromes

Classification	Subclassification	Example
Localization-related (focal, local, partial)	Idiopathic (with age-related onset)	Benign rolandic epilepsy
	Symptomatic	Post-traumatic epilepsy
	Cryptogenic	
Generalized	Idiopathic (with age-related onset)	Childhood absence epilepsy
	Cryptogenic or symptomatic	Lennox-Gastaut syndrome
	Symptomatic	Early myoclonic encephalopathy
Undetermined whether focal or generalized		Landau-Kleffner syndrome
Special syndromes		Febrile convulsions

(Modified from Commission on Classification and Terminology of the International League Against Epilepsy, 1989, with permission.)

or without secondary generalization (Hughes, 1986). It would therefore be classified as a localization-related (focal) symptomatic epilepsy syndrome. It is important to remember, however, that (1) a temporal relationship between a head injury and the presence of epilepsy does not prove that the injury caused the epilepsy, (2) most head injuries do not cause epilepsy, and (3) seizures due to a pre-existing epileptic condition may themselves cause head injuries.

Post-traumatic seizures are typically divided into three categories, defined by their timing relative to the head injury and distinguished by different natural histories (Jennett, 1974). *Immediate* post-traumatic seizures are those that occur within minutes of the injury. Immediate seizures are of no prognostic value for the subsequent development of epilepsy and will not be discussed further. *Early* post-traumatic seizures are those that occur after the immediate time frame but within the first week after injury. By definition early post-traumatic seizures are time-limited and can thus only loosely be classified as an epileptic syndrome. However, their occurrence is a risk factor for the development of *late* post-traumatic seizures, which occur more than 1 week after the injury. On the other hand, most patients with early post-traumatic seizures do not develop late epilepsy.

Differential Diagnosis

Not all paroxysmal neurologic events are seizures. In the head-injured patient, the differential diagnosis of post-traumatic seizures includes headaches, syncope, transient metabolic disturbances such as hypoglycemia, transient ischemic attacks, and sleep disorders (e.g., narcolepsy). Pseudoseizures (paroxysmal spells of psychological origin) can be difficult to diagnose in the head-injured patients and may realistically mimic true epileptic seizures. Pseudoseizures may occur on either a volitional (e.g., malingering, attention-seeking) or subconscious (e.g., conversion reaction) level. Aside from a placebo effect, they will not respond to standard anticonvulsant therapy but are often amenable to psychological intervention. Office diagnosis of pseudoseizures is often difficult, as they share many clinical features in common with epileptic seizures (Saygi et al., 1992). Accurate diagnosis often depends on recording an event by EEG, which can be carried out in an epilepsy monitoring unit with prolonged video-EEG recording (see below). Pseudoseizures are discussed in detail in Chapter 12.

As discussed in other chapters in this volume, head injury may produce a constellation of symptoms and signs, many of which are nonspecific (such as dizziness, transient memory loss or concentration difficulty, or rage attacks). These events should be considered to be nonepileptic until proved otherwise with supportive electrophysiologic or other clinical data. The diagnosis of epilepsy unfortunately still carries a stigma in our society, and to overdiagnose epilepsy probably causes more harm than to underdiagnose it. True epilepsy always declares itself in time.

FACTORS INFLUENCING POST-TRAUMATIC EPILEPSY

Our understanding of early and late post-traumatic epilepsy is based on observations from a number of large series of head-injured patients, many taken from military experience of the past century. While these series provide a vast number of cases to study, this retrospective manner of review has several important potential flaws, which should be kept in mind when analyzing the data. First, the series report head injuries of various severity, with some reports weighted more heavily toward (or based exclusively on) penetrating head wounds and others dealing primarily with closed head injuries. Studies involving primarily closed head injury will be reviewed here, unless otherwise noted. Second, irregular periods of follow-up were used in the studies, which may influence outcome statistics. Third, most of the studies were carried out prior to the development of modern neuroimaging techniques. Fourth, treatment was variable and was primarily carried out when many fewer antiepileptic drugs were available. Despite these drawbacks, the series reviewed here share a number of common views with respect to several important factors in the development of post-traumatic epilepsy. These are summarized in Table 11-3.

Early Seizures

Early post-traumatic epilepsy is thought to be a separate entity from late PTE for several reasons: (1) epilepsy occurs 30 times as often in the first week after injury than in weeks 2 through 8; (2) focal motor seizures are common in the first week after injury, less so in weeks 2 through 8, and rare after 3 months; and (3) less than one-third of patients with seizures in the first week after injury develop late PTE, but about 70 percent of those with seizures in weeks 2 through 8 do so (Jennett, 1973b). The overall incidence of early post-traumatic epilepsy is around 4 to 6 percent (Jennett and Lewin, 1960; Jennett, 1974; Jawahar et al., 1985). Several risk factors for the development of the early form have been identified.

TABLE 11-3. Risk factors in the Development of Early and Late Post-Traumatic Epilepsy

Form	Risk Factor
Early	Severity of injury Age at injury Loss of consciousness or amnesia > 24 h
Late	Severity of injury Age at injury Loss of consciousness or amnesia > 24 h Presence of early post-traumatic epilepsy

Severity of injury is a major determinant of early post-traumatic epilepsy. In the series of Jawahar et al. (1985), 1,005 head-injured patients (including those with mild, moderate, and severe injury) were followed. The presence of depressed skull fracture was associated with a 13 percent incidence of early PTE compared with 6 percent in those without fracture. The presence of an intracranial hematoma was associated with a 21 percent incidence, (which was even higher, 36 percent, in patients with subdural hematoma) compared with 4 percent incidence in those without hematoma. Focal neurologic signs, such as hemiparesis or dysphasia (implying some degree of structural brain injury) were associated with a 13 percent incidence of early post-traumatic epilepsy, compared with 3 percent in patients without neurologic signs.

Age is another major determinant of early post-traumatic epilepsy and also affects the subsequent development of late seizures. Children less than 5 years old, as compared with patients older than 5, are more likely to experience early seizures (11 versus 5 percent) (Jawahar et al., 1985); are more likely (13 versus 3 percent) to develop early seizures after trivial head injury (i.e., an injury in which coma or post-traumatic amnesia longer than 24 hours is not present) (Jawahar et al., 1985); but are less likely to subsequently develop late seizures (19 versus 26 percent) (Jennett, 1974). Children are more likely to have their first post-traumatic seizure in the first day after injury; 78 percent of children with early post-traumatic epilepsy had their first seizure in the first day, compared with 49 percent of adults. Over one-third of children have the first seizure within 1 hour of the injury (Jennett, 1973a). Children are about twice as likely to have status epilepticus in the early period, but it does not tend to be associated with the same degree of morbidity and mortality as in adults (Grand, 1974; Jennett, 1974).

Loss of consciousness and post-traumatic amnesia are signs of global central nervous system dysfunction. If these signs are present for more than 24 hours, the incidence of early post-traumatic epilepsy is 12 percent, compared with 3 percent if less than 24 hours (Jennett and Lewin, 1960). This factor is relevant only in adults, as in children the rates for more than and less than 24 hours are not significantly different (9.2 and 6.4 percent, respectively) (Jennett, 1973a).

Late Stage

Late post-traumatic epilepsy (seizures occurring more than 1 week after a head injury) has been reported in a number of large series, taken from both military (Caveness et al., 1979; Hughes, 1986; Nuutila and Huusko, 1972; Salazar et al., 1985; Walker and Jablon, 1958; Weiss et al., 1983) and civilian (Annegers et al., 1980; Black et al., 1975; Jawahar et al., 1985; Jennett and Lewin, 1960) populations. The pertinent findings of these series are summarized in Table 11-4.

Like early post-traumatic epilepsy, the late type is strongly correlated with the severity of the injury. The series presented in Table 11-4 bear this out. Those series derived from military experience (which tend to consist of more cases of penetrating head injuries) show an incidence of around 30 percent for late seizures while those based on civilian populations show a rate of 10 percent or less. The series of Jennett and Lewin (1960) from Oxford includes only cases of closed head injury and has an incidence rate of 10 percent. In this series severity of closed head injury also influenced the rate of late seizures; patients with intracranial hematoma had their risk increased to 29 percent.

The presence of early post-traumatic epilepsy and the duration of post-traumatic coma or amnesia are also significant factors in the development of late seizures. If seizures are present in the first week, the risk of late seizures is 29 percent, compared with 8 percent without early seizures (Jennett and Lewin, 1960). If post-traumatic coma or amnesia persists longer than 24 hours, the risk of late seizures is roughly doubled.

The series of Annegers et al. (1980) deserves special mention for several reasons. First, it is a large population-based study, which probably more realistically reflects post-traumatic epilepsy in the community at large than the military series. Second, the investigators rigorously applied definitions of seizure and epilepsy as given above and excluded patients with pre-existing epilepsy and those experiencing only a single seizure. Third, they divided all cases into severe (with brain contusion, intracerebral hematoma, or 24 hours of either amnesia or coma), moderate (skull fracture or 30 minutes to 24 hours of coma or amnesia), and mild (neither unconsciousness nor amnesia lasting longer than 30 minutes).

TABLE 11-4. Summary of Large Series of Post-Traumatic Epilepsy

Study	Population	No.	Nature of Injury	Incidence[a]	First Seizure[a]	Remission Rate[a]	Follow-up (Yr)
Nuutila and Huusko (1972)	M (WW II)	6,498	C,P	—	53% in 1 yr	13%	26–31
Walker and Jablon (1958)	M (WW II)	932	C,P	28	50% in 9 mo	—	7–8
Weiss et al. (1983)	M (V)	1,221	C,P	31	—	—	—
Caveness et al. (1979)	M (V)	1,030	C,P	28	67% in 1 yr	50%	5–10
Salazar et al. (1985)	M (V)	421	C	53	57% in 1 yr	50%	15
Hughes[b] (1986)	M (WW I,WW II,K,V)	7,303	C,P	34	—	—	—
Jennet and Lewin (1960)	C	1,000	C	10	50% in 1 yr	—	—
Annegers et al. (1980)	C	2,747	C,P	2	37% in 1 yr	—	5
Jawahar et al. (1985)	C	1,005	C,P	10	—	—	5

[a] Incidence is the incidence of late PTE. First seizure is the percentage of patients with their first (late) seizure within the given time. Remission rate is the percentage of patients with late PTE who became seizure free, over a specified follow-up time.

[b] The larger series of Hughes includes the series reported by Caveness et al.

Abbreviations: M, military; C, civilian; WW I, World War I; WW II, World War II; K, Korean War; V, Vietnam War; C, closed head injury; P, penetrating head injury.

Finally, this population of 2,747 patients was followed for 5 years, during which the incidence of late seizures was 11.5 percent in the severe injury group, 1.6 percent in the moderate group, and only 0.6 percent in the mild group (a rate identical to the incidence of epilepsy in the general population). Therefore, one can conclude that head injuries causing less than 30 minutes of unconsciousness or amnesia do not cause epilepsy. When considering the diagnosis of epilepsy in someone with a history of head injury of a mild nature, one must therefore carefully consider alternate (nonepileptic) diagnoses and use great caution when assigning a cause-and-effect relationship to the injury and the seizures.

The military and civilian series are in general agreement that roughly half of the late post-traumatic epilepsy patients will experience their first post-traumatic seizure within the first year (Table 11-4). If seizures have not developed by the fifth year after injury, they are unlikely to develop later. Most of the patients have partial seizures or partial seizures with secondary generalization (Hughes, 1986), probably related to the tendency for focal brain injury in head trauma.

PATHOPHYSIOLOGY

The basic mechanisms of human epileptogenesis are not completely understood, and the basic mechanisms of post-traumatic epilepsy are even less well understood. Given the heterogeneous nature of epilepsy, with its many potential causes and manifestations, it is likely that several pathophysiologic systems could be at work in the generation of epileptic seizures. On the other hand, the pathology of head trauma is known, and some insight into pathophysiology has been gained from animal models of epilepsy.

Pathology of Head Trauma

PTE is an acquired condition, resulting from injury to the brain's parenchyma. The degree of parenchymal damage depends to a large degree on the severity of the head injury, but even mild head injuries can be associated with pathologic changes (see Ch. 3). After cerebral contusion in humans, acute changes (seen within 3 hours) consist largely of astrocyte swelling followed by extravasation of red blood cells into the surrounding nervous tissue. Neuronal injury may be detected within 3 to 11 days and is followed by a phagocytic reaction as products of necrosis are removed (Bullock et al., 1991). More severe injuries may cause diffuse axonal injury (Strich, 1956). However, the precise nature and severity of injury needed to produce this pathologic condition and its relationship to the clinical findings of unconsciousness and amnesia remain controversial. Postmortem series of head-injured patients have revealed white matter degeneration, with the presence of microhemorrhage (Mendelow and Teasdale, 1983). Closed head injury with skull fracture is associated with thickening of the leptomeninges, with underlying gliosis and neuronal loss. In the absence of fracture, closed head injury may actually show more severe and widespread pathologic changes, probably because the force of impact has been centered in the brain rather than being absorbed by the skull. Leptomeningeal thickening and vascular reactions are seen, along with neuronal loss, gliosis, and hemosiderin deposition. Penetrating head wounds cause local tissue necrosis, with glial scarring and deposition of hemosiderin (Payan et al., 1970).

Seizure Generation

Which, if any, of these above pathologic changes may correlate with the generation of epileptic seizures? A leading possibility is that extravasation of red blood cells into brain parenchyma is epileptogenic. More specifically, the iron breakdown products of red blood cells have been shown to produce epileptic seizures in animals. Willmore et al. (1978), injected ferrous or ferric chloride into the sensorimotor cortex of rats and cats and produced spontaneously recurring epileptic electrical discharges and clinical seizures. The epileptic activity developed within 72 hours and persisted over the 6 weeks of the experiment. Clinical seizures did not occur in control animals injected with saline. Pathologic examination in these specimens revealed astrocyte proliferation, iron-filled macrophages, and neuronal changes; findings resembling those seen in patients with post-traumatic epilepsy. In a subsequent study using this model, Rubin and Willmore (1980) demonstrated that pretreatment of the animals with α-tocopherol, an antioxidant, blocked the development of the epileptic discharges. They then showed that the means by which this effect occurred was the prevention of lipid peroxidation and hypothesized that a cascade of post-traumatic events, including extravasation of heme, focal edema, activation of lipid peroxidase, generation of free radicals, and subsequent neuronal injury, may be responsible for the development of post-traumatic epilepsy (Willmore and Rubin, 1984).

Another model that has contributed greatly to our understanding of epileptogenesis is that of *kindling*. Kindling, first described by Goddard et al. in 1969, is a phenomenon whereby repeated transient electrical stimulation applied to the amygdala or hippocampus initially produces brief electrical afterdischarges, then later produces electrical and clinical seizures. The phenomenon has been described in many species, including rats, cats, baboons, and monkeys. Over time, the electrical and clinical seizures may occur independently of the electrical stimulation, and this process is easier to achieve the lower the animal phylogenetically (i.e., a rat will reach a state of spontaneous recurrent seizures after fewer stimuli than a baboon) (Wada, 1976). The demonstration of kindling in animals, including higher primates, has suggested a mechanism for the development or potentiation of epilepsy in humans. Pathologically, kindling is associated with neuronal loss in the hilar region of the hippocampus (Cavazos and Sutula, 1990) and with synaptic reorganization of the hippocampal mossy fibers (Cavazos et al., 1991). Similar changes have been seen in the human temporal lobe in specimens taken from patients with medically refractory seizures undergoing epilepsy surgery (Sutula et al., 1989), and kindling has been inferred from these findings. However, to date there is no direct evidence that kindling occurs in humans.

Another model of focal epilepsy is the kainic acid model. Kainic acid is an analogue of the excitatory amino acid neurotransmitter glutamate. Intraventricular injection of kainic acid in rats produces seizures of hippocampal origin, increased susceptibility to the effects of kindling, and hippocampal neuronal loss with mossy fiber synaptic reorganization. Sutula et al. (1992) showed that the morphologic (mossy fiber sprouting), electrophysiologic (susceptibility to kindling), and clinical (seizures) consequences of this model can be blocked if the animals are cotreated with phenobarbital. This finding has clear relevance to the prospect for treating human epilepsy. The relevance of this model to human post-traumatic epilepsy is not clear, but the involvement of excitatory neurotransmitters (including glutamate) has been hypothesized in brain injury (Sutula et al., 1992; Willmore, 1990). In future, antagonism of glutamate's action may play a role in preventing epilepsy following brain injury.

EVALUATION OF EPILEPSY

As epilepsy is a clinical syndrome and not a single disease entity, its diagnosis depends on the judicious application and integration of multiple sources of information. As such, there is no "standard" evaluation of epilepsy. This section discusses common tools in the diagnosis of epilepsy in general, with particular emphasis on post-traumatic epilepsy. The evaluation of epilepsy is summarized in Table 11-5.

Clinical Data

The heart and soul of epilepsy diagnosis are the clinical history and physical/neurologic examination. Any attempt to diagnose epileptic seizures without such information would be highly inaccurate. As discussed above, the differential diagnosis of epileptic seizures is large. Particular attention needs to be paid to the presence of any potential causative factors, such as birth injuries or past central nervous system infections. With respect to post-traumatic epilepsy, the precise nature of the injury should be ascertained. Was there significant loss of consciousness or amnesia? Was there an associated skull fracture or intracranial hemorrhage? How long after the injury did the presumed seizures start? If this interval is longer than several years, a cause-and-effect relationship between the injury and the seizures becomes more tenuous. Family history must be explored, seeking evidence of a genetic predisposition toward epilepsy. Information regarding other acute precipitants, including acute illness, use of prescription or illicit drugs, and alcohol use, should be sought.

The exact nature of the seizure(s) is critical in terms of making an accurate syndrome diagnosis. For example, a child having absence seizures (brief staring with unresponsiveness without prodromal aura or postictal confusion) after a head injury is far more likely to have an epileptic syndrome of genetic basis rather than post-traumatic epilepsy. Also, accurate seizure classification has treatment implications, as will be discussed below. One can usually not rely solely on the seizure history given by patients themselves, as they may be unaware of ongoing events during a complex partial or generalized seizure. Consequently, corroborating evidence from an eyewitness to the seizure, usually a family member, close friend, or co-worker, is important. Unfortunately, these individuals are generally not trained observers and may fail to register critical details of the event,

TABLE 11-5. Evaluation of Epilepsy

Data	Specific Queries, Tests
History	History of the seizures themselves (from patient and witness) Past history (e.g., febrile seizures, central nervous system infections, head trauma) Family history
General and neurologic examinations	Evidence of medical illness Localizing or lateralizing neurologic signs
Electrophysiologic testing	EEG (routine and/or sleep-deprived) Long-term video EEG monitoring Ambulatory EEG
Neuroimaging	Structural imaging (MRI, CT) Functional imaging (PET, SPECT)
Laboratory testing	Chemistry profile Antiepileptic drug levels

Abbreviations: PET, positron emission tomography; SPECT, single-photon emission computed tomography. See text for other definitions.

including its duration and the subject's movements or level of responsiveness. Instructing the patient or family to keep an event diary can be helpful. They should be asked to make notes on the date and time of events, what activity was observed, and what precipitating factors may have been involved. Also, missed or tardy medication doses can be noted. This information may make diagnosis more accurate and after the diagnosis of epileptic seizures has been established, may lead to rational treatment changes. For example, the physician may decide to increase the morning anticonvulsant dose if most of the seizures are found to occur in the late morning.

The definition of seizure given at the beginning of this chapter is based on an electrophysiologic phenomenon but is of limited practical use in the clinical setting because it is rare to obtain an EEG recording during the events in question. In fact, it is relatively rare for physicians to witness the events themselves. The clinical distinction between epileptic seizures and nonepileptic paroxysmal events is often a judgment call. Factors to consider before making the diagnosis of epilepsy include the following:

How stereotypical are the events? Epileptic seizures tend to be fairly stereotypical, whereas nonepileptic events may be more variable.

How long do they last? Epileptic seizures, with few exceptions, last for several seconds to a few minutes; it is rare for complex partial seizures to last for only a few seconds or longer than a few minutes. Events lasting longer than 5 minutes are more likely to be nonepileptic.

Do the events have a clear beginning and end? Epileptic seizures have relatively discrete onset and termination. Nonepileptic events may start insidiously, evolve over many minutes, and resolve gradually.

Is consciousness affected? By definition, complex partial and generalized tonic-clonic seizures involve some degree of impaired consciousness and often leave the patient with postictal confusion. If consciousness is never altered, the events are more likely to be nonepileptic.

Do the events arise out of sleep? Complex partial (epileptic) seizures occasionally originate in sleep. Pseudoseizures and other nonepileptic events of a volitional nature must arise from wakefulness.

The general physical examination is performed with an eye to evidence of other conditions, such as cardiac arrhythmia or syncope. The neurologic examination may disclose lateralizing or localizing signs (such as weakness or relex asymmetry) indicating focal dysfunction of the central nervous system.

Electrophysiologic Data

EEG is the primary electrophysiologic tool in the evaluation of epilepsy. When considering a diagnosis of epilepsy, the routine EEG may show either ictal findings (during the event itself) or interictal findings (between events). If one is fortunate enough to be recording the EEG during the clinical event, the concomitant presence of epileptic EEG changes can be diagnostic of an epileptic seizure. These EEG changes vary depending on the type of seizure, but complex partial seizures typically consist of focal or regional changes in cerebral activity. The electrographic characteristics of a seizure often include an increase in rhythmic activity, an increase in voltage, and a progression from higher- to lower-frequency activity. This activity may spread to adjacent brain areas. After the seizure, postictal slowing may be seen, usually in the area of the seizure. Interictal abnormality is a less specific finding than ictal changes, but the presence of focal or generalized paroxysmal activity (e.g., spikes, sharp waves, spike-wave complexes), occurring either singly or in bursts, will suggest a tendency to have seizures. However, one must use caution when making the leap from an epileptic interictal abnormality to the diagnosis of epilepsy. Many people have abnormal interictal paroxysmal activity on their EEG but never have seizures. Also, not all paroxysmal epileptiform ("shaped like an epileptic discharge") discharges imply abnormality. For example, vertex sharp waves and small sharp spikes are known to occur as normal or benign features of the drowsy or alseep EEG. Finally, EEG may record artifacts of noncerebral origin, which may mimic epileptiform discharges. The EEG should be interpreted only by a trained electroencephalographer. In summary, the EEG (particularly the interictal EEG) is never the sole diagnostic modality in epilepsy. The findings on the EEG must be interpreted in the context of the overall clinical picture.

The specific role of EEG in post-traumatic epilepsy is unclear. A number of large series (Jennett and van de Sande, 1975; Masquin and Courjon, 1963; Reisner et al., 1979; Walker and Jablon, 1958) have shown that the EEG is of no specific value either in predicting the risk of epileptic seizures after head injury or in gauging the rate of remission after the development of seizures. Only a single relatively small study (Courjon, 1970) found that the EEG held some positive prognostic value, although only if the EEG "normalized" after the occurrence of the first seizure. In summary, the EEG in post-traumatic epilepsy remains more a tool of diagnosis and classification than of prognosis.

Paroxysmal disturbances of behavior or consciousness are occasionally difficult to diagnose in the outpatient setting as they infrequently occur in the presence of the physician. Inpatient long-term video electroencephalography (VEEG) can be helpful in this situation as it provides for the continuous and prolonged acquisition of both clinical (video and audio) and electrophysiologic (EEG) data. The strengths of VEEG relative to routine EEG include:

1. The ability to make prolonged recordings (hours to weeks).
2. Recording of the event itself rather than interictal EEG.
3. Recording during full day/night cycles (some seizures of some patients occur exclusively at night, for example).
4. The ability to correlate behaviors (on video) with EEG changes.

Drawbacks of VEEG include cost (VEEG is considerably more expensive than routine EEG) and inconvenience, as patients must spend time in the hospital. Technical guidelines for the performance of VEEG as well as details on its indications have been published by the American Electroencephalographic Society (1994).

An alternative to inpatient VEEG monitoring is outpatient ambulatory electroencephalography (AEEG). Currently available systems can provide either continuous or event-related recording on cassette tape or digital storage media. After connection in the EEG laboratory, patients are free to go about their daily activities, which may be more likely to incite an event. The recording is then analyzed later in the EEG laboratory. AEEG shares with VEEG the advantages of prolonged recording, directly capturing a clinical event, and recording during the full diurnal cycle. Theoretically, it more closely simulates the patient's usual daily activities than does a stay in the hospital. It does have some major drawbacks, including:

1. Lack of technical oversight. If the recording fails or electrodes fall off, the recording may be rendered worthless. This may not be discovered until after the fact.
2. Limited numbers of EEG channels. Most AEEG systems provide only 8 or 16 channels of EEG (although some noncontinuous event recorders offer more). If the presumed seizure arises from areas not being recorded, it may not be detected.
3. Lack of corresponding clinical (video, audio) information.
4. High incidence of artifact. Because the study is performed outside the controlled setting of the EEG laboratory, it is prone to a variety of environmental and physiologic artifacts, which may mimic cerebral activity and may at times take on the hypersynchronous, rhythmic appearance of a seizure. Such studies

should be interpreted with caution by an experienced electroencephalographer.

Routine EEG, VEEG, and AEEG are compared in Table 11-6.

Structural Data

Insight into epilepsy, particularly the focal epilepsies, has been greatly enhanced by the advent of modern neuroimaging techniques, first computed tomography (CT) and then magnetic resonance imaging (MRI). Neuroimaging is discussed in detail in Chapter 5. The main value of imaging in epilepsy is the ability to show a structural cause for the seizures (e.g., stroke, tumor, migrational disorder, or mesial temporal sclerosis). The latter is a pathologic description, the MRI equivalent of which is hippocampal atrophy and increased hippocampal signal on T_2-weighted images. Mesial temporal sclerosis is the structural correlate of many cases of temporal lobe epilepsy, although not all cases of post-traumatic epilepsy arise from the temporal lobe. CT studies have been made of both the acute and chronic phases of head trauma. Acutely, CT abnormalities are seen in about one-half of the cases, including diffuse cerebral edema, focal hypodensity, and intracranial hemorrhage (D'Alessandro et al., 1982; D'Alessandro et al., 1988). Series of CT studies in post-traumatic epilepsy are limited in numbers of patients, but some evidence exists that an early CT showing abnormality (particularly intracranial hemorrhage) is a risk factor for the subsequent development of epilepsy. Late CT (many years after the injury) may be normal, or may show an area of focal cortical atrophy or porencephaly. The relationship of these abnormal findings to post-traumatic epilepsy is unclear. Large MRI studies in post-traumatic epilepsy have not been reported.

TABLE 11-6. Comparison Between Different EEG Modalities

Characteristic[a]	REEG	AEEG	VEEG
Ambulatory	−	++	+
Prolonged	−	++	++
Ictal recording	−	++	++
Interictal recording	++	−	+
Clinical observation	+	−	++
Interactive/flexible	++	−	+
Technical adequacy	++	−	++

[a] Scale is relative.

Abbreviations and Symbols: REEG, routine EEG; AEEG, ambulatory EEG; VEEG, video EEG; −, poor; +, good; ++, excellent.

Other Data

Laboratory data such as electrolyte profiles, liver enzymes, and urinalysis are often useful in detecting metabolic abnormalities that may either mimic or precipitate epileptic seizures.

TREATMENT

We treat epilepsy to prevent the occurrence of future seizures and to circumvent the complications that may ensue with seizures. In this respect post-traumatic epilepsy is like any other epileptic syndrome, and its treatment parallels that of epilepsy in general. There is no evidence to suggest that post-traumatic seizures should respond to treatment any differently than seizures of other structural cause (e.g., stroke, tumor).

Medical Therapy

The pharmacotherapeutic approach to epilepsy can be reduced to three basic questions: (1) whether or not to treat, (2) with what to treat, and (3) when to stop treatment. Given that only 5 to 10 percent at most of all head injury victims will develop epilepsy, one can ask whether it is reasonable to expose the other 90 to 95 percent to the expense and risks of antiepileptic drug therapy prophylactically. Also, one can ask whether there is any evidence that prophylactic drug therapy will prevent the development of epilepsy in those who are susceptible. Animal models suggest that prophylactic antiepileptic drug treatment can be effective. Willmore and Triggs (1994) showed that, in rats injected with ferrous chloride, treatment with phenytoin lowered the risk of subsequent development of seizures. In another model (cobalt-induced experimental epilepsy in the cat) Rapport and Ojemann (1975) showed that prophylactic phenytoin prevented the development of seizures as well.

This experimental evidence has not translated as well to the human experience, however. A number of studies have been published investigating prophylactic antiepileptic drug therapy in head injury, most using phenytoin and some using phenobarbital. Some showed effectiveness of the prophylactic treatment (Servit and Musil, 1981; Wohns and Wyler,

1979; Young et al., 1975), and some did not (McQueen et al., 1983; Rish and Caveness, 1973; Young et al., 1983). These studies can all be faulted for relatively small numbers of patients, short follow-up periods, or inadequate medication levels. A large, well-controlled trial of prophylactic phenytoin was reported by Temkin et al. in 1990. They demonstrated that phenytoin was effective in reducing the number of early post-traumatic seizures (within the first week after injury) but was ineffective in preventing the development of late seizures. Current standards of treatment suggest that antiepileptic drug therapy may be used in the early phase after head injury in those patients most susceptible to the development of seizures (e.g., those with penetrating head wounds, intracranial hematomas, or prolonged unconsciousness), but that such therapy can be withheld in the long run until the clear development of epilepsy (i.e., more than one seizure without acute precipitant).

These recommendations may change in the near future as the possible role of so-called neuroprotectant therapy (e.g., free-radical scavengers, lipid peroxidase inhibitors, glutamate antagonists) is investigated. However, at present there are no data supporting the prophylactic treatment of mild head injury with anticonvulsant medications.

Once epilepsy has occurred in the post-traumatic setting, the treatment issues involved are no different than with epilepsy of any other cause. Treatment now becomes a task of preventing future seizures so as to reduce the morbidity (and rare mortality) that can accompany them. Issues unique to the individual patient, such as job and lifestyle considerations, medication cost, and compliance with a daily medication regimen, must be considered when initiating therapy, but several general guidelines are helpful:

Verify the diagnosis. To as great a degree as possible, make sure epilepsy is the correct diagnosis. Nonepileptic conditions will not respond to antiepileptic drugs.

Choose a drug known to be effective for that patient's seizure type(s). Different drugs are effective against different types of seizures (see Table 11-7).

Use one drug (monotherapy) whenever possible. Exhaust all reasonable monotherapy possibilities before using polytherapy.

Use that dose of medication which controls the seizures but does not produce excessive side effects. This "therapeutic window" may be very narrow (or nonexistent) for some medications in some patients. For dosing guidelines, see Table 11-8.

Use plasma drug levels as guidelines. Realize, however, that some patients will experience control of seizures at or below the "low" end of the range, while others may require levels at or above the "high" end and yet not have side effects.

Details of pharmacotherapy of epilepsy have been reviewed by Scheuer and Pedley (1990).

When to stop therapy is another important issue. As Table 11-4 demonstrates, up to half of patients with post-traumatic epilepsy may go into remission over a period of several years. In general, when a person's seizures have not recurred for several years, it is reasonable to consider a trial without the drug. Data that may carry a favorable prognosis include young age at onset of seizures, low total number of seizures, normal neurologic examination, normal EEG, and absence of a definable cause (Callaghan et al., 1988; Pedley, 1988; Shinnar et al., 1985). Overall relapse rates in epilepsy are in the range of 30 percent (Pedley, 1988) but have not been specifically studied in post-traumatic epilepsy patients.

Surgical Therapy

Patients with medically uncontrolled seizures are potential candidates for epilepsy surgery provided that the origin of the seizures can be precisely localized and that the focus can be removed without untoward risk of permanent neurologic impairment. The presurgical evaluation, surgical procedures, and outcome measurements are detailed in a number of texts (Engel, 1993; Wyler and Hermann, 1994) and will not be repeated here. Epilepsy surgery in the post-traumatic setting may be more difficult, as a region rather than a discrete focus of epileptic abnormality is likely to exist or multiple independent epileptic foci may be present (David et al., 1970). Also, surgical outcome is best in the setting of epilepsy of mesial temporal onset. However, post-traumatic epilepsy is often of extratemporal origin arising, for example, from the frontal or parietal lobe (Payan et al., 1970). Still, a fair number of medically refractory post-traumatic epilepsy patients may experience relief of their seizures with surgery.

PROGNOSIS

Morbidity and Mortality

The potential for physical and emotional consequences of epilepsy drives our desire to treat the condition. Depending on the setting of their occur-

TABLE 11-7. Summary of First- and Second-Line Antiepileptic Drugs for Various Seizure Types

Type of Seizure	First-Line Drugs	Second-Line Drugs
Simple and complex partial	Phenytoin, carbamazepine, felbamate[a]	Valproic acid, gabapentin,[b] phenobarbital, primidone, lamotrigine[b]
Partial with secondary generalization	Phenytoin, carbamazepine, felbamate,[a] valproic acid	Gabapentin,[b] phenobarbital, primidone, lamotrigine[b]
Primary generalized seizures		
Tonic-clonic	Valproic acid, phenytoin, carbamazepine	Felbamate,[a] phenobarbital
Absence	Ethosoximide, valproic acid	
Myoclonic	Valproic acid	Felbamate[a]
Atonic	Valproic acid, felbamate[a]	

[a] Owing to reports of aplastic anemia associated with felbamate, the Food and Drug Administration and Wallace Laboratories (the manufacturer) advised in August 1994 that its use be suspended. The status of felbamate is currently uncertain.

[b] Monotherapy trials of gabapentin and lamotrigine in partial seizures are underway, and they may soon be considered first-line therapy in these types.

rence, seizures place the individual at risk for falls, burns, drowning, lacerations, and more. Automobile accident rates in people with epilepsy are slightly higher than in the general population (Hansotia and Broste, 1991) although still lower than for teenage male drivers. Subgroups of patients with epilepsy including those with recent or frequent seizures, may be at greater risk for vehicular accidents. This risk forms the basis for laws, which vary from state to state, amending a person's driving privileges until seizure-free for a specified time (usually 3 to 6 months). Epilepsy carries a risk of status epilepticus, which occurs in 1.3 to 16 percent of people with epilepsy at some time during their life (Delgado-Escueta et al., 1990). Staus epilepticus is associated with a significant risk of mortality, which was found to be 23.3 percent in the recent series of Towne et al (1994). A syndrome of sudden unexplained death has been recognized in people with epilepsy, with an estimated annual incidence of 1 to 2 per 1,000, which is probably re-

TABLE 11-8. Antiepileptic Drugs and Their Properties

Drug	Brand Name	Usual Daily Adult Dose (mg)	Therapeutic Serum Concentration (μg/ml)[a]	Toxicity[b]
Carbamazepine	Tegretol	400–1,600	4–12	Drowsiness, diplopia, ataxia, pancytopenia, hyponatremia, hepatic dysfunction
Felbamate	Felbatol	1,200–3,600	[c]	Aplastic anemia,[d] insomnia, weight loss, headache, nausea, dizziness
Gabapentin	Neurontin	900–2,400	[c]	Somnolence
Lamotrigine	Lamictal	300–500[e]	[c]	Dizziness, ataxia, somnolence, headache, diplopia, blurred vision, nausea, vomiting
Phenobarbital	Phenobarbital	60–200	10–30	Sedation, irritability, memory trouble, loss of concentration
Phenytoin	Dilantin	300–400	10–20	Drowsiness, ataxia, gingival hyperplasia, hirsutism, pancytopenia, hepatic dysfunction
Valproic acid	Depakote, Depakene	1,000–3,000	50–100	Nausea, weight gain, tremor, hepatic dysfunction, thrombocytopenia

[a] Reference values of the University of Iowa Hospitals and Clinics. Values will vary slightly for other laboratories.

[b] Lists are not all-inclusive. Other side effects may be encountered. All antiepileptic drugs have the potential to cause rash.

[c] Therapeutic range has not yet been clearly established.

[d] Owing to reports of aplastic anemia associated with felbamate, the Food and Drug Administration and Wallace Laboratories (the manufacturer) advised in August 1994 that its use be suspended. Its status is currently uncertain.

[e] A more gradual titration and lower target dose of lamotrigine are recommended in patients concomitantly taking valproic acid.

lated to a seizure triggering a lethal cardiac arrhythmia (Dasheiff, 1991). Medication noncompliance may be a risk factor.

Life expectancy has been shown to be significantly shorter in persons with head injuries as compared with the general population (Walker et al., 1971) and even shorter in those with post-traumatic epilepsy (Walker and Blumer, 1989). However, these studies were drawn from populations with military injuries and therefore may not accurately reflect the civilian head injury population.

Remission of Symptoms

Remission of PTE was briefly discussed earlier in the chapter. Considering all epilepsies, it is estimated that 70 to 80 percent of patients will eventually achieve remission (Sander, 1993). The approximately 50 percent remission rate in post-traumatic epilepsy is lower, probably because of chronic structural brain changes associated with moderate and severe head injuries. Prognostic factors have been reported in several series of post-traumatic cases (Caveness, 1963; Walker and Erculei, 1970; Weiss and Caveness, 1972). A greater number of seizures suggests a poor prognosis. About half of those who will remit will do so within 3 years of the injury. If seizures are continuing 5 to 8 years after the injury, they are unlikely to ever remit.

CONCLUSIONS

Head injury is the leading cause of acquired epilepsy in teenagers and young adults. Post-traumatic epilepsy can be divided into early and late forms, the major risk factor for each being the severity of head injury. PTE is least likely to occur after a mild head injury and may be no more likely in this group than in the general population. Recognition of other conditions that can mimic epilepsy is crucial, as treatment strategies and prognosis will differ. The evaluation and treatment of post-traumatic epilepsy parallels that of epilepsy in general. Prognosis of epilepsy after traumatic brain injury is variable. Precise favorable prognostic factors are not known for post-traumatic cases but based on series of general epilepsy cases may include a low total number of seizures, a normal neurologic examination, and a normal EEG. Some patients may achieve remission. In the near future novel preventive strategies, including inhibition of excitatory amino acid neurotransmitters and free-radical production, may be used.

REFERENCES

American Electroencephalographic Society Guideline Twelve: guidelines for long-term monitoring for epilepsy. J Clin Neurophysiol 11:88–110, 1994

Annegers JF: The epidemiology of epilepsy. p. 161. In Wyllie E (ed): The Treatment of Epilepsy: Principles and Practice. Lea & Febiger, Philadelphia, 1993

Annegers JF, Grabow JD, Groover RV et al: Seizures after head trauma: a population study. Neurology 30:683–689, 1980

Black P, Shepard RH, Walker AE: Outcome of head trauma: age and post-traumatic seizures. Proc Ciba Found Symp 34:215-216, 1975

Bullock R, Maxwell WL, Graham DI et al: Glial swelling following human cerebral contusion: an ultrastructural study. J Neurol Neurosurg Psychiatry 54:427–434, 1991

Callaghan N, Garrett A, Goggin T: Withdrawal of anticonvulsant drugs in patients free of seizures for two years. N Engl J Med 318:942–946, 1988

Cavazos JE, Golarai G, Sutula TP: Mossy fiber synaptic reorganization induced by kindling: time course of development, progression, and permanence. J Neurosci 11:2795–2803, 1991

Cavazos JE, Sutula TP: Progressive neuronal loss induced by kindling: a possible mechanism for mossy fiber synaptic reorganization and hippocampal sclerosis. Brain Res 527:1–6, 1990

Caveness WF: Onset and cessation of fits following craniocerebral trauma. J Neurosurg 20:570–583, 1963

Caveness WF, Meirowsky AM, Rish BL et al: The nature of posttraumatic epilepsy. J Neurosurg 50:545–553, 1979

Commission on Classification and Terminology of the International League Against Epilepsy. Proposal for revised clinical and electroencephalographic classification of epileptic seizures. Epilepsia 22:489–501, 1981

Commission on Classification and Terminology of the International League Against Epilepsy. Proposal for revised classification of epilepsies and epileptic syndromes. Epilepsia 30:389–399, 1989

Courjon J: A longitudinal electro-clinical study of 80 cases of post-traumatic epilepsy observed from the time of the original trauma. Epilepsia 11:29–36, 1970

D'Alessandro R, Ferrara R, Benassi G et al. Computed tomographic scans in posttraumatic epilepsy. Arch Neurol 45:42–43, 1988

D'Alessandro R, Tinuper P, Ferrara R et al. CT scan prediction of late post-traumatic epilepsy. J Neurol Neurosurg Psychiatry 45:1153–1155, 1982

Dasheiff RM: Sudden unexpected death in epilepsy: a series from an epilepsy surgery program and speculation on the relationship to sudden cardiac death. J Clin Neurophysiol 8:216–222, 1992

David M, Talairach J, Bancaud J: Post-traumatic epilepsies of multiple cortical origin. Epilepsia 11:49–58, 1970

Delgado-Escueta AV, Schwartz B, Abad-Herrera P: Status epilepticus. p. 251. In Dam M, Gram L (eds): Comprehensive Epileptology. Raven Press, New York, 1990

Engel J (ed): Surgical Treatment of the Epilepsies 2nd Ed. Raven Press, New York, 1993

Goddard GV, McIntyre DC, Leech CK: A permanent change in brain function resulting from daily electrical stimulation. Exp Neurol 25:295–330, 1969

Grand W: The significance of post-traumatic status epilepticus in childhood. J Neurol Neurosurg Psychiatry 37:178–180, 1974

Hansotia P, Broste SK: The effect of epilepsy or diabetes mellitus on the risk of automobile accidents. N Engl J Med 324:22–26, 1991

Hughes JR: Post-traumatic epilepsy in the military. Milit Med 151:416–419, 1986

Jawahar G, Peria-Thambi T, Natarajan M: Experience in post-traumatic early epilepsy. J Indian Assoc 83:199–202, 1985

Jennett, B: Trauma as a cause of epilepsy in childhood. Dev Med Child Neurol 15:56–62, 1973a

Jennett B: Epilepsy after non-missile head injuries. Scot Med J 18:8–13, 1973b

Jennett B: Early traumatic epilepsy: incidence and significance after nonmissile injuries. Arch Neurol 30:394–398, 1974

Jennett B, van de Sande J: EEG prediction of post-traumatic epilepsy. Epilepsia 16:251–256, 1975

Jennett WB, Lewin W: Traumatic epilepsy after closed head injuries. J Neurol Neurosurg Psychiat 23:295–301, 1960

Masquin A, Courjon J: Prognostic factors in posttraumatic epilepsy. Epilepsia 4:285–297, 1963

McQueen JK, Blackwood DHR, Harris P et al: Low risk of late post-traumatic seizures following severe head injury: implications for clinical trials of prophylaxis. J Neurol Neurosurg Psychiatry 46:899–904, 1983

Mendelow AD, Teasdale GM: Pathophysiology of head injuries. Br J Surg 70:641–650, 1983

Nuutila A, Huusko S: Epilepsy among brain-injured veterans 26 to 31 years following the injury. Scand J Rehabil Med 4:81–84, 1972

Payan H, Toga M, Berard-Badier M: The pathology of post-traumatic epilepsies. Epilepsia 11:81–94, 1970

Pedley TA: Discontinuing antiepileptic drugs. N Engl J Med 318:982–984, 1988

Rapport RL III, Ojemann GA: Prophylactically administered phenytoin. Arch Neurol 32:539–548, 1975

Reisner T, Zeiler K, Wessely P: The value of CT and EEG in cases of posttraumatic epilepsy. J Neurol 221:93–100, 1979

Rish BL, Caveness WF: Relation of prophylactic medication to the occurrence of early seizures following craniocerebral trauma. J Neurosurg 38:155–158, 1973

Rubin JJ, Willmore LJ: Prevention of iron-induced epileptiform discharges in rats by treatment with antiperoxidants. Exp Neurol 67:472–480, 1980

Salazar AM, Jabbari B, Vance SC et al: Epilepsy after penetrating head injury. I. Clinical correlates: a report of the Vietnam head injury study. Neurology 35:1406–1414, 1985

Sander JWA: Some aspects of prognosis in the epilepsies: a review. Epilepsia 34:1007–1016, 1993

Saygi S, Katz A, Marks DA, Spencer SS: Frontal lobe partial seizures and psychogenic seizures: comparison of clinical and ictal characteristics. Neurology 42:1274–1277, 1992

Scheuer ML, Pedley TA: The evaluation and treatment of seizures. N Engl J Med 323:1468–1473, 1990

Sérvit Z, Musil F: Prophylactic treatment of posttraumatic epilepsy: results of a long-term follow-up in Czechoslovakia. Epilepsia 22:315–320, 1981

Shinnar S, Vining EPG, Mellits ED et al: Discontinuing antiepileptic medication in children with epilepsy after two years without seizures. N Engl J Med 313:976–980, 1985

Strich SJ: Diffuse degeneration of the cerebral white matter in severe dementia following head injury. J Neurol Neurosurg Psychiatry 19:163–185, 1956

Sutula T, Cascino G, Cavazos J et al: Mossy fiber synaptic reorganization in the epileptic human temporal lobe. Ann Neurol 26:321–330, 1989

Sutula T, Cavazos J, Golarai G: Alteration of long-lasting structural and functional effects of kainic acid in the hippocampus by brief treatment with phenobarbital. J Neurosci 12:4173–4187, 1992

Temkin NR, Dikmen SS, Wilensky AJ et al: A randomized, double-blind study of phenytoin for the prevention of post-traumatic seizures. N Engl J Med 323:497–502, 1990

Temkin O: The falling sickness: A History of Epilepsy from the Greeks to the Beginnings of Modern Neurology. (2nd Ed.) Johns Hopkins University Press, Baltimore

Towne AR, Pellock JM, Ko D, DeLorenzo RJ: Determinants of mortality in status epilepticus. Epilepsia 35:27–34, 1994

Wada JA: The clinical relevance of kindling: species, brain sites and seizure susceptibility. pp. 369–386. In Livingston KE, Hornykiewicz O (eds): Limbic Mechanisms: the Continuing Evolution of the Limbic System Concept. Plenum Press, New York, 1976

Walker AE, Blumer D: The fate of World War II veterans with posttraumatic seizures. Arch Neurol 46:23–26, 1989

Walker AE, Erculei F: Post-traumatic epilepsy 15 years later. Epilepsia 11:17–26, 1970

Walker AE, Jablon S: A follow-up of head-injured men of World War II. Harvey Cushing Society Meeting, Washington, Apr. 1958

Walker AE, Leuchs HK, Lechtape-Gruter H et al: Life expectancy of head injured men with and without epilepsy. Arch Neurol 24:95–100, 1971

Weiss GH, Caveness WF: Prognostic factors in the persistence of posttraumatic epilepsy. J Neurosurg 37: 164–169, 1972

Weiss GH, Feeney DM, Caveness WF et al: Prognostic factors for the occurrence of posttraumatic epilepsy. Arch Neurol 40:7–10, 1983

Willmore LJ: Post-traumatic epilepsy: cellular mechanisms and implications for treatment. Epilepsia suppl. 3 31:S67–S73, 1990

Willmore LJ, Rubin JJ: Effects of antiperoxidants on $FeCl_2$-induced lipid peroxidation and focal edema in rat brain. Exp Neurol 83:62–70, 1984

Willmore LJ, Sypert GW, Munson JB: Recurrent seizures induced by cortical iron injection: a model of posttraumatic epilepsy. Ann Neurol 4:329–336, 1978

Willmore LJ, Triggs WJ: Effect of phenytoin and corticosteroids on seizures and lipid peroxidation in experimental posttraumatic epilepsy. J Neurosurg 60:467–472, 1984

Wohns RNW, Wyler AR: Prophylactic phenytoin in severe head injuries. J Neurosurg 51:507–509, 1970

Wyler AR, Hermann BP (eds): The Surgical Management of Epilepsy. Butterworth-Heinemann, Boston, 1994

Young B, Rapp R, Brooks WH et al: Posttraumatic epilepsy prophylaxis. Epilepsia 20:671–681, 1979

Young B, Rapp RP, Norton JA et al: Failure of prophylactically administered phenytoin to prevent early posttraumatic seizures. J Neurosurg 58:231–235, 1983

Young B, Rapp RP, Perrier D et al: Early post-traumatic epilepsy prophylaxis. Surg Neurol 4:339–342, 1975

Nonepileptic Events 12

John R. Gates
Mark A. Granner

Paroxysmal alterations of behavior or consciousness can occur in many different conditions and often pose a diagnostic challenge to the clinician. When the troublesome events occur in the setting of trauma, the diagnosis of post-traumatic epilepsy is seductively available. Epilepsy is indeed a significant consequence in some trauma cases, but it is not expected in cases of mild traumatic brain injury (TBI) (see Chapter 11). When the latter patients present with unusual events, nonepileptic etiologies should be strongly considered.

The prevalence of paroxysmal nonepileptic events is not well defined. Scott (1982) has estimated this as 5 percent of an outpatient epilepsy population, although some estimates are much higher. At the Minnesota Epilepsy group in St. Paul, where there are over 500 admissions processed annually in the pediatric and adult inpatient units, approximately 15 to 20 percent of the referred patients with medically refractory events have nonepileptic events. Further confounding the problem, some individuals have both nonepileptic and epileptic events, although the estimates of this association vary widely from 10 to 58 percent. (Desai et al., 1982; Gates et al., 1985; Lesser, 1985; Trimble, 1986). Unfortunately, there is no study clearly documenting the prevalence of nonepileptic events in patients with a history of head trauma or TBI.

HISTORY AND TERMINOLOGY

Historical descriptions of epilepsy and hysteria have often been closely intertwined (Trimble, 1986). In his Diseases of Women, Hippocrates distinguished between the clinical presentation of a nonepileptic event and epilepsy, the "sacred disease" (Tempkin, 1945). So did Ariatus, who divided epilepsy into ordinary and hysterical varieties (Wayne-Massey, 1982). These early Greek writers emphasized the uterine and therefore presumably feminine relationship with hysteria.

In 1684 Willis moved the origin of hysteria from the abdomen to the brain, thus clouding the distinction between epileptic and nonepileptic pathophysiology.

In the eighteenth and nineteenth centuries the French introduced the term *hysterical epilepsy,* implying a clear link between hysteria and epilepsy (Trimble, 1986). Briquet and later Charcot believed that hysterical epilepsy with mixed attacks was a form of hysteria, but others continued to raise the question of an intermediate disorder. Gower (1881), in a classic monograph, also emphasized the difference between the seizures of epilepsy and those of hysteria. In subsequent years most authors have been in strong agreement with Gower, and many have gone on to formulate tables of differential diagnoses to illustrate differences between those disorders (Trimble, 1986). The clinical recognition of these differences has displaced the treatment of epilepsy almost entirely into neurologic practice and the treatment of hysteria into psychiatry. This has led to practical difficulties in treating difficult cases that fall at the borderline between the two specialties.

As a consequence, a number of curious terms have been developed, of which two of the most popular are *pseudoseizure* and *pseudoepileptic seizure.* According to Gates and Erdahl (1993), these terms carry a pejorative connotation, implying that any seizure of nonepileptic origin constitutes a condition unrelated to true illness. The term *nonepileptic event* is less likely to alienate patients and their families and has been used to identify the disorders described in this chapter. Figure 12-1 shows the division of nonepileptic paroxysmal events into those of physiologic and psychogenic origin.

PHYSIOLOGIC NONEPILEPTIC EVENTS

Physiologic nonepileptic events include a broad spectrum of entities (Figure 12-2). Several of the possible etiologies are discussed in this section.

Syncope

Syncope is the nonepileptic physiologic event that is most often confused with epilepsy. As discussed by Andermann (1987), the mechanisms of syncope are quite diverse, ranging from cardiac arrhythmia to a simple vasovagal event (Aminoff et al., 1988; Driver and Selby, 1977; Fowler, 1984; Gastaut and Gastaut, 1958; Lai and Ziegler, 1983; Von Bernuth et al., 1982). The distinction of syncope from epilepsy is not trivial. For example, tonic and clonic movements of nonepileptic etiology can occur with syncope, and syncope can even produce seizures due to decreased cerebral perfusion. To further confound the clinician, seizures of temporal lobe origin may produce cardiac arrhythmias. Seizures most often result in sinus tachycardia, but profound bradycardia, and even cardiac asystole, have rarely been reported (Constantin et al. 1990). The prodrome of lightheadedness, clamminess, and sweatiness generally distinguishes vasovagal syncope from epilepsy. The distinction between syncope and seizure can be particularly difficult to make in children with apnea and breath-holding spells. However, the duration of the tonic or clonic phase in syncope is usually briefer, the tonic phase lasting only a few seconds, and there are usually only a couple of clonic jerks.

It can be difficult in the elderly to distinguish between syncope and epilepsy. For example, an elderly individual may sustain an unwitnessed event and afterward be found confused, on the floor. Syncope and seizures are both possible causes. The event may often reflect a complication of a pre-existing medical illness. For example, some patients with advanced diabetes may have an autonomic neuropathy. In these individuals prodromal symptomatology is often lacking, and the resultant paroxysm can be quite abrupt (Marble, 1985).

Paroxysmal Toxic Phenomena

Certain medications, for example hallucinatory agents such as atropine or illicit drugs, may produce abrupt behavioral changes that mimic the effects of epilepsy. Moreover, drugs such as cocaine, amphetamines, or alcohol are well known to cause seizures. Alcohol withdrawal seizures are not uncommon in

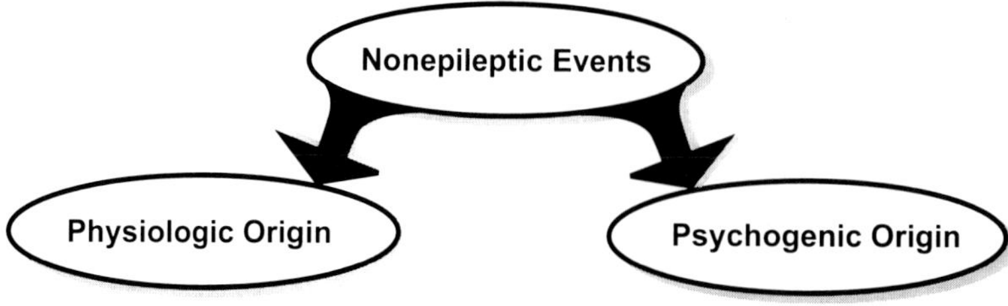

Fig. 12-1. The two distinct origins of nonepileptic paroxysmal events.

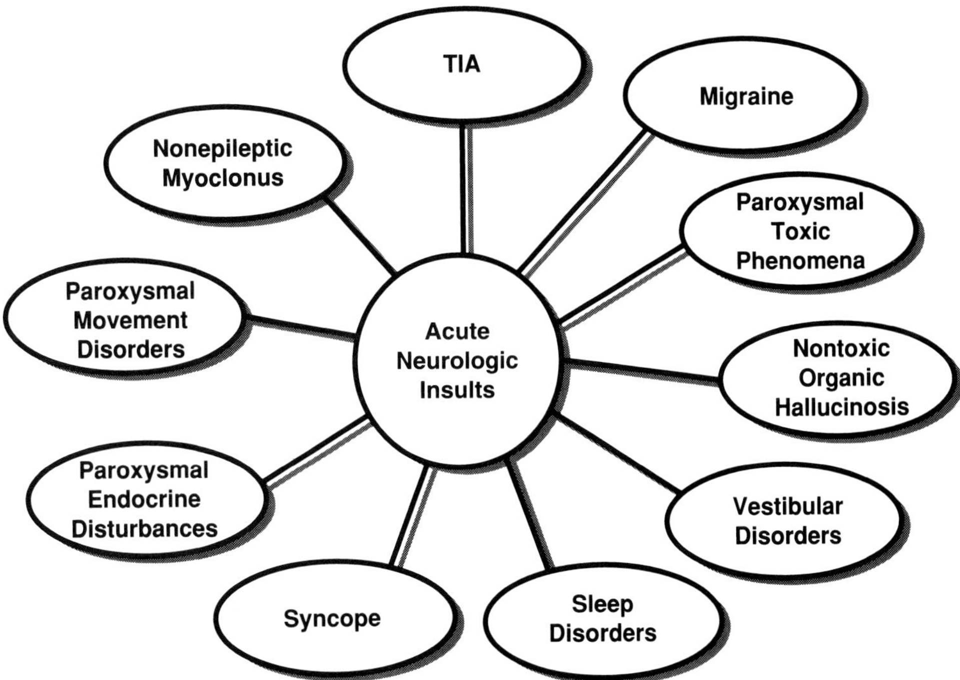

Fig. 12-2. Disorders that can be classified as physiologic nonepileptic events.

the 24 to 72 hours after cessation of alcohol abuse. Alcoholic hallucinosis or delirium tremens can also occur in the same time frame, and both of these conditions can be confused with complex partial epilepsy (Baker, 1994).

Sensory Deprivation

Nontoxic organic hallucinosis due to advanced sensory deprivation also must be kept in mind. Consider the older person with bilateral cataracts, hearing loss, neuropathy, or mild cognitive impairment. Such patients may experience paroxysmal phenomena, including formed visual hallucinations or fleeting dysesthesias, which could be confused with epilepsy. In these cases the past medical history and physical findings are often diagnostic. When the diagnosis remains uncertain, an electroencephalographic (EEG) recording during the clinical event may be helpful. It is important, however, not to be misled by the presence of sharp waves on the EEG, which are often seen in the absence of epileptic seizures (Doane et al., 1959; Heron et al., 1956; Heron, 1961).

Nonepileptic Myoclonus

Nonepileptic myoclonus must be distinguished from myoclonic seizures. A large spectrum of myoclonic disorders exist, with no uniform consensus on their classification (Marseille Consensus Statement, 1990; Przutek and Muhr, 1983). Myoclonus may be categorized anatomically as arising from the spinal cord, brainstem, diencephalon, or cerebral cortex. Myoclonus of cortical origin is generally considered to be epileptic while that of subcortical origin is not. The presence of epileptiform EEG abnormalities, occurring in synchronous fashion with the myoclonic jerks, is the signature of cortical origin.

Myoclonic epilepsy is generally inherited. When myoclonus arises in the setting of TBI, the injury is usually severe and associated with cerebral anoxia. Myoclonic seizures may respond to benzodiazepines or valproic acid. Subcortical myoclonus is often treated with the same drugs. Some myoclonic activity, such as sleep myoclonus, is normal and does not require treatment. Distinguishing between physiologic myoclonus and abrupt movements originating from a psychological condition is also critical, since the latter require very different treatment.

Sleep Disorders

Importantly, sleep disorders may be confused with epilepsy and in the setting of trauma might be confused with post-traumatic seizures. Three conditions deserve special comment. Night terrors (pavor nocturnus) occur in children and are often confused with epilepsy, as the child is usually unresponsive during the event. REM (rapid eye movement) behavior disorder is an uncommon disorder seen in middle-aged to elderly men. The hypothetical cause is a lack of motor inhibition, which supposedly allows these patients to act out their dreams. Lugaresi et al. (1986) have drawn attention to the paroxysmal nocturnal dystonias. These attacks are frequently stereotyped and often awaken the patient. When epilepsy coexists, this can confuse the picture. Some patients apparently also respond to carbamazepine or phenytoin. There are many other kinds of sleep disorders (see Ch. 14 for discussion of those related to TBI).

Paroxysmal Movement Disorders

Paroxysmal movement disorders can also be confused with epilepsy. Paroxysmal kinesigenic choreoathetosis is a dominantly inherited disorder in which the attacks are triggered by movement. The disorder responds to antiepileptic medications (Kertesz, 1967). Paroxysmal dystonia may also be a dominantly inherited disorder (Lance, 1977). The attacks generally last longer than those of paroxysmal kinesigenic choreoathetosis but unfortunately do not respond to antiepileptic drugs. Paroxysmal ataxia, a condition associated with perinatal encephalopathy (Vaamonde et al., 1990) also does not respond to drugs. The attacks in this condition may last minutes to hours. Multiple sclerosis can produce painful paroxysmal tonic spasms, which can be mistaken for epilepsy. Epileptic seizures may occur in multiple sclerosis patients but are not common (Matthews, 1958).

Transient Ischemic Attacks

Importantly, transient ischemic attacks (TIAs) can be confused with epilepsy. TIAs, however, tend to produce negative phenomena such as weakness, whereas epilepsy tends to produce positive phenomena such as muscle jerking. In practice, however, the distinction may be difficult. For example, dysesthesias due to ischemia of the primary sensory cortex can resemble a primary somatosensory seizure. Similarly, aphasia due to transient ischemia to Broca's or Wernicke's areas may resemble ictal or postictal aphasia. TIAs are most commonly seen in patients with cardiac disease and atherosclerosis. However, a TIA might occur in patients with head or neck trauma as a result of injury to the carotid or vertebral arteries, causing an arterial dissection.

An EEG evaluation can provide helpful information in the acute setting to help distinguish between a TIA and a seizure. A TIA may cause focal slowing on the EEG, even in the absence of a structural abnormality on computed tomography (CT) or magnetic resonance imaging (MRI). The location of the slowing depends on the arterial territory involved. This slowing often persists for several hours in TIA, a duration that generally exceeds the period for postictal slowing following an epileptic seizure. Obviously, if a paroxysm of epileptiform discharges is observed, the diagnosis of epilepsy is more likely. It should be kept in mind, however, that acute cerebral ischemia such as may occur with cortical emboli can produce a seizure.

Migraine

Migrainous phenomena are sometimes difficult to differentiate from epileptic events (Andermann, 1987; Andermann and Andermann, 1987). For example, migrainous and epileptic auras may include similar visual symptoms, such as scintillating lights. Similarly, basilar migraines may produce transient amnesia, which might be confused with the ictal or postictal state in complex partial seizures. Also, migraine and epilepsy are relatively common conditions and occasionally coexist in the same patient. (See Ch. 8 for discussion of post-traumatic migraine.)

Vestibular Disorders

Vestibular dysfunction can produce paroxysmal symptoms, including dizziness, vertigo, and lightheadedness. Furthermore, vestibular dysfunction can be caused by a concussion of the inner ear in head trauma cases (see Ch. 9). The symptoms may be misinterpreted as being of cerebral origin and misdiagnosed as simple partial or complex partial seizures. A key distinction is that vestibular symptoms and signs are often triggered by movements such as rolling over in bed, turning the head, or traveling in a car. Barany maneuvers may replicate the patient's symptoms and produce nystagmus, which is often rotatory in nature. Electronystagmography is also helpful. Post-traumatic seizures are generally not triggered by movement.

Acute Neurologic Insults

Very often in the setting of acute neurologic insults such as encephalitis or acute head injury, paroxysmal phenomena occur which can be misinterpreted as epilepsy. For example, decortication or decerebration, especially when associated with muscle rippling, can often be misinterpreted as an epileptic phenomena. Similarly, motor neuron release phenomena such as jaw, arm or leg clonus have been misinterpreted as epileptic by clinicians. Some neurologic conditions may even resemble a prolonged seizure state. For example, encephalitis patients sometimes have paroxysmal behavioral alternations that can be confused with nonconvulsive status epilepticus, which is, of course, a possible sequela of their condition. Careful interpretation of the neurologic examination and EEG record are essential to proper diagnosis in these cases.

Paroxysmal Manifestations of Endocrine Disturbances

Conditions such as pheochromocytoma or carcinoid syndrome can produce sudden onset of symptoms as in epilepsy. These endocrine disorders should be considered in patients with episodes of sudden flushing or rapid heart rate. Diabetes can result in hyperosmolar nonketotic hyperglycemia and produce focal neurologic dysfunction or seizures.

PSYCHOGENIC NONEPILEPTIC EVENTS

Psychogenic nonepileptic events comprise a heterogeneous group of disorders (Fig. 12-3) that may occur in patients with TBI. In this chapter DSM-IV categories (with their classification numbers) have been used to define these disorders (American Psychiatric Association, 1994).

Conversion Disorders

The largest group of patients within the psychogenic nonepileptic seizure category are those with conversion disorders (300.11). The symptoms in these patients may mimic the effects of brain trauma. For example, the classic Briquet patient may present with apparent hemiparesis of the nondominant side or paroxysmal episodes mimicking tonic-clonic seizures. According to DSM (Diagnostic and Statistical Manual of Mental Disorders)-IV, conflicts or other stressors are important triggers in such cases. The complications of systemic medical disease, adverse drug effects, culturally sanctioned behavior, and malingering must be excluded. Finally, the patient's symptoms or deficits should cause significant distress or impairment in social or occupational functioning.

Conversion disorders are more common in women than in men, especially younger to middle-aged women. One possible precipitant is sexual abuse (Rowan and Gates, 1993), and another is the death of a loved one. For example, the patient with a conversion disorder may have been a passenger in a car crash in which his or her spouse was killed. The time elapsed between the precipitation and presentation is often several years. Video-EEG may provide confirmation of nonepileptic events and further support the diagnosis of conversion disorder. Psychotherapy may be required before any underlying stressors or abuse is revealed.

Factitious Disorders

Conversion disorders must be distinguished from factitious disorders (300.19). Individuals with-a factitious disorder focus on being admitted to the hospital by feigning a variety of medical complaints. They may intentionally produce neurologic complaints resembling post-traumatic seizures.

The Munchausen-by-proxy syndrome can be construed as a factitious disorder. In this syndrome a parent exhibits psychopathology and creates difficulty by producing the symptoms or signs of a disease such as post-traumatic epilepsy in a child. Once this diagnosis is made, the inappropriate antiepileptic medications can be removed and the child will generally remain episode-free (Rowan and Gates, 1993). Unfortunately, this diagnosis can create turmoil in an already troubled family. Social services have to be on alert, and the child must sometimes be protected from the injurious parent.

Malingering

Malingering (V65.2) may also result in paroxysmal events that resemble post-traumatic seizures and should be distinguished from a conversion disorder. Malingering is the intentional production of false or grossly exaggerated physical or psychological symptoms motivated by external incentives such as "avoiding military duty, avoiding work, obtaining financial

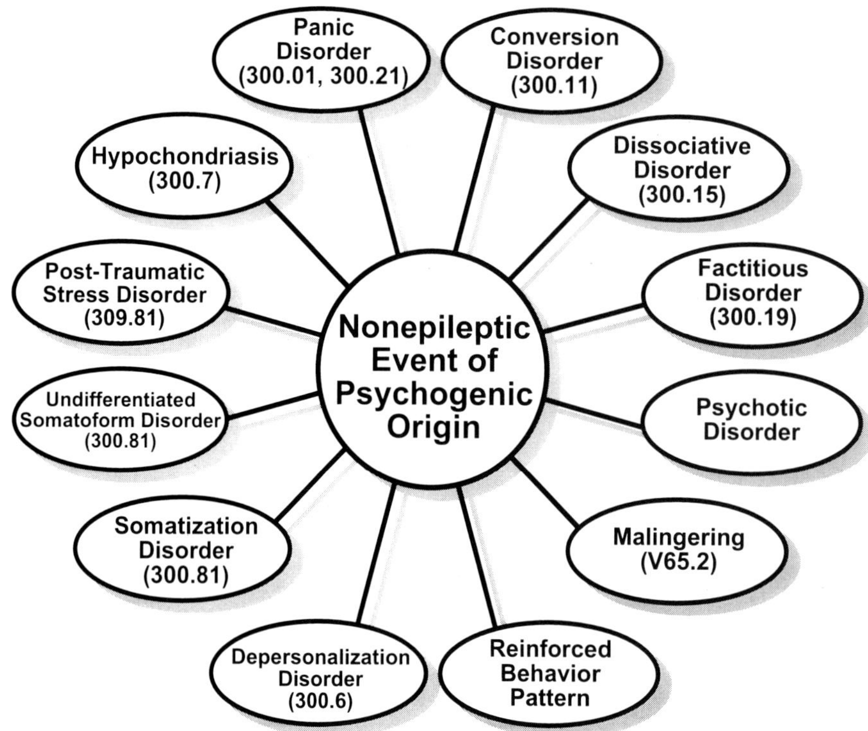

Fig. 12-3. Disorders that can be classified as psychogenic nonepileptic events.

compensation, evading criminal prosecution, or obtaining drugs'' (American Psychiatric Association, 1994) (see also Ch. 25).

Reinforced Behavior Pattern

A disorder that has eluded DSM classification to date is the reinforced behavior pattern observed in cognitively impaired individuals (Rowan and Gates, 1993; Savard et al., 1988). This condition has features of a factitious disorder (not otherwise specified, 300.19) in that patients appear to place themselves voluntarily in the sick role for secondary gain. The difference is that cognitively impaired individuals may not consciously appreciate the cause-effect relationship between the symptoms and the secondary gain. Some patients have pre-existing epilepsy, which may even be post-traumatic in origin, while others have observed the response to seizures in themselves or others. They may have learned that a paroxysmal event is a marvelous attention-getting device, which allows significant control over the environment. Behavior modification techniques should be employed with these patients.

Somatization and Somatoform Disorders

Somatization disorder and undifferentiated somatoform disorder (300.81) are also associated with paroxysmal events, which should not be confused with post-traumatic epilepsy. The hallmark of these disorders is multiple physical complaints that cannot be adequately explained by a general medical condition (American Psychiatric Association, 1994) despite a thorough investigation. The complaints should have been present for at least 6 months and not intentionally produced or feigned as in factitious or malingering disorders. Nonepileptic events are part of a larger picture, which includes a variety of other symptoms such as neurologic, cardiac, and gastrointestinal complaints. These patients require a step-by-step exhaustive diagnostic approach to address their presumed medical concerns.

Post-traumatic Stress Disorder

Patients with post-traumatic stress disorder (309.81) may experience a perceived threat of death or serious injury to themselves or others, along with a strong sense of fear, helplessness, or horror. Distressing and intrusive recollections may recur. Patients may even claim to be reliving their traumatic experience and act as if it were really happening. Although this might appear as a loss of awareness and compromised interaction with the environment, this is not epilepsy. The condition is overdiagnosed in the context of litigation (Lees-Haley, 1989; Rosen, 1995).

Hypochondriasis

Hypochondriasis (300.7) is a preoccupation with the idea that one has a serious disease and is due to misinterpretation of bodily sensations. This preoccupation persists despite normal medical evaluations. Patients may experience episodes of light headedness, tingling, or dizziness, which they believe are epileptic phenomena, despite multiple reassurances to the contrary. Patients who have hit their heads or been in a car crash may believe they have post-traumatic epilepsy. Very often these patients are anxious and depressed and have obsessive-compulsive personality traits. Psychosocial stressors may exacerbate the disorder as well.

Panic Disorder

Panic disorder with (300.21) or without (300.01) agoraphobia is characterized by recurrent, unexpected panic attacks. There may be persistent concern of future attacks and a significant change in lifestyle in response to these concerns. Panic disorder is not due to the effect of a drug, and other mental disorders must be excluded. It is also not an expected sequela of TBI. Symptoms include shortness of breath, a smothering sensation, dizziness, and feelings of depersonalization, derealization, or fear of being out of control. Any of these symptoms could be misinterpreted as a simple partial seizure.

Depersonalization Disorder

Depersonalization disorder (300.6) is characterized by the persistent or recurrent feeling of being detached from oneself. Mental functions, however, are intact. There is usually significant distress or impairment in social or occupational functioning. Depersonalization episodes may be misinterpreted as simple partial seizures.

Dissociative Disorder

Dissociative disorder (300.15) is characterized by a disruption in the usually integrated functions of consciousness, memory, identity, or perception of the environment (American Psychiatric Association, 1994). Some of the associated symptoms are distinctly non-neurologic, including confusion about one's identity in the face of a relatively clear sensorium or the assumption of a new identity. Because the disruption can occur quite suddenly, it might be misconstrued as epilepsy and in the setting of trauma as post-traumatic epilepsy. The differential diagnosis includes nonconvulsive status epilepticus.

MANAGEMENT OF NONEPILEPTIC EVENTS

The patient with nonepileptic seizures is often encountered in clinic with a history of unexplained paroxysmal events, which may include unresponsiveness, apparent involuntary limb movements, or subjective complaints such as dizziness, lightheadedness, tingling, word finding trouble, or memory lapses. An accurate history of the paroxysmal events is essential, as is a detailed history of any associated physical trauma. In difficult cases, video EEG monitoring can provide critical evidence to make the appropriate diagnosis. This study can be performed on an outpatient basis if the events are sufficiently frequent (Gates et al., 1991). If the events are relatively infrequent and the outpatient EEG tracing is equivocal, inpatient assessment may be needed. Our approach is exemplified in the following two case reports.

Case 1: Nonepileptic Physiologic Events

A 43-year-old man was referred for two episodes of sudden confusion, each lasting about 10 minutes. The first episode had occurred 2 months earlier and was poorly documented. In the second episode the man was talking to his wife on the telephone and was suddenly unable to produce the proper words. His wife thought he "was talking gibberish" and called for immediate medical assistance.

General medical and neurologic examinations were completely normal. The patient had struck his head on the windshield in a car crash 6 months earlier. He reportedly "saw stars" and had a small bruise over the left temple, but there was no loss of consciousness or amnesia and the patient did not seek medical attention. He had a mild headache that lasted for about 2 weeks, but this resolved and he returned to his job as a janitor within 3 days of the crash. The patient had a history of occasional headaches preceding the car crash. There was no history of epilepsy in the patient or his family. He drank alcohol on social occasions, did not smoke, and was not diabetic.

The patient had normal serum electrolytes, glucose, liver, and renal functions, vasculitis screen (antinuclear antibodies, rheumatoid factor, erythrocyte sedimentation rate), Lyme titers, VDRL (Venereal Disease Research Laboratory) and HIV (human immunodeficiency virus) tests. Magnetic resonance imaging (MRI) scan with T_1- and T_2-weighted images showed no evidence of a structural brain lesion. MRI angiography showed no abnormalities in the carotid, vertebral, or intracranial vessels. An electrocardiogram (ECG) showed nonspecific ST and T wave changes. Echocardiography showed no evidence of valvular disease or thrombus. However, the EEG was read as abnormal because of occasional right occipital spike discharges, suggesting a possible focal seizure tendency. His physician was impressed by the report and the trauma history and diagnosed him with post-traumatic seizures, which were then treated with phenytoin. Afterward, the patient reported drowsiness, irritability, unsteadiness, memory changes, a depressed mood, and trouble in performing his job. Neurologic referral was denied until a third episode occurred despite therapeutic anticonvulsant levels. Permission for further referral was finally obtained.

The patient was admitted for inpatient video EEG monitoring. Phenytoin was discontinued. On the second day the patient had one of his typical spells. This consisted of sudden onset of agrammatic speech, including neologisms, paraphasic errors, and difficulty in comprehending the instructions of the nurse. The corresponding EEG record showed slowing in the left hemisphere, prominent over the temporal area. However no ictal epileptiform activity was seen. These changes evolved over 20 minutes and were followed by a throbbing left-sided headache, photophobia, phonophobia, and nausea. A diagnosis of complicated migraine was made, and the patient was successfully treated with sumatriptan.

Discussion

This case illustrates several points. First, the patient gave an unimpressive history of brain trauma. Individuals with such a history are unlikely to develop post-traumatic seizures (see Ch. 11). Second, it is possible to have epileptiform EEG activity in the absence of epilepsy; migraine headaches have been associated with such tracings (Andermann and Andermann, 1987). Third, the inpatient video EEG can provide invaluable data to discriminate between epileptic and nonepileptic physiologic events, especially when the diagnosis is unclear. Such information may protect the patient from exposure to unnecessary drug treatment and its complications.

Case 2: Psychogenic Nonepileptic Events

A 44-year-old, right-handed, married woman was admitted for evaluation of paroxysmal episodes. At the age of 40 she was working on an assembly line when she fell backward and hit her occiput on a steel beam. She was dazed and had a laceration over the upper thoracic spine region. She complained of severe headaches for several days, as well as dizziness and stuttering speech. After the injury, the company physician examined her and diagnosed a mild concussion. On the next day she had an episode of apparent unresponsiveness and confusion, which lasted for several hours. She was evaluated by a neurologist, who discovered no abnormal findings on neurologic examination; EEG, MRI, and CT scans of the brain were normal. However, the patient persisted in having episodes. She was treated with carbamazepine, valproic acid, phenytoin, phenobarbital, chlorazepate, and diazepam without success over the next 4 years. She never returned to work.

At the time of referral, the patient was taking diazepam and valproic acid. She described three types of events. The first she described as her "quiet one." She would stare with a glazed look, drool, chew her lip, and not respond to command. She said she could hear people talking but not remember what was said. She denied urinary or fecal incontinence. These episodes could last for up to 15 minutes and their frequency ranged from weekly to daily. The second type of event was described as her "silent one." She would appear as if she were sleeping and not respond for 60 to 90 minutes. She had one or two of these episodes each week. The third event type was her "big one." These events began like her first episodes. However, the patient would also hit herself in the face with her right arm, claw her face with both hands, turn her head to the left, twist backward, and end up lying on her right side with her legs drawn up. These episodes were occurring on a daily to weekly basis and would tend to cluster, with four to nine events per cluster.

The patient was admitted, her medications were withdrawn, and video EEG was recorded for 7 consecutive days. She also received a comprehensive psychological and social assessment. All three types of her ictal events were captured on the video EEG for a total of 28 events. There was no evidence of an epileptiform EEG correlate for any event, which strongly militated against epilepsy. Similarly, serum prolactin levels, drawn following events of generalized motor activity or loss of consciousness, showed no elevation as compared with baseline interictal levels. Comprehensive psychological and neuropsychological evaluations, including personality and projective testing, strongly suggested a conversion disorder and depression.

The patient expressed surprise and disbelief at her diagnoses but appeared to accept the idea that these did not require antiepileptic drugs. With the support of her husband, she agreed to psychological therapy and counseling as a psychiatric inpatient. Discharge medications included desipramine 75 mg PO daily at bedtime, piroxicam 20 mg daily in the morning, and Premarin 1.25 mg daily in the morning. Two years later, she was having a rare nonepileptic event, and was still taking no antiepileptic drugs.

Discussion

Once the diagnosis of psychogenic nonepileptic events is made, referral to a psychiatrist, psychologist, or psychiatric social worker is often helpful. This team can function in coordination with the epileptologist for the treatment of inpatients. However, a multidisciplinary neuropsychiatric outpatient clinic would also be an appropriate setting. Particular attention should be paid to the possibility of depression (Gates et al., 1991). Anxiety disorders or personality disorders must also be considered. The treatment should be directed at the primary psychopathology (Glenn and Simonds, 1977; Linder, 1973). Specific stressors, reinforcers, antecedents, or consequences associated with the suspected nonepileptic event may be identified. If there is any question about the diagnosis, it is sometimes helpful for the patient's caregivers or family to view the videotaped events to decide if these are compatible with the episodes at issue. This is particularly important if suggestive techniques have been used in order to bring out the episodes. We prefer not to use such techniques since a breach of trust may result, which interferes with subsequent therapeutic interventions.

Serum prolactin levels can provide supporting evidence to discriminate between epileptic and nonepileptic events. Prolactin levels usually rise manyfold after epileptic seizures that impair consciousness, especially generalized tonic-clonic and complex partial seizures. The greatest diagnostic utility is gained if the prolactin level is determined within 15 minutes of the event, 4 hours after the event (to serve as a "postevent" baseline), and 24 hours after the event (to serve as a diurnal control). While a positive result (generally considered to be a threefold rise over diurnal control value) supports the diagnosis of epileptic seizures, one should be aware of false negative results, as prolactin levels will not rise after all seizures (Wyllie et al., 1984). Prolactin will not rise after syncope (Anzola, 1993) or nonepileptic psychogenic events (Trimble, 1978).

If patients prove to have mixed events (i.e., both epileptic and nonepileptic), these need to be clearly defined for the caregivers so that they know how to distinguish between episodes. The patient should also be clearly informed exactly why antiepileptic drugs are still being prescribed. In general, the events that precipitated the admission are nonepileptic, even if true epileptic seizures are ultimately uncovered upon reduction of medications during the diagnostic recording phase.

Some patients are relieved to have a definitive diagnosis of nonepileptic events while others react angrily. Consequently the diagnosis should be presented in a dignified way, with clear indication that there are many patients with similar problems. Patients should be reassured that the caregivers now understand the problem. Patients should be further encouraged by informing them that they will develop alternative coping skills that will make future nonepileptic events unnecessary. Patients will often exhibit an immediate decrease in the frequency of events.

PROGNOSIS OF NONEPILEPTIC EVENTS

The prognosis of nonepileptic physiologic events varies greatly as a function of the underlying physiologic etiology. There is a great deal of difference between the expected course of, for example, a fusiform aneurysm of the basilar artery and vasovagal syncope. With psychogenic nonepileptic events the results are also variable. Studies have reported favorable results in 25 to 87 percent of these patients (Doherty et al., 1993; Kristensen and Alving, 1992; Krumholz, 1983; Lancman et al., 1993; Lempert and Schmidt, 1990; Ljundberg, 1957; Meierkord et al., 1991; Ramani and Gumnit, 1982; Wyllie et al., 1991). Obviously the prognosis is a function of the natural history of the underlying psychopathology and the efficacy of current therapies. Another factor is the duration of the nonepileptic events, a shorter duration carrying a better prognosis (Gates et al., 1991).

CONCLUSION

Epilepsy is a sequela in some cases of TBI injury. However, it is not an expected sequela in cases of mild TBI. When the latter patients present with spells, nonepileptic etiologies should be strongly considered. Physiologic conditions that produce symptoms or signs resembling epilepsy include syncope, drug effects, migraine, and even normal sleep phenomena. Psychogenic nonepileptic events are associated with a heterogenous group of disorders that are classifiable by DSM IV criteria and include somatization disorder, conversion disorder, hypochondriasis, and malingering. The spells in these patients may represent a dysfunctional coping strategy or be motivated by secondary gain.

The diagnosis of nonepileptic events demands a thorough neurologic and medical evaluation and is sometimes difficult, especially if epileptic and nonepileptic events co-occur in the same patient. In difficult cases, a patient's events can be captured during prolonged video EEG recordings. Correlations of the simultaneous EEG and video records taken during the event provide the method of choice for determining the nature of the events in question. Serum prolactin levels can also be helpful.

Once the diagnosis is made, patients with physiologic nonepileptic events should receive the appropriate medical therapy. Those with psychogenic nonepileptic events can benefit from psychological counseling, termination of inappropriate antiepileptic drug therapy, and treatment of any possible underlying psychiatric condition. The prognosis depends on the underlying cause.

REFERENCES

American Psychiatric Association: Diagnostic and Statistical Manual of Mental Disorders. 4th Ed. American Psychiatric Association, Washington, 1994

Aminoff MJ, Scheiriman MM, Griffin JC, Herre JM: Electrocerebral accompaniments of syncope associated with malignant ventricular arrhythmias. Ann Intern Med 108:791–796, 1988

Andermann F: Clinical features of migraine-epilepsy syndromes. pp. 3–30. In Andermann F, Lugaresi E (eds): Migraine and Epilepsy. Butterworth (Publishers), Boston, 1987

Andermann E, Andermann F: Migraine-epilepsy relationships: epidemiological and genetic aspects. pp. 281–291. In Andermann F, Lugaresi E (eds): Migraine and Epilepsy. Butterworth (Publishers), Boston, 1987

Anzola GP: Predictivity of plasma prolactin levels in differentiating epilepsy from pseudoseizures: a prospective study. Epilepsia 34:1044–1048, 1993

Baker (ed): Clin Neurol 61:12–18, 1994

Constantin L, Martins JB, Fincham RW, Dagli RD: Bradycardia and syncope as manifestations of partial epilepsy. J Am Coll Cardiol 15:900–905, 1990

Desai BT, Porter RJ, Penry JK: Psychogenic seizures: a study of 42 attacks in six patients, with intense monitoring. Arch Neurol 39:202–209, 1982

Doane BK, Mahatoo W, Heron W, Scott TH: Changes in perceptual function after isolation. Can J Psychol 13:210–219, 1959

Doherty K, Mason S, Gates J: Psychogenic seizures (pseudoseizures), prognosis after inpatient evaluation. Epilepsia suppl. 6, 34:26, 1993

Driver MV, Selby PJ: Apparent epilepsy due to intermittent ventricular tachyarrthymia (Romano-Ward syndrome). Electroencephalogr Clin Neurophysiol 43:289, 1977

Fowler HL: Stokes-Adams attacks masquerading as epilepsy, case reports. Milit Med 149:680–681, 1984

Gastaut H, Gastaut Y: Etude electroencephalographique et clinique des convulsions anoxiques de l'enfant, leur situation dans le cadre des convulsions infantiles. Rev Neurol (Paris) 99:100–125, 1958

Gates JR, Erdahl P: Classification of non-epileptic events. pp. 21–30. In Rowan AJ, Gates JR (eds): Non-Epileptic Seizures. Butterworth-Heinemann, Boston, 1993

Gates JR, Luciano D, Devinsky O: The classification and treatment of non-epileptic events. pp. 251–263. In Devinsky O, Theodore WH (eds): Epilepsy and Behavior. Wiley-Liss, New York, 1991

Gates JR, Ramani V, Whalen S, Loewenson R: Ictal characteristics of pseudoseizures. Arch Neurol 42:1183–1187, 1985

Glenn TJ, Simonds JF: Hypnotherapy of a psychogenic seizure disorder in an adolescent. Am J Clin Hypn 19:245–249, 1977

Gower WR: Epilepsy. JA Churchill, London, 1881

Heron W: Cognitive and physiological effects of perceptual isolation. pp. 6–33. In Solomon P et al (eds): Sensory Deprivation, Harvard University Press, Cambridge, MA, 1961

Heron W, Doane BK, Scott TH: Visual disturbances after prolonged perceptual isolation. Can J Psychol 10:13–18, 1956

Kertesz A: Paroxysmal kinesigenic choreoathetosis: an entity within the paroxysmal choreoathetosis syndrome. Description of 10 cases, including 1 autopsied. Neurology 17:680–690, 1967

Kristensen O, Alving J: Pseudoseizures — risk factors and prognosis. Acta Neurol Scand 85:177–180, 1992

Krumholz A: Psychogenic seizures: a clinical study with follow-up data. Neurology 33:498–502, 1983

Lai CW, Ziegler DK: Repeated self induced syncope and subsequent seizure. Arch Neurol 40:820–823, 1983

Lance JW: Familial paroxysmal dystonic choreoathetosis and its differentiation from related syndromes. Ann Neurol 2:285–293, 1977

Lancman ME, Brotherton TA, Asconape JJ, Penry JK: Psychogenic seizures in adults: a longitudinal analysis. Seizure 2:281–286, 1993

Lees-Haley P: Malingering posttraumatic stress disorder on the MMPI. Forensic Rep 2:89–91, 1989

Lempert T, Schmidt D: Natural history and outcome of psychogenic seizures: a clinical study in 50 patients. J Neurol 237:35–38, 1990

Lesser RP: Psychogenic seizures. pp. 273–296. In Pedley TA, Meldrum BS (eds): Recent Advances in Epilepsy, Vol. 2. Churchill Livingstone, Edinburgh, 1985

Linder H: Psychogenic seizure states: a psychodynamic study. Int J Clin Exp Hypn 21:261–271, 1973

Ljundberg L: Hysteria: A clinical, prognostic and genetic study. Acta Psychiatr Neurol Scand Suppl 112:1–162, 1957

Lugaresi E, Cirignotta F, Montagna P: Nocturnal paroxysmal dystonia. J Neurol Neurosurg Psychiatry 49:375–380, 1986

Marble et al. (eds): Joslin's Diabetes Mellitus. Lea & Febiger, Philadelphia, p. 671

Marseille Consensus Statement: Classification of the progressive myoclonus epilepsies and related disorders. Ann Neurol 28:113–116, 1990

Matthews WB: Tonic seizures in disseminated sclerosis. Brain 81:193–206, 1958

Meierkord H, Will B, Fish D, Shorvon S: The clinical features and prognosis of pseudoseizures diagnosed using video-EEG telemetry. Neurology 41:1643–1646, 1991

Przutek H, Muhr H: Essential familial myoclonus. J Neurol 230:153–162, 1983

Ramani V, Gumnit RJ: Management of hysterical seizures in epileptic patients. Arch Neurol 39:78–81, 1982

Rosen GM: The Aleutian Enterprise sinking and posttraumatic stress disorder: misdiagnosis in clinical and forensic settings. Prof Psychol 26:82–87, 1995

Rowan AJ, Gates JR: Non-Epileptic Seizures. Butterworth-Heinemann, Boston, 1993

Savard G, Andermann F, Teitelbaum J, Lehmann H: Epileptic Munchhausen's syndrome: a form of pseudo-seizures distinct from hysteria and malingering. Neurology 38:1628–1629, 1988

Scott DF: Recognition and diagnostic aspects of nonepileptic seizures. pp. 21–34. In Riley TL, Roy A (eds): Pseudoseizures. Williams & Wilkins, Baltimore

Tempkin O: The Falling Sickness. Johns Hopkins University Press, Baltimore, 1945

Trimble MR: Serum prolactin in epilepsy and hysteria. Br Med J 2:1682, 1978

Trimble MR: Pseudoseizures. Neurol Clin 4:531–548, 1986

Vaamonde J, Muruzabal J, Artieda J, Obeso JA: Semiological peculiarities of familial paroxystic ataxia (FPA). Mov Disord 5:8–12, 1990

Von Bernuth G, Bernsau V, Gutheil H et al: Tachyarrhythmic syncopes in children with structurally normal hearts with and without QT prolongation in the electrocardiogram. Euro J Pediatr 138:206–210, 1982

Wayne-Massey E: History of epilepsy and hysteria. pp. 1–20. In Riley T, Roy A (eds): Pseudoseizures. Williams & Wilkins, Baltimore, 1982

Willis T: An essay on the pathology of the brain and nervous stock in which convulsive diseases are treated. Pordage S transl Leigh, Harper, Dring, 1684

Wyllie E, Friedman D, Luders H et al: Outcome of psychogenic seizures in children and adolescents compared with adults. Neurology 41:742–744, 1991

Wyllie E, Luders H, MacMillan JP, Gupta M: Serum prolactin levels after epileptic seizures. Neurology 34:1601–1604, 1984

Cervical Pain Syndromes 13

Warren Rizzo
Matthew Rizzo

Post-traumatic cervical spine pain can be the result of acute disruption of the osseous, ligamentous, muscular, or neural elements of the spine or of the imperfect healing of those tissues. This is especially true for the arthritic spine, which is functionally compromised and may already be painful. There also exist less well defined entities such as fibromyalgia, the myofascial pain syndrome, and post-traumatic cervical dystonia, whose functional or physical manifestations are pronounced but whose pathologic correlates are currently lacking. This chapter covers the various pain syndromes using the time to appearance of pain as a rough classification scheme. The main focus is on the patient with chronic or late-onset pain.

ANATOMY AND PHYSIOLOGY OF THE CERVICAL SPINE

In order to understand the mechanisms of cervical injury and pain the underlying anatomy should first be mastered. The anatomy of the cervical spine reflects its unique function in "support" of the special sense organs. It balances the weight of the head on the lateral articular facets of the atlas. The highly mobile cervical spine is in nearly constant motion, repositioning more than 600 times per hour (Bland, 1989; Bland and Boushey, 1989). Through or in close proximity to the cervical spine pass the spinal cord, major elements of the autonomic nervous system, and the vascular supply to the head and neck.

The cervical spine is composed of seven vertebrae (Fig. 13-1). The first two are extremely specialized and the other five tend to follow a typical pattern. Intervertebral discs are interposed between the bony elements and contribute to the more than 30 separate joints of the cervical spine. Ligaments, articular capsules, muscles, and fibrous and elastic tissues tie these bony elements together (Bland and Boushey, 1989; Carpenter, 1978; Harrison, 1978).

Typical Cervical Vertebrae

The typical cervical vertebra (C3 to C7) consists of an anterior body and a posterior arch formed by the pedicle and laminae (Fig. 13-2). The bodies of these vertebrae are small, reflecting the relatively low weight they bear. They are wider than they are deep, and the lateral edges of the superior surface of each body enlarges so that after the second decade of life

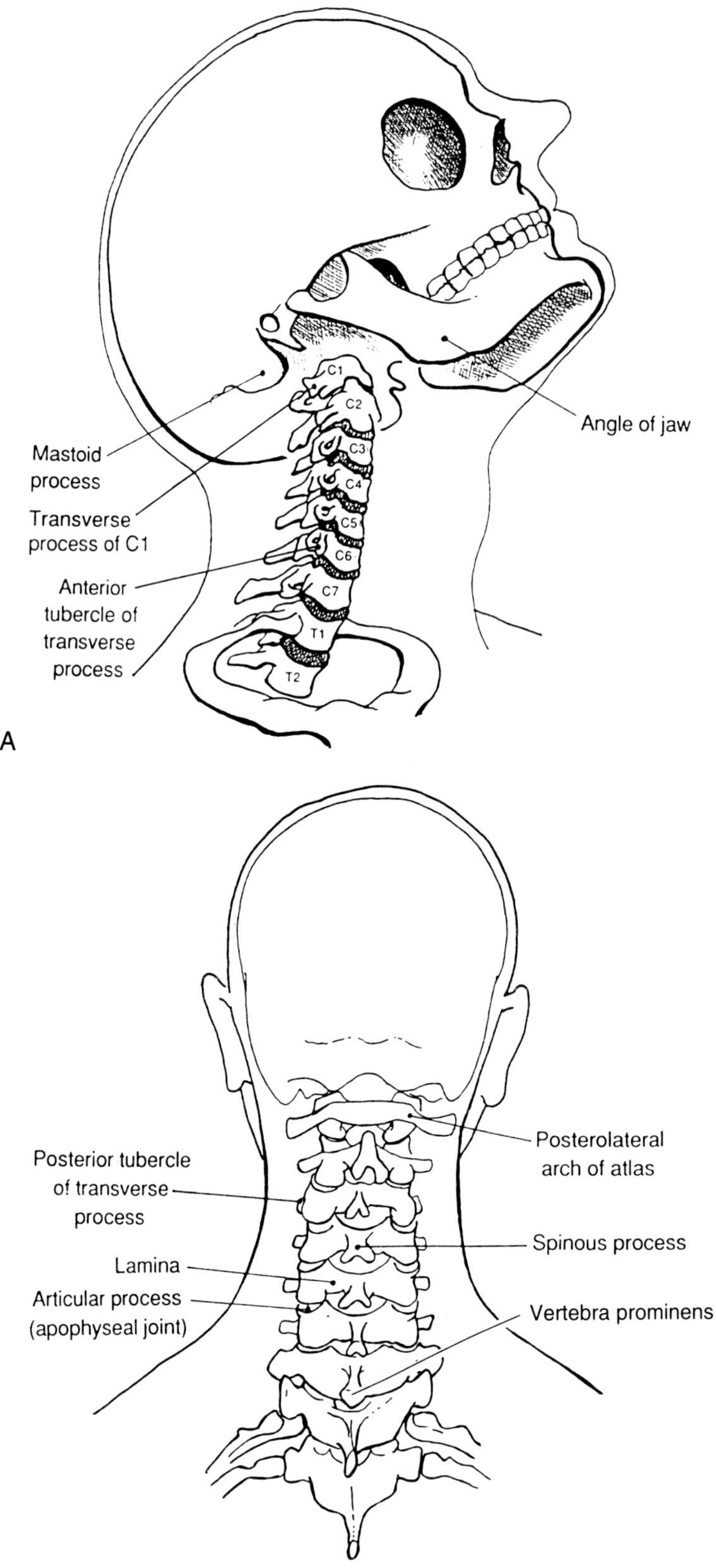

Fig. 13-1. (A) Anterolateral view of the cervical spine, showing the location of the seven cervical vertebrae, C1–C7, and accessible palpatation points. **(B)** Posterior view of the cervical spine and palpatation points. (Adapted from Olivier and Middlemarch, 1991, with permission.)

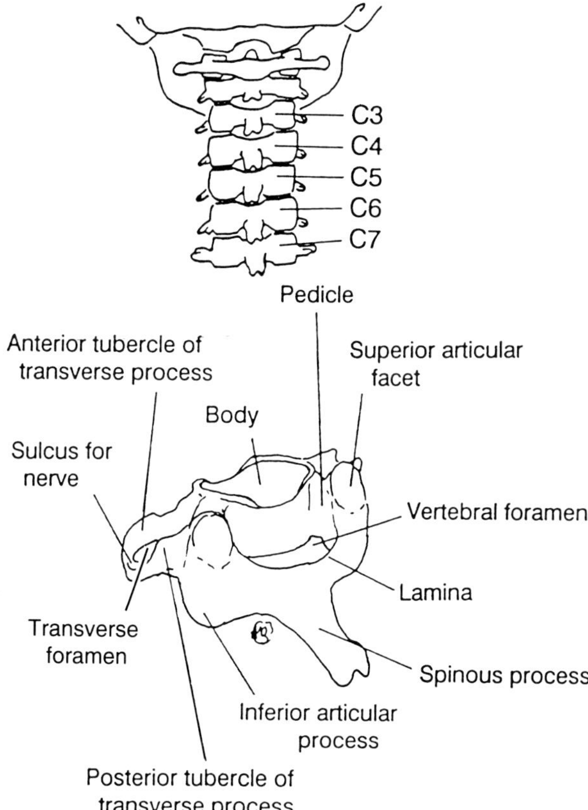

Fig. 13-2. The scheme for a typical cervical vertebra (C3–C7) is shown. The view is superior, posterior, and slightly rotated to the left. (Adapted from Bonsall, with permission.)

they each articulate with the vertebra above to form the uncovertebral joints, or joints of Luschka. There are also symphysis joints formed by the vertebral bodies and discs (below C2).

The pedicles arise from the posterolateral aspect of the vertebral body. The upper (superior) and lower (inferior) surfaces (facets) of the pedicles are beveled and form the apophyseal (zygapophyseal) joints (Fig. 13-3). These joints are diarthrodial and are covered by hyaline cartilage and bound by a loose capsule. When united, they form two bony shafts posterolateral to the vertebral body.

The laminae arise from the pedicles and project backward at a 45-degree angle to meet in the midline, where they form a bifid spinous process. In front of the facets, on the lateral surface of the pedicle, the transverse processes project anteriorly and downward. They are grooved on the superior surface, which permits the passage of the spinal nerves.

From C1 to C6 the transverse processes have a foramen, known as the transverse foramen (foramen transversarium), for the vertebral artery, its venous plexus, and the accompanying autonomic nerves. The transverse process terminates in an anterior and a posterior tubercle, which serve for the attachment of the anterior and posterior cervical muscles, respectively.

The C7 vertebra differs from the other typical cervical vertebrae in that the spinous process is elongated and no longer bifid. It is easily palpated at the base of the neck when held in full flexion, which is why it is also referred to as the *vertebra prominens.* The transverse process at this level also lacks the transverse foramen; the vertebral artery courses anteriorly.

The Atlas

The first cervical vertebra, or *atlas,* is the ring of bone that seats the skull (Fig. 13-4). Its architecture differs greatly from that of a typical vertebra. It has a rudimentary spinous process and no vertebral body, that having been "donated" to the axis. The lateral masses connect the anterior and posterior arches of the atlas. They correspond to the pedicles of the typical vertebrae and are covered superiorly and inferiorly by concave articular surfaces. The superior facets articulate with the occipital condyles of the skull. The inferior facets are rounder and face laterally to articulate with the axis.

The transverse processes permit the passage of the vertebral artery and associated structures. The transverse process of the atlas is not grooved, and the nerve roots exit posterior to the articular masses. The superior surface of the posterior arch of the atlas has an oblique groove, which accommodates the vertebral artery after it twists around the articular complex. This tortuous course ends with the passage of the arteries through the atlanto-occipital membrane.

The posterior surface of the anterior arch has a cartilage-lined facet, which articulates with the facet on the anterior surface of the odontoid process. This articulation is lined by synovium, which assumes importance in certain disease processes. Lateral to the articular facet, where the anterior arch joins the lateral masses, a bony prominence can be noted. This is the attachment of the transverse ligament.

The Axis

The second cervical vertebra, or *axis,* is characterized by the odontoid process (Fig. 13-5), a pivot for the atlas. The odontoid process articulates anteriorly

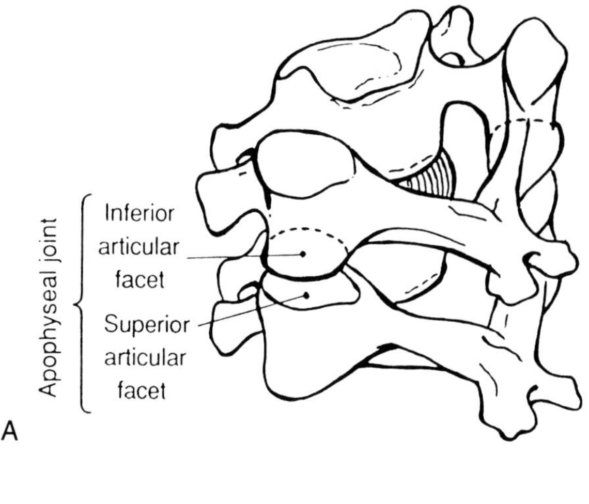

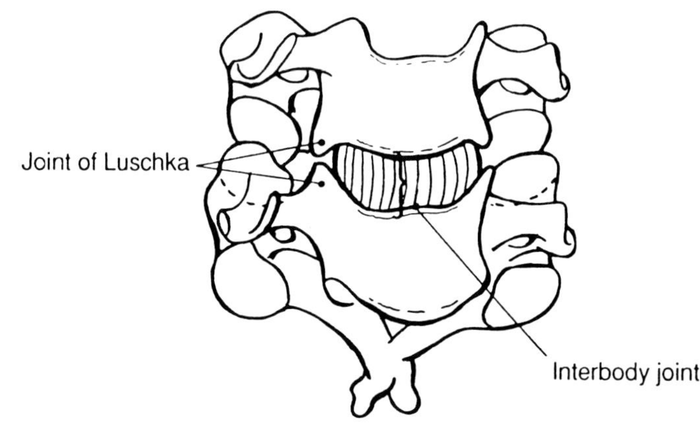

Fig. 13-3. The joints between the cervical vertebrae are shown. **(A)** An apophyseal (zygoaphyseal) joint is shown from a posterolateral view. **(B)** The joint of Luschka and interbody joint are shown from an anterolateral view. (From Olivier and Middlemarch, 1991, with permission.)

with the posterior surface of the anterior arch of the atlas and posteriorly is separated from the restraining transverse ligament by a bursa.

The apical ligament arises from the tip of the odontoid process, and the alar ligaments arise posterior to the apex. The superior articulating surfaces of the axis are lateral to the odontoid process and are convex. The inferior articulating surfaces assume the characteristics of the lower cervical vertebrae. The laminae join to form a bifid spinous process.

The axis lacks an intervertebral foramen, and the nerve roots lie posterior to the articular complex. The transverse processes are directed inferiorly. Because of the attitude of the transverse foramen, the vertebral artery must make a sharp upward and lateral bend to penetrate the transverse foramen of the atlas.

Intervertebral Discs

The intervertebral discs make up 25 percent of the height of the vertebral column. They are biconvex and wedge-shaped, the greatest width being anterior. This results in the normal cervical lordosis and the extreme flexibility of the cervical spine. Each disc is composed of an external annulus fibrosus and an internal nucleus pulposus. The annulus is composed of an intersecting series of fibrocartilaginous lamellae, which connect adjacent vertebrae. It is reinforced at its periphery by the anterior and posterior longitu-

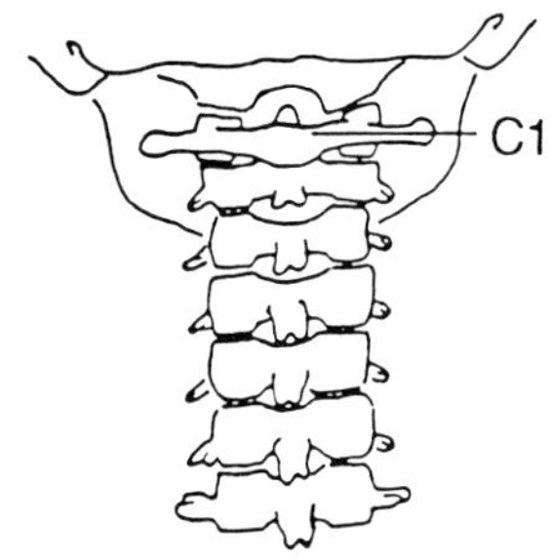

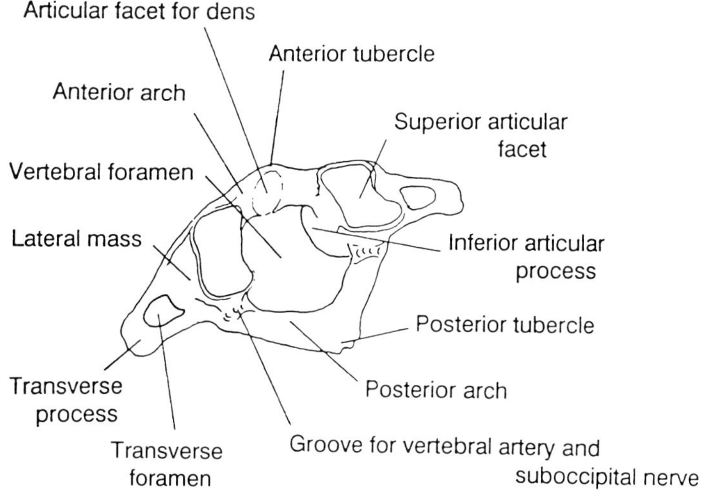

Fig. 13-4. The atlas, C1, is shown in schematic form (same vantage as Fig. 13-2). (From Bonsall, with permission.)

dinal ligaments. The nucleus pulposus lies eccentrically, just anterior of center, and is composed of a mesh of collagen fibers and water-rich proteoglycan gel. In spite of its being avascular, a considerable number of cells are suspended in its matrix. It has the remarkable ability to retain its water content in spite of applied pressure and consequently regains its original shape after deformation. Some authors believe that the nucleus pulposus is absent from the adult cervical spine (Giesler et al., 1983; Bland and Boushey, 1989), an important point when we discuss disc herniations.

Ligaments

The cruciform ligament holds the odontoid process tightly against the anterior arch of the atlas. It is composed of two fibrous bands, one of which is attached to the occipital bone and the body of the axis. The other, the transverse ligament, is more important in preventing sublimation of the odontoid.

The apical ligament attaches to the anterior rim of the foramen magnum and to the tip of the odontoid process. The alar ligaments connect the posterior aspect of the tip of the odontoid process to the margins of the foramen magnum. The continuation of the anterior longitudinal ligament connects the anterior arch of the atlas to the anterior margin of the foramen magnum.

The tectorial membrane is the continuation of the posterior longitudinal ligament, which blends with the dura mater at the base of the occipital bone. The posterior longitudinal ligament is located within the vertebral canal. It is firmly bound to each disc and is not attached to the posterior surface of the vertebral body. This ligament prevents hyperflexion of the vertebral column.

The anterior longitudinal ligament covers most of the anterolateral surface of the vertebral bodies. It is loosely attached to the annulus over which it passes. It is most strongly attached to the rim of the articular lip and merges with the periosteum of the vertebral

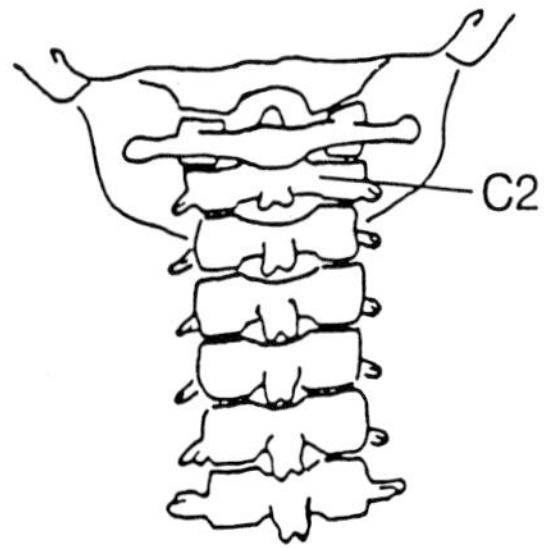

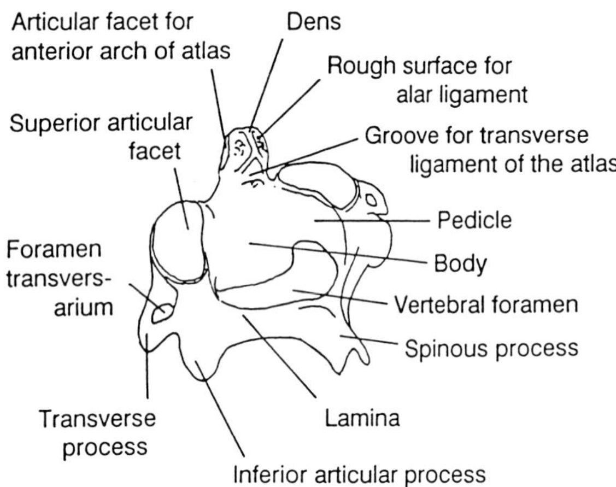

Fig. 13-5. The axis, C2, is shown in schematic form (same vantage as Fig. 13-1). (From Bonsall, with permission.)

body. The anterior longitudinal ligament limits extension of the vertebral column.

The ligamenta flava are paired, extremely elastic ligaments, which are attached to the anteroinferior surface of the superior lamina and the posterosuperior margin of the inferior lamina (Figs. 13-6 and 13-7). They extend from the roots of the spines laterally to the zygapophyseal joint and join with the fibers of the capsule. The ligamenta flava stretch and return to the relaxed state without buckling.

The fibrous intertransverse ligaments connect the transverse processes and are present in the cervical spine as a few tough bands (Fig. 13-6). The interspinous ligaments are situated medial to the paired interspinous muscles and connect adjoining spinous processes (Fig. 13-7). Their fibers are arranged obliquely, connecting the base of the superior vertebra to the superior ridge and apex of the next vertebra.

The supraspinal ligament is present in the cervical spine as the ligamentum nuchae (Fig. 13-7). This elastic ligament is tethered from the occipital protuberance to the spine of the seventh cervical vertebra. It extends anteriorly as a fibrous sheet and connects to the cervical spinous processes. It acts as a support of the head on the neck.

The Intervertebral Foramina

The vertebral foramina are small (0.5-cm) oval passages, whose boundaries are defined anterormedially by the intervertebral disc and posterolaterally by the zygapophyseal joint and the superior articular surface of the contiguous vertebra. The lateral opening of the passage is oriented slightly inferiorly. This space is occupied by the anterior and posterior nerve roots, the intervertebral veins and plexuses, the radicular arteries, and a projection of the epidural space. The anterior nerve root lies anterior and inferior to the posterior root and near the uncovertebral joint. The posterior root is situated in proximity to the zygapophyseal joint and the superior articular process of the next vertebra. The nerve roots occupy only one-third of the available foraminal space (Bland, 1987; Carpenter, 1978; Harrison, 1978). The exit of spinal roots C5 to T1 is shown in Fig. 13-8.

Movement of the Cervical Spine

The cervical spine moves in flexion, extension, lateral flexion, and rotation. The difference in length of the cervical vertebral canal between flexion and extension is 2 to 3 cm (Bland and Boushey, 1987). In flexion the cord moves up and tension is placed on the intrathecal nerve roots. In extension the opposite happens. Lateral flexion and rotation tend to occur together to some degree. The atlanto-occipital joints allow flexion and extension while the atlanto-axial joint allows rotation, mainly around the odontoid pivot. The muscles concerned with movement of the atlanto-occipital and atlanto-axial joints are listed in Table 13-1.

Extension of the head is limited by the entrapment of the posterior arch of the atlas between the occiput and the spinous process of the axis. Further extension occurs as the lower elements are recruited.

About 50 percent of cervical flexion is accounted for by the atlanto-occipital joint. The remaining movement is unevenly distributed in the remaining cervical spine, with the upper elements contributing the most. Flexion ceases as the posterior ligaments become taut and the tip of the odontoid process approximates the margin of the foramen magnum. Of the approximately 160 degrees of pos-

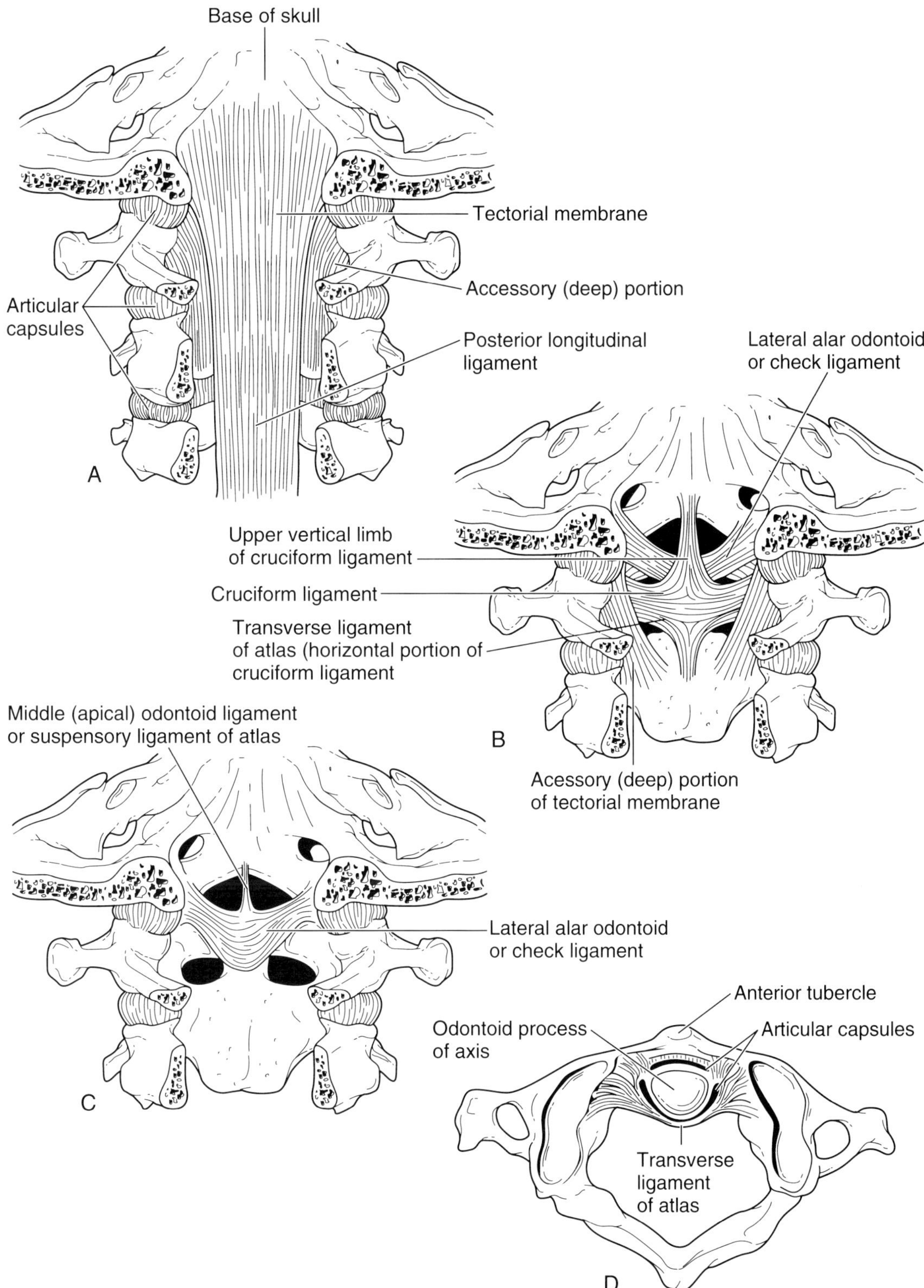

Fig. 13-6. The internal ligaments of the cervical spine. **(A)** Upper portion of spinal canal opened from behind by removal of spinous processes and portions of vertebral arches to expose ligaments on posterior aspect of vertebral bodies. **(B)** Principal portion of tectorial membrane removed to expose deeper ligaments. **(C)** Cruciform ligament removed to show deepest ligaments. **(D)** Atlanto-odontoid articulation viewed from above. (Adapted from Williams et al, 1989, with permission.)

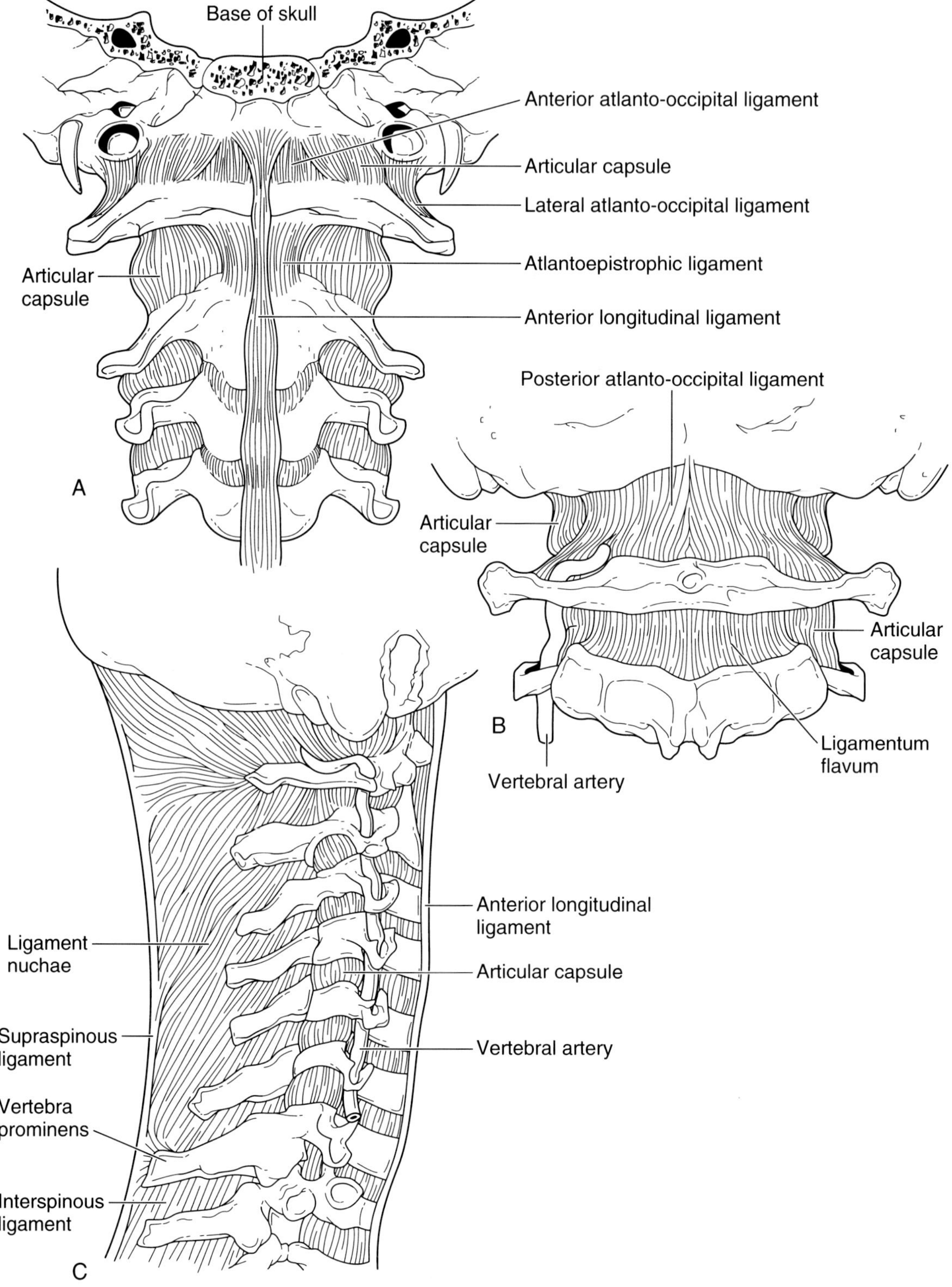

Fig. 13-7. The external ligaments of the cervical spine. **(A)** Base of skull and upper cervical vertebrae with ligaments viewed from in front. **(B)** Base of skull and upper cervical vertebrae with ligaments viewed from behind. **(C)** Base of skull and upper cervical vertebrae with ligaments viewed from the right side. (Adapted from Williams et al, 1989, with permission.)

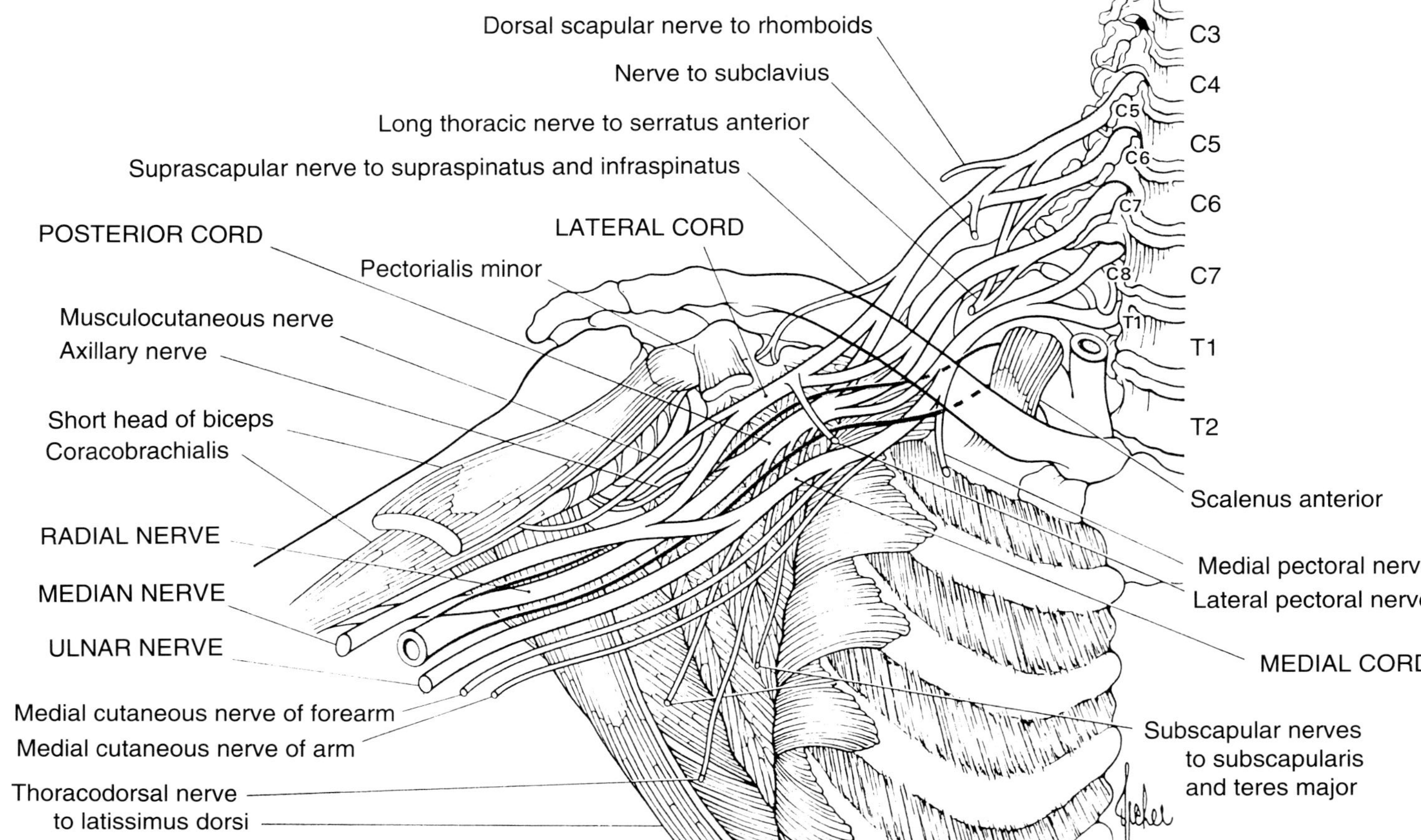

Fig. 13-8. The exit of the spinal roots from C5 to T1 is shown. Each root exits above the vertebra for which it is named. These roots form the cords of the brachial plexus and innervate the muscles that move the arm and shoulder girdle. (From Medical Research Council, 1976, with permission.)

TABLE 13-1. Muscles Concerned in Movements of the Atlanto-Occipital and Atlantoaxial Joints

Movement	Muscle
Flexion	Longus capitis Rectus capitis anterior Sternocleidomastoid (anterior fibers)
Extension	Semispinalis capitis Splenius capitis Rectus capitis posterior major Rectus capitis posterior minor Obliquus capitis superior Longissimus capitis Trapezius Sternocleidomastoid (posterior fibers)
Rotation and lateral flexion	Sternocleidomastoid Obliquus capitis inferior Obliquus capitis superior Rectus capitis lateralis Longissimus capitis Splenius capitis

(From Romaines, 1987, with permission.)

sible rotational movement, the atlanto-axial joints contribute about half, with the lower elements again contributing the other half.

Selective motion can occur between the atlas and the skull and between the atlas and the axis. The lower cervical vertebrae do not possess this capacity. The intervertebral discs also participate in cervical motion. Their elastic properties permit motion and act to limit excessive motion.

It is important to note that the diameter of the vertebral canal is not constant. During rotation and lateral flexion the axis narrows the canal diameter at the level of the axis by one-third. Fortunately, at the level of the atlas one-third of the vertebral canal is occupied by the odontoid and one-third by the spinal cord, and the remaining one-third is free space. The intervertebral foramina are also subject to changes in their diameters, increasing in flexion and decreasing in extension by approximately one-third. Normally there is enough free space to compensate without injuring the nerve root.

ACUTE TRAUMATIC PAIN

Acute traumatic cervical spine injury has many causes. These include car crashes, falls or falling objects, acts of violence, and sports, particularly diving and football. There are four basic types of injury: flexion, extension, compression (axial loading), and rotational (Osborn, 1994). The resultant lesion can be relatively minor as in neck sprain, or catastrophic as in fracture-dislocation with spinal cord transection. Avulsion of a cervical nerve root (usually C5 to T1) may also occur (e.g., owing to arm traction or shoulder depression with the head turned away as in a motorcycle crash). Because joint capsules, blood vessels, periosteum, tendons, ligaments, and dura are all heavily innervated, trauma to any of these structures, as well as to the cervical nerve roots or spinal cord, can produce painful sensations.

Acute therapy varies widely depending on the type of injury. The basic principles of immobilization and subsequent surgical reduction and stabilization of the vertebral elements apply to fracture cases with spinal cord or nerve root injury. Analgesics with narcotics and on occasion non-narcotic analgesics are indicated. Transcutaneous electrical nerve stimulation has been reported to relieve the acute pain of spinal cord injuries (Richardson et al., 1980), but agreement is not universal (Deyo et al., 1990; Langley et al., 1984; Nepomuceno et al., 1979).

Treatment of neck sprain or strain is conservative initially. Headaches should be evaluated and the possibility of a cerebral concussion considered (see Chs. 1 and 8). The associated symptoms include pain and stiffness in the muscles of the upper neck, especially on motion; headache, especially at the occiput; blurred vision; dizziness; and inability to concentrate. A cervical collar may be helpful and should be continued for 3 to 6 weeks. The patient should be placed at bed rest for a few days, but absolute immobility should be discouraged. Pain may be treated with mild analgesic or nonsteroidal anti-inflammatory drugs. Muscle relaxants are sometimes used, but not to great effect. Treatment with any of the physical modalities of heat, massage, or ultrasound may be added. Exercises and stretching are recommended as soon as pain permits. Any change in the clincial neurologic condition warrants further investigation. Motivated patients tend to improve. A debate centers on why any of these patients should develop chronic intractable pain (see Ch. 26).

SUBACUTE AND CHRONIC PAIN

There are several syndromes of subacute and chronic cervical pain. In many cases the relationship with a single acute traumatic event is often difficult to ascertain. This is particularly true in the "soft tissue" syndromes of myofascial pain and fibromyalgia (Bohr, 1995). A cause-and-effect relationship is even more difficult to prove, especially as the time between injury and onset of symptoms lengthens or if there are ancillary factors such as psychological distress or litigation. Cervical radiculopathy may be more readily traced to an acute event, but often it reflects a hereditary disposition combined with years of wear and tear causing cervical arthritis. Importantly, patients with pre-existing cervical arthritis, whatever the cause, are more prone to traumatic cervical injury. We discuss these issues below (see Fig. 13-8).

Cervical Disc Disease with Radiculopathy

Cervical disc disease accompanied by radiculopathy is seen in the aging population. In many cases it is difficult to assign the cause to a single acute traumatic event.

Radiculopathy refers to dysfunction and the sensation of pain along a nerve root due to root compression around the intervertebral foramen. This can be caused by an extruded disc or by osteophytic enlargement of the zygapophyseal joints. The first two cervical roots exit behind the articular facets, and radiculopathy of these nerves is unusual. Radiculopathy is much more likely at the level of C4 and below (see Fig. 13-8).

C3 Radiculopathy

The first cervical intervertebral disc is located between the second and third cervical vertebrae and would affect the third cervical root if it were to protrude. In reality, impingment at this spinal level is extremely unusual (Simeone, 1992). The third nerve root travels up the back of the head, and its involvement would cause paresthesias of the posterior cheek, possibly the ear, and the lateral portion of the neck. Pain in this area, if present, may be confused with tension headache (see Ch. 8). Vertebral artery insufficiency as well as trigeminal neuralgia is included in the differential diagnosis.

C4 Radiculopathy

Radiculopathy of the fourth cervical nerve root is also uncommon. Like C3 radiculopathy, it does not involve any motor deficit. Pain is a prominent symptom, involving the midneck to the shoulders and down to the scapula. Even though the phrenic nerve exits at this level, diaphragmatic weakness does not seem to occur.

C5 Radiculopathy

Radiculopathy affecting the fifth cervical nerve root produces a numbness over the top of the shoulder and halfway down the lateral aspect of the arm. This "epaulet" distribution is specific for the C5 nerve root. The sensory dysfunction may extend down the radial side of the forearm and hand. The radiculopathy has a prominent motor component, which affects the deltoid muscle and to a lesser extent the infraspinatus, supraspinatus, and biceps muscles. The biceps reflex may be diminished or absent.

C6 Radiculopathy

Radiculopathy affecting the sixth cervical nerve root is the second most common form. Pain is present on the lateral side of the arm and radial surface of the forearm and extends into the thumb and index finger. Numbness may also be present at the tips of the thumb and index finger. Muscle weakness involves the biceps, extensor carpi radialis, extensor pollicis, supinator, and serratus anterior. The biceps reflex may provide an important clue in the diagnosis and is usually absent early.

C7 Radiculopathy

Impingement at the C6-C7 level produces a radiculopathy at the level of the seventh cervical nerve root. The sensory component involves pain radiating across the posterior shoulder and down the posterior arm and forearm to the fingertips. Numbness of the middle and ring as well as the index finger is present. The triceps is principally involved, and the triceps reflex may be lost. The pectoralis major, extensors of the wrist and fingers, pronator, and latissimus dorsi may be weak. As with all radiculopathies, extension of the neck can exacerbate the pain and weakness, and in this case pain may even be reported in the upper thoracic spine. The differential diagnosis includes medial epicondylitis, triceps tendinitis, and bronchial carcinoma.

C8 Radiculopathy

Nerve root compression at the C8 level has a profound effect on the functioning of the hand. The sensory disturbance is a cutaneous hypesthesia of the fifth finger and the ulnar half of the ring finger. The patient may complain of pain in the back at the inferior level of the scapula, the medial aspect of the arm, and the forearm. The triceps, extensor carpi ulnaris, and wrist flexors may be involved. The interosseous muscles of the hand are innervated by this root. Weakness involving these muscles results in an inability to perform those activities that require a strong grip such as holding a pen or using a hammer. The differential diagnosis of conditions affecting this level would include thoracic outlet obstruction compressing the lower trunk of the brachial plexus, cervical rib, Pancoast tumor, angina of cardiac origin, and ulnar neuropathy. The pattern of deficits associated with cervical radiculopathy is summarized in Table 13-2 and Figure 13-9.

Pain Features

The pain associated with nerve root compression is abrupt, appearing over minutes to hours and reaching its full intensity in a few days. It is usually appreciated in the neck, shoulder, arm, forearm, or hand and is dependent on the nerve root involved. The pain is often severe, with an aching or shooting quality, sometimes likened to that of an electric shock. A herniated disc may be compressing the nerve root against the vertebral lamina. As a rule, the larger the herniation, the more severe the pain and the more extensive its radiation. The pain is initially constant during the day. At night most patients will have frequent interruptions in their sleep, and many cannot lie flat and choose to sleep in a chair. Any change in position of the head will exacerbate the pain, extension being the action most likely to exacerbate paresthesias and increase discomfort. Lateral flexion and rotation will also increase the symptoms associated with cervical radiculopathy.

On examination of the patient, the clinician should attempt to discover which positions exacerbate the pain symptoms either through observation of the patient's posture and movements or by gentle repositioning of the head until the symptoms are reproduced. This is done to give the examiner an indication of the side and approximate level of the lesion. An interesting antalgic position is often assumed by patients with C8 lesions. They commonly rest their forearms or wrists on top of their heads and may also tilt the head away from the affected side. A "frozen shoulder" may be associated with cervical disc radiculopathy at any level but is more commonly seen with C5-C6 disease. The neck pain and weakness of the deltoid muscle will limit the activity of that shoulder. This may then allow the muscles and ligaments to shorten. Once the original condition has subsided, the patient continues to experience pain and limitation in the range of motion in that shoulder, at which time the diagnosis can be made.

In general the diagnosis of cervical radiculopathy from disc protrusion is both clinical and radiologic. The type of radiologic intervention is based on the symptoms encountered. Plain films, computed tomography (CT) with or without contrast, magnetic resonance imaging (MRI) with or without contrast, and even myelography may be necessary at some time in the evaluation. Electromyography may also be helpful. These techniques are discussed in more detail in the section, *Diagnostic Methods*.

TABLE 13-2. Manifestations of Cervical Radiculopathy

Cervical Nerve	Sensory Manifestations	Motor Manifestations
C3	Paresthesias or pain of the ear, cheek, and lateral neck	None
C4	Pain in midneck and shoulders	Phrenic nerve involvement rare
C5	Numbness over top of shoulder and lateral aspect arm "epaulet"	Deltoid, biceps, infraspinatus, supraspinatus
C6	Pain in lateral arm, radial forearm; numbness in tip of thumb and index finger	Biceps, wrist extensors, thumb extensor, and supinator weakness
C7	Pain across posterior shoulder, arm, forearm to fingers; numbness in second, third, and fourth fingers	Triceps, pectoralis, wrist and finger extensor weakness
C8	Pain in back at scapula, medial level of arm, and forearm; numbness of fourth and fifth fingers	Triceps, wrist extensor and flexor weakness, profound

(From Patton, 1977, with permission.)

Management

Management of cervical radiculopathy is initially conservative. This approach is not based on the results of prospective, double-blind, placebo-controlled studies of cervical disc disease, which are lacking (Block, 1987), but rather on empirical data and common practice. As with all therapeutic interventions, the patient should be educated about the disease process and allowed to assist in decision making.

The first step is to immobilize the neck and place the patient at bed rest. This removes many of the compressive forces acting on the cervical spine and prevents activities that may contribute to the pain. Immobilization can be accomplished with a soft cervical collar, which holds the head in a neutral or slightly flexed position. The patient should not be fitted with a collar that forces the chin up and the neck in painful extension.

The longest lasting "immobilization" of the bony elements is accomplished by strong cervical musculature. Exercises to that end can be initiated early and are limited by the appearance of pain and reproduction of symptoms. These exercises should be aimed at strengthening the cervical paravertebral musculature and increasing the range of motion. The recommended exercise is dependent upon the patient's symptoms and past exercise history. It is usually sufficient to initiate therapy with isometric neck exercises and progress as the patient's condition allows.

Medication can be used to soothe the pain, relieve the inflammation, and promote muscle relaxation. Analgesia can be obtained with codeine, 30 to 60 mg every four hours, or its equivalent. Nonsteroidal anti-inflammatory drugs are used on the assumption that the mechanical compression by the disc causes a secondary inflammation of the nerve. This assumption has not been proved by any convincing studies. Any of the class can be used, as none has been proved to be superior. In the patient in whom peptic ulceration has been or is a problem, there are newer preparations that have less gastrointestinal toxicity, although they are still not approved for this purpose.

Muscle relaxants can help relieve the painful muscle spasms that may be caused by the pain and in turn increase the pain. Cyclobenzaprine, methocarbamol, and carisoprodol are commonly used. Diazepam should be used with caution because of its tendency to cause depression. These medications may be helpful for a limited period of time, usually several weeks, and should be discontinued if the effects are not striking.

The use of traction is still contested, some claiming it is undoubtedly effective and others concluding that it is ineffective and possibly harmful (Bland, 1987; Harris, 1977). The clinician may attempt to predict the effect of cervical spine traction in relieving pain or paresthesias by first performing the distraction test. With the patient sitting, the examiner places one hand, palm up, under the chin and the other hand behind the occiput. The examiner then lifts the head, thereby removing the compressive force of the head and distracting the intervertebral foramina. If the patient experiences relief with disappearance of symptoms, traction may be of benefit. Traction can be performed with the patient either seated or supine, intermittently or continuously, and can be manual, mechanical, or performed at home. The type of traction used is the result of a detailed clinical evaluation and is therefore tailored to the individual patient.

Many patients appreciate the beneficial effects of heat. Transfer of heat to the cervical area can be accomplished by heat packs or wet compresses, hot showers, and diathermy using microwaves or ultrasound. Other physical therapy methods include massage, manipulation, and the use of a transcutaneous electrical nerve stimulation (TENS) unit. There are also advocates of the use of trigger or tender point injection in the patient with radiculopathy. This technique is discussed in further detail in the section, *Myofascial Pain Syndrome.*

Soft Tissue Cervical Pain Syndromes

Acute trauma may injure the soft tissues of the neck, causing reduced mobility and pain, as in whiplash. In the absence of neurologic or radiographic abnormalities, recovery is expected. Some patients, however, report chronic pain and are diagnosed with chronic soft tissue injury. Two conditions that are sometimes invoked in these cases are the myofascial pain syndrome (MFS) and the fibromyalgia syndrome (FMS). These conditions share several features. Both are associated with painful musculotendinous structures, including those of the cervical region. Both must be distinguished from occipital neuralgia and other forms of head and neck pain (see Ch. 8). Also, there is controversy regarding the true nature of both conditions (Bohr, 1995): Are they manifestations of localized pathologic states or are

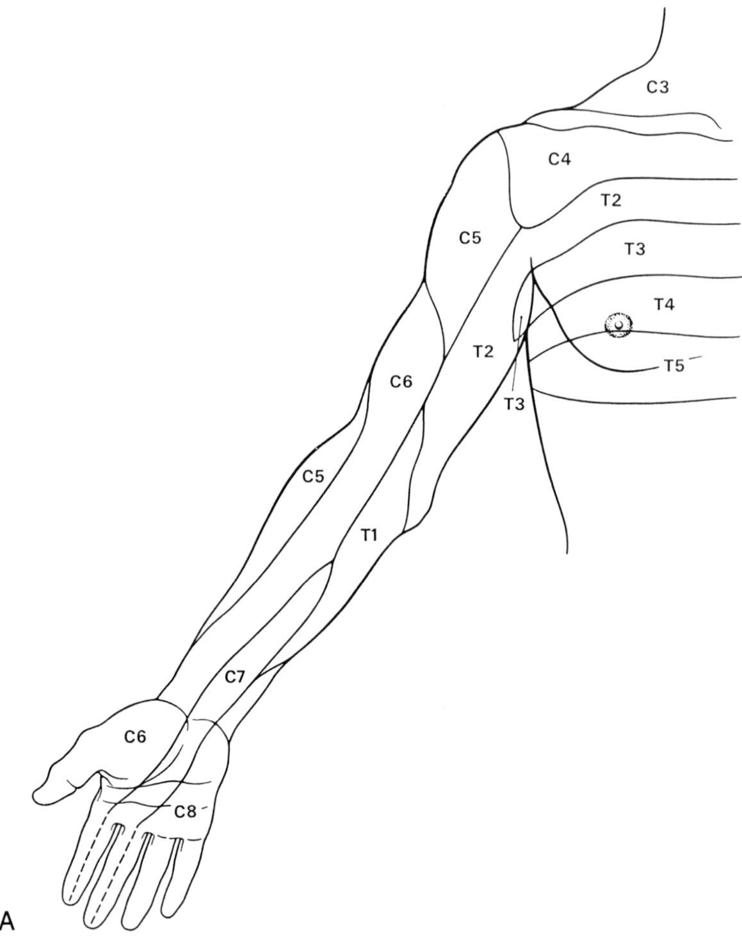

Fig. 13-9. The patterns of cutaneous sensory loss with cervical radiculopathy in the anterior **(A)** and posterior **(B)** aspect of the upper limb. (From Medical Research Council, 1976, with permission.) (*Figure continues.*)

they psychophysiologic or psychosomatic phenomena? Some of the patients may meet DSM (Diagnostic and Statistical Manual of Mental Disorders) IV criteria for somatoform or conversion disorders, or there may be psychological stressors, coded on axis 4 (American Psychiatric Association, 1994). As will be seen, the management can be difficult. MPS, FMS, and another poorly understood syndrome associated with cervical, post-traumatic cervical dystonia, are reviewed below.

Myofascial Pain Syndrome

MPS is characterized by musculoskeletal pain referred from "trigger points" to areas more or less distant from those points (Friction, 1990). The latter zones of referral do not correspond to the usual dermatomal or myotomal patterns but are located throughout the musculoskeletal system including the cervical region (Fig. 13-10). Travell and Simons (1983) have defined the location of these trigger points and their zones of referral based on the examination of over 1,000 patients.

Trigger points may result from acute trauma, chronic microtrauma, or undefined stimuli (Travell and Simons, 1983). Holmes et al. (1989) have emphasized the pathophysiologic importance of structural asymmetry or muscle imbalance. The requisite finding in an area defined as a trigger point is the presence of a localized contraction of the deep muscle fibers or bundle of fibrous tissue. This focus will, when active and irritated, produce the sensation of pain or discomfort locally and in a specific referred

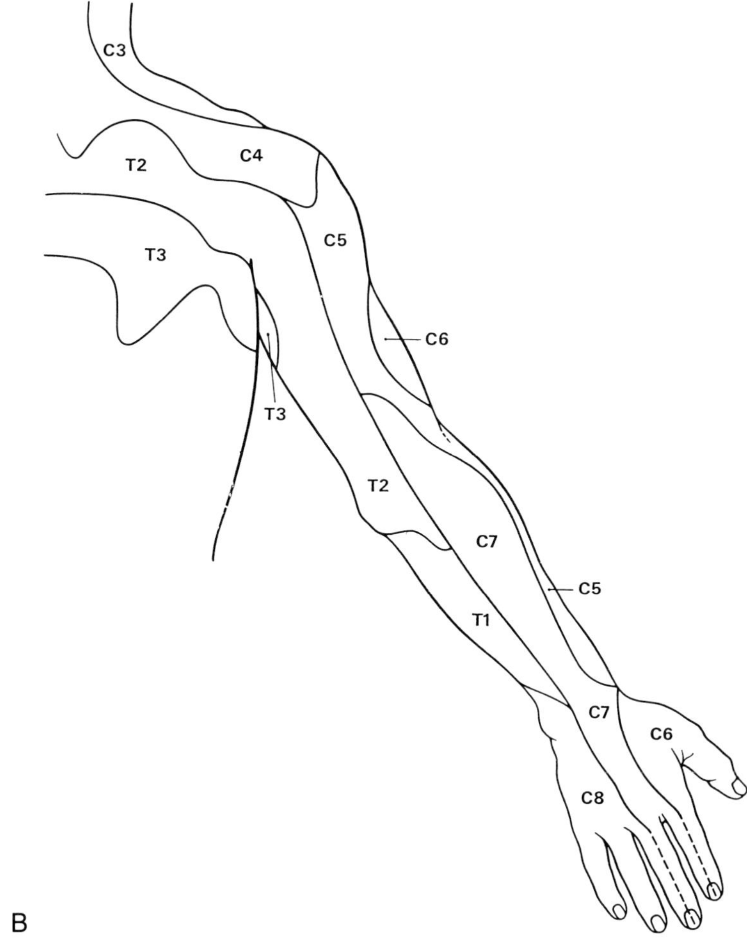

Fig. 13-9. (*Continued*).

area. The patient reacts characteristically to the palpation of the trigger point by withdrawal from the stimulus, which is accompanied by a pained facial expression and possibly even a verbal response. This is known as the *jump sign*. Another finding is shortening of the involved muscle when the band containing the trigger point is "snapped" by the examiner. This response is referred to as the *local twitch response*. The involved muscle may show weakness, easy fatigability, stiffness, and especially decreased range of motion. The specificity of these findings and the interexaminer reliability for demonstrating MPS phenomena have been questioned (Bohr, 1995).

An important diagnostic feature in MPS is that treatment of the trigger point will ameliorate the pain located at that point as well as in the zone of referral (Travell and Simons, 1983). According to Arroyo (1966), electromyography (EMG) may show a burst of electrical activity when the trigger point is needled, but no such activity is apparent in the surrounding muscle. This abnormal response is reportedly abolished by local anesthetics, spinal anesthesia, and trigger point elimination (Travell, 1976).

Histologic studies in MPS have produced a variety of findings, but none is consistent. Yunus (1989) reported loss of cross-striations, fatty infiltration, and increased numbers of both fibrocytic and sarcolemmal nuclei. Others have reported the accumulation of acid mucopolysaccharides, myofibrillar degeneration, and occasional lymphocytic inflammatory infiltration (Awad, 1973). Ragged red fibers and "motheaten" fibers were seen by light microscopic analysis in trapezius muscle biopsies from MPS patients (Bengtsson et al., 1986b). Bengtsson et al. (1986a)

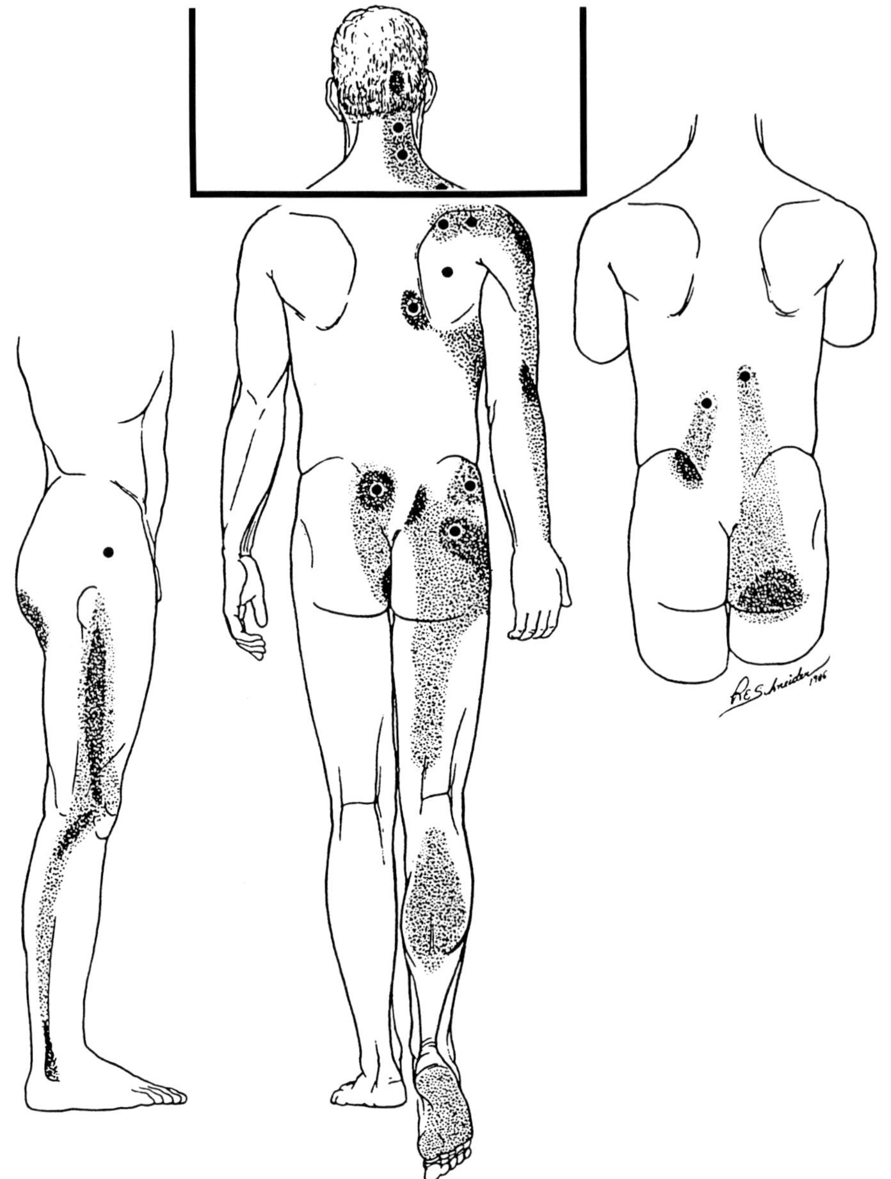

Fig. 13-10. Myofascial trigger points and zones of pain referral are shown in a posterior view. The trigger points of the posterior cervical region are depicted within the box. An occipital zone of referral is depicted by crosshatching. (From Sheon et al., 1987, with permission.)

also studied the muscle energy metabolism from 15 patients. They found an increase in the levels of adenine monophosphate and creatine and a decrease in the levels of adenine di- and triphosphate and phosphocreatine. According to those authors this is indicative of an ongoing energy depletion in those fibers. Attempts have also been made to incorporate the findings in MPS into more central models of pain (see Ch. 8).

The classic symptom of MPS is deep, aching pain present at rest. This phase may then progress to pain present only with specific movements and also characterized by pain-free intervals. The latent phase is manifested by tenderness and stiffness of involved muscles and a decreased range of motion of that part.

Psychological symptoms are myriad in MPS and can include depression, anxiety, anger, and frustration. Multiple somatic complaints include gastrointestinal distress; paresthesias; visual, auditory, and vestibular disturbances; excessive sweating; muscle twitching; skin flushing; and swelling. There also appears to be an increased incidence of disorders such as low back pain, neck pain, peptic ulcer disease, and migraine headaches (Berry, 1967; Gold and Lipton, 1975). Patients report poor sleep, poor posture, poor dietary habits, and lack of exercise. There can also be medication dependencies and noncompliance, which further contribute to the establishment of a chronic pain state (Moldofsky et al., 1975).

Management

The basic management of MPS includes (1) exlusion of a serious systemic disease as the source of pain; (2) patient education, including emphasis of the importance of self-help; (3) modification of inciting or aggravating factors; and (4) relief from pain. An interested, informed, educated, and motivated patient has a better chance of breaking free of the chronic pain cycle. Success also demands that the clinician have a thorough knowledge of the patient and identify the location of all active trigger points.

Therapy consists of many counterstimulation techniques aimed at inactivating painful trigger points. Noninvasive methods include massage, moist heat or ice pack application, cold spray, diathermy, ultrasound, or acupressure. Electrical stimulation of the trigger point with TENS, direct current stimulation of muscle, or electroacupuncture has been employed. Invasive procedures include trigger point injection with local anesthetic, corticosteroids, or saline as well as dry needling and acupuncture. The relief provided by most available techniques is temporary. Lasting relief requires the identification and elimination of any contributing factors (medical, psychological, or psychiatric) and rehabilitation with muscle stretching and strengthening.

Two of the most common techniques of counterstimulation are the spray-and-stretch technique and trigger point injections. The former directs a spray of refrigerant, such as dichlorofluoroethane, at the skin overlying a trigger point. At the same time the area is passively stretched. This technique is described in detail by Travell and Simons (1983).

Failure to respond to spray-and-stretch may justify the trigger point injection, a technique used in both MPS and FMS. Therapeutic action may be related to the mechanical disruption of the trigger point and not to the action of any injected substance (Lewit, 1979). This may explain the beneficial effects that patients also have with acupuncture.

The injection technique requires accurate identification of the trigger point. The skin is cleaned with antiseptic scrub. The needle is then inserted quickly to minimize the discomfort at the level of the skin. The use of a topical refrigerant spray may also help. The location of the needle tip is ensured by provoking the twitch response in the trigger point or by increasing the pain in the zone of reference. An anesthetic agent, often in combination with a steroid, is used. The clinician will know if the location was indeed appropriate because the patient should note rapid relief from pain. The muscle is then passively stretched, care being taken not to provoke a reactive spasm. A series of repeated injections may be required in one trigger point or in several separate points. Relief may last a few hours to a few months.

Another therapeutic strategy in MPS involves physical "reeducation" of affected muscles. The key is to encourage the patient to perform active and passive stretching exercises aimed at increasing the range of motion of stiff and tight muscles. Neck stretching must take into consideration any coexisting limitations in range of motion due to cervical degenerative arthritis, disc disease, or an ankylosing condition, as well as normal physiologic limitations.

Muscle reconditioning by progressive strengthening and postural exercises is another approach in the treatment of MPS. Factors that may be contributing to muscle tension need to be eliminated. These factors include poor posture (including behavior such as shoulder hunching), cradling the phone on the shoulder, or struggling at a work station that is placed too high or too low.

Patients with refractory MPS may need a series of therapeutic interventions (Friction et al., 1982). In this situation a team of providers, each specialized in a diverse facet of the patient's problem, may be called upon to assist in treatment in the setting of a pain clinic. The core of providers usually consists of a physician, a psychologist, and a physical therapist. A key element in this approach is the self-care philosophy. The patient is made an active participant in the healing process and is counseled by the staff, but is reponsible for making any progress.

Fibromyalgia Syndrome

FMS is characterized by widespread musculoskeletal pain, with tender areas in well defined and reproducible locations. Fibrositis is an earlier term that is some-

TABLE 13-3. Comparison of Myofascial Pain Syndrome and Fibromyalgia Syndrome

	Myofascial Pain Syndrome	Fibromyalgia Syndrome
Tender point characteristics	Point tenderness with area of referred pain	Defined areas of local tenderness without referral
Distribution of pain	Usually only one body region	Diffuse both above and below the diaphragm
Aggravating factors	Local trauma, overuse, strain	Weather change, overuse, fatigue
Local response	Twitch response on stroking	No response
Pathologic findings	Usually none	

times used to describe the same symptom complex (Bohr, 1995). FMS shares several features with MPS, but there are also important differences (see Table 13-3). The presence of tenderness on palpation of at least 11 tender points out of a possible 18 is necessary for diagnosis. The widespread pain is chronic, symmetric, and often noted in the low back, neck, shoulders, hips, knees, and hands.

Headaches are a common complaint and are typically fronto-occipital. They are more consistent with tension headaches; however, a minority of patients will have migraine-like headaches (see Ch. 8). Interestingly, the presence of a sleep disturbance is considered a sine qua non by some clinicians. Wolfe et al. (1990) studied 293 patients with fibromyalgia. Compared with 265 controls, they found a higher incidence of fatigue, sleep disturbances, and paresthesias, but the presence of these factors did not provide greater diagnostic sensitivity or specificity. The authors also failed to find significant differences to justify any distinction between primary or secondary FMS.

There is no consistent pathologic finding in FMS. Moldofsky et al. (1975) claimed a disturbance of stage 4 sleep, characterized in EEG tracings by superimposition of an alpha rhythm on the slower delta rhythm. In fact, Moldofsky and Scarisbrick (1976) reported that they could induce aching and fatigue in six sedentary subjects by inducing alpha intrusion in stage 4 sleep. When alpha intrusion was induced in three trained athletes, the symptoms did not appear. However, this electroencephalographic (EEG) finding is not unique to FMS and has been seen in psychiatric patients (Hauri, 1973) as well as in healthy individuals (Scheuler et al., 1988).

Investigation of the tender points by light microscopy has revealed little evidence of inflammation (Kalyan-Raman et al., 1984). Electron microscopy performed by the same group showed more frequent findings, including myofibrillar lysis, glycogen accumulation, and papillary projections; yet, these same findings were present in asymptomatic healthy controls (Yunus et al., 1989a).

Metabolic activity in the muscle surrounding the tender points in fibrositic patients is reportedly deficient in high-energy phosphates (ATP, ADP, and phosphocreatine) as compared with control groups and to muscle without tender points in the same FMS patient (Bengtsson and Henriksson, 1986). Oxygen electrode maps of the trapezius and brachioradialis muscle in FMS and healthy controls showed possible defects in the microcirculation around tender points (Lund et al., 1986). These findings have been interpreted to indicate that the muscle in fibrositis is ischemic.

EMG abnormalities in FMS are inconsistent or lacking (Kraft et al., 1968; Stokes et al., 1988). Perhaps a more central mechanism is involved. Such a mechanism has not been as yet discovered and may simply represent an unwillingness and not an inability. FMS patients typically see themselves as being weak and fatigued. Poor conditioning and/or reduced effort becomes especially evident when patients with fibrositis are exercised. When 25 women with FMS were exercised to volitional exhaustion with maximum oxygen uptake at exhaustion used as the measure of fitness, the majority performed worse than sedentary controls (Bennett et al., 1989). Improvement in aerobic conditioning appears to have a beneficial effect in the treatment of fibrositis (McCain, 1986).

The role of a psychopathologic process remains a paramount question in FMS. Previously, patients were labeled with the term "psychogenic rheumatism." In line with this view FMS patients were compared with rheumatoid and other arthritics by Payne et al. (1982). On Minnesota Multiphase Personality Inventory (MMPI) testing, all FMS patients had abnormalities on the hypochondriasis and hysteria scales. Such MMPI findings have also been noted elsewhere (Ahles et al., 1984; Wolfe et al., 1984).

Smythe (1984) argued that the characteristics displayed by these patients on MMPI are common to any chronic pain patients. Yet, the differences between those with rheumatoid arthritis and those with fibrositis cannot be ignored. Both groups have chronic pain, yet the fibrositic group seem to be more concerned with their symptoms, with increased somatization, hysteria, and hypochondriasis. It is this interest that renders fibrositic patients more difficult to treat.

A possible precipitant in the development of FMS is noted in only about 50 percent of patients (Goldenberg, 1987). The patient may report a traumatic event, either physical or emotional, or a medical illness, especially a flu-like syndrome, but no well-defined cause is established. Some patients, however, can identify a concurrent condition that may help explain some of their symptoms. Examples include rheumatoid arthritis, low back pain, anxiety, and depression.

Management

Management strategies of FMS have many pitfalls and low success rates. One study reported that only 5 percent of FMS patients had sustained remission of all their symptoms at a 3-year follow-up (Felson and Goldenberg, 1986). It seems that even the most comprehensive therapeutic interventions are unlikely to succeed. The patient is often tense, anxious, and skeptical. Thus, the first important step is to assure the fibromyalgic patient that no life-threatening or crippling illness is present. Once the diagnosis of FMS has been made, the routine ordering of serologies or blood tests (rheumatoid factor, antinuclear antibodies, complete blood count, or erythrocyte sedimentation rate) becomes unnecessary and even counterproductive. Patients who continue to go to the laboratory for one venipuncture after another can hardly be faulted if they do not believe in the benign nature of their condition. In addition, patients should also be educated about the possible physiologic basis of the disease and the importance of aggravating factors, both physical and psychological. They should be encouraged to explore all possible factors underlying their complaints. At the same time, patients should also be encouraged toward self-reliance.

Psychological or psychiatric counseling and even biofeedback techniques may be helpful in some cases (Ferraccioli et al., 1987). Behavioral changes must be made with the patient setting realistic goals. The chronic pain patient cannot be expected to become immediately functional simply because the physician has decreed it so. Taking a short walk or preparing a simple meal may be all that can be expected at first. Another cornerstone in the treatment of FMS is the restoration of physical fitness. This can be accomplished by increasing the patient's aerobic capacity through cardiovascular fitness training. McCain et al. (1989), in a 20-week study, noted decreased pain over tender points when patients randomized to a cardiovascular fitness program were compared with the group randomized to a flexibility exercise program. Exercise may aid in the return of restorative sleep, perhaps through an increase in the production of endogenous opioids.

The medical treatment of FMS has met with modest success. The mainstay drugs for musculoskeletal pain appear to be no more effective than placebo (Yunus et al., 1989b). Use of narcotic analgesics is to be avoided. The use of tricyclic drugs seems to have been prompted by the description of the phase 4 sleep disturbance identified by Moldofsky et al. (1975). These drugs may improve sleep by increasing the levels of biogenic amines at the level of the central nervous system (CNS) synapses (Willner, 1985). Amitriptyline (25 to 50 mg at night) may help reduce pain and promote sleep (Carette et al., 1986; Goldenberg, 1987). Cyclobenzaprine (10 to 40 mg at night) may provide similar benefits (Bennett et al., 1988). Imipramine, nortriptyline, doxepin, and trazadone have been used in FMS (in small doses of 10 to 40 mg at bedtime), but their efficacy is not established. Drowsiness and behavioral changes are two side effects that may limit the use of all the aforementioned drugs (see also Ch. 17).

Tender point injection by the technique already described for treatment of myofascial trigger points can be beneficial in the appropriately chosen fibromyalgic patient. This patient should have only a few well-identified painful, tender points. The effects of the injection may last from the duration of the local anesthetic up to several months.

Nonmedicinal therapeutic interventions abound in FMS. Many of the same concepts that govern the management of MPS are applicable. Muscle strengthening and stretching have been advocated. Acupuncture, behavioral therapy, hypnosis, and relaxation training are claimed to produce a beneficial effect. Experience with the use of TENS units in chronic low back pain patients has been extrapolated to suggest its use in FMS. However there are, as yet, no good studies that support the use of any of these modalities in FMS and their use depends on the basis and experience of the practitioner.

Post-Traumatic Cervical Dystonia

Post-traumatic cervical dystonia, also known as post-traumatic torticollis, represents the other end of the soft tissue pain syndrome clinical spectrum from FMS. Whereas in the latter the physical manifestations of the illness are difficult to appreciate, in cervical dystonia the physical aberration is readily apparent. The factors common to both are that even minor trauma reportedly precipitates the onset of spasm and the underlying pathophysiology is unknown.

Truong et al. (1991) reported six cases of torticollis precipitated by neck trauma. In five of the six cases the radiologic investigation by CT, MRI, or myelography did not reveal any evidence of fracture, subluxation, or disc disease. All patients complained of pain immediately after the episode, and the torticollis began within 1 to 4 days of the trauma. These patients differed from those with idiopathic torticollis in several ways. In idiopathic disease the patient can usually turn away from the affected side without difficulty. However, the post-traumatic patient has a decreased range of motion in all directions. The post-traumatic group did not have the morning improvement seen in the idiopathic group nor did they have the worsening of the symptoms usually seen with activity. They also differed from psychogenic torticollis patients, whose symptoms are inconsistent and incongruous over time. Goldman and Ahlskog (1993) found similar results. It appears that the muscular contraction is driven by an as yet unexplained central command.

Treatment of post-traumatic torticollis may not respond to the usual antitorticollis medications. These include benzodiazepines, trihexyphenidyl, baclofen, and botulinum toxin injection. Selective denervation may be an alternative in refractory cases.

Post-Traumatic Spinal Cord Pain Syndromes

Spinal Cord Injury

Chronic intractable pain in spinal cord-injured patients is associated with paralysis, sensory disturbances, or autonomic nervous system dysfunction. In a study by Nepomuceno et al. (1979), pain or some other unpleasant sensation was reported by 75 percent of patients. Approximately 50 percent of patients used the term pain to describe the sensation, while 33 percent described it as an ache, 20 percent as soreness, cramps, or pressure, and 12 percent as suffering. The painful sensation may be described as a burning, stinging, cramping, stabbing, tingling, or numbness. Most patients manifest pain within 6 months of injury, only a small percentage reporting its onset after 1 year. Only 20 percent of cervical spine-injured patients complained of neck pain. Pain is also referred to the upper extremities, trunk, and lower extremities. The relationship between the anatomic extent and location of cord injury and the severity of the pain is highly variable. Exacerbating factors include inactivity, tension, overexertion, and even "the weather." The pathophysiology of the pain is believed to be central in origin.

Chronic neuropathic pain from spinal cord injury may arise from areas where scarred, deafferented nervous tissue is located. Arachnoiditis and tethering of the dorsal horn may also develop in these areas. Alterations of the normal neurophysiology may cause abnormal neuronal firing, sprouting, altered neuropeptide concentration, ephaptic spread from sympathetic to pain fibers, and possibly a disturbance in the inhibitory pain pathways that terminate in the dorsal horn, more specifically the dorsal root entry zone or the substantia gelatinosa (Balazy, 1992).

Therapy

Management of chronic intractable spinal cord injury pain should be directed to the probable central mechanism of pain (see also Ch. 8). Antidepressants, anticonvulsants, and antipsychotics are the most commonly used centrally acting medications. Controlled scientific studies in support of the use of these medications are lacking, and many specialists believe that they produce no real pain relief (Britel and Umlauf, 1986). However, patients often report a subjective improvement in their pain, and a trial with one of these medications seems worthwhile. Narcotic use in these patients is controversial. Methadone is the narcotic of choice because it produces minimal cognitive dulling and it has a relatively long half-life. The addiction potential in patients treated for such pain has been reported to be low (Green and Coyla, 1989). However, narcotics in general should be reserved for the reliable patient who can abide by a regimen for their use in an appropriate clinical setting.

A variety of physical modalities are also incorporated in the treatment strategies of the spinal cord-injured patient. Physical and occupational therapy can restore a certain level of independence, which can only improve the patient's psychological status. Range-of-motion and stretching exercises can prevent contractions and reduce spasticity.

Another mode of therapy is TENS, which, like almost all interventions aimed at pain control, has both proponents and opponents (Hachen, 1977; Rawlings et al., 1989). The presumed mechanism of therapy is stimulation of large-diameter type A fibers, which activate the inhibitory pain interneurons in the dorsal root entry zone, thereby inhibiting the pain impulse. If conservative therapy is ineffective, neurosurgical modalities can be attempted. These treatments consist of nerve blocks and neuroablative and neuroaugmentative procedures. Continuous intrathecal analgesia has also been used in refractory cases.

Dorsal root entry zone ablation has received some attention. The substantia gelatinosa, or dorsal root entry zone, is believed to be responsible for the processing of sensory information and transferral of that information to secondary pain or tract neurons. The creation of a lesion in this area is thought to block effectively the abnormal generation of impulses created by the deafferented state (Alexander et al., 1991). Dorsal column stimulation has been proposed as a treatment alternative, but its value has been debated (Megylio et al, 1989). In these patients, as in any who have chronic pain, a multidisciplinary approach has met with some success.

Cystic Myelopathy

Cystic myelopathy, also known as delayed cystic degeneration or post-traumatic syringomyelia, often presents as acute recurrent pain. Arnold-Chiari malformations, tumor, arteriovenous malformations and arachnoiditis are other possible causes of syringomyelia. An intramedullary cavity (a syrinx) may develop at the level of spinal cord injury and expand cephalad (Balazy, 1992; Laha et al., 1975; Yashon, 1986). In the cervical region these cavities usually manifest as loss of pinprick and thermal sensation with preservation of touch in a capelike distribution over the shoulders and arms. Other manifestations include progressive wasting of the arms and hands, spasticity, Horner syndrome, Charcot's arthropathy (Rhoades et al., 1983), severe orthostatic hypotension (Maynard, 1984), and paroxysmal loss of consciousness (McComas et al., 1983). The incidence of cystic myelopathy is estimated at 1 to 1.5 percent (Rossier et al., 1983).

Development of intramedullary cystic cavities has been reported as early as 4 months (Barnett and Jousse, 1973) or as late as 16 years following injury (White et al., 1977). Important factors include arachnoiditis and tethering of the cord to the spinal canal. Hemorrhage tracking upward from the site of injury may also play a role. Diagnosis is confirmed by CT (with or without metrizamide) or MRI (Balazy, 1992). Therapy is surgical, with shunting of the cystic fluid via a catheter into the subarachnoid space or peritoneum. Appropriately timed surgery may restore lost function.

TRAUMA AND THE ARTHRITIC SPINE

Trauma to the arthritic cervical spine as opposed to the healthy spine is more likely to cause structural damage, pain, and functional compromise. The very nature of the arthritic disease causes a decrease in normal range of motion, stiffening and shortening of the supporting soft tissues, weakening of the involved musculature, and varied degrees of aberrant calcification or ossification. These processes render the spine less able to absorb or dissipate the applied traumatic forces, resulting in more severe injury. The main diseases to consider are osteoarthritis, rheumatoid arthritis, and the seronegative spondyloarthopathies.

Osteoarthritis

Osteoarthritis of the cervical spine is characterized by involvement of the zygapophyseal joints, joints of Luschka, and intervertebral discs. The basic pathophysiologic lesion is destruction of the articular cartilage, sclerosis of the subchondral bone, formation of subchondral cysts, and production of osteophytes. The trigger to these events has not yet been completely defined. There may be an alteration of the microenvironment at the cellular level of the chondrocyte, which precipitates these changes. This mechanism is suspected in ochronosis, or calcium pyrophosphate dihydrate deposition disease. Genetic factors are also important. Primary generalized osteoarthritis shows a dominant pattern of inheritance in women and a recessive pattern in men. This entity affects the hands, cervical spine, knees, and feet while

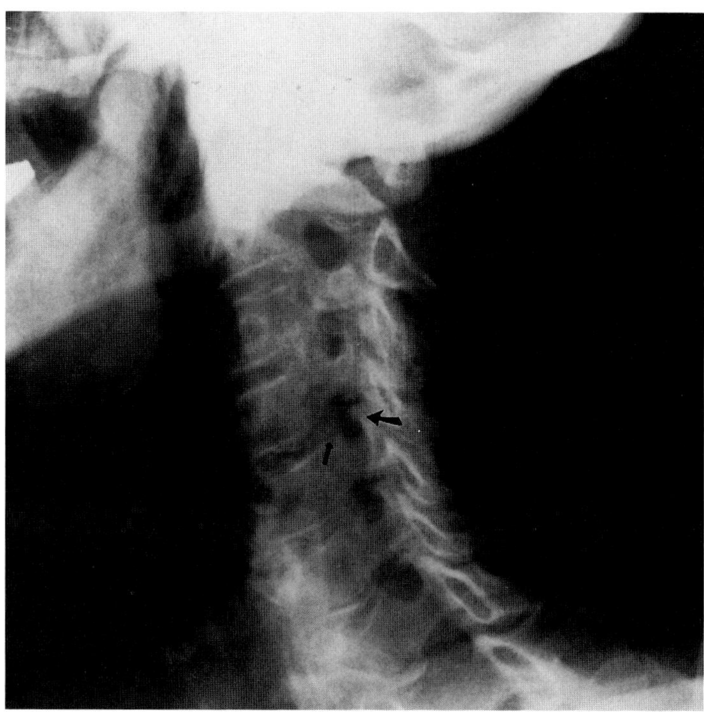

Fig. 13-11. Cervical spine radiographs. Left oblique view in a 78-year-old man shows an uncinate spur at C5 (*small black arrow*) and a zygoapophyseal spur at the superior facet of C5 (*curved arrow*), causing narrowing of the foramina for the left C6 nerve root. The patient had neck pain. (Courtesy of Tereasa Simonson, M.D.)

apparently ignoring other joints. The diversity of presentation indicates that many other factors exist, which still await discovery. Osteoarthritis of the cervical spine is nearly universal in people over the age of 70 (Bland, 1987). It is complicated by the presence of osteoporosis in postmenopausal women, who are prone to vertebral compression fractures. The number of people who can be expected to present with symptoms is impressive.

Cervical osteoarthritis may manifest as attacks of neck pain, often unilateral, with frequent alterations of posture or position. The pain, usually severe, will persist for several days to a week, with resolution occurring within 10 days. Ligaments, tendons, muscles, or the joint capsule can be implicated as the source of pain. The patient may awaken with stiffness, decreased range of motion, and crepitus. The cervical segment is usually straightened and muscle spasm is present. The superior segment of the cervical spine is likely to express osteoarthritis of the facet joints more often, while the inferior segment is likely to suffer from intervertebral disc disease (Bland, 1987). Anterior osteophytes arise at disc margins and are likely to be asymptomatic. Facet osteophytes arise posteriorly and may cause impingement of the nerve root, producing a radiculopathy that affects only the posterior root (Bland and Boushey, 1989). Facet osteophytes can also cause compression of the vertebral artery. Symptoms include dizziness, vertigo, headaches, transient ischemic attacks, and autonomic symptoms (see the discussion of headaches due to sympathetic injury in Ch. 8). Posterior osteophytes of the posterior disc margins may grow into the spinal canal and if of sufficient dimension can cause compression of the spinal cord. Bland and Boushey (1989) claim that myelopathy is probably more common than radiculopathy, especially in older men. Neurologic symptoms and signs are extremely variable and difficult to classify (Bland, 1987). Both upper and lower extremity symptoms can be prominent, and spasticity is common.

The occurrence of traumatic injury in a patient who already suffers from osteoarthritis renders diagnosis and management even more difficult. The possibility of acute ligamentous, tendon, bone, or neural injury is investigated through a complete history and

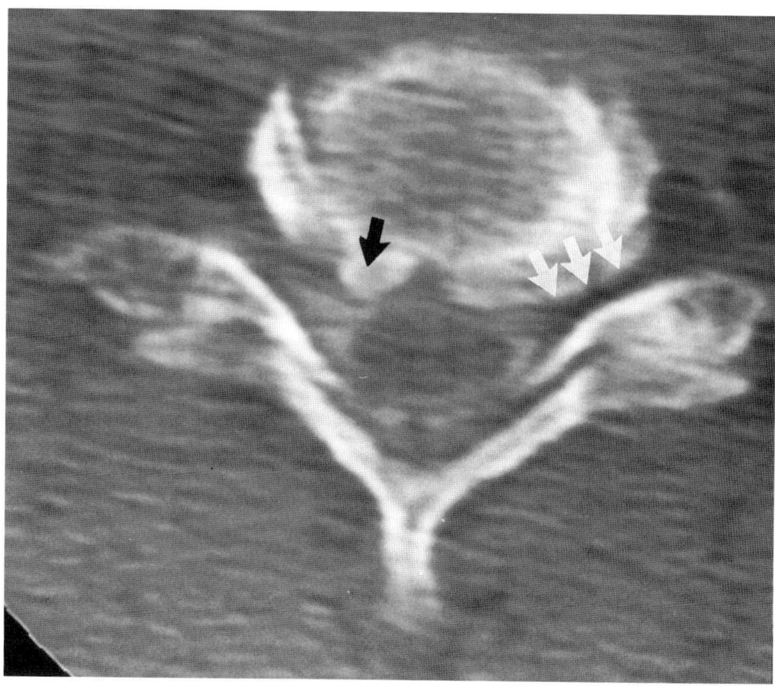

Fig. 13-12. CT myelogram at C6-C7 level in a 53-year-old man. The black arrow shows the location of a marginal osteophyte on the right (left side of picture). At the open arrows, uncinate hypertrophy narrows the neural foramina for the left C7 nerve root. (Courtesy of Tereasa Simonson, M.D.)

physical examination to determine what is new. A detailed description of past symptoms is obtained, and based on that information appropriate diagnostic modalities are used. The basic avenues of arthritis management are education, rehabilitation, exercise, and medication. Calcium replacement is an important preventive measure in women with osteoporosis.

Rheumatoid Arthritis

Rheumatoid arthritis aggressively attacks the upper segments of the cervical spine. Severe involvement can leave the spine unstable and therefore more prone to traumatic consequences. The basic lesion is an inflammatory proliferation of the synovial lining membrane of the joint. The pannus then enzymatically attacks the joint structure, leaving it eroded and weak.

In rheumatoid spondylitis the most conspicuous involvement is at the C1-C2 level. The odontoid process is partially covered with a synovial membrane, as are the lateral facet joints and the atlanto-occipital joints. Erosion of any of these structures can predispose to one or more patterns of subluxation. Anteroposterior, lateral, rotatory, superior, and subaxial subluxation are all seen.

One of the most memorable and frightening experiences in spine medicine is to watch as a rheumatoid patient's head slides forward up on the neck during flexion. This effect makes it understandable how even the slightest forces of acceleration or deceleration can produce spinal cord compression, which can cripple or even kill such a patient. The inferior portion of the cervical spine can be affected by spondylodiscitis, vertebral end plate erosion, or posterior element disease. Subluxations are also seen, and modest forces can again produce severe traumatic sequelae (Halla et al., 1989).

If the estimates of the prevalence of rheumatoid arthritis (up to 1.5 percent of the population) are accurate (Zvafler, 1993), there is a significant risk in quite a large number of people. Recognition of cervical spine instability should be followed by prompt surgical consultation for fusion. The patient should be informed of the dangers inherent in the condition, and use of external supportive devices (collars) should be encouraged when traveling. If the inflammatory process is active, appropriate treatment should be initiated or referral made. The medical treatment of active rheumatoid arthritis has included corticosteroids, gold salts, penicillamine, hydroxy-

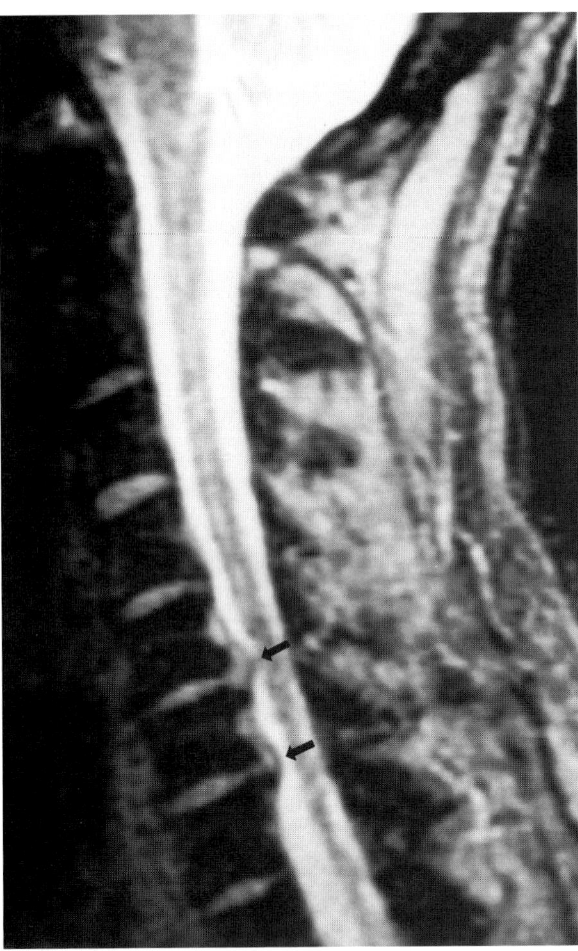

Fig. 13-13. T2-weighted saggital MRI in a 45-year-old man showing posterior disc herniation with mild cord effacement at C5-C6 and C6-C7 levels (*black arrows*). The patient complained of neck pain. (Courtesy of Tereasa Simonson, M.D.)

chloroquine, and immunosuppressants such as azothioprine and cyclophosphamide.

Seronegative Spondyloarthropathies

The term *seronegative spondyloarthropathy* refers to a group of diseases that produce axial skeletal involvement in the absence of rheumatoid factor. The prototype disease is ankylosing spondylitis. This is characterized by sacroiliitis and bridging osteophytosis, which begins in the lumbosacral spine and progresses cephalad. The end result is fusion of the spine into an immobile mass, the "bamboo spine." The pathophysiologic lesion is an inflammatory enthesopathy, in which ligaments attach to bone. Reiter syndrome and psoriatic arthritis may present a similar picture. Danger arises in ankylosing spondylitis when the head is rapidly accelerated or decelerated on the neck. Fractures through the calcified ligaments as well as dislocation or displacement are possible. Neurologic injury is common, and mortality is almost 35 percent (Murray and Persellin, 1981). Travel need not be prohibited, but patients should be aware of the dangers they face and plan accordingly. The practitioner must pay heed to the cervical spine, and neurologic symptoms should be thoroughly investigated.

DIAGNOSTIC METHODS

The appropriate diagnostic pathway in cervical spine injury depends on the patient's symptoms, the clinician's diagnostic suspicion, and whether the investigation is conducted in the acute or chronic phase. Several useful techniques are available.

The radiographic investigation of the cervical spine should begin with plain films. Standard views include the anteroposterior view, the frontal open mouth (odontoid) view, lateral views (full flexion, neutral, and extension), and 45-degree oblique view, both left and right. The frontal view is best at showing the uncovertebral joints. The open mouth view affords a view of the atlantoaxial joint and the lateral masses of the atlas. The lateral view, which should include the whole spinal segment and the intervertebral discs, as well as the zygapophyseal joints, allows the best assessment of the posture of the neck. The oblique views are used to investigate the neural foramina and less effectively, the zygapophyseal joints.

Plain films reveal any change in curvature of the cervical spine, flattening or reversal in curvature being seen in muscle spasm. Changes in an intervertebral disc can be noted as a decrease in the intervertebral space, long-standing changes being noted by the presence of marginal osteophytes. Osteoarthritis presents changes at the level of the zygoapophyseal joints, disc margins, and uncovertebral joints (Fig. 13-11). Rheumatoid subluxation of the odontoid is evaluated with open mouth views. The presence of erosions of the zygoapophyseal joints and the lack of osteophytes favor rheumatoid arthritis over osteoarthritis. The presence of syndesmophytes bridging the vertebral bodies suggests ankylosing spondylitis. Zygapophyseal fusion and paravertebral ossifications may indicate advanced disease.

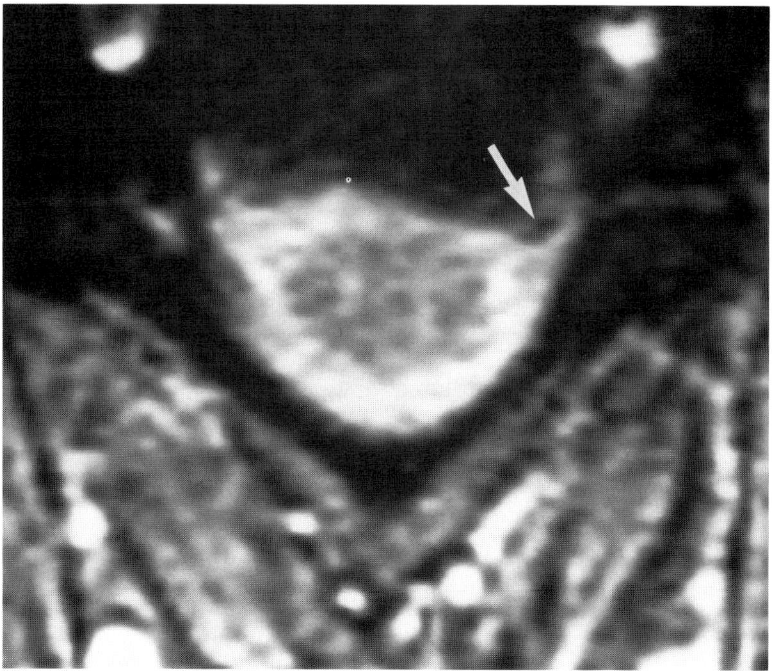

Fig. 13-14. T_2-weighted axial MRI at the C3-C4 level shows a characteristic left uncinate spur (*white arrow*) (right side of picture). The spur appears dark. The patient presented with neck pain. (Courtesy of Tereasa Simonson, M.D.)

CT can be used as the next step when the diagnosis of cervical spine pathology remains uncertain (Fig. 13-12). CT imaging is also used to investigate the extent of disease and to aid in planning surgical or medical intervention. CT imaging is able to demonstrate osseous injury such as marginal fractures and to accurately define the volumes of the spinal canal. Subluxations of the bony elements or stenosis can be diagnosed, as can the presence of intraspinal masses. Encroachment on the spinal cord by either soft or hard tissue can be seen. The lateral recesses of the spinal cord and the neural foramina are visualized, and narrowing or obstruction is noted. Utilizing myelography in combination with CT scanning can enhance resolution quality (Figure 13-12). CT is also an excellent means for evaluating bone mineral content in the cancellous bone, thereby providing a means for the diagnosis and follow-up of osteoporosis or osteomalacia.

MRI is now ubiquitously available. Kent et al. (1994) have reported a study on the efficacy of MRI in neuroimaging, and their findings have been used by the American College of Physicians (1994) as a guideline. MRI has become the preferred modality for the investigation of radiculopathies, malignancies, spinal cord injury, and rupture of the cervical ligaments. The neural column can be imaged without the need for intrathecal injection of contrast medium (Figs. 13-13 to 13-15), although paramagnetic contrast materials such as gadolinium chelates may improve the detection of pathology. In cervical myelopathy the clinical neurologic findings correspond to the areas of neurologic injury on MRI. In disc disease the loss of signal intensity indicates degeneration, although the correlation of signal loss and back pain syndromes is not always clear. The incidence of bulging or herniated discs has been as high as 20 percent of a population of middle-aged asymptomatic patients and more than 50 percent of asymptomatic patients over the age of 64 (Teresi et al., 1987). Many of these individuals have no complaints. The profound implication is that we now have a diagnostic modality so sensitive that it can detect pathology in the patient who has no disease.

Myelography is much less common than it used to be, but it remains extremely useful in certain settings (see Fig. 13-12). For example, some patients are too large to fit into CT or MRI machines or object to the

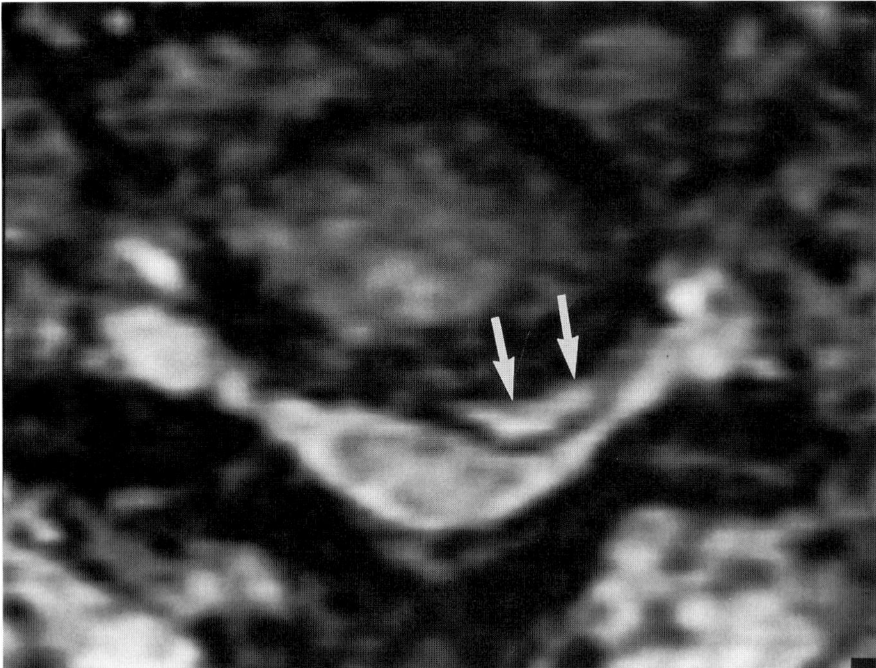

Fig. 13-15. T_2-weighted axial MRI at the C5-C6 level shows a left posterolateral disc herniation (*white arrows*). The disc appears relatively bright compared with the bone and similar in brightness to CSF (Cf. Fig. 13-14). This 45-year-old man had a left C6 radiculopathy. (Courtesy of Tereasa Simonson, M.D.)

latter procedures owing to claustrophobia. Myelography also allows the collection of cerebrospinal fluid samples, which is important for certain diagnoses.

Electrodiagnostic evaluation (Kimura, 1989) of the patient with cervical spine pain is reserved for patients with equivocal radiologic findings or significant physical findings but atypical symptoms. One technique is EMG, which samples the electrical activity in muscle fibers using a needle probe. A short burst of electrical activity is noted when the probe is inserted into normal muscle. This insertional activity is pathologically increased in denervated conditions.

Muscle that has been liberated from neural control by death of the axon will also develop the tendency to contract spontaneously. The EMG changes may take 1 to 2 weeks to become detectable. In the case of cervical radiculopathy, abnormalities (positive sharp waves and fibrillation potentials) will develop in the appropriate cervical paraspinous or arm muscles (see Table 13-2), providing valuable evidence of injury. However, the origin of EMG abnormalities may present a puzzle in a patient who has already had spine surgery. Finally, we note that while EMG findings have been reported in MPS, the procedure is not useful in practice.

Nerve conduction studies can be performed on accessible nerves along which two points are available for placement of the electrodes. Conduction velocities, amplitudes, and distal latencies in the nerve can then be obtained. Both the motor and sensory components of a mixed nerve, such as the median or ulnar nerve, are available for investigation. Focal compression of a traumatized nerve may produce localized slowing or blocks in conduction. The findings can help reveal an unexpected source of pain referred to the neck.

The investigation of spinal reflexes by the study of the H reflex and the F wave may provide information about the most proximal segments of the nerve or spinal roots (Kimura, 1989). The H reflex is produced by the submaximal stimulation of a mixed motor-sensory nerve. The motor response is not produced, but a motor contraction is produced after a period of increased latency. This reflex is dependent on the activation of anterior horn cells by sensory impulses.

The F wave is produced by the supramaximal stimulus of the motor-sensory nerve. The motor fibers that can conduct back toward the anterior horn cells are activated, and they stimulate the forward-conducting neurons, producing a response. Prolonged latencies of the H and F waves are taken as evidence of disease in the proximal segments of the nerves or the spinal roots (Kimura, 1989).

CONCLUSION

The investigation of the patient with post-traumatic cervical spine pain should proceed in a systematic manner. A thorough knowledge of cervical musculoskeletal and neuroanatomy is essential. The source of pain should be vigorously sought in cases of acute injury. The patient who has had a period of relative improvement and then an exacerbation of the previous symptoms or the appearance of new symptoms presents the greatest diagnostic challenge. An accurate history and physical examination must be repeated, with particular emphasis on the nature of the pain, its location, radiation triggers, relievers, and prior therapies. In our litigious society the examiner should note not only patient's complaints but also how they are expressed. Any inconsistencies or incongruities should be noted. A methodical approach with attention to the neurologic and then osseous, ligamentous, and finally soft tissue structures will usually produce a diagnosis.

REFERENCES

Ahles TA, Yunus MB, Railey SD et al: Psychological factors associated with primary fibromyalgia syndrome. Arthritis Rheum 27:1101, 1984

Alexander E III, Nashold BS Jr, Rossitch E Jr: Dorsal root entry zone surgery for pain management: an update. Pain Manag 4:15, 1991

American College of Physicians: Position paper: Magnetic resonance imaging of the brain and spinal cord: a revised statement. Ann Intern Med 120:872, 1994

American Psychiatric Association: (DSM Diagnostic and Statistical Manual of Mental Disorders IV). Washington, 1994

Arroyo DJ: Electromyography in the evaluation of reflex muscle spasm. J Fla Med Assoc 53:29, 1966

Awad EA: Interstitial myofibrositis: hypothesis of the mechanism. Arch Phys Med Rehabil 54:449, 1973

Balazy TE: Clinical management of chronic pain in spinal cord injury. Clin J Pain 8:102, 1992

Barnett HJM, Jousse AT: Nature, prognosis and management of posttraumatic syringomyelia. p.154. In Barnett HJM, Foster JB, Hudgson P (eds): Syringomyelia. WB Saunders, Philadelphia, 1973

Bengtsson A, Henriksson KG: Scand J Rheumatol 16:97, 1986

Bengtsson A, Henriksson KG, Larsson J: Reduced high-energy phosphate levels in the painful muscles of patients with primary fibromyalgia. Arthritis Rheum 29:817, 1986a

Bengtsson A, Henriksson KG, Larsson J: Muscle biopsy in fibromyalgia: light microscopical and histochemical findings. Scand J Rheumatol 15:1, 1986b

Bennett RM, Clark SR, Goldberg L et al: Aerobic fitness in patients with fibromyalgia: a controlled study of respiratory gas exchange and xenon clearance from exercising muscle. Arthritis Rheum 32:454, 1989

Bennett RM, Gatter RA et al: A comparison of cyclobenzaparine and placebo in the management of fibrositis. Arthritis Rheum 31:1535, 1988

Bland JH: Differential diagnosis and specific treatment. p.186. In Disorders of the Cervical Spine: Diagnosis and Medical Management. WB Saunders, Philadelphia, 1987

Bland JH: The cervical spine: from anatomy to clinical care. Med Times 117:9:15, 1989

Bland JF, Boushey DR: Anatomy and biomechanics. p.9. In Disorders of the Cervical Spine: Diagnosis and Medical Management. WB Saunders, Philadelphia, 1987

Block R: Methodology in clinical back pain trials. Spine 12:430, 1987

Bohr, TW: Fibromyalgia syndrome and myofascial pain syndrome. Do they exist? Neurologic Clinics 13:365, 1995

Bonsall A: Flash Anatomy Flashcards: The Bones. Flash Anatomy, Inc. Santa Ana, CA

Britel CW, Umlauf R: Problem survey in an SCI outpatient clinic population: a case for multifaceted, ongoing care. Arch Phys Med Rehabil 67:654, 1986

Carette S, McCain GA, Bell DA et al: Evaluation of amytriptyline in primary fibrositis: a double blind placebo controlled study. Arthritis Rheum 29:655, 1986

Carpenter MB: Spinal cord: gross anatomy and internal structure. p.44. In Core Text of Neuroanatomy. 2nd Ed. Williams & Wilkins, Baltimore, 1978

Deyo RA, Walsh NE, Martin DC et al: A controlled trial of transcutaneous nerve stimulation (TENS) and exercise for chronic low back pain. N Engl J Med 322:1627, 1990

Felson DT, Goldenberg DL: The natural history of fibromyalgia. Arthritis Rheum 29:655, 1986

Ferraccioli G, Ghirelli L, Scita F et al: EMG-biofeedback training in fibromyalgia syndrome. J Rheumatol 14:820, 1987

Friction JR: Myofascial pain syndrome. p.109. In Friction JR, Essam A (eds): Advances in Pain Research and Therapy. Vol 17. Raven Press, New York, 1990

Friction J, Kroening R, Haley D et al: Myofascial syndrome of the head and neck: a review of clinical characteristics in 164 patients. Oral Surg Oral Med Oral Pathol 60:615, 1982

Giesler WO, Jousse AT, Wynne-Jones M et al: Survival in traumatic spinal cord injury. Paraplegia 21:364, 1983

Gold S, Lipton J: Sites of psychophysiologic complaints in MPD patients: II. Areas remote from the orofacial region. J Dent Res 54:165, 1975

Goldenberg D: Fibromyalgic syndrome: an emerging but controversial condition. JAMA 257:2782, 1987

Goldman S, Ahlskog JE: Post-traumatic cervical dystonia. Mayo Clin Proc 68:443, 1993

Green J, Coyla M: Methadone use in the control of nonmalignant chronic pain. Pain Manag 2:241, 1989

Hachen HJ: Physiological, neurophysiological and therapeutic aspects of chronic pain. Preliminary results with transcutaneous electrical stimulation. Paraplegia 78:353, 1977

Halla JT, Hardin JG et al: Involvement of the cervical spine in rheumatoid arthritis. Arthritis Rheum 32:652, 1989

Harris W: Cervical traction: review of the literature and treatment guidelines. Phys Ther 57:8, 1977

Harrison RJ: The vertebral column. p.85. In Romanes CJ (ed): Cunningham's Textbook of Anatomy. 11th Ed. Oxford University Press, London, 1978

Hauri P, Hawkins DR: Electroencephalogr Clin Neurophysiol 34:233, 1973

Holmes GP, Kaplan JE, Gantz NM: Ann Intern Med 108:387, 1988

Kalyan-Raman UP, Kalyan-Raman K, Yunus MB et al: Muscle pathology in primary fibromyalgia syndrome: light microscopic, histochemical and ultrastructural study. J Rheumatol 11:808, 1984

Kent DL, Haynor DR, Longstretg WT Jr et al: The clinical efficacy of magnetic resonance imaging in neuroimaging. Ann Intern Med 120:856, 1994

Kimura J: Electrodiagnosis in Diseases of Nerve and Muscle: Principles and Practice. 2nd Ed. FA Davis, Philadelphia, 1989

Kraft GH, Johnson EW, LaBan MM: The fibrositis syndrome. Arch Phys Med Rehabil 49:155, 1968

Kraus JF, Franti CE, Riggins RS et al: Incidence of traumatic spinal cord lesions. J Chronic Dis 28:471, 1975

Laha PK, Malik HG, Langville RA: Posttraumatic syringomyelia. Surg Neurol 4:519, 1975

Langley BG, Sheppeard H, Johnson M et al: The analgesic effects of transcutaneous electrical nerve stimulation and placebo in chronic pain patients: a double blind non-crossover comparison. Rheumatol Int 4:119, 1984

Lewit K: The needle effect in the relief of myofascial pain. Pain 6:83, 1979

Lund N, Bengtsson A, Thorborg P: Muscle tissue oxygen pressure in primary fibromyalgia. Scand J Rheumatol 15:165, 1986

Maynard FM: Posttraumatic cystic myelopathy in motor incomplete quadriplegia presenting as progressive orthostasis. Arch Phys Med Rehabil 65:30, 1984

McCain GA: Role of fitness training in fibrositis/fibromyalgia syndrome. Am J Med 81:73, 1986

McCain GA, Bell DA, Mai FM et al: A controlled study of the effects of a supervised fibromyalgia. Arthritis Rheum 31:1135, 1989

McComas CF, Fost JL, Schocehet SS Jr: Posttraumatic syringomyelia with paroxysmal episodes of unconsciousness. Arch Neurol 40:322, 1983

Megylio R, Cioni B, Rossi GF: Spinal cord stimulation in the treatment of chronic pain, a 9 year experience. J Neurosurg 70:519, 1989

Moldofsky H, Scarisbrick P: Induction of neurasthenic musculoskeletal pain syndrome by selective sleep stage deprivation. Psychosom Med 38:35, 1976

Moldofsky H, Scarisbrick P, England R: Musculoskeletal symptoms and non-REM sleep disturbance in patients with "fibrositis" syndrome and healthy subjects. Psychosom Med 37:341, 1975

Murray G, Persellin R: Cervical fracture complicating Ankylosing Spondylitis. Am J Med 70:1033, 1981

Nepomuceno C, Fine PR, Richards JS et al: Pain in patients with spinal cord injury. Arch Phys Med Rehabil 60:605, 1979

Oliver J, Middlemarch A: Functional Anatomy of the Spine. Butterworth-Heinemann, Oxford, 1991

Osborn A: In Patterson AS (ed): Diagnostic Neuroradiology. Mosby Press, St. Louis, 1994

Patton J: Neurological Differential Diagnosis. Harold Stark Ltd. London, 1977

Payne TC, Leavitt F, Garron DC et al: Fibrositis and psychological disturbance. Arthritis Rheum 25:213, 1982

Rawlings CCE III, Rossitch E Jr, Nashold BS Jr: The use of limited DREZ lesions for intractable pain. Pain Manag 2:315, 1989

Rhoades CE, Neff JR, Rengachary SS et al: Diagnosis of posttraumatic syringohydromyelia presenting as neuropathic joints. Report of two cases and review of the literature. Clin Orthop 1980:182, 1983

Richardson RR, Meyer PR, Cerullo LJ: Transcutaneous electrical stimulation in musculoskeletal pain of acute spinal cord injuries. Spine 5:42, 1980

Romaines GJ: Muscles concerned in movements of the atlanto-occipital and atlanto-axial joints. In Romaines GJ (ed): Cunningham's Textbook of Anatomy. 11th Ed. Oxford University Press, London, 1977

Rossier AB, Foo D, Naheedy MH et al: Radiography of posttraumatic syringomyelia. AJNR 4:637, 1983

Scheuler W, Kubicki S, Marquardt J: In Koella WP, Obal F et al (eds): Sleep '86. Gustav Fischer Verlag, Stuttgart, 1988

Sheon RP, Moscowitz RW, Goldberg VM: Soft Tissue Rheumatic Pain. Recognition, Management, and Prevention. Lea & Febiger, Philadelphia, 1987

Simeone FA: Cervical disc disease with radiculopathy. p.553. In Rothman RH, Simeone FA (eds): The Spine. 3rd Ed. WB Saunders, Philadelphia, 1992

Smythe HA: Problems with the MMPI. J Rheumatol 11:417, 1984

Stokes MJ, Cooper RG, Edwards RHT: Normal muscle strength and fatigability in patients with effort syndromes. Br Med J 297:1014, 1988

Teresi LM, Lufkin RB, Reicher MA et al: Asymptomatic degenerative disc disease and spondylosis of the cervical spine: MR imaging. Radiology 164:83, 1987

Travell JG: In Bronica J, Albe-Fessard D (eds): Advances in Pain Research and Therapy. p.919. Vol 1. Raven Press, New York, 1976

Travell JG, Simons DG: Myofascial Pain and Dysfunction: the Trigger Point Manual. Williams & Wilkins, Baltimore, 1983

Truong DD, Dubinsky R, Hermanowicz N et al: Posttraumatic torticollis. Arch Neurol 48:221, 1991

White JC, Kneisley LW, Rossier AB: Delayed paralysis after cervical fracture-dislocation. J Neurosurg 46:512, 1977

Williams PL, Warwick R, Dyson M, Bannister LH: Gray's Anatomy. 37th Ed. Churchill Livingstone, New York, 1989

Willner D: Antidepressants and serotonergic neurotransmission: an integrative review. Psychopharmacology (Berlin) 85:387, 1985

Wolfe F, Cathey MA, Kleinheksel SM et al: Psychological status in primary fibrositis and fibrositis associated with rheumatoid arthritis. J Rheumatol 11:500, 1984

Wolfe F, Smythe HA, Yunus MB et al: The American College of Rheumatology 1990 criteria for the classification of fibromyalgia: report of the Multicenter Criteria Committee. Arthritis Rheum 33:160, 1990

Yashon D: In Spinal Injury. p.333. 2nd Ed. Appleton & Lange, East Norwalk, CT, 1986

Youmans JC: In Neurological Surgery. p.1075. Vol 2. WB Saunders, Philadelphia, 1973

Yunus MB, Kalyan-Raman VP, Masi AT et al: Electron microscopic studies of muscle biopsy in primary fibromyalgia syndrome: a controlled and blinded study. J Rheumatol 16:97, 1989

Yunus MB, Masi AT, Aldag JC: Short term effects of ibuprofen in primary fibromyalgia syndrome: a double blind placebo controlled study. J Rheumatol 16:527, 1989b

Zvaifler NJ: p 723. In McCarty, DJ, Koopman WJ (eds): Arthritis and Allied Conditions. 12th Ed. Lea and Febiger, Philadelphia, 1993

Sleep Disorders

14

Mark W. Mahowald
Maren L. Mahowald

The field of sleep medicine has recently established itself as a distinct discipline. The rich and complex spectrum of sleep disorders requires active involvement of neurologists, psychiatrists, pulmonologists, pediatricians, otolaryngologists, physiatrists, behavioral psychologists, and nurses. As sleep is an active and integral component of central nervous system (CNS) function, traumatic brain injury (TBI) may result in substantial abnormalities of sleep/wake function. Consideration of sleep disorders in patients with TBI is important: head trauma results in the hospitalization of 500,000 individuals in the US annually and causes permanent disability in 90,000 with severe and complicated social, medical, and personal consequences (Gennarelli et al., 1989; Goldstein, 1990). Despite the large number of TBIs effects on sleep are mentioned only briefly if at all in recent sleep medicine and rehabilitation medicine textbooks.

REVIEW OF NORMAL SLEEP

There are three states of mammalian consciousness: wakefulness, non–rapid eye movement (NREM) sleep, and rapid eye movement (REM) sleep. Each of these states has its own distinct neuroanatomic, neurophysiologic, and neuropharmacologic mechanisms and behavioral features (Aserinski and Kleitman, 1953; Jones, 1994; Steriade and Hobson, 1976; Vertes, 1984). Most of the state-determining mechanisms that result in the declaration of a given state depend on the brainstem (especially the pons) and basal forebrain regions. No single anatomic site is responsible for all the manifestations of a given state. Neurophysiologic and behavioral features of one state may intrude into another state, or states may oscillate rapidly, resulting in bizarre clinical phenomena (Mahowald and Schenck, 1991). It is important to remember that sleep and coma are *not* on a continuum. Sleep differs from coma in that it is: physiologic, recurrent, and reversible (Aldrich, 1991).

DETERMINANTS OF SLEEPINESS/ALTERNESS

A number of different physiologic variables combine to determine the level of sleepiness-alertness at any given point in time. The two most important are homeostatic and chronobiologic (i.e., circadian). The homeostatic factor is related to the duration of prior wakefulness: the longer the duration of waking, the greater the pressure to sleep. In animals and humans the chronobiologic factor is determined by the "biologic clock" located in the suprachiasmatic nucleus of the hypothalamus. The biologic clock has an inherent rhythm that is entrained by the environmental light-dark cycle. Proof that the suprachiasmatic nucleus is the biologic clock is compelling: (1) its lesions in humans and animals result in a random, irregular wake/sleep pattern; and 2) when lesions of this nucleus are produced in one strain of hamster with a given wake/sleep cycle and the animal is then transplated with the suprachiasmatic nucleus of another strain with a different cycle, the recipient develops the cycle of the donor (Ralph et al., 1990).

There are major changes in the sleep-wake pattern across the lifetime of an individual. Age-related changes include (1) changes in the overall sleep-wake cycle pattern and (2) changes in the distribution of sleep stages within the sleep period.

Sleep/Wake Cycle Patterns

The timing and duration of the sleep-wake pattern within the 24-hour day change with age. At birth, on the average about 16 to 18 hours per day are spent in sleep, and sleep is distributed irregularly. There is a gradual consolidation of sleep into a long, nocturnal period, with a morning and afternoon nap in the first few months. At about 4 years of age there is a single nocturnal sleep period and a single afternoon nap period. By age 6 there is a single nocturnal sleep period with no naps (Webb, 1989). The timing of the major sleep period is somewhat variable, so that some individulas are early-to-bed, early-to-rise "larks" and some are late-to-sleep, late to rise "owls" (Kripke et al., 1979). This variation in the timing of the sleep. is in part genetically determined.

The amount of sleep per 24-hour day rapidly diminishes to about 7.5 to 8 hours by late childhood and then remains relatively constant. It should be remembered that although the average total sleep time is 7.5 to 8 hours, the range is normal adults is from 4 to 10 hours (Kripke et al., 1979). As with the timing of the major sleep period, the total sleep requirement appears to be genetically determined on an individual basis. The tendency for afternoon sleepiness persists and is a function of the underlying biologic clock. This explains the propensity for dozing off in the early to midafternoon. With advancing age, sleep phase tends to advance to an earlier time of sleep onset in the 24-hour period, and the intensity of the sleep phase is reduced (Hofman and Swaab, 1993; Witting et al., 1994).

Changes in Distribution of Sleep Stage Within the Sleep Period

In utero it is likely that almost all sleep is REM sleep (Rigatto et al., 1986). At birth, about 50 percent of sleep is REM. The percentage of sleep that is REM then decreases to 20 to 25 percent by age 3 to 5 years. This percentage persists for the remainder of the life span. In infancy there is a large percentage of slow-wave sleep, the deepest stage of NREM sleep, which diminishes to about 25 percent during adolescence (Williams et al., 1974). After adolescence there is a gradual reduction of slow-wave sleep to very low percentages in senescence (Bliwise, 1994; Carskadon and Dement, 1994). The generators of the patterns of distribution of REM and NREM within sleep are not known. Multiple sleep-promoting factors have been proposed, and some have been identified. Their roles in the determination of state are extremely complex and incompletely understood (Inoue, 1989; Kreuger and Obal, 1993).

EVALUATION OF SLEEP/WAKE COMPLAINTS

Sleep-wake disorders are prevalent in the general population and could be expected to persist following TBI. Furthermore, as discussed below, TBI likely results in a number of sleep-wake complaints. Such complaints, whether pre-existing or following TBI, can be evaluated by both clinical and sleep laboratory techniques.

The initial evaluation of sleep complaints begins with a thorough sleep history and physical examination. Particular attention should be paid to the cardiopulmonary, neurologic, and psychiatric examinations. A meticulous history of sleep-wake function must be detailed. Corroborating information from bed partners, other family members, co-workers, or caregivers is usually required for a complete and accurate assessment of sleep behaviors. Prolonged sleep/wake diaries completed by the patient or observer may give an at-a-glance overview of wake/sleep patterns not obviously apparent by clinical history.

If the sleep-wake disturbance is bothersome and cannot be diagnosed by history alone, procedures to obtain objective information regarding the quality, quantity, and/or timing of sleep should be performed.

Polysomnography

The technology used for the diagnosis of sleep disorders employs standard electrophysiologic recording systems (Guilleminault, 1982). The basic polysomnography format has been standardized and includes, continuous monitoring of eye movements, at least one channel of electroencephalography (EEG) (usually C3/A2 or C4/A1), respiratory parameters (at minimum, airflow), electrocardiography (ECG), submental electromyography (EMG), and anterior tibialis EMG. Multiple respiratory parameters must be monitored to evaluate sleep-disordered breathing: (1) airflow (thermistors, thermocouples, or expired carbon dioxide sensors); (2) respiratory effort (strain gauges, inductance plethysmography, impedance pneumography, endesophageal pressure, intercostal EMG); and (3) gas exchange (oximetry). Other parameters may be monitored as clinically indicated, such as extensive EEG for parasomnias, esophageal pH for gastroesophageal reflux, or penile tumescence for erectile function. The American Electroencephalographic Society, Ad Hoc Committee on Polysomnographic Guidelines (1991) has outlined specific polysomnographic recording techniques, and sleep stage scoring techniques have been standardized (Rechtschaffen and Kales, 1968).

By recording an all-night polysomnogram, sleep can be accurately quantified and sleep stages fully characterized. It is also possible to determine the presence of (1) sleep architecture disruption, (2) cardiopulmonary abnormalities, (3) sleep-related motor activity, and (4) other sleep-associated disorders. Visual scoring and interpretation of polysomnograms is the currently accepted standard. The reliability of computer-aided systems to evaluate sleep disorders awaits objective, published verification (Lesch and Spire, 1990). The complex nature of normal and abnormal sleep, together with complexities of the physiologic recording equipment (artifacts and maintenance of the recording signals) are challenging (Mahowald and Schenck, 1991; Mahowald et al., 1991). It is unknown whether computerized scoring systems will be valid for studying the changes in EEG and sleep patterns associated with TBI.

Multiple Sleep Latency Test

The multiple sleep latency test (MSLT) is a standardized and well validated measure of physiologic sleepiness. The parameters monitored are the same as for basic polysomnography—usually two eye movement and two EEG (central and occipital) channels, in addition to ECG, airflow, and submental EMG. The MSLT consists of four or five 20-minute nap opportunities offered at 2-hour intervals (Carskadon et al., 1986). The MSLT is designed (1) to quantitate sleepiness by measuring how quickly an individual falls asleep on sequential naps during the day (Roehrs et al., 1989) and (2) to identify the abnormal occurrence of REM sleep during a nap. For each nap, the latency between "lights out" and sleep onset is recorded. Pathologic ranges of sleep latency have been carefully defined. A mean latency of 5 minutes or less indicates severe excessive sleepiness. The number of naps during which REM sleep appears is also noted. Many factors can affect sleep latency during the daytime, including prior sleep deprivation, sleep continuity, age, time of day, and medication (American Sleep Disorders Association, 1992). Proper interpretation requires a preceding night polysomnogram to measure the quality and quantity of sleep obtained immediately prior to the MSLT. The MSLT is a most useful tool in quantifying daytime sleepiness and in differentiating the subjective complaints of "sleepiness," "tiredness," and "fatigue."

Actigraphy

Analysis of sleep diaries may be insufficinet to verify a tentative diagnosis in patients with suspected sleep-wake cycle abnormalities. In such cases, definitive objective data may be obtained by actigraphy, a recently developed technique to record activity during waking and sleep, which supplements the subjective sleep log. An actigraph is a small wrist-mounted device, which records the activity plotted against time, usually for 1 or 2 weeks. There are different models of actigraphs, whose principles are reviewed elsewhere (Tryon, 1991). When data collection has been completed, the results are transferred into a personal computer, where software displays activity versus time. Figures 14-1 and 14-2 show actigraphic reports and demonstrate how the rest/activity pattern is apparent at a glance. There is direct correlation between the rest/activity recorded by the actigraph and the wake/sleep pattern as determined by polysomnography (Brown et al., 1990a; Brown et al., 1990b).

EFFECT OF TBI ON SLEEP-WAKE FUNCTION

Neuropathology

The mechanisms of brain injury are very complex. Direct blows to the head are not necessary; severe TBI may occur simply from cranial acceleration/deceleration injuries. Shearing injuries in direct and indirect TBI produce pathologic changes which are often very diffuse, affecting multiple portions of the CNS including the brainstem (Adams, 1992). Since sleep-wake generation is dependent on the proper functioning of multiple levels of the nervous system, particularly the brainstem, basal forebrain, and hypothalamus, many severe TBIs could be expected to affect at least some of the structures involved in sleep/wake declaration and function.

Increased Intracranial Pressure

Intracranial pressure (ICP) normally has circadian or sleep-state determinants, being increased during sleep. The ICP increases were noted to occur during REM sleep (DiRocco et al., 1975; Gucer and Viernstein, 1979; Hirsch et al., 1978; Pierre-Kahn et al., 1978; Renier et al., 1982) and were formerly attributed to sleep-related carbon dioxide retention. The change in ICP is now thought to be related to a diurnal increase in blood volume. The increased ICP during sleep may be exaggerated in patients whose ICP is already elevated (Cooper and Hulme, 1969; Furuse et al., 1979; Munari and Calbucci, 1981; Ueno et al., 1986; Yokota et al., 1989a; Yokota et al., 1989b). Cerebral blood flow, which may be compromised in the setting of increased ICP, may be monitored by the transcranial Doppler ultrasound technique (Goh et al., 1992; Newell et al., 1992). In TBI patients with nocturnal decompensation of ICP, severe bradycardia and systemic arterial hypertension were inaccu-

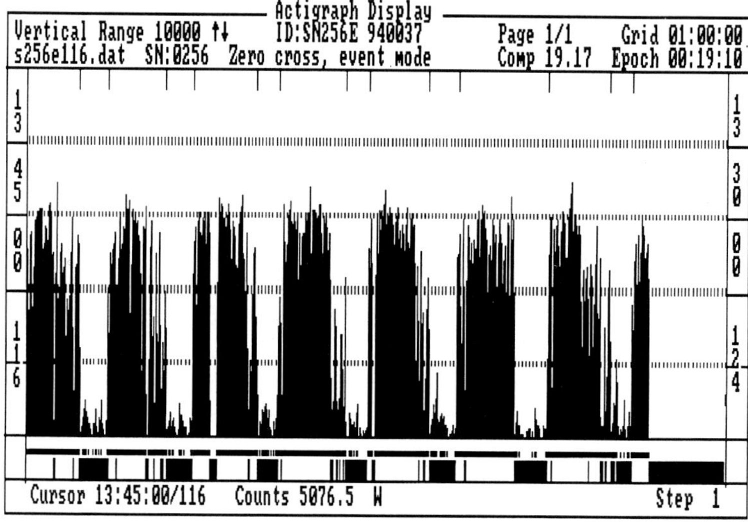

Fig. 14-1. Sample of actigraphic report: vertical bars represent activity levels plotted over seven consecutive 24-hour periods. An apparently normal cycling of rest/activity (sleep/wake) is displayed.

SINGLE PLOT OF DATA

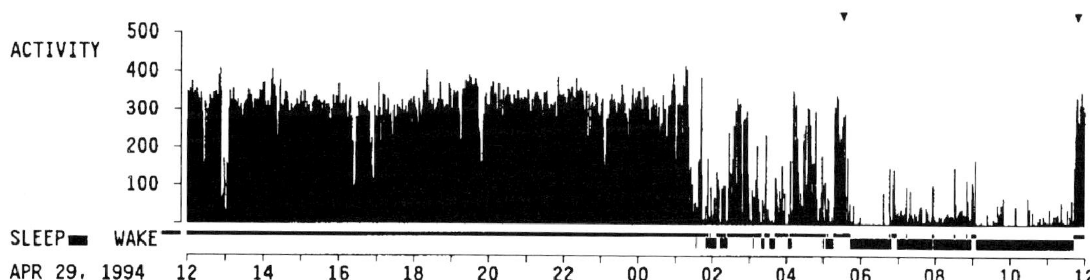

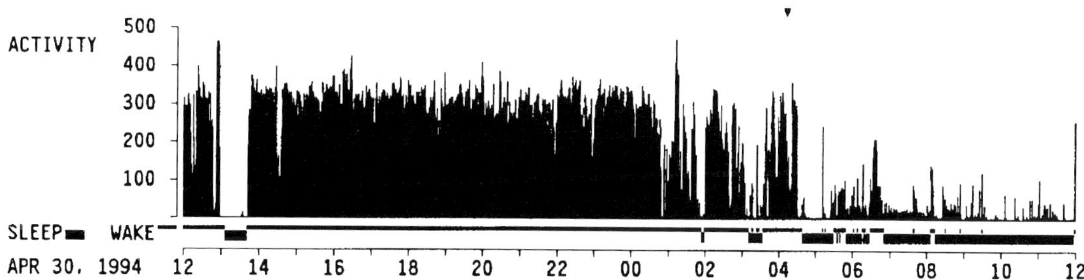

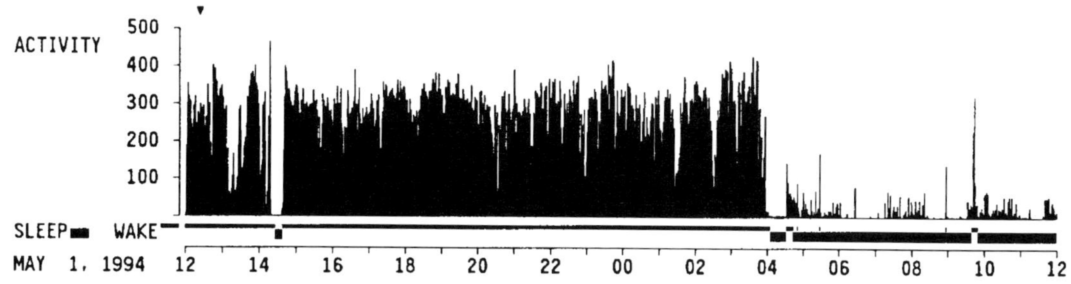

Fig. 14-2. Closer examination of each 24-hour period reveals that although the cycling is normal, the timing of the sleep period is abnormal, with a striking delay in the onset of the sleep period until 4 to 6 A.M..

rate predictors of the increased ICP (Marshall et al., 1978).

Secondary CNS Injury

Acute TBI may be associated with apnea and hypotension which individually result in additional secondary CNS damage, increasing morbidity and mortality from severe head injury (Chestnut et al., 1993). It must be remembered that sleep-disordered breathing identified following TBI may have been present prior to the TBI, may have resulted from the neurologic injury, or may be due to associated nonneurologic (cervical spine, thoracic cage, cardiopulmonary) injuries. It is important to detect and treat obstructive sleep apnea because it causes severe sleep fragmentation, sleep-related hypoxia, and/or hypercapnia, which may interfere with recovery from TBI. Another important reason to identify and treat this disorder is that there may be marked episodic increases in ICP during the apneic episodes (Doyle and Tami, 1991; Jennum and Borgesen, 1989; Kuchiwaki et al., 1988; Sugita et al., 1985). This is particularly relevant for those TBI patients who may already have increased ICP secondary to their head injury.

Sleep Studies in Severe TBI

There have been numerous reports of the presence or absence of normal polygraphic sleep patterns as an indicator of the extent or severity of brain injury and as a predictor of recovery from TBI. Given the fact that multiple levels of the CNS are necessary to generate and coordinate the sleep-wake cycle, it should follow that the more abnormal are the sleep-wake patterns in a TBI patient, the more extensive is the damage to the CNS. Conversely, the more normal the sleep-wake cycle, the greater the likelihood that the integrity of the CNS has been maintained, and perhaps the better the outcome. Many of the commonly cited studies are compiled in Table 14-1.

Sleep has been reported in a variety of ways: subjective report, limited EEG monitoring, and formal polysomnographic recording. There is no objective confirmation of insomnia or excessive daytime sleepiness in studies reporting those complaints. It is difficult to compare these studies, as the selection criteria, methods of monitoring, and outcome measures are quite variable, as was the severity of TBI and interval between TBI and study. By definition there are no behavioral manifestations of sleep-wake cycling in comatose patients; however, electrophysiologic evidence of sleep/wake is seen as various stages of NREM sleep reappear, followed by episodes of REM sleep. It may be tentatively concluded that the early appearance of wake/sleep cycling generally but not invariably indicates a better prognosis. The same may be said for the correlation (again, incomplete) between the preservation or reappearance of REM sleep and cognitive recovery. Although it has been suggested that this supports the postulated role of REM sleep in memory, it could just as easily indicate that the better the return of brain function, the better the memory.

There have been studies employing neurophysiologic measures other than sleep as prognosticators in TBI. One of the most comprehensive is that of Rae-Grant et al. (1991), who found a high correlation between Glasgow Outcome Scale score and a number of EEG criteria, including sleep spindles and EEG reactivity and variability (Rae-Grant et al., 1991; Tsukokawa et al., 1990). EEG reactivity was also found to be prognostically significant in another study by Synek (1988).

Despite the importance of nighttime sleep and daytime altertness on daytime function and performance, studies of psychosocial outcome of severe head injury have made no mention of either objective or subjective findings regarding sleep (Bond, 1975).

Sleep Studies in Minor Head Injury

There are virtually no objective studies of sleep-wake function in minor head injury patients. In one subjective questionnaire study, Levin et al. (1987) listed "sleep disturbance" as a subscale of the "emotional disturbance" category. In another questionnaire survey of 75 patients following minor head injury, sleep interruption and impaired sleep quality were reported. The percentage experiencing sleep-wake complaints was not stated, and no objective studies were performed (Parsons and Ver Beek, 1982). In still another study of minor head injury, about 20 percent of patients reported subjective "dysfunction of sleep and rest" (Dikmen et al., 1986).

All objective EEG sleep studies in TBI to date have been performed on patients with severe TBI, and the outcome variables have been generally gross. Given the broad spectrum of EEG changes attendant on acute severe TBI and the variable rate of recovery, it is questionable whether further EEG sleep study of this acute and severely affected population will be fruitful. These studies are very expensive in terms of both time and money. Attention may be better directed to evaluation of sleep-wake functioning in the patient who has recovered sufficiently from TBI to participate in a rehabilitation program.

Regrettably, the objective study of sleep-wake functioning and cycling in those patients who have regained consciousness and who are candidates for rehabiltation has never been addressed. It is clear that insomnia, excessive daytime sleepiness, and shifts in the timing of the sleep-wake cycle are common following TBI and should be expected to pose severe impediments to rehabilitation programs. There is some clinical suggestion (without objective verification) that the complaints of disturbed sleep and impaired attention during wakefulness may change as the patient progresses (Kowatch, 1989). These complaints may be confounded or exacerbated by the routines employed in most rehabilitation and chronic care facilities. For instance, the practice of putting patients to bed at the same time, usually very early, is more for the convenience of the staff than in the best interest of the patients. Imposing such constraints upon a patient's sleep-wake cycle may result in sleep-onset "insomnia" or early morning awakenings, leading to unnecessary administration of medication. Such practices could be expected to exacerbate circadian abnormalities.

Chronopharmacology

The circadian timing of administraction of a wide variety of (and, perhaps all) medications and other therapies such as x-ray irradiation may have profound effects upon their efficacy and toxicity (Halberg, 1969; Moore-Ede, 1973; Radzialowski and Bousquet, 1968; Reinberg, 1967). There is compelling evidence of the importance of considering the time of circadian cycle in drug administration in other conditions such as cancer chemotherapy, use of anesthetics and antiepileptic drugs, and steroid administration (Koren et al., 1992). There have been no studies to date on the circadian considerations of drugs used in the treatment of TBI. It is likely that chronopharmacologic considerations will prove to be of importance in TBI.

SPECIFIC SLEEP DISORDERS

Hypersomnia

Sleep Apnea

Since obstructive sleep apnea is prevalent in the general population, 4 percent of female and 9 percent of male patients on the TBI rehabilitation service could be expected to have this disorder prior to the trauma (Young et al., 1993). TBI may cause obstructive sleep apnea by altering respiratory control systems. (Chokroverty, 1994). Furthermore, many patients with TBI have also sustained noncerebral injuries that would predispose to this condition. Obstructive sleep apnea may result from injury, burns, or surgery to the upper airway (Robertson et al., 1985; Sher, 1990). It may also result from simple nasal obstruction (Olsen et al., 1981) or nasal packing used for treatment of upper airway problems (Johannessen et al., 1992). Sleep-disordered breathing is particularly prevalent in patients with cervical spinal cord lesions, which may be associated with some degree of loss of central respiratory muscle control. In one series, 10 of 22 unselected adult patients with stable spinal cord injury were found to have sleep apnea (Short et al., 1992). Another study showed significant sleep-disordered breathing in a group of quadriplegic patients in whom there was a low clinical suspicion for sleep-disordered breathing (Cahan et al., 1993). Persistence of sleep-disordered breathing in patients with traumatic tetraplegia has been documented in a longitudinal study (Back and Wang, 1994). This has important therapeutic implications. It should also be remembered that many patients on the rehabilitation service are given drugs (sedative/hypnotics, myorelaxants, and analgesics) that may exacerbate sleep-disordered breathing (Sanders, 1994). To make matters worse, many patients who are relatively immobile tend to gain weight, a known risk factor for the development of obstructive sleep apnea.

Sleep-disordered breathing is readily diagnosed by formal sleep studies. There are a number of treatment options, including nasal continuous positive airway pressure (Powell et al., 1994) and upper airway surgery (Powell et al., 1994).

Narcolepsy and Idiopathic CNS Hypersomnia

Narcolepsy and idiopathic CNS hypersomnia are two conditions characterized by excessive daytime sleepiness in the absence of sleep deprivation or any identifiable abnormality during sleep such as obstructive sleep apnea (Aldrich, 1990; Guilleminault, 1994; Mitler et al., 1990). Well documented narcolepsy or idiopathic CNS hypersomnia following head injury is very uncommon (Billiard et al., 1993). The lack of documentation relates to the fact that many older reports were based on clinical criteria, did not utilize objective methods such as formal sleep studies, and

TABLE 14-1. Sleep Wake Abnormalities as Predictors of TPI Severity and Outcome

Author/Yr	Selection Criteria	Number of Subjects	Age	Coma Scale	Duration of Coma	Interval: TBI Evaluation	Subjective/ Objective	Outcome Measures	Findings	Comments
Bergamasco et al., 1968a	Traumatic coma Exclude coma "depasse" Exclude akinetic mutism	20 ("both sexes")	3–66 years (no mean)	Clinical/EEG (Fischgold & Mathis, 1959)	3–218 days	"Generally" began 48–72 hours following TBI, recorded at intervals until clinical resolution or death	EEG - longitudinal. Daily/nightly until clinical resolution (lethal or not) (9/20 died); Determined "slow phase" (NREM) and "rapid phase" (REM) (called biphasic when both phases were present and monophasic when only "slow phase was present." These were not considered to be normal sleep (?nonreactive to stimulation?)	"Recovered" vs. "dead"	Preservation of typical polysomnographic sleep patterns or organized circadian activity was a favorable prognostic finding	
Bergamasco et al., 1968b	Appear to be same subjects as those of Bergamasco (1968) above but with 18 rather than 20 subjects	18								
Bricolo et al., 1968	Posttraumatic coma	22	4–67 years (mean, median N/A) of "both sexes"	Four degrees (Fischgold & Mathis) (apallic, coma vigil, and akinetic mutism were classified independently)	15 days to over 1 year	More than 15 days	One all-night and "short-lasting" clinical electropolygraphic examinations in all (12 once, 4 twice, 6 three times). Sleep classified in 4 main phases	"Improved, no changes, impairment"	"A certain relation between presence and degree of organization of the sleep patterns and degree of consciousness impairment was apparent." ". . . the better the organization of sleep, the greater the chance of a favorable outcome." There were exceptions	
Lessard et al., 1974	10 coma subjects	8 post-traumatic, 2 drug ingestion	Sex, age N/A	"Grade I–III not otherwise specified	N/A	N/A	EEG sleep patterns and period analytical characteristics of the EEG to follow cyclic variations during sleep	"Recovered" vs. "died"—not otherwise specified	2 with cyclic EEG variations regained "full consciousness", 1 died. Of 7 who did not show such variations, 6 died	

Bergamasco et al., 1977	Prolonged post-traumatic coma in various stages of the "apallic syndrome"	46 (appears to include 18 cases reported above); appears to represent a summation of the literature without details. 8 subjects were monitored until "recovery or exitus."	N/A	N/A	N/A	N/A	N/A	N/A	"In cases where the bioelectric reorganization of nocturnal sleep does not take place or takes place to an incomplete degree, there is usually a poor clinical evolution, even if it is long-lasting."	No individual data are available to support the conclusions
Alexandre et al., 1979	Severe head injuries operated on for intra- or extra-cerebral expanding lesions	20	N/A	Clinical coma scale, brainstem level	? within 1 week	? within 1 week	Nocturnal polygraphic recordings in acute phase, during PTA, every 2 months thereafter	Sleep parameters, neuropsychological testing (WAIS, Raven Corsi, Kimura, Token tests)	There was a correlation between the return of REM sleep and cognitive outcome. REM was normal initially in all who were free from cognitive deficits: none with initial severe REM alterations had normal performance 14 months later.	Scanty tabular data to support conclusions
Billiard et al., 1979	Severe head trauma with brainstem dysfunction acutely	9 (8 male)	26.8 years (+5.05) median 20 years	Clinical - not stated	N/A	37–111 days	Divided into two groups: one with normal NREM REM paterns (5 subjects), the other with no NREM and uncertain or absent REM (4 subjects)	N/A (in French)	"At the chronic stage of post-traumatic comas a 24-hour polygraphic recording supplies no definite information with regard to the prognosis."	Found that the synchronization of sleep with dark periods was lost in 7/9 cases.
Ron et al., 1980	TBI	9 (8 male)	Mean 22.5 (16–36)	N/A	0.5–16 weeks	1–6 mo	EEG sleep stage: 4–7 recording nights over 5–8 weeks Average period of followup 38 wks (22–52)	Independence, locomotion, cognition	The sleep-waking rhythm not useful long-term measure of prognosis There was a correlation between REM sleep and cognition (high in 7, low in 2)	
Rumpl et al., 1979	Closed traumatic head injuries with secondary brainstem dysfunctions	113 (? sex distribution)	6–74 years (mean/ median N/A)	6 neurologic stages (Gerstenbrand and Lucking, 1970)	N/A	Few hours to 7 days	EEG recordings (time of day/ night not specified)	EEG pattern with clinical level of brainstem dysfunction	"The variety of EEG patterns, especially 'sleep or sleeplike' activities and alternating patterns decreased with the grade of rostrocaudal deterioration."	Sleep EEG patterns were mentioned, but sleep per se was not studied.

(*Continued*)

TABLE 14-1 (*continued*). Sleep Wake Abnormalities as Predictors of TPI Severity and Outcome

Author/Yr	Selection Criteria	Number of Subjects	Age	Coma Scale	Duration of Coma	Interval: TBI Evaluation	Subjective/ Objective	Outcome Measures	Findings	Comments
Hansotia et al., 1981	Coma of varied etiology	370 (22 with "spindle coma" [8 TBI])	1–69 years (mean/ median N/A)	N/A	Within 3 days of onset of coma	N/A	EEG recordings (duration, time of day/night not specified)	Clinical evaluation: level of consciousness; ocular movements; respiration; limb movement: spontaneous and following stimulation	"The occurrence of sleep spindles in successive records, or improved organization of sleep patterns in successive EEGs, bore no relationship to outcome." "EEG features of sleep in the form of spindles, V waves, or K complexes and their reactivity did not predict outcome"	Study limited to 22 subjects with EEGs with the spindle pattern of sleep (spindle coma)
Alexandre et al., 1983	100 surviving with "more or less impairment" of 178 severely head-injured patients (76 died, 2 remained in persistent vegetative state	178 (functional outcome only on 100 survivors) Nocturnal polysomnograms performed on 40 subjects	N/A	Glasgow coma scale and Plum and Posner, Bricolo	N/A	"As soon as possible after injury"	EEG "as soon as possible after admission, repeated 'frequently' " Sleep EEG (on 40 subjects) "as soon as possible after admission and periodically thereafter and every 2 months after discharge)	Multiple neuropsychological tests 1 and 2 years after injury	EEG: diphasic with spindles had best outcome There was a high correlation between abolition of deep NREM and REM sleep and severe residual cognitive deficits. "REM sleep abolition entailed some degree of neuropsychological decay in 87.5%"	3 subjects with no REM sleep at follow-up had no residual cognitive deficits.
George and Landau-Ferey, 1986	Severe head trauma	?16? (sex not mentioned) It is virtually impossible to ascertain how many subjects were studied and whether the 6 and 12-mo studies were on the same subjects as the 1 mo studies or whether it was a different group	Divided into two groups: ?10 young (15–25 years old) and ?6 adult (35–45 years old) (means/median N/A)	Four clinical levels (cortical, diencephalic, mesodiencephalic, mesencephalic)	Means of 3 groups 16–21 days	N/A	Sleep EEG pattern	"Recovery was assessed as soon as the patient regained normal consciousness, speech, and adapted movements." Not further specified	"The lower the initial level of brain stem dysfunction, the greater the sleep disturbances were."	

Askenasy and Rahmani, 1988	Penetrating craniocerebral trauma	20	19–31 years (mean, median N/A)	No mention of coma or initial clinical status	N/A	Polysomnogram 3 months after injury	2 nights of polysomnography 3 months following injury	Neurologic examination, neuropsychological evaluation, rehabilitation surveys every 3 months	65% had sleep disturbances (45% insomnia, 20% hypersomnia) Insomnia pattern has a more severe prognosis than hypersomnia. Coma longer than 7 h and intracerebral hemorrhage were determining factors in producing insomnia. "There is a relationship between fragmented sleep, polyphasic sleep cycles, and recovery from brain damage."	No data (sleep or clinical) are given to support the stated conclusions.
Cohen et al., 1992	Two groups of TBI subjects: 1 hospitalized 2 discharged	 22 (16 male) 77 (57 male)	 Median 29 years Median 26 years	 N/A N/A	 6.5 (1–60) days 12 (1–60) days	 3.5 mo (no range) 29.5 mo (24–36 mo)	Sleep questionnaire	Motor deficits, communicative skills, cognitive and behavioral performance. Rehabilitation outcome only in discharged subjects	Hospitalized group: 72.7% reported sleep disturbances (82% insomnia, 14% excessive sleepiness) Discharged group: 52% reported sleep disturbances (8% insomnia, 73% excessive sleepiness)	In both groups, age and duration of coma were not significantly associated with sleep complaints. Discharged subjects with sleep complaints had significantly poorer occupational outcome.
Alster et al., 1993	Trauma and nontrauma patients	29 (? 14 TBI)	18–90 (mean 52.5) 19 male, 10 female)	Glasgow coma scale on day of recording	0.5–66 days	1–76 days	Physiological response to sound stimulus (increase in EMG, change in EEG frequency, and appearance of sharp waves or k-complex) temperature rhythm	"Good, deficit, vegetative, death"	A physiologic response to a sound stimulus was the best predictor for outcome. All exhibited a 24-h circadian temperature rhythm, but it was out of phase with the environment.	This is not a "sleep" study per se, but it does use the k-complex (an indicator of arousal during sleep) as a response to auditory stimulation and does address circadian temperature rhythms

did not employ HLA typing. The recently described very high association of a specific HLA type of narcolepsy may help identify such cases in the future (Aldrich, 1990). The absence of the expected HLA type may speak for "symptomatic" or acquired narcolepsy. The documentation of narcolepsy associated with nontraumatic lesions of the diencephalon suggest that TBI (possible interacting with genetic predisposition) may result in narcolepsy (Aldrich and Naylor, 1989). One case reported as post-traumatic more likely represented the spontaneous development of narcolepsy following head injury; the degree of trauma was mild, the interval between injury and onset of symptoms was 18 months, and the HLA typing indicated a genetic predisposition to narcolepsy (Good et al., 1989). Another more convincing case is that of a young man with onset of symptoms during the first month following a more severe head injury (Maccario et al., 1987). A single case of TBI resulting in cataplexy (without objective studies) has been reported (Sadowski, 1981). A careful study of 20 patients with objectively evaluated post-traumatic hypersomnia revealed multiple causes, including sleep-disordered breathing, nonspecific objective hypersomnia, and two cases of subjective but not objective hypersomnia (Guilleminault et al., 1983). The multiple etiologies that have been identified mandate objective study of the complaint or observation of hypersomnia in TBI. Data now available indicate that there are multiple possible causes of post-TBI hypersomnia, which must be characterized by objective polysomnography and MSLT because the treatments are diagnosis-specific. The hypersomnia of narcolepsy and idiopathic CNS hypersomnia usually responds well to stimulant medication (American Sleep Disorders Association, Standards of Practice Committee, 1994; Guilleminault, 1994).

Kleine-Levin Syndrome

The Kleine-Levin syndrome is characterized by periodic hypersomnia lasting days to weeks and occurring at intervals of days to years, with intervening normal wake/sleep function and alertness. The classic form is idiopathic and seen most commonly in adolescent boys but may affect both sexes and all age groups. The periodic hypersomnia may be associated with hyperphagia and hypersexuality and likely represents recurrent hypothalamic dysfunction. Many cases are not associated wtih hyperphagia or hypersexuality (Smolik and Roth, 1988). This syndrome has been reported following mild head injury. The post-traumatic form, like the idiopathic, may respond to lithium (Gill et al., 1988).

Sleep-Wake Cycle Abnormalities

The sleep-wake cycle in mammals is determined by the suprachiasmatic nucleus. Given the fact that this is a neurologic structure, it would be expected that TBI affecting it might result in severe abnormalities of the sleep-wake cycle (Okawa et al., 1986). Although circadian dysrhyhmias have most important rehabilitation implications, they have been virtually ignored in TBI research. A single case of delayed sleep phase syndrome following a very minor head injury (5-minute loss of consciousness) has been reported. There were no subjective (behavioral ratings or sleep logs) or objective confirmatory studies (Patten and Lauderdale, 1992). In one study of severely head-injured patients, Billiard et al. (1979) found that in seven of nine there was a reversal of the normal circadian rhythmicity. In another study, a large percentage of comatose TBI patients demonstrated a persistent 24-hour temperature cycle, which was advanced or delayed from the usual sleep-wake cycle by a number of hours. This study suggested that the biologic clock is resilient but may become "reset" relative to the environment following TBI (Alster et al., 1993). Perhaps chronobiologic abnormalities are far more common in TBI patients than is generally appreciated. Identification of cycle abnormalities is most important, as these disorders could be expected to severely impede rehabilitation and there are a number of effective treatment options available.

Visual dysfunction may occur in patients with TBI, and when the injury is severe, blindness may ensue (see Ch. 10). The majority of blinded individuals have abnormal sleep-wake cycles (Sack and Lewy, 1993). Some patients who have pregeniculate blindness (lesions anterior to the suprachiasmatic nucleus) as a result of TBI could be expected to develop abnormalities of the sleep wake cycle.

Circadian Rhythms and Psychiatric Disorders

There is a striking relationship between circadian rhythms and certain psychiatric disorders, particularly seasonal affective disorder, primary depression, and bipolar affective disorder (Kupfer et al., 1990; Rosenthal and Blehar, 1989; Wehr, 1990). Appreciation of this relationship may be relevant in the rehabilitation of TBI patients with major neuropsychological problems, either premorbid or post-traumatic. It is likely that there is a high incidence of premorbid psychosocial disorders in patients wtih TBI resulting from high-risk behaviors such as recklessness or alcohol or illicit drug abuse. (A more in-depth discussion of this topic is presented in Ch. 2.)

Treatment Modalities

Many patients with incapacitating sleep-wake cycle disorders will benefit from accurate diagnosis and appropriate treatment. The mainstays of treatment are sleep hygiene programs, phototherapy and chronotherapy. In addition, promising new pharmacologic treatments are on the horizon.

Chronotherapy

In chronotherapy the desirable total sleep time is determined by sleep logs during a "free-running" period. The patient then delays or advances sleep onset by a few hours every day, sleeping only the predetermined number of hours until the desired sleep onset time is reached. Thereafter strict adherence to the "new" sleep-wake schedule should be maintained (Czeisler et al., 1981; Moore-Ede et al., 1983; Weitzman et al., 1981). The method requires several days of free time and can be derailed if sleeping quarters cannot be kept dark and quiet during the several daytime sleeps required (Rosenthal et al., 1990). Such a regimen may be difficult to carry out in the setting of intensive care, rehabilitation, and long-term care facilities.

Phototherapy

It has recently been discovered that exposure to bright light at strategic times of the sleep-wake cycle results in a shift of the underlying rhythm. This affords an opportunity to treat circadian dysrhythmias very effectively (O'Connor et al., 1994). The timing of the phototherapy and its duration depend on diagnosis and individual response. The patient is exposed to a bright light, furnishing an illuminance of more than 2,500 lux at a prescribed distance. Fluorescent lights are commonly used. Distance from the light is critical in determining the illuminance. Indoor ambient light is of insufficient intensity to have an effect on the human biologic clock. The lack of exposure to light of sufficient intensity of patients confined to bed or indoors during periods of rehabilitation may encourage circadian dysrhythmias. Much remains to be learned regarding these variables and the effectiveness of phototherapy in the clinical setting (Lewy and Sack, 1988; Terman, 1994). Dramatic results in a series of children with severe non-TBI brain damage are encouraging (Guilleminault et al., 1993).

Adverse effects of phototherapy include headache, eyestrain, excessive advance of sleep onset, and precipitation of mania in bipolar individuals (Kripke, 1991; Schwitzer et al., 1990). For patients with a history of eye disorders, an ophthalmologist should be consulted before beginning treatment (Terman et al., 1990). Light units should be safety-tested electrically and should include devices to screen ultraviolet (Terman et al., 1991). Photosensitization by certain medications (such as tetracycline) should be kept in mind (Roberts et al., 1992).

Pharmacologic Manipulations

Pharmacologic manipulation of biologic rhythms is still in its developmental phase. Preliminary data suggest that a number of medications may affect biologic rhythms. These include: benzodiazepines (Alvarez et al., 1992; Ozaki et al., 1989; Turek, 1988; Turek and Losee-Olson, 1987), vitamin B_{12} (Ohta et al. 1991a; Ohta et al. 1991b; Okawa et al., 1990; Tshjimaru et al., 1992), tricyclic antidepressants, monoamine oxidase inhibitors, and lithium (Hallonquist et al., 1986). None is of proven efficacy for any given clinical chronobiologic application. There have been no systematic studies of the use of these agents in TBI-associated sleep/wake cycle disturbances.

Another promising pharmacologic agent is melatonin, a hormone secreted by the pineal gland. This secretion is suppressed by exposure to light, is entrained by the light-dark cycle, and is coupled to the sleep-wake cycle and to the circadian cortisol rhythm. Melatonin is a valuable marker of the underlying sleep-wake cycle. It is likely that this substance plays an important role in biologic rhythms, and there is evidence that administration of exogenous melatonin may alter the biologic rhythm (Erlich and Apuzzo, 1985; Lewy et al., 1985; Lewy et al., 1992). The presence of melatonin receptors in the suprachiasmatic nucleus in humans suggests its importance in biologic rhythms (Reppert et al., 1988).

Insomnia

No studies specifically address the association between TBI and insomnia. Insomnia is a symptom of many different conditions and not a disorder in and of itself. The major categories include psychophysiologic (conditioned), psychiatric, medical condition-related, and drug-induced (Zorick, 1994). These predisposing conditions are present in many TBI patients during the period of rehabilitation. It should also be remembered that persistent insomnia affects 30 percent of the adult population and therefore will be a pre-existing condition in many TBI patients (Gallup Organization, 1991). Once the factors contributing to insomnia are identified in a given case, specific effective behavioral and/or pharmacologic therapies may be undertaken (Walsh and Mahowald, 1991). Newer nonbenzodiazepine sedative-hypnotics may prove most useful (Maarek et al., 1992; Merlotti et al., 1989).

Parasomnias

Parasomnias are undesirable motor or behavioral events that occur exclusively or predominantly during the sleeping state. These may result in potentially injurious and violent behaviors or disruption to caregivers or ward-mates (Mahowald and Ettinger, 1990; Schenck et al., 1989). They may even present in the hospital/intensive care setting (Schenck and Mahowald, 1991). Many different conditions may present with such bothersome or injurious sleep-period-related behaviors (Mahowald and Ettinger, 1990). These conditions are undoubtedly present in the TBI population, but virtually no systematic studies are available to indicate whether they are more common following TBI than in the population at large. Only a few parasomnias will be mentioned.

Rhythmic Movement Disorder

Rhythmic movement disorder is characterized by stereotypic rhythmic head and/or body rocking. This behavior is usually seen during the transition from wake to sleep but may actually arise from any stage of sleep and may persist for protracted periods of time (Mahowald and Thorpy, 1994). A single case of this disorder has been described in association with a global encephalopathy and frontal lobe dysfunction following a severe closed head injury. This case was successfully treated with imipramine (Drake, 1986).

Disorders of Arousal

Disorders of arousal occur on a spectrum: confusional arousals, sleepwalking, and sleep terrors. They appear to have a genetic component. Contrary to conventional teaching, they are usually not associated with significant psychiatric conditions even when persisting into or beginning during adulthood (Mahowald and Ettinger, 1990; Schenck et al., 1989). There are no studies addressing TBI and disorders of arousal. In some cases the TBI may have resulted from a pre-existing disorder of arousal, which led to the injurious behavior (e.g., frenzied sleepwalking).

Nocturnal Seizures

Post-traumatic seizures are a well known but relatively uncommon sequel to TBI (Yablon, 1993). See Chs. 11 and 12). There is no information on predominatly or exclusively nocturnal seizures following TBI, but is is plausible that a causal relationship exists in some cases. The bizarre manifestations of some nocturnal seizures should be kept in mind. These seizures often masquerade as other parasomnias. Postictal confusion (poriomania) may mimic a number of other parasomnias (Mahowald and Schenck, 1993).

REM Sleep Behavior Disorder

REM sleep behavior disorder is a recently described condition in which the anticipated atonia of REM sleep is absent, hypothetically allowing patients to "act out their dreams," often with violent or injurious results (Schenck et al., 1986). The disorder may result from TBI. Given the diverse neurologic conditions associated with it, it is likely that the disorder is more common following TBI than the statistics would indicate. It is important to identify REM sleep behavior disorder, as it is readily diagnosable by formal sleep studies, which reveal the absence of somatic muscle atonia that normally accompanies REM sleep (Schenck et al., 1993). The disorder responds exquisitely to clonazepam (Schenck and Mahowald, 1990).

Psychiatric Conditions

There are a number of "psychiatric" conditions associated with troubled sleep. These include nocturnal panic, post-traumatic stress disorder, and psychogenic dissociative states (e.g., multiple personality disorder, which in a case reported by Sandel et al. [1990] was at first misdiagnosed as being due to TBI). These conditions may be triggered by emotional or physical trauma, which suggests that they may occur in the TBI population (Mahowald and Schenck, 1993). However, there are few studies available.

Dreaming

The cessation of dreaming has been reported following TBI. This alteration in oneiric (dreaming) activity may be related to impairment of visual memory (Humphrey and Zangwill, 1951). In one study of 10 patients reporting decreased or absent dreaming following head injury, there was no correlation between the dream change complaint and the amount of time spent in REM sleep (Prigatano et al., 1982). This may reflect the fact that much dream mentation occurs during NREM sleep (Cavallero et al., 1992; Foulkes, 1993). Another study questioned the common belief that dream recall is reduced following severe head injury. It found, rather, a change in the content (more threatening, fewer with sexually manifest content) but not in the overall incidence (Benyaker et al., 1988). More studies of larger numbers of subjects are needed.

Hallucinations

In keeping with the concept of state dissociation, it must be kept in mind that waking hallucinations may actually be the manifestation of sleep-dreaming intruding into wakefulness (Mahowald and Schenck, 1991). Clearly, waking hallucinations do not necessarily indicate major psychiatric disorders (Asaad and Shapiro, 1986; Carter, 1992). Treatment of organic hallucinations with haloperidol is often effective (Horvath et al., 1989).

SLEEP DISORDERS AS A CAUSE OF TBI

Sleep disorders not only may result from TBI but may actually cause it. The true consequence of sleep disorders and sleepiness, with particular reference to accidents on the highway and in the workplace, is now known, and the figures are staggering. In the United States alone in 1990 it is estimated that 200,000 motor vehicle crashes were due to falling asleep at the wheel (National Commission on Sleep Disorders Research, 1992) (see Chs. 2 and 4). Statistics on motor vehicle accidents clearly indicate that fall-asleep crashes are more prevalent in patients with untreated obstructive sleep apnea and narcolepsy (Broughton et al., 1983; Findley et al., 1991; Haraldsson et al., 1992). This undoubtedly holds true for other sleepy populations such as shift workers. Frequent falling asleep on the job has been well documented in night shift workers (Akerstedt, 1991), as have sleep episodes occurring in pilots while "at the stick" (Moore-Ede, 1993). The potential for TBI in this setting is obvious. Violent parasomnias, particularly sleepwalking, sleep terrors, and REM sleep behavior disorder have resulted in significant injury, and it is likely that TBI may result (Schenck et al. 1989). Just as in the multiple personality disorder case cited above, it must be remembered that any sleep disorder following TBI may have been preexisting, and may have, in fact, even caused the TBI. Given the known consequences of sleepiness due to sleep disorders and sleep deprivation, the American public, employers, and policymakers must consider these conditions as a significant *cause* of TBI. Sleepiness and sleep disorders can no longer be discounted as a "minor annoyance."

SUMMARY AND DIRECTION FOR THE FUTURE

Review of available literature indicates that although much is known about the nature of sleep and sleep/wake cycling, there is a striking lack of specific information regarding sleep and sleep/wake disorders in patients with TBI (both as cause and consequence). Given the huge numbers of TBI patients and the prevalent and incapacitating nature of sleep/wake disorders, much work needs to be done. Most sleep disorders can be readily diagnosed, with effective therapeutic implications. Their identification and treatment in the TBI population will have important and exciting rehabilitation ramifications. There are critical scientific lessons to be learned from this population, and more significantly, there are substantial therapeutic implications.

REFERENCE

Adams JH: Head injury. pp. 106–152. In Adams JH, Duchen LW (eds): Greenfield's Neuropathology 5th Ed. Oxford University Press, New York, 1992

Akerstedt T: Sleepiness at work: effects of irregular work hours. pp. 129–152. In Monk TH, (ed): Sleep, Sleepiness and Performance. John Wiley & Sons, Chichester, England, 1991

Aldrich MS: Narcolepsy. N Engl J Med 323:389–394, 1990

Aldrich MS: Cardinal manifestations of sleep disorders. pp. 418–425. In Kryger MH, Roth T, Dement WC (eds):

Principles and Practice of Sleep Medicine WB Saunders, 1994

Aldrich MS, Naylor MW: Narcolepsy associated with lesions of the diencephalon. Neurology 39:1505–1508, 1989

Alexandre A, Colombo F, Nertempi P, Bendetti A: Cognitive outcome and early indices of severity of head injury. J Neurosurg 59:751–761, 1983

Alexandre A, Rubini L, Nertempi P, Farinello C: Acta Neurochir Suppl (Wien) 28:188–192, 1979

Alster J, Pratt H, Feinsod M: Density spectral array, evoked potentials, and temperature rhythms in the evaluation and prognosis of the comatose patient. Brain Inj 7:191–208, 1993

Alvarez B, Dahlitz MJ, Vignau J et al: The delayed sleep phase syndrome: clinical and investigative findings in fourteen subjects. J Neur Neurosurg Psychiatry 55:665–670, 1992

American Electroencephalographic Society, Ad Hoc Committee on Polysomnographic Guidelines; American Electroencephalographic society guidelines for the polygraphic assessment of sleep-related disorders (polysomnography). J Clin Neurophysiol 9:88–96, 1991

American Sleep Disorders Association; The clinical use of the multiple sleep latency test. Sleep, 15:268–276, 1992

American Sleep Disorders Association, Standards of Practice Committee: Practice parameters for the use of stimulants in the treatment of narcolepsy. Sleep 17:348–351, 1994

Asaad G, Shapiro B: HAllucinations: theoretical and clinical overview. Am J Psychiatry, 143:1088–1097, 1986

Aserinski E, Kleitman N: Regularly occurring periods of eye motility, and concomitant phenomena during sleep. Science, 118:273–274, 1953

Askenasy JJM, Rahmani L: Neuropsycho-social rehabilitation of head injury. Am J Phys Med Rehabil 66:315–327, 1988

Bach JR, Wang T-G: Pulmonary function and sleep disordered breathing in patients with traumatic tetraplegia: a longitudinal study. Arch Phys Med Rehabil 75:279–284, 1994

Benyakar M, Tadir M, Groswasser Z, Stern MJ: Dreams in head-injured patients. Brain Inj 2:351–356, 1988

Bergamasco B, Bergamini L, Bricolo A, Dolce G: Studies in sleep during the apallic syndrome. Monographien aus dem Gesamigebiete der Psychiatrie. Psychiatry Ser 14:155–159, 1977

Bergamasco B, Bergamini L, Doriguzzi T: Clinical value of the sleep electroencephalographic patterns in post-traumatic coma. Acta Neurol Scand, 44:495–511, 1968a

Bergamasco B, Bergamini L, Doriguzzi T, Fabiani D: EEG sleep patterns as a prognostic criterion in post-traumatic coma. Electroencephalogr Clin Neurophysiol 24: 374–377, 1968b

Billiard M, Carlander B, Ondze B, Besset A: Post-traumatic hypersomnia associated with cataplexy, hypnagogic hallucinations, sleep paralysis and disturbed nocturnal sleep but not with SOREM episodes and HLA DR2. Sleep Res 22:171, 1993

Billiard M, Negri C, Badly-Milliner M et al: Organisation du sommeil chez les sujets atteints d'inconscience post-traumatique chronique. Rev Electroencephalogr Neurophysiol Clin 9:149–152, 1979

Bliwise DL: Sleep in normal aging and dementia. Sleep 16:40–81, 1993

Bond MR: Outcome of severe damage to the central nervous system. (pp. 141–157). Porter R, Fitzsimons DW (eds): Ciba Found Symp 34 (new series): Elsevier, New York, 1975

Bricolo A, Gentilomo A, Rosadini G, Rossi GF: Long-lasting post-traumatic unconscousness. A study based on nocturnal EEG and polygraphic monitoring. Acta Neurol Scand 44:512–532, 1968

Broughton R, Ghanem Q, Hishikawa Y et al: Life effects of narcolepsy: relationships of geographic origin (North American, Asian, or European) and to other patient and illness variables. Can J Neurol Sci 10:100–104, 1983

Brown A, Smolensky M, D'Alonzo G et al: Circadian rhythm in human activity objectively quantified by actigraphy. pp. 77–83. In Hayes DK (ed): Chronobiology: Its Role in Clinical Medicine, General Biology, and Agriculture (Part A), John Wiley & Sons, New York, 1990a

Brown AC, Smolensly MH, D'Alonzo GE, Redman DP: Actigraphy: a means of assessing circadian patterns in human activity. Chronobiol Int 7:125–133, 1990b

Cahan C, Gothe B, Decker M et al: Arterial oxygen saturation over time and sleep studies in quadriplegic patients. Paraplegia 32:172–179, 1993

Carskadon MA, Dement WC: Normal human sleep: an overview. pp. 16–25. In Kryger MH, Roth T, Dement WC (eds): Principles and Practice of Sleep Medicine. WB Saunders, Philadelphia, 1994

Carskadon MA, Dement WC, Mitler MM et al: Guidelines for the multiple sleep latency test (MSLT): a standard measure of sleepiness. Sleep 9:519–524, 1986

Carter JL: Visual, somatosensory, olfactory, and gustatory hallucinations. Psychiatr Clin North Am 15:347–358, 1992

Cavallero C, Cicogna P, Natale V et al: Slow wave sleep dreaming. Sleep, 15:562–566, 1992

Chestnut RM, Marshall LF, Klauber MR et al: The role of secondary brain injury in determining outcome from severe head injury. J Trauma 34:216–222, 1993

Chokroverty S: Sleep, breathing, and neurological disorders. pp. 295–335. In Chokroverty S (ed): Sleep Disorders Medicine. Butterworth-Heinemann, Boston, 1994

Cohen M, Oskenberg A, Snir D et al: Temporally related changes of sleep complaints in traumatic brain injured patients. J Neurol Neurosurg Psychiatry, 55, 313–315, 1992

Cooper R, Hulme A: Changes of the EEG, intracranial pressure and other variables during sleep in patients with intracranial lesions. Electroencephalogr Clin Neurophysiol 27:12–22, 1969

Czeisler CA, Richardson GS, Coleman RM et al: Chronotherapy: resetting the circadian clocks of patients with delayed sleep phase insomnia. Sleep 4:1–21, 1981

Dikmen S, McLean A, Temkin N: Neuropsychological and psychosocial consequences of minor head injury. J Neurol Neurosurg Psychiatry 49:1227–1232, 1986

DiRocco C, McLone DG, Shimoji T, Raimondi AJ: Continuous intraventricular cerebrospinal fluid pressure recording in hydrocephalic children during wakefulness and sleep. J Neurosurg 42:683–689, 1975

Doyle KJ, Tami TA: Increased intracranial pressure and blindness associated with obstructive sleep apnea. Otolaryngol Head Neck Surg 105:613–616, 1991

Drake ME, Jr: Jactatio nocturna after head injury. Neurology, 36, 867–868, 1986

Erlich SS, Apuzzo MLJ: The pineal gland: anatomy, physiology, and clinical significance. J Neurosurg 63:321–341, 1985

Findley LJ, Weiss JW, Jabour R: Drivers with untreated sleep apnea. A cause of death and serious injury. Arch Intern Med 151:1451–1452, 1991

Fischgold H, Mathis P: Obnubilations, comas et stupeurs. Electroencephalogr Clin Neurophysiol Suppl, 11, 1959

Foulkes D: Dreaming and REM sleep. J Sleep Res 2:199–202, 1993

Furuse M, Ikeyama A, Mabe H et al: Relationship between rapid variations in intracranial pressure and changes in respiratory pattern during postoperative monitoring. Neurol Med Chir (Tokyo) 19:9–16, 1979

Gallup Organization: Sleep in America. The Gallup Organization, Princeton, NJ, 1991

Gennarelli TA, Champion HR, Sacco WJ et al: Mortality of patients with head injury and extracranial injury treated in trauma center. J Trauma, 29:1193–1201, 1989

George B, Landau-Ferey J: Twelve months follow-up by night sleep EEG after recovery from severe head trauma. Neurochirugia (Stuttg) 29:45–47, 1986

Gerstenbrand F, Lucking CH: Die akuten traumatischen Hirnstammschaden. Arch Psychiatrie Nervenkr 213: 264–281, 1970

Gill RG, Young JPR, Thomas DJ: Kleine-Levin syndrome: report of two cases with onset of symptoms precipitated by head trauma. Br J Psychiatry 152:410–412, 1988

Goh D, Minns RA, Pye SD, Steers AJW: Cerebral blood-flow velocity and intermittent intracranial pressure elevation during sleep in hydrocephalic children. Dev Med Child Neurol 34:676–689, 1992

Goldstein M: Traumatic brain injury: a silent epidemic. Ann Neurol 27:327, 1990

Good JL, Barry E, Fishman PS: Posttraumatic narcolepsy: the complete syndrome with tissue typing. J Neurosurg 71:765–767, 1989

Gucer G, Viernstein LJ: Intracranial pressure in the normal monkey while awake and sleep. J Neurosurg 51:206–210, 1979

Guilleminault C: Sleeping and Waking Disorders: Indications and Techniques. Addison-Wesley, Menlo Park, CA, 1982

Guilleminault C: Idiopathic central nervous system hypersomnia pp. 562–566. In Kryger MH, Roth T, Dement WC (eds): Principles and Practice of Sleep Medicine. WB Saunders, Philadelphia, 1994

Guilleminault C, Faull KF, Miles L, van den Hoed J: Posttraumatic excessive daytime sleepiness: a review of 20 patients. Neurology 33:1584–1589, 1983

Guilleminault D, McCann CC, Quera-Salva M, Cetel M: Light therapy as treatment of dyschronosis in brain impaired children. Eur J Pediatr 152:754–759, 1993

Halberg F: Chronobiology. Annu Rev. Physiol. 31: 675–725, 1969

Hallonquist JD, Goldberg MA, Brandes JS: Affective disorders and circadian rhythms. Can J Psychiatry, 31:259–272, 1986

Hansotia P, Gottschalk P, Green P, Zais D: Spindle coma: incidence, clinicopathologic correlates, and prognostic value. Neurology, 31:83–87, 1981

Haraldsson P-O, Carenfelt C, Tingvall C: Sleep apnea syndrome symptoms and automobile driving in a general population. J Clin Epidemiol, 45:821–825, 1992

Hirsch JC, Pierre-Kahn A, Hirsch JF: Experimental study of intracranial pressure during rapid eye movement sleep in the chronic cat. Neurosci Lett 7:245–249, 1978

Hofman MA, Swaab DF: Diurnal and seasonal rhythms of neuronal activity in the suprachiasmatic nucleus of humans. J Biol Rhythms, 8:283–295, 1993

Horvath TB, Siever LJ, Mohs RC, Davis K: Organic mental syndromes and disorders. pp. 599–641. In Kaplan HI, Sadock BJ (eds): Comprehensive Textbook of Psychiatry. Williams & Wilkins, Baltimore, 1989

Humphrey ME, Zangwill OL: Cessation of dreaming after brain injury. J Neurol Neurosurg Psychiatry, 14: 322–325, 1951

Inoue S: Biology of Sleep Substances. CRC Press, Boca Raton, FL, 1989

Jennum P, Borgesen SE: Intracranial pressure and obstructive sleep apnea. Chest, 95:279–283, 1989

Johannessen N, Jensen PF, Kristensen S, Juul A: Nasal packing and nocturnal oxygen desaturation. Acta Otolarynol Suppl (Stockh) 492:6–8, 1992

Jones BE: Basic mechanisms of sleep-wake states. pp. 145–162. Kryger MH, Roth T, Dement WC (eds): Principles and Practice of Sleep Medicine WB Saunders, Philadephia 1994

Koren G, Ferrazzini G, Sohl H et al: Chronopharmacology of methotrexate pharmacokinetics in childhood leukemia. Chronobiol Int 9:434–438, 1992

Kowatch RA: Sleep and head injury. Psychiatr Med 7:37–41, 1989

Kreuger J, Obal F Jr: A neuronal group theory of sleep function. Sleep factor theory. J Sleep Res 2:63–69, 1993

Kripke DF: Timing of phototherapy and occurrence of mania. Biol Psychiatry 29:1156–1157, 1991

Kripke DF, Somons RN, Garfinkel L, Hammond EC: Short and long sleep and sleeping pills: is increased mortality associated? Arch Gen Psychiatry, 36:103–116, 1979

Kuchiwaki H, Takada S, Ishiguri H et al: Pressure wave with apnea evaluated by sleep level in patient with ventricular dilation. Neurol Res 10:105–111, 1988

Kupfer DJ, Monk TH, Barchas JD: Biological Rhythms and Mental Disorders. Guilford Press, New York, 1988

Lesch DR, Spire J-P: Clinical electroencephalography. pp. 13–31. In Thorpy MJ (ed): Handbook of Sleep Disorders. Marcel Dekker, New York, 1990

Lessard CS, Sances A Jr, Larson SJ: Period analysis of EEG signals during sleep and post-traumatic coma. Aviat Space Environ Med 45:664–668, 1974

Levin HS, Mattis S, Ruff RM et al: Neurobehavioral outcome following minor head injury: a three-center study. J Neurosurgery, 66:234–243, 1987

Lewy AJ, Ahmed S, Latham Jackson JM, Sack RL: Melatonin shifts human circadian rhythms according to a phase-response curve. Chronobiol Int 9:380–392, 1992

Lewy AJ, Sack RL: Intensity, wavelength, and timing: three critical parameters for chronobiologically active light. pp. 197–217. In Kupfer DJ, Monk TH, Barchas JD (eds): Biological Rhythms and Mental Disorders. Guilford Press, New York, 1988

Lewy AJ, Sack RL, Singer CM: Melatonin, light and chronobiological disorders. pp. 231–252. In Everd D, Clark S (eds): Photoperiodism, Melatonin, and the Pineal (Ciba Found Symp 117). Pitman, London, 1985

Maarek L, Cramer P, Attali P et al: The safety and efficacy of zolpidem in insomniac patients: a long-term open study in general practice. J Int Med Res 20:162–170, 1992

Maccario M, Ruggles KM, Meriwether MW: Post-traumatic narcolepsy. Milit Med 152:370–371, 1987

Mahowald M, Schenck C: Status dissociatus—a perspective on states of being. Sleep 14:69–79, 1991

Mahowald MW, Ettinger MG: Things that go bump in the night—the parasomnias revisited. J Clin Neurophysiol 7:119–143, 1990

Mahowald MW, Iber C, Walsh JK: Evaluation of obstructive sleep apnea: considerations and caveats. Operative Tech Otolaryngol Head Neck Surg 2:73–80, 1991

Mahowald MW, Schenck CH: Parasomnia purgatory—the epileptic/non-epileptic interface. pp. 123–139. In Rowan AJ, Gates JR (eds): Non-Epileptic seizures. Butterworth-Heineman, Boston, 1993

Mahowald MW, Thorpy MJ: Rhythmic movement disorder and other childhood parasomnias. In Kryger MH, Roth T, Dement WC (eds): Principles and Practice of Pediatric Sleep Disorders. WB Saunders, Philadelphia

Marshall LF, Smith RW, Shapiro HM: The influence of diurnal rhythms in patients with intracranial hypertension: implications for management. Neurosurgery 2:100–102, 1978

Merlotti L, Roehrs T, Koshorek G et al: The dose effects of zolpidem on the sleep of healthy normals. J Clin Psychopharmacol 9:9–14, 1989

Mitler MM, Hajdukovic R, Erman M, Koziol JA: Narcolepsy. J Clin Neurophysiol 7:93–118, 1990

Moore-Ede M: The Twenty-Four-Hour Society. Addison-Wesley, Reading, MA, 1993, pp. 81–96

Moore-Ede MC: Circadian rhythms of drug effectiveness and toxicity. Clin Pharmacol Ther, 14:925–935, 1973

Moore-Ede MC, Czeisler CA, Richardson GS: Circadian timekeeping in health and disease. Part 2. Clinical implications of circadian rhythmicity. N Engl J Med, 309:530–536, 1983

Munari C, Calbucci F: Correlations between intracranial pressure and EEG during coma and sleep. Clin Neurophysiology Electroencephalogr 51:170–176, 1981

National Commission on Sleep Disorders Research: Wake up America: A National Sleep Alert. DHHS Publication No. 61353. U.S. Government Printing Office, Washington, 1992

Newell DW, Aaslid R, Stooss R, Reulen HJ: The relationship of blood flow velocity fluctuations to intracranial pressure B waves. J Neurosurg, 76:415–421, 1992

O'Connor KA, Mahowald MW, Ettinger MG: Circadian rhythm disorders. pp. 369–379. In Chokroverty S (ed): Sleep Disorders Medicine. Butterworth-Heinemann, Boston, 1994

Ohta T, Ando K, Iwata T et al: Treatment of persistent sleep-wake schedule disorders in adolescents with methylcobalamin (vitamin B12). Sleep 12:414–418, 1991a

Ohta T, Iwata T, Kayukawa Y et al: Daily activity and persistent sleep-wake schedule disorders. Prog Neuropsychopharmacol Biol Psychiatry 16:529–537, 1991b

Okawa M, Mishima K, Nanami T et al: Vitamin B_{12} treatment for sleep-wake rhythm disorders. Sleep, 13:15–23, 1990

Okawa M, Takahashi K, Sasaki H: Disturbance of circadian rhythms in severely brain-damaged patients correlated with CT findings. J Neurol, 233:274–282, 1986

Olsen KD, Kern EB, Westbook PR: Sleep and breathing disturbance secondary to nasal obstruction. Otolaryngol Head Neck Surg, 89:804–810, 1981

Ozaki N, Iwata T, Itoh A et al: A treatment trial of delayed sleep phase syndrome with triazolam. Jpn J Psychiatry Neurol 43, 51–55, 1989

Parsons LC, Ver Beek D: Sleep-awake patterns following cerebral concussion. Nurs Res 31:260–264, 1982

Patten SB, Lauderdale WM: Delayed sleep phase disorder after traumatic brain injury. J Am Acad Child Adolesc Psychiatry 31:100–102, 1992

Pierre-Kahn A, Gabersek V, Hirsch J-F: Intracranial pressure and rapid eye movement sleep in hydrocephalus. Childs Nerv Syst 2:156–166, 1976

Powell NB, Guilleminault C, Riley RW: Surgical therapy for obstructive sleep apnea. pp. 706–721. In Kryger MH,

Roth T, Dement WC (eds): Principles and Practice of Sleep Medicine. WB Saunders, Philadelphia, 1994

Prigatano GP, Stahl ML, Orr WC, Zeiner HK: Sleep and dreaming disturbances in closed head injury patients. J Neurol Neurosurg Psychiatry 45:78–80, 1982

Radzialowski FM, Bousquet WF: Daily rhythmic variation in hepatic drug metabolism in the rat and mouse. J Pharmacol Exp Ther. 163:229–238, 1968

Rae-Grant AD, Barbour PJ, Reed J: Development of a novel EEG rating scale for head injury using dichotomous variables. Electroencephalogr Clin Neurophysiol 79: 349–357, 1991

Ralph MR, Foster RG, Davis FC, Menaker M: Transplated suprachiasmatic nucleus determines circadian period. Science, 247:975–978, 1990

Rechtschaffen A, Kales A: A Manual of Standardized Terminology: Techniques and Scoring System for Sleep Stages of Human Subjects. UCLA Brain Information Service/Brain Research Institute, Los Angeles, 1968

Reinberg A: The hours of changing responsiveness or susceptibility. Perspect Biol Med 11:111–126, 1967

Renier D, Sainte-Rose C, Marchac D, Hirsch J-F: Intracranial pressure in craniostenosis. J Neurosurg 57:370–377, 1982

Reppert SM, Weaver DR, Rivkees SA, Stopa EG: Putative melatonin receptors in a human biological clock. Science 242:78–81, 1988

Rigatto H, More M, Cates D: Fetal breathing and behavior measured through a double-wall plexiglas window in sheep. J Appl Physiol 61:160–164, 1986

Roberts JE, Reme CE, Dillon J, Terman M: Exposure to bright light and the concurrent use of photosensitizing drugs. N Engl J Med, 326:1500, 1992

Robertson CF, Zuker R, Dabrowski B, Levison H: Obstructive sleep apnea: a complication of burns to the head and neck in children. J Burn Care Rehabil 6:353–357, 1985

Roehrs T, Zorick F, Wittig R et al: Predictors of objective level of daytime sleepiness in patients with sleep-related breathing disorders. Chest, 95:1202–1206, 1989

Ron S, Algom D, Hary D, Cohen M: Time-related changes in the distribution of sleep stages in brain injured patients. Electroencephalogr Clin Neurophysiol 48:432–441, 1980

Rosenthal NE, Blehar MC: Seasonal Affective Disorders and Phototherapy. Guilford Press, New York, 1989

Rosenthal NE, Joseph-Vanderpool JR, Levendosky AA et al: Phase-shifting effects of bright morning light as treatment for delayed sleep phase syndrome. Sleep 13:354–361, 1990

Rumpl E, Lorenzi E, Hackl JM et al: The EEG at different stages of acute secondary traumatic midbrain and bulbar brain syndromes. Electroencephalogr Clin Neurophysiol 46:487–497, 1979

Sack RL, Lewy AJ: Human circadian rhythms: lessons from the blind. Ann Med 25, 303–305, 1993

Sadowski S: Post-traumatic cataplexy. Can Med Assoc J 126:1150–1151, 1982

Sandel ME, Weiss B, Ivker B: Multiple personality disorder: diagnosis after a traumatic brain injury. Arch Phys Med Rehabil 71:523–525, 1990

Sanders MH: Medical therapy for sleep apnea. pp. 678–693. In Kryger MH, Roth T, Dement WC (eds): Principles and Practice of Sleep Medicine. WB Saunders, Philadelphia, 1994

Schenck CH, Bundlie SR, Ettinger MG, Mahowald MW: Chronic behavioral disorders of human REM sleep: a new category of parasomnia. Sleep, 9:293–308, 1986

Schenck CH, Hurwitz TD, Mahowald MW: REM sleep behavior disorder: an update on a series of 96 patients and a review of the literature. J Sleep Res 2:224–231, 1993

Schenck CH, Mahowald MW: A polysomnographic, neurologic, psychiatric and clinical outcome report on 70 consecutive cases with REM sleep behavior disorder (RBD): sustained clonazepam efficacy in 89.5% of 57 treated patients. Cleve Clin J Med suppl. 57:10–24, 1990

Schenck CH, Mahowald MW: Injurious parasomnias affecting patients on intensive care units. Intensive Care Med 17, 219–224, 1991

Schenck CH, Milner DM, Hurwitz TD et al: A polysomnographic and clinical report on sleep-related injury in 100 adult patients. Am J Psychiatry 146:1166–1173, 1989

Schwitzer J, Neudorfer C, Blecha HG et al: Mania as a side effect of phototherapy. Biol Psychiatry 28:523–524, 1990

Sher AE: The upper airway in obstructive sleep apnea syndrome: pathology and surgical management. pp. 311–335. In Thorpy MJ (ed): Handbook of Sleep Disorders. Marcel Dekker New York

Short DJ, Stradling JR, Williams SJ: Prevalence of sleep apnoea in patients over 40 years of age with spinal cord lesions. J Neurol Neurosurg Psychiatry, 55:1032–1036, 1992

Smolik P, Roth B: Kleine-Levin syndrome: ethnopathogenesis and treatment. Acta Univ Carol Med Monogr (Praha) 128:1–94, 1988

Steriade M, Hobson JA: Neuronal activity during the sleep-waking cycle. Prog Neurobiol 6:155–376, 1976

Sugita Y, Iijima S, Teshima Y et al: Marked episodic elevation of cerebrospinal fluid pressure during nocturnal sleep in patients with sleep apnea hypersomnia syndrome. Electroencephalogr Clin Neurophysiol 60:214–219, 1985

Synek VM: Prognostically important EEG coma patterns in diffuse anoxic and traumatic encephalopathies in adults. J Clin Neurophysiol 5:161–174, 1988

Terman M: Light therapy. pp. 1012–1029. In Kryger MH, Roth T, Dement WC (eds): Principles and Practice of Sleep Medicine. WB Saunders, Philadelphia

Terman M, Reme CE, Rafferty B et al: Bright light therapy for winter depression: potential ocular effects and theoretical implications. Photochem Photobiol 51:781–793, 1990

Terman M, Williams JB, Terman JS: Light therapy for winter depression: a clinician's guide. In Keller PA (ed) Innovations in Clinical Practice: A Source Book. Vol. 10. Professional Resource Exchange, Sarasota FL, 1991

Tryon WK: Activity Measurement in Psychology and Medicine. Plenum Press, New York, 1991

Tshjimaru S, Kideaki E, Honma G et al: Effects of vitamin B_{12} on the period of free-running rhythm in rats. Jpn J Psychiatry Neurol 46:225–226, 1992

Tsubokawa T, Yamamoto T, Katayama Y: Prediction of outcome of prolonged coma caused by brain damage. Brain Inj 4:329–337, 1990

Turek FW: Manipulation of a central circadian clock regulating behavioral and endocrine rhythms with a short-acting benzodiazepine used in the treatment of insomnia. Psychoneuroendocrinology 13:217–232, 1988

Turek FW, Losee-Olsen S: Entrainment of the circadian activity rhythm to the light-dark cycle can be altered by a short-acting benzodiazepine, triazolam. J Biol Rhythms 2, 249–260, 1987

Ueno H, Shima K, Chigasaki H, Ishii S: Oscillation of intracranial pressure and sleep. Clin Neurol Neurosurg 88:163–168, 1986

Vertes RP: Brainstem control of the events of REM sleep. Prog Neurobiol 22:241–288, 1984

Walsh JK, Mahowald MW: Avoiding the blanket approach to insomnia. Postgrad Med 20:211–224, 1991

Webb WB: Development of human napping. pp. 31–51. In Dinges DF, Broughton RJ, (eds): Sleep and Alertness: Chronobiological, Behavioral, and Medical Aspects of Napping. Raven Press, New York, 1989

Wehr TA: Effects of wakefulness and sleep on depression and mania. pp. 42–86. In Montplaisir J, Godbout R, (eds): Sleep and Biological Rhythms. Basic Mechanisms and Applications to Psychiatry. New York: Oxford University Press, 1990

Weitzman ED, Czeisler CA, Coleman RM et al: Delayed sleep phase syndrome. A chronobiological disorder with sleep-onset insomnia. Arch Gen Psychiatry 38:737–746, 1981

Williams RL, Karacan I, Hursch CJ: Electroencephalography (EEG) of Human Sleep. John Wiley & Sons, New York, 1974

Witting W, Mirmiran M, Bos NPA, Swabb DF: The effect of old age on the free-running period of circadian rhythms in rat. Chronobiol Int 11:103–112, 1994

Yablon SA: Posttraumatic seizures. Arch Phys Med Rehabil 74:983–1001, 1993

Yokota A, Matsuoka S, Ishikawa T et al: Overnight recordings of intracranial pressure and electroencephalography in neurosurgical patient. Part I: Intracranial pressure waves and their clinical correlations. University of Occupational and Environmental Health, Japan 11:371–381, 1989a

Yokota A, Matsuoka S, Ishikawa T et al: Overnight recordings of intracranial pressure and electroencephalography in neurosurgical patients. Part II: Changes in intracranial pressure during sleep. University of Occupational and Environmental Health, Japan 11:383–391, 1989b

Young T, Palta M, Dempsey et al: The occurrence of sleep-disordered breathing among middle-age adults. N Engl J Med 328:1230–1235, 1993

Zorick F: Overview of insomnia. pp. 483–485. In Kryger MH, Roth T, Dement WC (eds): Principles and Practice of Sleep Medicine. WB Saunders, Philadelphia, 1994

Psychiatric Conditions 15

William R. Yates

DIAGNOSIS OF PSYCHIATRIC DISORDERS IN TRAUMATIC BRAIN INJURY

Importance of Psychiatric Assessment and Treatment

The physical manifestations of traumatic brain injury (TBI) often dominate the early clinical picture. However, later in the rehabilitation process psychosocial issues often emerge as the most significant factors in producing a poor outcome (Dikmen et al., 1993). Emotional symptoms related to TBI can be chronic and produce significant distress many years after the injury. Cognitive and psychiatric disorders may cause more problems in rehabilitation than the physical complications of trauma (Levin, 1987) and are a significant burden for family members (Rappaport et al., 1989). Psychiatric symptoms and disorders are common in both the early and late periods of rehabilitation. Clinicians can improve the outcome of TBI by attending to the accurate assessment and treatment of psychiatric syndromes. This chapter reviews diagnosis, classification, and treatment of psychiatric disorders commonly associated with TBI.

Psychiatric Risk Factors for Trauma

Some psychiatric disorders increase risk for TBI. Substance abuse increases risk for head trauma through multiple mechanisms. Acute alcohol intoxication produces impaired coordination, sedation, and impaired judgment. Additionally, intoxication may promote aggressive behaviors resulting in assault and reckless driving. The extent and mechanism of head trauma risk with drugs other than alcohol are less well studied. However, cocaine abuse appears to play a significant role in the drug-related risk for all types of trauma (Lindenbaum et al., 1989).

The prevalence of premorbid alcohol and drug use disorders among victims of TBI is high. In a series of 322 patients evaluated with TBI, 70 percent had a history of alcohol abuse, drug abuse, or both (Drubach et al., 1993). The risk of significant TBI is related not only to the diagnosis of alcohol abuse but to the state of intoxication itself. In a series of patients admitted for traumatic brain injuries, 32 percent were found to be intoxicated at the time of admission (Edna, 1982). Average blood alcohol level among these patients was 220 mg/dl (the usual definition of intoxication is 100 mg/dl). Head trauma patients often present for emergency treatment at the times of high population rates for drinking and intoxication (11 PM to 3 AM on weekends).

The association of alcohol and drug abuse with TBI has significant pathophysiologic, outcome, and treatment implications. Some of these issues will be considered later in this chapter.

An additional psychiatric disorder associated with trauma and head trauma is premorbid antisocial personality disorder. By definition antisocial personality disorder is associated with "irritability and aggressiveness, as indicated by repeated physical fights or assaults" and "reckless disregard for safety of self or others" (American Psychiatric Association, 1994). Persons with antisocial personality disorder appear to be at higher risk for dangerous driving behavior and motor vehicle crashes (Yates et al., 1987) Antisocial personality is also associated with alcohol and drug abuse. The combination of antisocial personality disorder and a substance abuse presents a particularly high-risk combination for trauma.

The increased prevalence rates for substance abuse and alcohol abuse in TBI patients have clinical importance. First, the association increases the chance that clinicians treating TBI encounter these patients. Second, the clinician's expertise in detecting, diagnosing, and treating these psychiatric disorders is likey to affect subsequent overall outcome.

Mechanisms of Psychiatric Disorder in Head Trauma

Multiple factors influence the risk for psychiatric disorders in the TBI patient. Figure 15-1 summarizes some of the pathways to co-morbid psychiatric disorder following head injury. The first step in understanding the relationship between TBI and co-morbid psychiatric disorder is to determine the time of onset of each condition. As noted in the previous section, some psychiatric disorders increase the risk for head trauma. Many of these psychiatric disorders are likely to continue as the subject of clinical focus after head trauma.

When there is a new onset of a psychiatric disorder following head trauma, various mechanism may be responsible for the disorder (Fig. 15-1). Many post-TBI psychiatric disorders are related to the severity of the initial head trauma, as indicated by the length of post-traumatic amnesia (Lishman, 1968) or the Glasgow Coma Scale (GCS) score. The extent of personality change associated with TBI appears linked to the length of post-traumatic amnesia (Steadman and Graham, 1970). Specific psychiatric disorders also appear to be related to the site of TBI.

Psychological factors also play an important role in the development of psychiatric disorder following TBI. The stress of a significant injury can produce psychological symptoms and psychiatric disorders. The stress associated with TBI may be quite variable and related to associated factors such as any physical disfigurement, loss of marital/social/work roles, development of seizure disorder, and financial factors. Premorbid personality traits may interact with the stress of TBI. This interaction can produce exacerbation of premorbid personality traits or development of a new psychiatric disorder.

The mechanism of psychiatric disorder in TBI may relate to the temporal presentation of the disorder and the TBI. Those psychiatric disorders occurring close to the episode of trauma often have a physiologic basis, while those with a late onset, often after 6 months or more, often have a primary psychological mechanism. Dunlop et al. (1991) studied a series of 193 TBI patients of whom 34 experienced a progressive, deteriorating psychiatric course 6 months or more following TBI. Deterioration was associated with head trauma due to assault and with prior history of alcohol abuse but not with length of post-traumatic amnesia or CT brain scan findings. The deterioration group demonstrated significantly more agitation, withdrawal, mood lability, and depression than the group who showed improvement.

However, the time of onset is not a perfect guide in separating physiologic from psychological mechanisms. Psychological factors can operate early after trauma and physiologic factors can continue to play a role for a long time after injury. Many psychiatric disorders may be the result of a combination of physiologic and psychological factors.

Classification of Psychiatric Disorder in Head Trauma

The spectrum of psychiatric conditions following TBI is extensive and can include nearly the entire range of psychiatric disorders. Symptoms produced can include delusions, hallucinations, agitation, mood changes, anxiety, sleep disruption, disturbance of sexual function, and personality change. To classify such changes and to consider other differential diagnoses it is important to understand the current classification scheme used by psychiatrists.

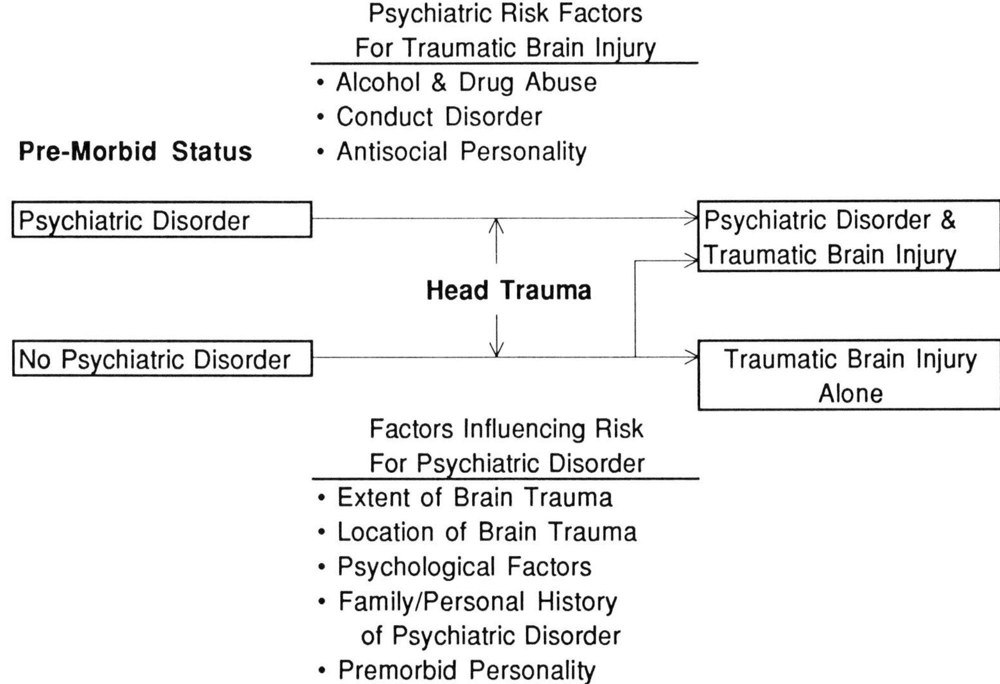

Fig. 15-1. Pathways to co-morbid psychiatric disorder in traumatic brain injury.

The American Psychiatric Association has been involved in refining the diagnostic criteria for psychiatric disorders. The most recent versions of these efforts culminated with the publication of DSM (Diagnostic and Statistical Manual of Mental Disorders)-IIIR in 1987 (American Psychiatric Association, 1987) and with the publication of DSM-IV in 1994 (American Psychiatric Association, 1994). The method of classification of psychiatric syndromes related to organic factors changed significantly between DSM-IIIR and DSM-IV. DSM-IIIR used the term *organic* to designate psychiatric disorders related to a physical factor. In DSM-IV the organic section has been deleted. In replacement, psychiatric disorders due to physical factors such as head trauma are now classified within the primary psychiatric syndrome categories such as psychotic disorders, mood disorders, and anxiety disorder. Because of the changes in classification strategies and in nomenclature, a review of the terminologies as related to head trauma patients is warranted.

Table 15-1 summarizes the changes in DSM-IV that affect classification of psychiatric disorders related to TBI. This table demonstrates the tendency to increase specificity and detail of diagnoses related to medical conditions such as head trauma. Of particular note is the expanded subtype classification for anxiety disorder and personality change associated with head trauma. Specific diagnostic groups and nomenclature are reviewed later in this section.

Psychiatric Diagnosis in the Postconcussive Syndrome

The postconcussive syndrome may include psychiatric symptoms of sufficient severity to require psychiatric attention. Since this syndrome produces a multitude of physical and psychiatric symptoms, psychiatric classification is best targeted to the primary psychiatric symptom, which is defined as the most severe symptom or the one causing the most impairment of personal, social, or occupational functioning. Psychiatric symptoms that may occur as part of the postconcussive syndrome include insomnia, irritability, emotional lability, depression, memory and attention problems, restlessness/anxiety, and post-traumatic stress disorder. Post-traumatic stress disorder is characterized by a pathologic anxiety response to a severe stressor. The traumatic event is persistently re-experienced and accompanied by avoidance behavior and increased arousal.

Brown et al. (1994) proposed that a DSM-IV category called *postconcussional disorder* be developed.

They documented the frequency of a cognitive, psychological, and behavioral syndrome related to mild head injury. Despite this proposal there is no single category to designate the effects of mild brain injury in DSM-IV. Postconcussional disorder is listed in DSM-IV as an appendix category worthy of further study. Specific clinical problems related to mild brain injury can be classified in DSM-IV by using existing categories. Such classification depends on the primary symptom related to the clinical presentation.

A suggested DSM-IV classification for problems associated with the postconcussive syndrome is listed in Table 15-2. Again, not all patients with postconcussive syndrome and psychiatric symptoms would necessarily receive a psychiatric diagnosis. The presence of the symptom is insufficient to diagnose a disorder. The psychiatric disorder classification should be limited to those with persistent, severe, and impairing symptoms. These patients are the ones most likely to benefit from psychiatric assessment and consideration of a medication trial. Suggested medication approaches to the treatment of psychiatric syndromes in TBI are covered later in this chapter.

PSYCHIATRIC DISORDERS FOLLOWING TBI

Psychotic Disorders

Clinical Presentation

Psychosis is a relatively rare phenomenon but quite clinically important when it occurs following TBI. TBI psychotic features tend to develop a paranoid theme. In lesser degrees this could simply be noticed as suspiciousness or ideas of persecution or suspected marital infidelity. The occurrence of frank psychosis is relatively rare, probably in the range of 2 to 10 percent of patients (Lishman, 1987).

Achte et al. (1991) studied a series of war veterans from Finland. Of 10,000 veterans suffering significant head trauma, 3,000 suffered from a psychiatric disturbance, with 750 (7.5 percent of the 10,000) developing psychosis. Delusional, paranoid, and affective psychotic states were the most common. Many psychotic symptoms resolved spontaneously with time. However 40 to 60 percent of psychotic disorder persisted longer than 5 years. Achte et al. reported that the head trauma was classified as moderate or severe, although preliminary reports did not state how severity was measured or what diagnostic criteria were used for psychotic disorders.

The role of early life brain trauma in producing adult psychotic disorders is receiving continuing attention. Gureje et al. (1994) studied a series of Nigerian patients with schizophrenia. Adult schizophrenic patients had higher rates of perinatal injury or head trauma than control manic psychotic adults (62 versus 8 percent).

Psychomotor agitation is often considered a symptom of some forms of psychosis. Post-TBI agitation is a syndrome of "episodic motor or verbal behavior which interferes with patient care or clearly requires physical or chemical restraint to prevent damage to persons or property" (Brooke et al., 1992). In a study of 100 consecutive TBI patients admitted to a trauma unit, 11 showed evidence of agitation for up to 4 weeks following TBI. Restlessness (defined as behavior interfering with staff but not meeting agitation criteria) was present in a greater number of admission (35 percent). Subjects in this study had a Glasgow coma scale (GCS) score of less than 8 at the time of admission to the emergency room.

DSM-IV Classification

The designation 293.xx Psychotic Disorder Due to Head Trauma is an appropriate diagnosis in many TBI patients with psychotic symptoms. For this diagnosis, psychotic conditions must follow TBI and the injury must be thought to produce the symptoms through a direct physiologic mechanism (American Psychiatric Association, 1994). Prominent hallucinations or delusions must be present and must not occur only in the context of a delirium. *Psychotic disorder due to head trauma* is subtyped according to the predominant symptom: 293.81 *with delusions* or 293.82 *with hallucinations.*

Differential Diagnosis

Primary psychotic disorders such as schizophrenia and mania must be ruled out. Primary psychotic disorders are more frequently associated with a personal or family history of psychotic disorders. The quality of auditory hallucinations may be helpful in differentiating schizophrenia from *psychotic disorder due to head trauma.* Schizophrenic hallucinations are more likely to involve multiple voices carrying on a complex conversation. *Substance-induced psychotic disorder* should also be ruled out. A urine drug screen provides assistance in documenting possible contributions of illicit drug use to psychotic phenomenology. When it is clinically impossible to differentiate primary, substance-induced, and TBI-related factors,

TABLE 15-1. Classification of Psychiatric Disorders Due to Traumatic Brain Injury

DSM-IIIR Classification		DSM-IV Classification
293.00 *Delirium*	⟶	293.00 *Delirium due to head trauma*
294.10 *Dementia*	⟶	294.10 *Dementia due to head trauma*
		293.xx *Psychotic disorder due to head trauma*
293.81 *Organic delusional disorder*	⟶	293.81 With delusions
293.82 *Organic hallucinosis*	⟶	293.82 With hallucinations
293.83 *Organic mood disorder* Manic Depressed Mixed	⟶	293.83 *Mood disorder due to head trauma* With depressive features With major depressive-like episode With manic features With mixed features
294.80 *Organic anxiety disorder*	⟶	293.89 *Anxiety disorder due to head trauma* With generalized anxiety With panic attacks With obsessive-compulsive symptoms
310.10 *Organic personality disorder* Explosive subtype	⟶	310.10 *Personality change due to head trauma* Labile type Disinhibited type Aggressive type Apathetic type Paranoid type Other type Combined type
294.80 *Organic mental disorder NOS*	⟶	625.80 Female hypoactive sexual desire due to head trauma
	⟶	608.89 Male hypoactive sexual desire due to head trauma
	⟶	607.84 Male erectile disorder due to head trauma
	⟶	780.xx *Sleep disorder due to head trauma*
	⟶	780.52 Insomnia subtype
	⟶	780.54 Hypersomnia subtype
	⟶	780.59 Parasomnia subtype

TABLE 15-2. Postconcussive Symptoms, Diagnosis, and Treatment

Predominant Symptom Causing Impairment	DSM-IV Classification	Possible Therapeutic Agents
Apathy/anergia	Personality change due to head trauma/apathetic subtype	Methylphenidate Dextroamphetamine Protriptyline
Insomnia	Sleep disorder due to head trauma/insomnia subtype	Trazodone Lorazepam Clonazepam
Irritability/anger	Personality change due to head trauma/aggressive type	Propranolol Amantidine
Emotional lability	Personality change due to head trauma/labile type	Fluoxetine Nortriptyline Trazodone
Depression	Mood disorder due to head trauma/with depressive features	Fluoxetine Nortriptyline
Anxiety/restlessness	Anxiety disorder due to head trauma/with generalized anxiety	Buspirone Trazodone

the residual diagnosis of *psychotic disorder not otherwise specified* can be used.

Mood Disorders

Clinical Presentation

Mood disorders are the most extensively studied sequelae of TBI. Depression complicates recovery in up to 25 percent of patients (Silver, 1991), while up to 15 percent of TBI patients attempt suicide in the 5-year period after injury (Brooks et al., 1986). Jorge et al. (1993a) studied the phenomenology of depressive states in a series of TBI patients. DSM-IIIR criteria for major depression appeared to be satisfactory to make the diagnosis of depression in the TBI patient. Early in the course of depression, poor self-attitude and anergia were characteristic symptoms. Later, depressed patients were likely to have early morning awakening and concentrations problems. They noted very few cases of "masked" depression (depressive syndrome in the absence of a report of depressed mood).

The clinical presentation of mood disorder in TBI may have an early or a delayed onset (Jorge et al., 1993b). Acute-onset depressive episodes appear to be related to the site of the trauma in the brain, while delayed depressive episodes appear to be linked to psychological mechanisms. Left dorsolateral frontal lesions and/or left basal ganglia lesions were associated with the highest rates of depressive episodes (Federoff et al., 1992). The site of brain trauma was determined by computed tomography (CT) scans rated by neurologists using operationalized criteria. The neurologists were blind to the patients psychiatric status. The authors concluded that depressive symptoms result from "interruption of biogenic amine-containing neurons as they pass through the basal ganglia or frontal subcortical white matter."

Manic syndromes have also been reported to follow TBI. Jorge et al. (1993d) studied a series of 66 patients following head trauma. Subjects were eligible if they met GCS criteria for mild, moderate, or severe brain injury. The majority of subjects met criteria for moderate brain injury. Six patients (9 percent) met criteria for mania at some point in the 1 year of follow-up. CT scans were rated for diffuse and mass lesions by brain location according to guidelines proposed by the Traumatic Coma Data Bank. Temporal lobe lesions predicted a manic episode, while severity of injury and personal/family psychiatric history did not predict such an episode. Manic episodes tended to brief, lasting on the average only 2 months and were not related to severity of brain lesion. Subcortical injury appears to be linked to manic and mixed manic-depressive states in TBI (Starkstein et al., 1991).

Mood disorders in TBI may not be limited to the patient suffering the injury. Linn et al. (1994) examined the effect of TBI on the mood of spouses in a study of married couples. They found that 73 percent of spouses of TBI patients reported depressive symptoms 6 years following the injury. Wives were particularly likely to develop depressive symptoms when their husbands experienced TBI. This study underlines the need to consider the familial and social implications of TBI.

DSM-IV Classification

When TBI is believed to be the primary physiologic factor in a depressive episode the DSM-IV classification would be 293.83 *mood disorders due to head trauma* (American Psychiatric Association, 1994). Subtype classifications for this category include *with depressive features, with major depressive-like episode, with manic features,* and *with mixed features.* When full major depression is present, the major depressive-like episode designation is appropriate. If only mood lability is present, *with depressive features* could be used. (Additionally, with lability a prominent symptom, the diagnosis of *personality change due to head trauma,* labile subtype, should be considered.)

Differential Diagnosis

Sadness commonly follows any significant injury, especially if the injury is associated with loss of function. Major depression can be distinguished from sadness by the extent and persistence of the depressed mood with accompanying fatigue, sleep disturbance, guilt, self-deprecation, and suicidal thoughts. Other medical causes of depression deserve review in the TBI patient. Adjustment disorder with depressed mood may mimic major depression, but is usually less severe and without the full complement of major depressive symptoms. Prescription, over-the-counter, and illicit drugs and alcohol can produce depressive symptoms and need consideration before attributing a depressive episode to TBI. Patients with TBI may be more vulnerable to adverse central nervous system (CNS) effects of licit and illicit drugs, including a drug-induced depressive response. (Gualtieri, 1990).

Anxiety Disorders

Clinical Presentation

There has been limited study of anxiety disorders in TBI. Jorge et al. (1993c) examined the frequency, course, and clinical correlates of generalized anxiety disorder in a series of 66 TBI patients. Generalized anxiety disorder is characterized as a disorder of excessive anxiety and worry that a person finds difficult to control, which is accompanied by at least three of the following symptoms: restlessness, easy fatigability, poor concentration, irritability, muscle tension, and sleep disturbance (American Psychiatric Association, 1994). Generalized anxiety criteria were met in 11 percent of TBI subjects. All generalized anxiety disorder subjects also met criteria for major depressive disorder, but 15 percent of the subjects met major depressive disorder criteria without concurrent generalized anxiety disorder. The authors hypothesized that major depression following TBI could be subtyped into those with and those without generalized anxiety.

Other features of anxiety can occur following TBI. Post-TBI anxiety appears more common when the traumatic event is especially frightening (Lishman, 1987). Patients may develop preoccupation with the event, frightening dreams, and phobic avoidance of things that may be associated with the event (McMillan, 1991). Obsessive-compulsive symptoms may also develop following TBI. McKeon et al. (1984) described a case series of four patients developing obsessive-compulsive disorder following acute brain injury. Of note, in all these cases the obsessional symptoms developed within 24 hours of the trauma with no premorbid history of obsessional disorder.

DSM-IV Classification

DSM-IV allows for the classification of TBI-related anxiety under the *anxiety disorders due to general medical conditions* format (American Psychiatric Association, 1994). Anxiety that is considered directly related in a physiologic manner to TBI would be designated as *anxiety disorder due to head trauma.* This diagnosis is more likely when anxiety symptoms emerge soon after trauma in an individual with no premorbid anxiety history and no family history of psychiatric disorder. The anxiety disorder can be subtyped according to the predominant anxiety presentation: *with generalized anxiety, with panic attacks,* or with *obsessive-compulsive symptoms.*

Differential Diagnosis

Primary anxiety disorders must be ruled out before making a diagnosis of *anxiety disorder due to head trauma.* Additional considerations in the differential diagnosis include substance-induced anxiety disorder and adjustment disorder with anxious or anxious and depressed mood. When the mechanism of anxiety symptoms is unclear, the category of *anxiety disorder not otherwise specified* can be used.

Sleep Disorders

Clinical Presentation

There has been limited study of the effects of TBI on sleep despite the high rates of sleep complaints in patients with TBI. Cohen et al. (1992) interviewed a series of TBI patients who were classified into recent onset (median 3.5 months from injury) and remote onset (median 29.5 months from injury). Rates of sleep complaints were high in both groups (72.7 percent in the recent and 51.9 percent in the remote group). Of note, the type of sleep complaint varied by the recency of trauma. Disorders of sleep initiation were more common in the recent group, while disorders of excessive somnolence were more common in the remote group (see Ch. 14).

DSM-IV Classification

Many patients with TBI have sleep complaints but would not merit a DSM-IV diagnosis for a sleep disorder. Diagnostic classification as a sleep disorder should be limited to cases that are severe enough to generate independent clinical attention. When severe sleep disturbances come to clinical attention, an appropriate designation would be 780.xx *sleep disorder due to a general medical condition.* The last two-digit coding would be reserved for the sleep disorder subtypes: 780.52 *Insomnia subtype,* 780.54 *hypersomnia subtype,* 780.59 *parasomnia subtype,* 780.59 *mixed subtype.*

Differential Diagnosis

Various causes for sleep complaints in the TBI patient should be reviewed. Patients may actually have a primary sleep disorder such as obstructive sleep apnea. Sleep complaints are common with a variety of mood, anxiety, and substance use disorders. A full psychiatric review of systems is needed when patients have a sleep complaint. Many prescription and over-the-counter medications produce changes in sleep patterns. High daily caffeine intake may also be related to sleep disturbance.

Sexual Disorders

Clinical Presentation

Symptoms of sexual dysfunction can be noted after TBI. These symptoms can be grouped into changes in sexual interest or performance and the development of inappropriate or unusual sexual behaviors. A syndrome of apathy can extend to apathy in sexuality, with diminished desire and reduced frequency of sexual intercourse. Impotence can also develop after TBI. Finally, inappropriate sexual behavior and speech have been noted, especially in patients with significant frontal lobe dysfunction. This can include suggestive remarks or unwanted sexual advances toward health professionals. Increased interest in pornography has also been noted (Lishman, 1989).

DSM-IV Classification

When sexual apathy is a target of evaluation and interest, the appropriate classification comes under the sexual dysfunction due to head trauma category. The subclassification would 608.89 Male (or 625.80 Female) *hypoactive sexual desire due to head trauma.* Male impotency following TBI would be denoted by 607.84, *male erectile disorder due to head trauma.*

Inappropriate sexual behavior problems can be clinically important enough for diagnosis. Inappropriate sexual behaviors believed to be due to frontal lobe damage would be designated as *personality change due to head trauma—disinhibited type.*

Differential Diagnosis

Disorders of sexual desire can be primary (i.e., present prior to head trauma or unrelated to the injury). Medications can have significant effect on sexual interest and performance. A variety of causes for impotence should be reviewed, including vascular disorders, diabetes, and psychological disorders impairing male sexual function.

Personality Change Due to Head Trauma

Clinical Presentation

There is substantial evidence that TBI contributes to changes in personality. Personality disorder is defined as "an enduring pattern of inner experience and behavior that deviates markedly from the expectations of the individual's culture, is pervasive and inflexible, has an onset in adolesence or early adulthood, is stable over time, and leads to distress or impairment" (American Psychiatric Association, 1994). DSM-IV defines 11 categories of primary personality disorder: paranoid, schizoid, schizotypal, antisocial, borderline, histrionic, narcissistic, avoidant, dependent, obsessive-compulsive, and personality disorder not otherwise specified. Patients experiencing TBI have demonstrated elevations on narcissistic, antisocial, and passive-aggressive measures (Tuokko et al., 1991).

Using the standard Minnesota Multiphasic Personality Inventory (MMPI) nomenclature, 58 brain-injured patients (duration of coma $<$ 24 hours in 72 percent, 1 to 7 days in 11 percent, and $>$ 7 days in 17 percent) demonstrated elevations on scales 1 (hypochrondriasis), 2 (depression), 3 (hysteria), 7 (psychathenia), 8 (schizophrenia) (Gass and Russell, 1991). Other studies support the association of brain injury with features of hysteria as described by Charcot (Eames, 1992). There is also some evidence to suggest minor head trauma is associated with greater MMPI personality pathology than severe head trauma (Leininger et al., 1991). This may be due to the increased health-seeking behavior in mild head trauma patients with personality psychopathology.

Personality disorders are believed to be the result of complex interactions between environmental and genetic factors. Personality changes due primarily to TBI receive a specific classification, *personality change due to head trauma.*

TBI may play a significant role in personality disorders thought to be due to other environmental and genetic forces. Van Reekum et al. (1993) studied a sample of 48 veterans with a diagnosis of borderline personality disorder. A control sample of psychiatric patients was matched with the borderline personality disorder group. The prevalence rate for a history of TBI in the borderline personality disorder group was 37.5 percent compared with 4.0 percent in the psychiatric controls. This study suggests that TBI may play a significant unrecognized role in the etiology of some primary personality disorders. However, retrospective studies such as this are unable to demonstrate causality. An alternate explanation for findings in the Van Reekum et al. study is that borderline personality disorder increases the risk for TBI.

The personality changes associated with head trauma can be grouped into three categories: active, passive, and other syndromes. A recent review outlined the types of personality changes associated with TBI in subjects with a GCS score of 12 or less (Prigatano, 1992). Active personality characteristics documented in the literature include irritability, agitation, belligerence, anger, episodic violent behavior, impulsiveness, restlessness, socially inappropriate behavior, emotional lability, sensitivity to noise, suspiciousness, and paranoia. Passive personality traits documented include aspontaneity, loss of interest in the environment, loss of drive or initiative, and easy fatigability.

Other syndromes that have been described include childishness, helplessness, and lack of awareness of behavioral limitations. Childishness is characterized as self-centered behavior, overtalkativeness, and insensitivity to others. The helplessness syndrome seen after brain injury produces a need for active supervision and repetitive assistance with each step to complete a complex task.

DSM-IV Classification

The DSM-IV category 310.10 *personality change due to head trauma* represents an appropriate designation for the effects of TBI on personality. This category is defined as a "persistent personality disturbance that is judged to be due to the direct physiological effects of a general medical condition" (American Psychiatric Association, 1994). This personality disturbance must be a change from the patient's previous personality pattern. DSM-IV includes a significant increase in the number of subtype classifications for this category, which include labile, disinhibited, aggressive, apathetic, paranoid, other, and combined. An individual subtype designation is used if the subtype captures the predominant feature of the personality change.

Differential Diagnosis

Clinicians need to determine the premorbid personality of patients in order to assess accurately any change due to TBI. This can be done by asking friends or family members about the patient's usual personality traits. These traits can be often ascertained by asking open-ended questions such as: What was this patient's personality like prior to the injury? Was he an emotional person? Did she have many friends and tend to trust others? Did he have a sense of humor? Was she easy to anger? What did he do when he became angry? Finally, it can be helpful to ask close family members to describe any changes in the patient that they have noticed since the injury.

Other diagnoses associated with TBI can mimic personality change. Psychotic disorder, mood disorder, and anxiety disorder can produce changes in personality. If these disorders affect personality, it is best to simply make the psychotic, mood, or anxiety disorder diagnosis and omit any personality change designation. Alcohol, drug abuse, and some prescription drugs prescribed postinjury can adversely affect personality. A review of the patient's alcohol, drug, and prescription use helps prevent misclassification of an adverse effect due to drugs or medications as personality change.

Substance Use Disorders

Clinical Presentation

The role of substance use disorders in raising the risk of TBI has already been noted. Concurrent alcohol abuse histories and intoxication at the time of TBI have important consequences. Many studies document the negative effect of current alcohol abuse in the presentation, pathology, and oucome of TBI.

Gurney et al. (1992) studied the effect of concurrent alcohol intoxication on the clinical presentation and course of TBI patients. In a series of 520 patients diagnosed in the emergency room with brain injury, 37 percent were intoxicated (>100 mg/dl blood alcohol). Intoxicated subjects were more likely to require intubation, to require placement of an intracranial pressure bolt, to develop respiratory distress requiring ventilatory support, and to develop pneumonia.

Alcohol abuse appears to influence the risk for more extensive brain injury with trauma. Ronty et al. (1993) compared multiple physiologic and anatomic parameters in a series of patients with head injury. Patients with alcohol abuse demonstrated greater volumes of cranial hemorrhage. In 1 year of follow-up, brain atrophy in the alcohol abuse group was more pronounced. Serial quantitative electroencephalographic (EEG) measures were slower to normalize in the group with alcohol abuse. The study of alcohol abuse in head trauma often involves the clinical problem of discriminating the brain effects of chronic alcohol use from the effects of the TBI. Some neuropsychological strategies provide assistance in discriminating the brain effects due to these two causes (Mearns and Lees-Haley, 1993).

Alcohol abuse adversely affects the rehabilitation and outcome of TBI patients. Brooks et al. (1989)

studied the effects of alcohol abuse and of intoxication at the time of injury and the duration of post-traumatic amnesia in a series of subjects. Alcohol consumption at the time of injury proved to be a significant predictor of later memory deficits. This effect occurred even if the period post-traumatic amnesia was brief. Ruff et al. (1990) also examined the effect of intoxication at the time of injury on the pathophysiology of TBI. Intoxication at the time of injury predicted poor global outcome when other variables were controlled and also was associated with development of a brain mass lesion.

DSM-IV Classification

One strategy for accurately diagnosing substance abuse problems in the brain-injured population is to screen all patients for substance abuse. Fuller et al. (1994) examined four different screening measures for alcohol abuse in a series of patients with TBI. The CAGE questionnaire (Ewing, 1984) and the Brief Michigan Alcoholism Screening Test (Pokorny et al., 1972) were both found to be reliable and valid instruments. Clinicians may want to consider using screening instruments to address difficult diagnostic issues associated with alcohol abuse.

Differential Diagnosis

Substance abuse criteria are relatively straightforward. Once the diagnosis of substance abuse is confirmed, the role of such abuse in contributing to mood, anxiety, or personality symptoms needs to be reviewed.

Adjustment Disorders

Clinical Presentation

There has been very limited study of the prevalence and presentation of adjustment disorders in TBI. The usual response to a severe medical illness and trauma can certainly include sadness, nervousness, withdrawal, anger, and irritability. When these symptoms persist, become pervasive, and impair function, including rehabilitation, the diagnosis of adjustment disorder should be considered. Adjustment disorder symptoms classically emerge immediately after the stressor and tend to diminish with time as the patient adjusts to the stress experience.

DSM-IV Classification

309.9 *Adjustment disorder* is defined as "the development of clinically significant emotional or behavioral symptoms in response to an identifiable psychosocial stressor or stressors" (American Psychiatric Association, 1994). By definition the patient's response to the stressor is clinically significant when it produces distress that is in excess of what would be considered the usual response to a similar stressor or when there is significant impairment in social or occupational functioning. Adjustment disorder with depressed mood can be subtyped according to the predominant symptom. These subtypes include *with depressed mood, with anxiety, with mixed anxiety and depressed mood, with disturbance of conduct,* and *with mixed disturbance of emotions and conduct.*

Differential Diagnosis

Of primary concern in the differential diagnosis of adjustment disorder is to separate the condition from a normal and usual response to a stress such as TBI. Personality disorders are often typified by maladaptive responses to stress. Adjustment disorder is not diagnosed when the patient's emotional and behavioral response is consistent with previous responses and part of a personality style. A more significant mood disorder or anxiety disorder needs to be considered when mood and anxiety symptoms predominate in the post-TBI period.

TREATMENT OF PSYCHIATRIC DISORDER IN TBI

Efforts to improve the outcome for the TBI patient constitute the process of rehabilitation. Volpe and McDowell (1990) reviewed the literature on the value of cognitive rehabilitation on outcome for TBI patients. They summarized some therapeutic interventions that may improve outcome, including treatment of seizures, interaction with a peer group, general encouragement by a team of health professionals, treatment of co-morbid depression, and patient and family education about the degree of impairment and how to deal with it. Their review suggested limited evidence that specific cognitive rehabilitation actually improves the natural history and outcome of TBI.

Of note, a significant part of the rehabilitation process falls within the domain of psychiatric treatment. The psychiatric goals of treatment in TBI are very similar to those for non-TBI patients. These goals include reduction in distressing psychiatric symptomatology, along with minimization of impairment in social, work, and family functioning. These goals can be defined and pursued best in the context of a multidisciplinary, individualized treatment plan for the TBI patient (Weinstein et al., 1994). Treatment team members may include neurologists, neuropsychologists, occupational therapists, physical therapists, social workers, nurses, psychiatrists, and psychologists. Individual patients may not need services from all the team members. However, a comprehensive evaluation process should involve multiple team members to help in the development of individual rehabilitation treatment plans.

Family assessment and follow-up is an important part of rehabilitation. Children of parents with TBI experience significant negative effects (Pessar et al., 1993). In a study of a series of 24 parents with TBI, 10 had children who developed significant behavior problems in the period after the injury. These problem behaviors included deteriorating parent-child relationships, acting-out behaviors, and the development of an emotional disturbance. Caregivers of patients with TBI experience significant depression and anxiety in the context of the rehabilitation process (Kreutzer et al., 1994).

Psychotherapy

The approach to the psychotherapy of TBI patients is influenced by several factors, including the specific psychiatric disorder identified and the extent of cognitive impairment associated with the TBI. Patients with no or very limited cognitive impairment are likey to benefit from psychotherapy approaches that have been validated as effective in non-TBI patients. Individual cognitive-behavior therapy as well as interpersonal psychotherapy has research documentation of effectiveness for a variety of mood and anxiety disorders. There are no studies of these models in TBI patients, but similar efficacy is likely in those with normal verbal and abstraction skills.

When cognitive impairment is significant, limited goals for psychotherapy can be set. Many psychotherapeutic principles require rather complex cognitive and abstract processes. When the individual is unable to use complex cognitive strategies, some forms of psychotherapy (e.g., psychodynamic psychotherapy) are inappropriate. Behavioral approaches are more suited to the cognitively impaired population. Several studies suggest that behavioral strategies may be effective in patients with TBI.

Uomoto and Broadway (1992) studied a behavioral and family approach to dealing with anger control problems in patients with TBI. Subjects were taught a method of self-talk, with time out for periodic anger. Family members were recruited to assist in the behavioral management by identifying environmental cues and assisting the subjects to use self-control methods. Simple behavioral management approaches can often be successfully used and negate the need for psychopharmacologic intervention.

Becker and Vakil (1993) describe behavioral psychotherapy for patients suffering from frontal lobe deficits due to TBI. Specific behavioral techniques can be targeted for the frontal lobe deficit syndromes of disinhibition and adynamia. A series of stages are required for providing behavioral psychotherapy. These include (1) establishment of a therapeutic alliance; (2) diagnostic evaluation; (3) selection of the problem to be treated; (4) behavioral intervention; (5) working through resistance to change; and (6) generalizing and internalizing adaptive change.

Substance Abuse Management

Alcohol use often decreases after a significant TBI. However, a significant number of TBI patients continue to abuse alcohol during the rehabilitation process. Kreutzer et al. (1991) found that 28 percent of a series of patients in rehabilitation continued to abuse alcohol, and 4 percent reported continued use of illicit drugs. A significant percentage (10 percent) also reported arrests for crime in the rehabilitation period. Obviously, ongoing assessment of the role of alcohol, drug use, and antisocial behavior is important in monitoring rehabilitation and outcome.

Substance abuse treatment for TBI patients often gives disappointing results. The cognitive impairment associated with TBI may reduce the effectiveness of traditional treatment approaches to substance abuse. Experience of TBI patients with Alcoholics Anonymous has not been favorable (Sparadeo et al., 1990). Many major rehabilitation centers are developing substance abuse treatment programs for patients with TBI. These programs modify existing approaches to the specific needs of the cognitively impaired patients. Various models of treatment have been described (Langley et al., 1990). These models often employ some common substance abuse treatment strategies, including education, behavior therapy, relapse prevention, and comprehensive aftercare programming.

Psychopharmacologic Intervention

Clinical experience and research studies provide a base of knowledge for the pharmacologic treatment of psychiatric disorders in the TBI patient. There is significant evidence of efficacy for various drug treatment approaches. However, the efficacy of drug treatment for psychiatric disorders in TBI patients may be less than for the equivalent functional psychiatric syndromes. Yates et al. (1991) examined the outcome of treatment for depression due to general medical conditions, including head trauma. A series of 50 patients (3 with head trauma) referred for psychiatric consultation were identified as having a depression due to an organic factor. A control series of patients were identified with depression and a medical disorder not believed to be causally related to the mood disorder. Despite similar histories of treatment with antidepressant medication, patients with organic depressive disorders demonstrated poorer response to treatment than the control group. Only 11 percent of depressives with an organic etiology recovered completely in 4 years of follow-up. This compares with a 58 percent complete recovery rate in depressed patients without organic etiologies (odds ratio, 13.0, 95 percent confidence interval, 1.5 to 100). Despite this relative lack of efficacy, pharmacologic approaches may often be critical for some individual patients.

Postconcussive Syndrome

Pharmacologic treatment of the postconcussive syndrome is targeted to the primary psychiatric symptom. The majority of patients with this syndrome do not need psychotropic treatment, which should be limited to patients with severe and persistent symptoms. Generally, persistent symptoms will be present for at least 6 months. Treatment guidelines for the various postconcussive syndrome symptoms have been suggested by Gualteri (1993).

Persistent cognitive and physiologic symptoms of memory impairment, concentration difficulties, anergia, and fatigue may be responsive to a trial of psychostimulants. Psychostimulant trials are relatively safe. Additionally, beneficial effects often emerge within 24 to 72 hours of therapy initiation. This rapid onset of therapeutic effect contrasts with a delayed effect noted for other types of psychotropic agents such as the tricyclic antidepressants. Two medications are available for psychostimulant trials: methylphenidate (Ritalin), 10 to 30 mg bid or dextroamphetamine, 5 to 15 mg bid. Psychostimulant trials should begin at about half the lowest suggested dosage and be increased over the initial 2 to 3 days based on the patient's tolerance for and therapeutic response to the agents. Adverse effects to monitor include restlessness, irritability, and insomnia. Psychostimulants are contraindicated in patients with a history of alcohol dependence, drug dependence, or antisocial personality. Patients with these disorders are at risk for stimulant misuse and the development of drug-seeking behavioral problems. There is some disagreement about the effectiveness of psychostimulants in this population (see Ch. 17). More placebo-controlled studies are necessary to document efficacy.

Another concern in treating TBI patients with psychostimulants is increased seizure risk. The Physicians Desk Reference (1994) notes an increased risk of seizure with stimulants such as methylphenidate. However, one case series study is reassuring about seizure risk in TBI patients. Wroblewski et al. (1992) retrospectively studied 30 consecutive patients with severe TBI and seizures who received a medication trial with methylphenidate. Overall, they noted a trend toward decreased seizure frequency in this series, although four patients did have an increased seizure rate with methylphenidate. Three of these patients were also taking tricyclic antidepressant, a class of agents also known to increase seizure risk.

One alternative to psychostimulants for anergia and attentional problems is protriptyline. Protriptyline is a tricyclic antidepressant known to be more stimulating than traditional antidepressants such as imipramine. Wroblewski et al. (1993) summarized their experience with protriptyline in eight patients with TBI. Using doses in the lower portion of the recommended range (10 to 60 mg daily) they reported significant activating effects. This case series is remarkable in that a significant number of patients responding to protriptyline had failed to respond to methylphenidate and other antidepressant agents before responding to protriptyline.

Patients with persistent severe insomnia associated with the postconcussive syndrome may benefit from a trial of trazodone 50 to 150 mg hs (at bedtime). Trazodone, a sedating heterocyclic antidepressant, has a significant effect on sleep. It has the advantage of often maintaining efficacy over prolonged periods.

This effect appears superior to that seen with benzodiazepine hypnotics. The primary adverse effect of trazodone is the risk for priapism in male patients. Although rare, this possible effect should be reviewed with patients prior to administration. If trazodone is not used, benzodiazepines can be tried, especially if the goal is short-term resolution of sleep problems. Lorazepam, 0.5 mg to 1 mg hs can be tried. This agent has the advantage of generic dosing at low cost. An alternate benzodiazepine for insomnia would be clonazepam, 0.5 mg to 1 mg hs. Clonazepam's longer half-life would be preferred if the patient suffers from daytime anxiety symptoms in addition to insomnia. Benzodiazepines need close monitoring for evidence of disinhibition of behavior. Disinhibition presents a higher risk in patients with TBI than in the general population.

Psychotic Disorders

Postcoma agitation can be a significant clinical problem. When conservative behavioral techniques do not eliminate risk to the patient or treatment team, acute pharmacologic intervention is appropriate. Antipsychotic or benzodiazepine agents are the agents of choice for acute control of agitation. Haloperidol can be used orally, intramuscularly, or for emergencies, intravenously. Lorazepam also can be used for acute sedation and is available for oral, intramuscular, and intravenous use. Control of agitation in TBI and other delirious states can often be achieved by use of haloperidol, lorazepam, or a combination of the two (Goldstein and Haltzman, 1993). Once acute agitation is controlled, it may be preferrable to maintain control with a nonsedating agent. Options for maintenance control of agitation include amantadine (100 to 400 mg daily), carbamazepine (blood levels of 4 to 14 μg/ml), valproic acid (blood levels of 50 to 150 μg/ml), or lithium (blood levels of 0.6 to 1.2 mEq/L).

For late-onset psychotic disorders (emergence of psychosis after at least 6 months), antipsychotic agents are often necessary. A haloperidol trial is a reasonable first-line choice beginning at 1 mg/day and titrating as tolerated and to response. Young males, those most likely to experience TBI, may be especially sensitive to dystonic reactions with antipsychotics such as haloperidol. An alternate agent to consider would be risperidone at 2 to 6 mg daily. Risperidone is a newer antipsychotic, which has limited study in TBI populations. However, it may be better tolerated with less induction of parkinsonian rigidity.

Mood Disorders

Several antidepressant agents have been used to treat emotional lability following TBI. Agents reported to be helpful have included amitriptyline (Schiffer et al., 1985), levodopa (Udaka et al., 1984), and most recently, fluoxetine (Sloan et al., 1992). The fluoxetine study examined six patients with brain injury (five poststroke patients and one TBI patient), who were distressed by embarrassing emotionalism. All six patients received a trial of fluoxetine 20 mg daily. All six are reported to have had significant improvement, as determined by using an observer rating scale for lability. Fluoxetine was reported to have been tolerated well in these patients and has the advantage of less anticholinergic effect than standard tricyclic antidepressants.

For TBI patients with a full major depressive disorder, a variety of treatment options are available. Cassidy (1989) reported moderate to marked improvement in depression following TBI in five of nine patients receiving a trial of fluoxetine. Selective serotonin re-uptake inhibitors such as fluoxetine, paroxetine, and sertraline are reasonable first-line antidepressant agents in TBI. Tricyclic antidepressants can also be used but have the disadvantage of anticholinergic effects and possible seizure problems. Successful treatment has also been reported with tricyclics, primarily nortriptyline (Ross and Rush, 1981). Nortriptyline has one of the lowest anticholinergic profiles of the antidepressants and can be monitored for therapeutic serum drug levels.

For medication-resistant depression, a trial of electroconvulsive therapy can be considered (Silver et al., 1991). This modality is absolutely contraindicated only for space-occupying lesions of the brain. However, TBI patients with depression may be more vulnerable to temporary memory impairment induced by this treatment. Temporary memory impairment can be minimized by decreasing the frequency of treatments or using unilateral electroconvulsive therapy.

Anxiety Disorders

Anxiety disorders following TBI can produce significant distress and impairment, which may require considering a pharmacologic treatment approach. Although benzodiazepine drugs promptly reduce a anxiety symptoms, chronic benzodiazepine treatment causes several problems. First, the possibility of acute withdrawal and possible withdrawal seizure is present, especially with the short-acting benzodiazepines. Second, benzodiazepines can impair cognitive function and reduce memory function. This can be a significant problem in the TBI patient population.

For generalized anxiety disorder, several treatment options deserve consideration. Buspirone at 15 to 60 mg daily is well tolerated, with some evidence of efficacy in this population (Gualtieri, 1991). Buspirone appears to lack an antipanic effect. Antidepressant drugs have significant antianxiety and antipanic effects. Tricyclics sometimes produce significant anxiolytic effects at doses lower than the antidepressant dose. Doxepin at 25 mg to 50 mg can be helpful as a sleep aid and an anxiolytic for generalized anxiety. For patients with significant obsessional symptoms, selective serotonin re-uptake inhibitors are probably the drugs of choice.

Personality Change

Control of anger and its behavioral consequences is an important goal of the rehabilitation process. The Federal Drug Administration (FDA) has not approved any specific medication for the treatment of aggressive behavior. Despite this lack of endorsement, clinicians have an extensive list of antiaggression pharmacologic agents that can be considered for subjects with TBI. Pharmacologic interventions should be reserved for severe behavioral disorders that have not responded to behavioral therapy. In such patients clinicians may want to begin with agents with which they have the most experience and begin a sequential trial until a suitable agent and dose schedule are discovered.

Lithium and carbamazepine have some support as antianger and antiaggressive agents (Patterson, 1988; Worrall et al., 1975). Both these agents require dose titration with therapeutic serum level monitoring to avoid the toxic effects of elevated serum drug levels.

Amantadine (a dopamine agonist) has recently also received attention for control of anger and aggressive behavior in TBI. Chandler et al. (1988) presented an early report of two aggressive TBI patients who responded to a trial of amantidine at 400 mg/day. A later report documented the results of amantidine treatment of 30 TBI patients (Gualtieri et al., 1989), 19 of whom were reported to have responded unequivocally. However, 5 of the 19 were unable to tolerate the drug. Amantadine is reported to have a fairly rapid onset of action (4 to 7 days).

ß-Adrenergic blocking agents also appear to lower levels of irritability and reduce agitation. Although studied more extensively in the management of dementia, ß-blockers can reduce aggressive behaviors in TBI (Yudofsky, 1981). Propranolol at 80 to 400 mg can be used with monitoring of blood pressure and pulse rate. Alternatively, pindolol at 40 to 60 mg daily can be used.

CONCLUSION

TBI frequently produces psychiatric disorders. The type of psychiatric symptoms produced by brain trauma is diverse and can include psychotic, affective, anxiety, and personality changes. Clinicians need to pay attention to the timing and severity of psychiatric symptoms along with premorbid status to make an accurate diagnosis. Psychiatric co-morbidity in TBI patients can produce significant distress and additional impairment in work and social roles. Psychologic and pharmacologic treatment modalities are available to reduce suffering and disability. Although a significant amount of literature exists for using pharmacologic agents in this population, the number of randomized, placebo-controlled studies is quite limited. Accurate diagnosis and aggressive treatment of psychiatric syndromes can significantly improve outcome for many patients with TBI.

REFERENCES

Achte K, Jarho L, Kyykka T, Vesterinen E: Paranoid disorders following war brain damage. Psychopathology 24:309–315, 1991

American Psychiatric Association: Diagnostic and Statistical Manual of Mental Disorders. 3rd Ed, Revised. American Psychiatric Association, Washington, 1987

American Psychiatric Association: Diagnostic and Statistical Manual of Mental Disorders, 4th Ed, (DSM-IV). American Psychiatric Association, Washington, 1994

Becker ME, Vakil E: Behavioral psychotherapy of the frontal-lobe-injured patient in the outpatient setting. Brain Inj 7:515–523, 1993

Brooke MM, Questad KA, Patterson DR, Bashak KJ: Agitation and restlessness after closed head injury: a prospective study of 100 consecutive admissions. Arch Phys Med Rehabil 73:320–323, 1992

Brooks N, Campsie L, Symington C: The five year outcome of severe blunt head injury: a relative's view. J Neurol Neurosurg Psychiatry 49:764–770, 1986

Brooks N, Symington C, Beattie A et al: Alcohol and other predictors of cognitive recovery after severe head injury. Brain Inj 3:235–246, 1989

Brown SJ, Fann JR, Grant I: Postconcussional disorder: time to acknowledge a common source of neurobehavioral morbidity. J Neuropsychiatry 6:15–22, 1994

Cassidy JW: Fluoxetine: a new serotonergically active antidepressant. J Head Trauma Rehabil 4:67–69, 1989

Chandler MC, Barnhill JL, Gualtieri CT: Amantadine for the agitated head-injury patient. Brain Inj 2:309–311, 1988

Cohen M, Oksenber A, Snir MJ et al: Temporally related changes of sleep complaints in traumatic brain injured patients. J Neurol Neurosurg Psychiatry 55:313–315, 1992

Dikmen S, Machamer J, Temkin N: Psychosocial outcome in patients with moderate to severe head injury: 2-year follow-up. Brain Inj 7:113–124, 1993

Drubach DA, Keely MP, Winslow MM, Flynn JPG: Substance abuse as a factor in the causality, severity, and recurrence rate of TBI. Md Med J 42:990–993, 1993

Dunlop TW, Udvarhelyi GB, Stedem AF et al: Comparison of patients without emotional/behavioral deterioration during the first year following TBI. J Neuropsychiatry Clin Neurosci 3:150–156, 1991

Eames P: Hysteria following brain injury. J Neurol Neurosurg Psychiatry 55:1046–1053, 1992

Edna T: Alcohol influence and head injury. Acta Chir Scand 148:209–212, 1982

Ewing J: Detecting alcoholism: the CAGE questionnaire. JAMA 252:1905–1907, 1984

Federoff JP, Starkstein SE, Forrester AW et al: Depression in patients with acute TBI. Am J Psychiatry 149:918–923, 1992

Fuller MG, Fishman CA, Taylor CA, Wood RB: Screening patients with traumatic brain injuries for substance abuse. J Neuropsychiatry 6:143–146, 1994

Gass CS, Russell EW: MMPI profiles of closed head trauma patients: impact on neurological complaints. J Clin Psychol 47:253–260, 1991

Goldstein MG, Haltzman SD: Intensive care. In Stoudemire A, Fogel B (eds): Psychiatric Care of the Medical Patient. Oxford University Press, New York, 1993

Gualtieri T: The neuropharmacology of inadvertent drug effects in patients with traumatic brain injury. J Head Trauma Rehabil 5:32–40, 1990

Gualtieri CT: Buspirone for the behavioral problems of patients with organic brain disorders. J Clin Psychopharmacol 11:280–281, 1991

Gualtieri CT: TBI. p. 517. In Stoudemire A, Fogel BS (eds): Psychiatric Care of the Medical Patient, Oxford University Press, New York, 1993

Gualtieri T, Chandler M, Coons TB, Brown LT: Amantadine: a new clinical profile for TBI. Clinical Neuropharmacol 12:258–270, 1989

Gureje O, Bamidele R, Raji O: Early brain trauma and schizophrenia in Nigerian patients. Am J Psychiatry 151:368–371, 1994

Gurney JG, Rivara FP, Mueller BA et al: The effects of alcohol intoxication on the initial treatment and hospital course of patients with acute brain injury. J Trauma 33:709–713, 1992

Jorge RE, Robinson RG, Arndt S: Are there symptoms that are specific for depressed mood in patients with TBI? J Nerv Ment Dis 181:91–99, 1993a

Jorge RE, Robinson RG, Arndt SV et al: Comparison between acute- and delayed-onset depression following TBI. J Neuropsychiatry 5:43–49, 1993b

Jorge RE, Robinson RG, Starkstein SE, Arndt SV: Depression and anxiety following TBI. J Neuropsychiatry 5:369–374, 1993c

Jorge RE, Robinson RG, Starkstein SE et al: Secondary mania following TBI. Am J Psychiatry 150:916–921, 1993d

Kreutzer JS, Gervasio AH, Camplair PS: Primary caregivers' psychological status and family functioning after TBI. Brain Inj 8:197–210, 1994

Kreutzer JS, Wehman PH, Harris JA et al: Substance abuse and crime patterns among persons with TBI referred for supported employment. Brain Inj 2:177–187, 1991

Langley M, Lindsay W, Lam C, Prickly D: A comprehensive alcohol abuse treatment programme for persons with TBI. Brain Inj 4:77–86, 1990

Leininger BE, Kreutzer JS, Hill MR: Comparison of minor and severe head injury emotional sequelae using the MMPI. Brain Inj 5:199–205, 1991

Levin HS: Neurobehavioral sequelae of head injury. pp. 442–463, In Cooper PR (ed): Head Injury.

Lindenbaum GA, Carrol SF, Daskal I, Kapusnick R: Patterns of alcohol and drug abuse in an urban trauma center: the increasing role of cocaine abuse. J Trauma 29:1654–1658, 1989

Linn RT, Allen K, Willer BS: Affective symptoms in the chronic stage of TBI: a study of married couples. Brain Inj 8:135–147, 1994

Lishman WA: Brain damage in relation to psychiatric disability after head injury. Br J Psychiatry 114:373–410, 1968

Lishman WA: Head Injury. p. 137. In Organic Psychiatry. 2nd Ed. Blackwell Scientific Publications, Oxford, 1987

McKeon J, McGuffin P, Robinson P: Obsessive-compulsive neurosis following head injury. A report of four cases. Br J Psychiatry 144:190–192, 1984

McMillan TM: Post-traumatic stress disorder and severe head injury. Br J Psychiatry 159:431–433, 1991

Mearns J, Lees-Haley PR: Discriminating neuropsychological sequelae of head injury from alcohol-abuse-induced deficts: a review and analysis. J Clin Psychol 49:714–720, 1993

Patterson JF: A preliminary study of carbamazepine in the treatment of assaultive patients with dementia. J Geriatr Psychiatry Neurol 1:21–33, 1988

Pessar LF, Coad ML, Linn RT, Willer BS: The effects of parental TBI on the behaviour of parents and children. Brain Inj 7:231–240, 1993

Physicians Desk Reference. Medical Economics Data Production, Montvale, NJ, 1994

Pokorny AD, Miller BA, Kaplan HB: The Brief MAST: a shortened version of the Michigan Alcohol Screening Test. Am J Psychiatry 129:342–345, 1972

Pritigano GP: Personality disturbances associated with traumatic brain injury. J Consul Clin Psychol 3:360–368, 1992

Rappaport M, Herrero-Backe C, Rappaport ML: Head injury outcome up to ten years later. Arch Phys Med Rehabil 70:885–892, 1989

Ronty H, Ahonen A, Tolonen U et al: Cerebral trauma and alcohol abuse. Eur J Clin Invest 23:182–187, 1993

Ross ED, Rush J: Diagnosis and neuroanatomical correlates of depression in brain-damaged patients. Arch Gen Psychiatry 38:1344–1354, 1981

Ruff RM, Marshall LF, Klauber MR et al: Alcohol abuse and neurological outcome of the severely head injured. J Head Trauma Rehabil 5:21–23, 1990

Schiffer RB, Herndon RM, Rudick RA: Treatment of pathologic laughing and weeping with amitriptyline. N Engl J Med 312:1480–1482, 1985

Silver JM, Yudofsky SC, Hales RC: Depression in TBI. Neuropsychiatry, Neuropsychol Behav Neurol 4:12–23, 1991

Sloan RL, Brown KW, Pentland B: Fluoxetine as a treatment for emotional lability after brain injury. Brain Inj 4:315–319, 1992

Sparadeo FR, Strauss D, Barth JT: The incidence, impact, and treatment of substance abuse in head trauma rehabilitation. J Head Trauma Rehabil 5:1–8, 1990

Starkstein SE, Federoff P, Bethier ML, Robinson RG: Manic-depressive and pure depressive states after brain lesions. Biol Psychiatry 29:149–158, 1991

Steadman JH, Graham: Head injuries: an analysis and follow-up study. J R Soc Med 63:23–28, 1970

Tuokko H, Vernon-Wilkinson R, Robinson E: The use of the MCMI in the personality assessment of head-injured adults. Brain Inj 5:287–293, 1991

Udaka F, Yamao S, Nagata H: Pathologic laughing and crying treated with levo-dopa. Arch Neurol 41:1095–1096, 1984

Uomoto JM, Brockway J: Anger management training for brain injured patients and their family members. Arch Phys Med Rehabil 73:674–679, 1992

Van Reekum R, Conway CA, Gansler D et al: Neurobehavioral study of borderline personality disorder. J Psychiatry Neurosci 18:121–129, 1993

Volpe BT, McDowell FH: The efficacy of cognitive rehabilitation in patients with TBI. Arch Neurol 47:220–222, 1990

Weinstein CS, Seidman LJ, Ahern G, McClure K: Integration of neuropsychological and behavioral neurological assessment in psychiatry: a case example involving brain injury and polypharmacy. Psychiatry 57:62–76, 1994

Worrall EP, Moody JP, Naylor GJ: Lithium in non-manic depressives: Antiaggressive effect and red blood cell lithium values. Br J Psychiatry 150:685–689, 1975

Wroblewksi B, Glenn MB, Cornblatt R et al: Protriptyline as an alternative stimulant medication in patients with brain injury: a series of case reports. Brain Inj 7:353–362, 1993

Wroblewski BA, Leary JM, Phelan AM et al: Methylphenidate and seizure frequency in brain injured patients with seizure disorders. J Clin Psychiatry 53:86–89, 1992

Yates WR, Noyes R, Petty F, Brown K: Risk factors associated with motor vehicle accidents in alcoholics. J Stud Alcohol 48:586–590, 1987

Yates WR, Wesner R, Thompson R: Organic mood disorder: a valid consultation diagnosis? J Affective Disord 22:37–42, 1991

Yudofsky S, Williams D, Gorman J: Propranolol in the treatment of rage and violent behavior in patients with chronic brain syndromes. Am J Psychiatry 138:218–220, 1981

Unexplained Neurologic Complaints

16

Roger Kathol

One of the problems faced by neurologists in the evaluation of their patients is to determine whether the presenting symptoms are the result of a neurologic disease or occur as voluntary simulation or involuntary production of symptoms. This problem is relevant to the evaluation of patients with putative head injury and postconcussive syndrome as well as other neurologic populations. This chapter outlines from the viewpoint of the practicing neurologist the potential etiologies from which symptoms may become manifest and provides a systematic approach to patient evaluation when neurologic disease is not readily apparent. This will ensure appropriate diagnosis and suggest treatment strategies for such patients by neurologists and by mental health specialists to whom the patient may be referred.

Since the diagnostic classification system used in psychiatry does not allow predictive statements about patients once they have received a somatoform diagnosis (psychiatric diagnosis categorizing patients with somatic symptoms without evidence of medical illness), with the exception of somatization disorder, a simplified etiologic approach to the assessment and labeling of these patients will be taken. Communication with psychiatric colleagues remains important; therefore, a comparison of the categorization presented in this chapter and that provided by the Diagnostic and Statistical Manual of Mental Disorders (DSM-IV) (American Psychiatric Association, 1994) will be given.

DEFINITION OF UNEXPLAINED NEUROLOGIC COMPLAINTS

For purposes of this chapter, unexplained neurologic complaints will include those symptoms and/or signs presented by the patient that do not have an adequate explanation based on organic or physical illness. Although many of the criteria provided in (DSM-IV) for somatoform disorders include comments about the relationship of unexplained symptoms to life events, psychosocial stresses, or psychological difficulties, the definition provided above does not include etiologic implications since most remain unproven. Using this definition allows the development of a differential diagnosis for neurologic unexplained complaints that does not assume psychiatric illness to be necessarily the cause.

Differential Diagnosis

Although patients presenting with unexplained neurologic complaints are all categorized by DSM-IV as having one of several psychiatric syndromes

TABLE 16-1. Psychiatric Explanation of Unexplained Neurologic Complaints Using DSM-IV

Somatoform disorders
- Somatization disorder
- Conversion disorder
- Pain disorder
- Hypochondriasis
- Somatoform disorder, not otherwise specified

Factitious disorder
Other psychiatric syndromes (associated somatic symptoms)
- Anxiety disorders
- Affective disorders
- Psychotic disorders

Malingering (not a mental disorder)

listed in Table 16-1, DSM-IV does not include several important potential etiologies for the development of these symptoms in all patients, nor does it predict outcome based on the category into which the patient has been placed. For this reason, an alternative approach to assessing patients with unexplained somatic complaints has been developed which should help to identify good and poor prognosis patients as well as to direct the therapeutic approach taken to the patient based on information provided by the literature (Table 16-2).

One of the most commonly overlooked reasons for the development of unexplained neurologic complaints is seen in the patient who does not understand normal bodily sensations. These patients recognize, much as medical students during their training, common minor normal bodily sensations and think that these could constitute serious disease. These patients do not have a psychiatric illness that leads them to seek attention for the unexplained symptoms but merely have a health concern about which they have inadequate knowledge to recognize the benign nature of the symptoms. For instance, a patient could present to a neurologist with concerns about tremor after heavy exercise. Of course, this could be associated with a neuromuscular disease; however, it most likely is related to normal tremors that develop after exercise due to muscle fatigue (Gilroy and Meyer, 1979).

TABLE 16-2. Differential Diagnosis for Unexplained Neurologic Complaints

Normal concern about physiologic bodily sensations
Unrecognized neurologic illness
Psychiatric explanation
- Pithiatism (Kathol et al., 1983a; Lewis and Berman, 1965; Whitlock, 1967) (hypersuggestibility)
  - Isolated symptom or symptom complex
  - Several current or past somatic symptoms
- Psychiatric syndromes
  - Depression
  - Anxiety
  - Psychosis
  - Other psychiatric syndromes
- Conscious production
  - Malingering
  - Factitious disorder

"Persistent" unexplained neurologic complaints
- No evidence suggesting a neurologic or psychiatric cause

The second possible explanation for unexplained complaints is an unrecognized neurologic condition. Follow-up studies confirm that 20 to 60 percent of patients presenting to physicians with conversion symptoms have coexisting medical illness, such as patients with pseudoseizures who also have an underlying seizure disorder (Kathol et al., 1983; McKegney, 1967; Raskin et al., 1966; Slater and Glithero, 1965; Stefansson et al., 1976). In 10 to 25 percent of patients with unexplained complaints, a physical condition will ultimately be found as a cause for the symptoms with which they present. The reasons that neurologic conditions can be overlooked during the initial examination is that they may be too early in their course to permit accurate diagnosis through either neurologic examination or testing procedures. Alternatively, they could be the result of a benign neurologic condition, which is not considered a serious enough threat to pursue an aggressive workup to document its presence. Of course, the neurologic condition finally diagnosed may not have been considered during the initial workup, and thus appropriate tests will not have been performed.

When a neurologic symptom cannot be readily associated with a specific neurologic disorder, neurologists must consider the possibility that a psychiatric condition is contributing to the development of the symptoms. There are several ways in which this can occur. First, it could be the result of hypersuggestibility or pithiatism. Second, it could be due to an unrecognized psychiatric syndrome such as depression or anxiety. Finally, it could be due to voluntarily produced symptoms, such as can occur with factitious disorder or malingering. The first and last of these possible psychiatric causes for unexplained neurologic complaints are more likely to occur in patients presenting with dramatic neurologic complaints such as paralysis, blindness, or aphonia, while the second could also present with less dramatic neurologic complaints such as dizziness, headache, or weakness, etc. In patients with head injury or postconcussive syndrome, all three have to be considered. Voluntarily induced symptoms are covered in greater detail in Chapter 25.

DSM-IV includes a number of somatoform disorders that can be subsumed under the general category of hypersuggestibility. Key characteristics of those likely to be seen by neurologists are listed in Table 16-3 to allow communication with psychiatric consultants. Although these have been used in the diagnostic classification system in psychiatry for a number of years, the only somatoform disorder with predictive validity is somatization disorder, which provides a reproducible approach to diagnosis; allows predictive statements about risk factors, usual time of onset of symptoms, natural history, and outcome; and gives practical information about a cost-effective approach to treatment. While the DSM-IV listings of the other somatoform disorders provide descriptions of how unexplained neurologic complaints can present, they do not provide useful predictive capabilities or therapeutic approaches that have proven efficacy.

There are many theoretical hypotheses about how unexplained neurologic complaints can occur (Table 16-4). For the purposes of this chapter it is not possible to explore each of these hypothetical considerations. However, it is useful to recognize that hypersuggestibility is a reasonable explanation consistent with these hypotheses of the production of unexplained neurologic complaints. This was first described by Babinski (1909, 1988), who coined the term *pithiatism,* which means "caused by suggestion, cured by persuasion." The concept of pithiatism actually follows evidence about what happens in these patients more closely than does Freud's conversion hypothesis, which has been touted since about the early 1940s as the principal cause for unexplained neurologic complaints (Lazare, 1981). Support for this comes from the fact that patients with hysterical symptoms have been found to be more suggestible than those in the normal population or those with other psychiatric conditions (Bliss, 1984; Speigel et al., 1982; Speigel

TABLE 16-4. Some Etiologic Hypotheses for the Development of Unexplained Neurologic Complaints

Exaggeration
Genetics
Manipulation
Fear of disease
Dissociation
Hostility
Repression
Attention seeking
Learned responses
Masked anxiety or depression
Corticofugal inhibition
Amplification
Secondary gain
Denial
Psychic to physical conversion
Poor understanding of the human body and its sensations
Conversion of psychic conflict into physical symptoms
Poor communication between the left and right brain

TABLE 16-3. Important Characteristics of the Somatoform Disorders in DSM-IV That May Be Seen by Neurologists

Conversion disorder: Unconscious development of one or more, usually pseudoneurologic, symptom related to psychological factors which causes distress or impaired function
Hypochondriasis: Unconsciously developed fear of 6 months duration about having a disease, which is not alleviated by medical reassurance and which causes distress or impaired function
Pain disorder: Pain related to psychological factors, which causes distress or impaired function
Somatization disorder: Early onset of multiple, unconsciously developed somatic complaints in multiple organ systems, which result in treatment or impaired function
Somatoform disorder not otherwise specified: Unconsciously developed unexplained somatic symptom of less than 6 months duration
Disease hierarchy: Somatization disorder preempts conversion disorder, which preempts hypochondriasis and somatoform disorder not otherwise specified; pain disorder cannot be diagnosed if somatization disorder is present in the absence of a medical illness
Symptom overlap: Somatization disorder and pain disorder; conversion disorder and pain disorder

and Fink, 1979). Patients with unexplained neurologic complaints also have a higher incidence of friends or relatives demonstrating behaviors in the organ system of dysfunction (Cloninger, 1986; Kathol et al., 1983c), a situation described by Babinski as "contagion" (Kessel, 1960; Shepherd et al., 1966). Furthermore, the neurologic examination in which nonphysiologic abnormalities are identified is often subjective, such as the visual field examination and the testing of sensation and strength. Finally, patients who present with unexplained neurologic complaints usually respond to reassurance that no serious neurologic disease is present and that the symptoms are likely to resolve with time (Kathol et al., 1983a). This is particularly true if symptoms have been present for only a short time because the patient has not become so attached to the symptoms that it would be an embarrassment for them to disappear.

Although conversion disorder is more commonly used as an explanation for unexplained neurologic complaints, it does not appear to have as much evidential support as the pithiatic hypothesis. Patients with unexplained neurologic complaints frequently do not have identifiable stress or psychological trauma preceding the onset of symptoms (Kathol et al., 1983b; Lewis and Berman, 1965; Whitlock, 1967). There have been no early life experiences (parental loss, abuse, etc.) that predictably lead to the development of unexplained neurologic complaints (Pitts et al., 1965). Secondary gain is not a useful diagnostic feature (Kellner, 1991; Lewis and Berman, 1965; Pitts et al., 1965; Whitlock, 1967). Gaining insight into the unexplained neurologic complaints has not led to resolution of symptoms as had been hoped or hypothesized by the proponents of this explanation (Kathol et al., 1983a; Ladee, 1966; Thomas, 1978). In fact, there is some evidence that dynamic psychotherapy not only does not help symptom resolution but may contribute to worsening of the patient's condition (Ladee, 1966).

While descriptions in terms of the entities hypochondriasis, conversion disorder, pain disorder, and somatoform disorder not otherwise specified have limited predictive power, somatization disorder stands alone as a somatoform condition that is helpful to recognize. Patients with somatization disorder present repeatedly with a variety of complaints in multiple organ systems, not the least of which is the nervous system. The usefulness of this diagnosis lies not so much in identifying the etiology of complaints, since they largely can be attributed to hypersuggestibility, but in the outcome that can be expected from these patients over time. Patients with somatization disorder are most commonly females, with an onset of symptom complaints in the teens to early twenties. The complaints span the organ systems and lead to many tests, many physicians, many surgeries, and the use of many medications. For these patients, a greater danger than unidentified physical illness is iatrogenically caused disorders from the aggressive evaluations they receive or the interventions that well-meaning practitioners provide in an attempt to alleviate their symptoms. Since a specific approach has been demonstrated to provide cost-effective care without increasing the risk of missed medical conditions, it is important to recognize these patients as a special category under the general heading of somatoform disorders or, in the differential diagnosis proposed in this chapter, hypersuggestibility.

The second important item in the psychiatric differential diagnosis for unexplained neurologic complaints is the presence of a psychiatric syndrome that could cause symptoms. The most common of these are depression and anxiety, which frequently have associated somatic complaints (Cadoret et al., 1980; Katon et al., 1982; Kellner, 1986; Kellner, 1988). Since the approach to these patients will be directed at the underlying psychiatric condition rather than the somatic complaint itself, it is important to recognize the presence of these syndromes. Because these psychiatric conditions are so common and so costly to the medical system and national economy, nonpsychiatrist physicians, both generalists and specialists, are now being provided with an expanding literature showing that they can effectively identify and treat patients with depression and anxiety. For those neurologists who have up to this point chosen not to address these two psychiatric conditions, recently published guidelines for depression in primary care (Depression Guideline Panel, 1993a, 1993b, 1993c) and Panic Disorder in the Medical Setting (Katon, 1989) can be used as resources for understanding how to identify and treat patients presenting with these conditions in whom the presenting symptoms are neurologic in origin.

Finally, it is important to recognize that voluntarily produced symptoms are possible explanations for the development of neurologic symptoms. In the psychiatric nomenclature there is an arbitrary distinction between factitious disorder, in which patients are producing the unexplained symptoms for purposes of obtaining medical care, and malingering, in which patients are producing the symptoms for secondary gain. The former constitutes a psychiatric diagnosis, while the latter is largely an accusation of intentional deception. These potential etiologies for unexplained neurologic complaints should be considered in the differential if the symptoms occur in a medicolegal context, if there is a marked discrepancy between clinical presentation and objective findings, if the patient exhibits a lack of cooperation with diagnostic efforts, or if compliance with medical management and the psychosocial history suggest the presence of antisocial or borderline personality disorder. All of these are risk factors for voluntarily produced symptoms (Folks and Houck, 1993).

Patients who present with voluntarily induced neurologic signs or symptoms can be some of the most difficult to diagnose and can be uncomfortable for the physician to deal with. A high index of suspicion is required. Willingness by the neurologist to perform special testing, which can be time-consuming and redundant in order to uncover signs and symptoms is also necessary. When the workup is complete and the diagnosis is established, the neurologist must additionally confront the patient with the findings, at best an unpleasant task. There are serious medical, legal, ethical, and social considerations in performing this important function, which many practitioners would prefer to avoid but which are of tremendous importance to the patient and to society.

Outcomes

Follow-up is one of the most critical aspects of care in patients presenting with unexplained neurologic complaints because many patients who have what are recognized as functional neurologic complaints also have underlying objective organic pathology. In fact, it is better to think of the complaints of patients as occurring in two separate dimensions, functional and organic, rather than in a single dimension as is commonly conceptualized (i.e., organic versus functional). This helps the neurologist to recognize that coexistence of organic disease with a psychological condition frequently affects symptom severity, functional impairment, and outcome.

It is well to recognize that unidentified neurologic disease can ultimately be uncovered as a cause of the unexplained neurologic complaints. It is also important to recognize that some patients with unexplained neurologic complaints in the absence of a neurologic disorder will have a good outcome with reassurance alone, while others can be expected to have a more protracted course (Kathol et al., submitted 1995a, submitted 1995b). Patients with poor prognoses can be identified by the presence of two of the three following clinical features: (1) numerous unexplained complaints, (2) impairment disproportional to physical disease, and (3) a history of psychiatric illness (Kathol et al., submitted 1995b). Patients who have none or only one of these clinical features can be expected to have symptom resolution, less impairment at presentation and follow-up, decreased psychiatric illness, lower use of medical care, and greater satisfaction with the care provided.

The importance of recognizing this distinction is that patients who fall into the good outcome category can usually be treated by the neurologist without need for referral. Patients with an anticipated poor outcome may benefit to a greater extent by psychiatric evaluation and/or psychosocial intervention. Patients with a poor prognosis also require special attention to the aggressiveness of the evaluation by the neurologist who is trying to uncover the etiology of the complaints with which the patient presents. These patients are a greater risk for iatrogenic worsening of symptoms or the development of new symptoms in response to the interventions or aggressive diagnostic assessments made. From a neurologic standpoint, a better approach to these patients is to complete a basic neurologic evaluation (i.e., neurologic history and examination and then follow-up). Expensive or invasive specialized testing should only occur in those situations in which objective evidence for a neurologic disorder can be identified or in which the diseases under consideration are potentially damaging to the patient if not recognized early.

RECOGNITION OF UNEXPLAINED NEUROLOGIC COMPLAINTS

History

As with all patients presenting with neurologic difficulties, it is important to identify the type of symptoms, their onset, their progression, aggravating factors, response to interventions, etc. in order to gain an adequate appreciation of the patient's problem. In head injury patients it would be important to know whether the patient was unconscious and if so for how long, whether it was an open or closed injury, what neurologic abnormalities or test findings were present at the time of injury, information about preexisting central nervous system (CNS) disease, etc. Usually during this process it is possible to determine whether the symptoms are characteristic of a specific neurologic syndrome or whether inconsistencies exist that require further clarification. It is often helpful to obtain further information from an additional informant, particularly if inconsistencies exist or the symptoms do not follow a course that would be expected from the diagnoses under consideration.

If the patient has had previous workups by neurologists or other physicians, it is important to obtain records from them concerning the patient's presentation and the evaluations performed. This can help to unravel quickly the uncertainty about the diagnoses that are entertained and can help to direct further workup and treatment. When reviewing outside information, it is important to remain as objective as possible, since many patients who suffer from undiagnosed neurologic conditions can present a histrionic or manipulative history with exaggeration of symptoms in order to "persuade" the neurologist that additional testing should be performed.

Physical/Neurologic Examination

A thorough neurologic evaluation is required, particularly of the section of the body in which dysfunction has been complained about or demonstrated, regardless of whether the neurologist believes that the symptoms are related to a neurologic condition. This is true even if the symptom presentation is blatantly nonphysiologic. By completing an examination, the neurologist may uncover organic components contributing to a mainly functional presentation. The examination is also necessary to provide reassurance. The patient has to recognize that the physician has performed an adequate evaluation to feel comfortable that physical disease is not contributing to the development of symptoms—otherwise reassurance is unlikely to be effective.

Some patients present a confusing, complicated history. In these patients the neurologic examination can help to sort out objective from subjective changes and physiologic inconsistencies. This requires a careful systematic approach to the evaluation, using different test procedures for the same dysfunctional aspect of the patient's examination. This is one of the areas in which testing the same sensory and motor system in a variety of ways is important. For instance, weakness of the lower extremities can be assessed by (1) direct muscle strength examination; (2) observation of strength in the same muscle groups by watching the patient get up from a chair, squat, etc.; and (3) assessment of physiologic changes that would be expected with various causes for weakness, such as muscle wasting, fasciculations, or hyperreflexia. Persistence of abnormality is also extremely important when patients are seen in follow-up examination. Care, however, must be taken in this situation that frequent and/or sudden shifts in neurologic findings are not to be expected in the condition under consideration, as can occur with multiple sclerosis or temporal lobe epilepsy, in both of which abnormalities can be intermittent. There are also several tricks to performing the neurologic examination, which make it difficult for the patient to conceal normal function of the affected area. These are illustrated and reviewed elsewhere (Weintraub, 1977). All these techniques can help to clarify the consistency of the symptoms and signs presented by the patient that are necessary to make a diagnosis.

In patients in whom the neurologic examination cannot clarify the etiology of symptom presentation, it is appropriate to progress to testing procedures that may reveal confirmatory evidence of a neurologic disease. These tests include electroencephalography; nerve conduction studies; electromyography; visual, auditory, or somatosensory evoked potentials; and formal visual field testing. Imaging studies, including angiograms, magnetic resonance imaging (MRI), and computed tomography (CT), may also be useful in uncovering objective abnormalities that cannot be delineated on neurologic examination. Single-photon emission computed tomography (SPECT) and positron emission tomography (PET) show promise for future testing of physiology during function but are now experimental.

Both basic and aggressive diagnostic procedures are driven not only by the patient's presentation and the diagnoses under consideration (their potential danger to the patient and treatability) but also by the way in which the patient presents to a neurologist, by the patient's history, by the number and type of symptoms with which the patient presents, and by a prior history of psychiatric difficulties. For instance, patients in whom the etiology of the symptoms is unclear after history and neurologic examination and patients with not more than two unexplained symptoms (both in the history and in review of the chart), with impairment proportional to the symptoms, and with no psychiatric history (with an anticipated good prognosis) may be candidates for more invasive and/or aggressive testing if there is concern about a serious neurologic disorder but there is significant cost or risk associated with the evaluation. On the other hand, patients with an anticipated poor socioeconomic outcome but who are at no greater and perhaps less risk for the ultimate identification of an organic condition as previously described may best be handled by providing reassurance and follow-up rather than by a costly or dangerous workup.

Neuropsychological Testing

Many neurologists use results from neuropsychological testing as a means of assessing whether a presenting symptom is organic or functional. The Minnesota Multiphasic Personality and Inventory (MMPI) is commonly used in this context, as a frequent part of neuropsychological test batteries (Hathaway and McKinley, 1943). It is a well standardized testing instrument for assessing personality function but has several limitations when used to distinguish organic from functional symptoms. First, the MMPI was not standardized on a neurologically ill population, and therefore the interpretation of results must be done with caution if the patient in whom testing is done is neurologically impaired (Osborne, 1985). Since neurologic illness is one of the two possibilities when assessing for a neurologic or functional cause for symptom development, the results of the MMPI must be interpreted in this context. For instance, the hypochondriasis scale on the MMPI may be elevated in a neurologically ill patient, because some items endorsed for hypochondriasis are the same as those that would be endorsed by a patient with a neurologic condition (weakness, worry about health, bodily change, etc.) Most neuropsychologists interpret the results of the MMPI in patients with neurologic difficulties with adjustments related to the clinical history. This depends to some extent on the background and expertise of the neuropsychologist in working with patients with neurologic disease, and caution is required in utilizing results from the MMPI.

The MMPI has been restandardized in a contemporary population (Colligan et al., 1984). During the standardization process it became evident that the old standards tend to overdiagnose psychopathology because of the change in cultural norms during the past 50 years. Also, standard interpretation of the MMPI uses a conceptual framework about psychiatric conditions that has changed considerably during the intervening years (Colligan, 1985). Therefore, terms used to reflect psychiatric disorders in the MMPI interpretation are often different from those currently used in the field of psychiatry. Physician-centered or psychologist-centered clinical evaluation may be preferable to the MMPI for identifying patients more likely to have a psychological contribution to their neurologic complaints.

Another common practice among neurologists and neuropsychologists is to use depression or anxiety screening instruments to identify patients with depression or anxiety contributing to symptom onset. This practice also has some limitations, since again the instruments have not been standardized in a neurologically ill population. Furthermore, these instruments do not identify syndromatic depression or anxiety (American Psychiatric Association, 1994) (i.e., those patients in whom treatment can be expected to result in improvement, not only of the anxiety or depression but also of the somatic complaints associated with them). Although the symptom screening scales can be used to identify those patients in whom depression and anxiety are more likely to be present or can be helpful in following patients over time for improvement of recognized depression and/or anxiety syndromes, they were not intended to be used for the diagnosis of these psychiatric syndromes. Again, it is necessary for the neurologist to perform an adequate diagnostic assessment for these syndromes or to refer the patient for evaluation by a psychiatric consultant.

Treatment

If a neurologic disease or dysfunction from head trauma or postconcussive syndrome is not considered a likely cause for the patient's symptomatology, treatment is dictated by the principal category in which the patient's symptoms are explained on a psychiatric basis. First, if the patient has a depressive or anxiety syndrome, these conditions would be the target for alleviation, not only of the anxiety and depression but also of the unexplained neurologic complaints. This is particularly true when the complaints are of a nonspecific nature such as headaches, weakness, or dizziness. Current practice suggests that neurologists should be as well equipped to treat uncomplicated anxiety and depression as are mental health professionals (Depression Guideline Panel, 1993a, 1993b, 1993c; Katon, 1989). Usually the approach taken will be to provide antidepressant or antianxiety medications, which have been shown to be effective in alleviating symptoms in up to 90 percent of patients presenting with these psychiatric conditions although some patients may require several medication trials. Alternatively, for patients who present a complicated symptom picture or severe psychiatric symptoms or who have demonstrated nonresponse to treatment, referral to a mental health specialist can be initiated. Some patients with depression and anxiety prefer not to take medications but to have their symptoms treated with psychotherapy. In this case, the neurologist should identify a mental health practitioner who provides time-limited psychotherapy, particularly cognitive-behavioral, interpersonal, or behavioral therapy, for patients with depression since these approaches have proved to be effective (Depression Guideline Panel, 1993b). Even if the patient is referred to a mental health practitioner for therapy, the neurologist or other primary care provider should follow the patient to ensure improvement. If it does not occur, other therapy such as medication may be necessary.

For patients in whom hypersuggestibility is considered the most likely cause of symptom development, reassurance (Sapira, 1972) is the most important clinical intervention that can be provided (Table 16-5). Examination is the first step in providing this therapy because patients who have not been appropriately examined will be unlikely to respond to reassurance that no serious disease is present, since they recognize that the physician does not adequately understand the symptoms. When reassurance is given, not only should patients be told that no serious disease is present, but they should also be told that the symptoms will improve with time. It is often helpful to give a framework for this improvement, since this provides a socially acceptable way for the symptom to resolve and also uses suggestion in removing the symptom as rapidly as possible. In most situations, symptoms that have a relatively short duration can be eliminated by suggestion over a short time, while symptoms that have been present for a longer period are less likely to resolve quickly and require a more gradual approach to their improvement. Sometimes nonspecific interventions such as physical therapy, eye exercises, or nonsteroidal anti-inflammatory drugs can provide a sufficient excuse for symptoms to resolve as predicted. Nonspecific therapies, however, have to be used with caution, since providing them can reinforce the patient's notion that an underlying neurologic condition is indeed present or otherwise treatment would not be given.

TABLE 16-5. Reassurance Steps for the Patient With Unexplained Neurologic Complaints

Step 1. Examine patient
Step 2. Suggest that no serious neurologic disease is present
Step 3. Educate patient about the nature of the symptoms
Step 4. Suggest that the symptom will get better with time
  a. Duration of symptom 1 day: improvement within a day
  b. Duration of symptom 3–4 days: improvement in 1–2 days
  c. Duration of symptom 1 week: improvement in 4–5 days
  d. Duration of symptom longer than several weeks: improvement in 1–3 weeks
Step 5. Encourage patient to return to regular activities
Step 6. Provide nonspecific treatment, if warranted
Step 7. Follow the patient

It is important to suggest in a nonhostile, nonjudgmental fashion that the symptom will improve rapidly. There is no useful purpose in telling hypersuggestible patients that you think they are putting the symptom on or that it is all in their minds. A better approach is to acknowledge that the patient is experiencing the symptom. This can be followed by the statement that a variety of things, including emotional factors or misinterpretation of bodily sensations, can lead to these "real" symptoms. It is sometimes useful to share with the patient how emotional factors can contribute to development of symptoms by talking about tension headaches, dizziness with anxiety through hyperventilation, etc. The worst thing is for the patient to get into an adversarial situation with the physician, such that the patient has to prove that the symptom is real by its maintenance and/or persistence. The patient then becomes invested in the symptom, and resolution is less likely to occur.

Other facets of reassurance include educating patients about the possible causes of their symptoms and how they have been assessed, instructing them to return to all readily performed activities since this will not cause further impairment, and follow-up. The last of these is one of the most important aspects of reassurance because most patients are afraid that their symptom will not improve and then they will have nowhere to go for help. Follow-up alleviates that concern and makes it more likely that the symptom will improve.

Reassurance may be the only therapy that is needed for many patients to have symptom resolution and return to normal functioning, particularly those patients with the anticipated good outcome previously described. Patients with multiple unexplained somatic complaints, as identified in those with somatization disorder (American Psychiatric Association, 1994) or subsyndromic somatization disorder (Escobar et al., 1991; Kirmayer et al., 1991), require additional interventions because the outcome is less likely to be positive. These are patients in whom either symptoms do not resolve adequately or symptoms resolve only to be replaced by other symptoms, which require further evaluation. For these patients, several steps in addition to providing reassurance can be helpful in minimizing morbidity associated with neurologic evaluations and/or therapeutic interventions as well as in decreasing the cost of health care utilization (Table 16-6).

Since these patients present with a myriad of somatic complaints, neurologic complaints being only one among several other categories, it is usually appropriate for non-neurologists to follow these patients over time. Usually, this is a primary care physician rather than a psychiatrist because these patients see their problems as medical rather than psychiatric. It is important for one physician to follow these patients since that practitioner will be most likely to detect organic conditions that do occur because of familiarity with the patient. Furthermore, in many situations an alliance can be developed between these patients and the primary physician, which minimizes medical morbidity through a willingness by the patient to accept the physician's recommendations for limited interventions or testing in exchange for continuity of care. This approach can be helped by explaining to patients that they are at as great risk from the diagnostic and therapeutic procedures used as from the disorders under consideration.

TABLE 16-6. Treatment of Patients with Somatization Disorder

Step 1.	Reassurance (see Table 16-5)
Step 2.	One physician to coordinate care
Step 3.	More frequent routine return visits (limit to 15 to 20 minutes)
Step 4.	Nonspecific therapy (e.g., dietary change, exercise, volunteer activity, hobbies, travel)
Step 5.	No medication, procedures, or surgery unless *objective* evidence of neurologic illness is identified on basic examination
Step 6.	If psychiatric symptoms (depression, anxiety, etc.) are to be treated with medication, close evaluation of target symptoms is necessary

In most situations patients with unexplained symptoms come to the neurologist in referral for evaluation of symptoms that the primary physician does not feel comfortable in evaluating. Special attention is required by the neurologist to establish the number and type of other symptoms that the patient has. After completion of the neurologic history and examination, additional testing should not be performed unless objective evidence of abnormality has been identified or the patient is in the good outcome category. In these patients further testing may be necessary to clarify symptoms. This approach prevents overutilization of resources, decreases the likelihood of false positive tests, and encourages the use of follow-up as a means of assessing whether objective neurologic disease may occur. It may be necessary for the neurologist to see the patient in follow-up consultation to ensure that no new neurologic symptoms develop that would warrant additional testing and/or intervention.

The approach to the treatment of patients with voluntarily induced symptoms from factitious disorder is empathic confrontation. These patients can present in two clinically meaningful ways. First, patients who are otherwise not personally, socially, or economically impaired by other psychiatric conditions may present with isolated symptoms. Examples include health care workers who take medications, such as anticoagulants, to produce the appearance of physical disease. Patients recovering from head trauma may also falsify symptoms in order to obtain compensation. These patients represent a more reprehensible group in situations where litigation is often pending or underway. Although the legal implications with these patients are substantial, they are beyond the scope of this chapter. More information related to this can be found in the handbook by Appelbaum and Gutheil (1991) (see also Ch. 25).

Patients with single feigned symptoms, in addition to receiving empathic confrontation and support, should be encouraged to consider employment in a non-health-related field to reduce the likelihood that they will use medication and medical supplies in their self-injurious behavior. It is also helpful, with the patient's permission, to inform family or those close to the patient that the problem was self-induced.

Again, this makes it less likely that patients will have a repeat of their clinical difficulties.

The second way in which patients with factitious disorders can present is with repeated self-injurious behaviors (Folks and Houck, 1993). This typically occurs in persons with underlying borderline, histrionic, or antisocial personality disorder. In most situations these patients require the additional assistance of mental health professionals to provide social support and crisis intervention. Certainly, more of these patients present to non-neurologists, since their self-injurious behavior is in the form of ingestion of foreign objects, intoxication with medications or toxins, self-inflicted injuries, or the introduction of foreign objects into various bodily orifices.

Malingerers should also be confronted in an empathic but firm way and informed that their behavior is an unacceptable approach to dealing with their life circumstances. These patients often deny that they did anything to themselves despite irrefutable evidence to the contrary. They then leave the hospital against medical advice or abscond from the clinic. It is very important to document the evidence for malingering during clinical evaluations, since medicolegal controversies often arise in these situations.

Consultation/Referral to Mental Health Professionals

Most patients who present with unexplained neurologic complaints do not view their problems as psychiatric in nature. They are more concerned about neurologic illness and therefore are unsatisfied with referral to mental health specialists for nonspecific intervention. For this reason many patients who present with unexplained neurologic complaints are dealt with from start to finish by the neurologist or primary physician in charge of their care. It is therefore important to have a strategy to deal with these patients that is the most likely to provide symptom improvement (Fig. 16-1).

Despite the fact that most patients with unexplained neurologic complaints limit their medical treatment to non-mental health personnel, it does not mean that mental health personnel cannot contribute to the care of individuals with unexplained neurologic complaints. Certainly, patients who present with complicated psychiatric symptoms that contribute to the neurologic symptoms are appropriate for referral to the mental health sector for psychological support and/or the initiation of interventions that are likely to adequately address psychiatric syndromes. Furthermore, patients with psychosocial problems that are contributing to the development of symptoms may benefit by short-term psychotherapeutic intervention that specifically targets the psychosocial problems rather than the neurologic problems of the patient. The mental health specialists to whom they are referred should recognize that insight-oriented therapies have not been shown to be effective and in some cases can lead to worsening of the patient's medical symptoms over time (Kellner, 1991; Ladee, 1966; Thomas, 1978).

It is also important to recognize that most mental health professionals do not perform neurologic examinations on the patients with whom they come into contact. This necessarily limits their ability to provide reassurance concerning the symptoms with which the patients are presenting. Therefore, reassurance will need to be provided by the neurologist rather than by a mental health professional.

CONCLUSION

Unexplained neurologic complaints in association with head trauma or other situations encountered in practice occur quite frequently. Patients who present with these require a basic neurologic examination since the differential diagnosis includes undiagnosed neurologic disease. Functional contributions can be conveniently ascribed to hypersuggestibility, psychiatric syndromes such as anxiety and depression, or voluntary induction. Each of these causes for the development of functional symptoms require a different intervention by the neurologist or other health care professional. Those with hypersuggestibility require reassurance and follow-up. Hypersuggestibility patients with multiple complaints additionally require limitation of aggressive evaluations and interventions and more imaginative nonspecific therapies for control of their frequent and persistent unexplained complaints. Patients with symptoms developing secondary to psychiatric syndromes require treatment of the psychiatric syndrome for resolution of the somatic symptoms. Finally, those who have voluntarily induced neurologic signs or symptoms should be treated with empathic confrontation and support. Although referral of these patients to mental health professionals may be appropriate to assist the neurologist in dealing with psychiatric syndromes and/or psychosocial issues, the majority of these patients will

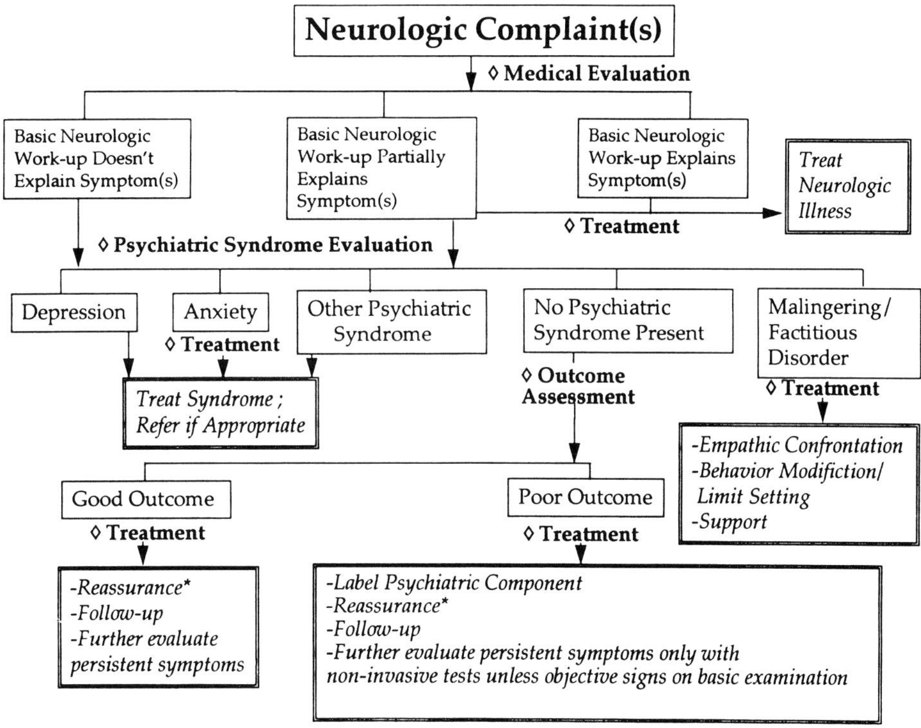

Fig. 16-1. Systematic approach to assessing patients with neurologic complaints. *, see Table 16-5; ◊, action item.

receive the majority of their care from neurologists or other primary care physicians.

ACKNOWLEDGMENTS

The author wishes to thank Bonnie Eicher for assistance in the preparation of this manuscript.

REFERENCES

American Psychiatric Association: Diagnostic and Statistical Manual of Mental Disorders. 4th Ed. American Psychiatric Association Press, Washington, 1994

Appelbaum PS, Gutheil TG: Clinical Handbook of Psychiatry and the Law. Williams & Wilkins, Baltimore, 1991

Babinski J: Démembrement de l'hysterie traditionelle. Pithiatisme. Sem Med 29:3–8, 1909

Babinski J: Dismembering of traditional hysteria-pithiatism. Psychiatr Med 6:1–16, 1988

Bliss EL: Hysteria and hypnosis. J Nerv Ment Dis 172: 203–206, 1984

Cadoret RJ, Widmer RB, Troughton EP: Somatic complaints: harbinger of depression in primary care. J Affective Disord 2:61–70, 1980

Cloninger CR: A unified biosocial theory of personality and its role in the development of anxiety states. Psychiatr Dev 3:167–226, 1986

Colligan RC: History and development of the MMPI. Psychiatr Ann 15:524–533, 1985

Colligan RC, Osborne D, Swenson WM, Offord KP: The aging MMPI: development of contemporary norms. Mayo Clin Proc 59:377–390, 1984

Depression Guideline Panel: Depression in Primary Care: Vol 1. Detection and Diagnosis. 124. 1st Ed. U.S. Dept. of Health and Human Services, Agency for Health Care Policy and Research. Public Health Service. U.S. Government Printing Office, Washington, 1993a

Depression Guideline Panel: Depression in Primary Care: Vol 2. Treatment of Major Depression. 175. 1st Ed. U.S. Dept. of Health and Human Services. Agency for Health Care Policy and Research. Public Health Service. U.S. Government Printing Office, Washington, 1993b

Depression Guideline Panel: Depression in Primary Care: Detection, Diagnosis, and Treatment. 21. 1st Ed. U.S. Dept. of Health and Human Services. Agency for Health Care Policy and Research. Public Health Service. U.S. Government Printing Office, Washington, 1993c

Escobar JI, Swartz M, Rubio-Stipec M, Manu P: Medically unexplained symptoms: distribution, risk factors, and comorbidity. pp. 63–78. In Kirmayer LJ, Robbins JM (eds): Current Concepts of Somatization: Research and Clinical Perspectives. American Psychiatric Association, Washington, 1991

Folks DG, Houck CA: Somatoform disorders, factitious disorders, and malingering. pp. 267–288. In Stoudemire A, Stoudemire FBS (eds): Psychiatric Care in the Medical Patient. Oxford University Press, New York, 1993

Gilroy J, Meyer JS: Medical Neurology. 3rd Ed. Macmillan, New York, 1979

Hathaway SR, McKinley JC: Manual for the Minnesota Multiphasic Personality Inventory. The Psychological Corp., New York, 1943

Kathol RG, Cox TA, Corbett JJ et al: Functional visual loss: I. A true psychiatric disorder? Psychol Med 13:307–314, 1983a

Kathol RG, Cox TA, Corbett JJ et al: Functional visual loss: II. Psychiatric aspects in 42 patients followed for 4 years. Psychol Med 13:315–324, 1983b

Kathol RG, Cox TA, Corbett JJ, Thompson HS: Functional visual loss: a follow-up of 42 patients. Arch Ophthalmol 101:729–735, 1983c

Kathol RG, Noyes R, Carney C, Fisher M: I. Structured outcomes assessment of organic and functional indicators in patients with unexplained somatic complaints. (Submitted for publication) 1995a

Kathol RG, Noyes R, Carney C, Fisher M: II. Simple clinical outcomes assessment of patients presenting with unexplained somatic complaints in primary care. (Submitted for publication) 1995b

Katon W: Panic Disorder in the Medical Setting. 135. 1st Ed. U.S. Government Printing Office, Washington, 1989

Katon W, Kleinman A, Rosen G: Depression and somatization: a review. Part I. Am J Psychiatry 72:127–135, 1982

Kellner R: Somatization and Hypochondriasis. Praeger, Westport, CT, 1986

Kellner R: Anxiety, somatic sensations, and bodily complaints., pp. 213–237. In Noyes R, Roth M, Burrows GD (eds): Handbook of Anxiety. Elsevier, New York, 1988

Kellner R: Treatment approaches to somatizing and hypochondriacal patients. pp. 159–179. In Kirmayer LJ, Robbins JM (eds): Current Concepts of Somatization: Research and Clinical Perspectives, American Psychiatric Press, 1991

Kessel WIN: Psychiatric morbidity in a London general practice. Br J Prev Soc Med 14:16–18, 1960

Kirmayer LJ, Robbins JM: Introduction: concepts of somatization pp. 1–20. In Kirmayer LJ, Robbins JM (eds): Current Concepts of Somatization: Research and Clinical Perspectives. American Psychiatric Association, Washington, 1991

Ladee GA: Hypochondriacal Syndromes. Elsevier, New York, 1966

Lazare A: Current concepts in psychiatry. N Engl J Med 305:745–748, 1981

Lewis WC, Berman M: Studies of conversion hysteria. I. Operational study of diagnosis. Arch Gen Psychiatry 13:275–282, 1965

Lipowski ZJ: Somatization: a borderland between medicine and psychiatry. Can Med Assoc J 135:609–614, 1986

McKegney FP: The incidence and characteristics of patients with conversion reactions. I. A general hospital consultation service sample. Am J Psychiatry 124(4):128–131, 1967

Osborne D: The MMPI in medical practice. Psychiatr Ann 15:534–541, 1985

Pitts FN, Meyer J, Brooks M, Winokur G: Adult psychiatric illness assessed for childhood parental loss, and psychiatric illness in family members—a study of 748 patients and 250 controls. Am J Psychiatry 121:1–10, 1965

Raskin M, Talbott JA, Meyerson AT: Diagnosis of conversion reactions: predictive value of psychiatric criteria. JAMA 197:102–106, 1966

Sapira JD: Reassurance therapy. Ann Intern Med 77: 603–604, 1972

Shepherd M, Cooper B, Brown AC, Katon AC: Psychiatric Illness in General Practice. Oxford University Press, London, 1966

Slater ETO, Glithero E: A follow-up of patients diagnosed as suffering from "hysteria." J Psychosom Res 9:9–13, 1965

Speigel D, Detrick D, Frischolz E: Hypnotizability and psychopathology. Am J Psychiatry 139:431–437, 1982

Speigel D, Fink R: Hysterical psychosis and hypnotizability. Am J Psychiatry, 136:777–781, 1979

Stefansson JG, Messina JA, Meyerowitz S: Hysterical neurosis, conversion type: clinical and epidemiological considerations. Acta Psychiatr Scand 53:119–138, 1976

Thomas KB: The consultation and therapeutic illusion. Br Med J 1:1327–1328, 1978

Tyrer P: The Role of Bodily Feelings in Anxiety. Oxford University Press, London, 1976

Weintraub MI: Hysteria: a clinical guide to diagnosis. Clin Symp 29(6):1–31, 1977

Whitlock FA: The aetiology of hysteria. Acta Psychiatr Scand 43:144–162, 1967

Medications and Their Effects

17

Carla Zeilmann
Paul J. Perry
Robert G. Robinson

The goal of this chapter is to review the pharmacotherapeutic treatment options for the short- and long-term sequelae of closed head injury. Standard therapies are discussed, as well as trials of drugs used to treat complications of head injury. Clinically significant drug interactions for the major drugs are listed in Tables 17-1 to 17-15, and Table 17-16 lists all drugs discussed and their brand names (see Appendix at end of chapter).

ACUTE PHARMACOTHERAPY OF CLOSED HEAD INJURY AND ITS EFFICACY

Overview

Several principles underpin medical treatment in acute closed head injury, and constant monitoring is required (Marshall, 1988). Initially the patient's head should be elevated to 30 degrees and be facing straight ahead, not to the left or right, as this can cause venous obstruction, which will increase the intracranial pressure (ICP). Head elevation can help lower ICP. Since extreme hyperventilation may produce excess vasoconstriction, it is important to monitor arterial carbon dioxide pressure (P_aCO_2). The patient, if necessary, should be intubated with controlled ventilation to maintain a P_aCO_2 of 27 to 30 mmHg, which will cause moderate intracerebral arterial vasoconstriction. Because of their central nervous system (CNS) respiratory depressant activity, sedatives and muscle relaxants must often be used with intubation. Fluid balance should be maintained, with appropriate intravenous fluids. It is important to keep systolic blood pressure between 100 and

160 mmHg, as hypo- or hypertension can be damaging. Additionally, hyperthermia (fever) can be injurious to the patient, so temperature must be maintained at a normal level. Ventricular drainage can be initiated if ICP is high, or mannitol 0.25 to 1g/kg every 3 to 6 hours can be used if drainage fails or is not available.

Management of Acute Closed Head Injury

Airway Management

After initial assessment of the severity of injury, protection and control of the airway is the first priority. If the Glasgow Coma Scale (GCS) score is greater than 8, airway management requires only supplemental oxygen. Otherwise, early intubation is recommended. An arterial oxygen pressure (P_aO_2) above 80 and a P_aCO_2 of 27 to 30 mmHg obtained with moderate hyperventilation are the target blood gas values. Below a P_aCO_2 of approximately 25 mmHg, there is too little blood flow to the brain and therefore swelling of the brain will increase (Ropper, 1994). The most efficient means to treat cerebral edema and increased ICP is with hyperventilation. Normally the effect of hyperventilation is obvious within 2 to 30 minutes. The patient may require succinylcholine up to 1 mg/kg IV to be successfully intubated. The effect lasts only 6 to 10 minutes, so if prolonged paralysis of the intercostal muscles is required, pancuronium bromide is the agent of choice, since it has a half-life of approximately 110 minutes in contrast to succinylcholine's extremely short half-life. The initial pancuronium dose is 0.08 mg/kg IV followed by 0.01 to 0.1 mg/kg IV as needed. In patients requiring a neuromuscular blocking agent as an adjunctive agent to increase compliance during assisted ventilation, it is critical to carefully monitor the patient's vital signs, since disconnection of the ventilator will cause rapid death. Prolonged paralysis may become necessary if the patient is fighting hyperventilation.

Hypotension

Approximately one-third of all patients with severe closed head injuries have hypoxia, and significant pulmonary shunting occurs in more than half (Marshall, 1988). Thus initial treatment should begin at the scene of injury. Moderate levels of hypotension can cause ischemic brain damage. Thus maintenance of normal blood pressure is imperative. Systolic blood pressure should be maintained between 100 and 120 mmHg with pressor agents or with antihypertensives if the patient is hypertensive (Ropper, 1994). The patient should be volume-replenished, and a blood pressure of at least 100 mmHg should be maintained. Hypertonic saline or pressor agents may be needed in the presence of severe hypotension. Available pressor agents are epinephrine, norepinephrine, isoproterenol, dopamine, and dobutamine. Dopamine and dobutamine are the preferred pressor agents because the other drugs cause vasoconstriction of the cerebral arteries, which results in a reduction of cerebral blood flow. Dopamine, which is usually preferred, acts at low, moderate, and high doses, respectively, at the D_1-dopaminergic, β_1-adrenergic, and α_1-adrenergic receptors located in the peripheral autonomic nervous system. At an infusion rate of 0.5 to 2.0 μg/kg/min, it acts on D_1 receptors and increases renal blood flow and urine output. At doses of 5 to 10 μg/kg/min, its β_1 effects increase heart contractility and cardiac output, with minimal effects on heart rate, blood pressure, or systemic vascular resistance. Dose rates greater than 20 μg/kg/min exert α_1-adrenergic effects and increse diastolic blood pressure, mean arterial pressure, systemic vascular resistance, and pulmonary capillary wedge pressure. Dopamine at doses greater than 5 μg/kg/min is used to increase cardiac output and mean arterial pressure. The drug should be started at this dose and titrated upward until the desired response is achieved. Dopamine-related adverse drug reactions that require monitoring include hypertension, tachycardia, tachyarrythmia, and ischemia. Dobutamine is a relatively specific β_1-agonist with minimal actions on the other adrenergic receptors. Dose rates of 5 to 10 μg/kg/min increase cardiac output. Dobutamine-related adverse reactions include arrhythmias, hypertension, myocardial ischemia, and tachycardia. Epinephrine, norepinephrine, and isoproterenol are usually reserved for refractory cases, as they cause an increased incidence of adverse reactions (Teich and Chernow, 1985).

Hypertension

Hypertension is most efficiently treated with diuretics, β-blockers, angiotensin-converting enzyme (ACE) inhibitors, or intermittent doses of barbitutates. Other antihypertensive drugs, including calcium channel blockers, may increase ICP and therefore are contraindicated. Although 15 percent of closed head injury patients experience hypertension, it appears transient for most patients. Hypertension is still significant since it ultimately affects survival and may cause perpetuation of the brain injury. Following a brain injury, patients are in a hyperdynamic state, which includes hypertension, tachycardia, increased cardiac output, and increased cardiac work. There may also be an increase in catecholamines, which may correspond to the severity of head injury. Propranolol is considered the treatment of choice for hypertension in the injured brain owing to its mechanisms of activity, which include direct cardiac effects, blockage of presynaptic β-receptors, and possibly direct CNS effects (Labi and Horn, 1990). Propranolol 1 to 3 mg is administered by slow intravenous push, at a rate not to exceed 1 mg/min. The dose may repeated after 5 minutes, since an intravenously injected dose produces peak levels within 1 minute and is undetectable within 5 minutes. The dose should thereafter not be repeated more than once every 4 hours. Propranolol may cause unwanted cognitive or affective side effects due to its lipophilicity and ability to penetrate into the CNS. Thus, use of less lipophilic β-blockers, such as atenolol, nadolol, timolol, or acebutolol, in order to lower the incidence of CNS side effects could be considered. However, only atenolol is available in a parenteral dosage formulation. Additionally, the only recommended injectable dose (i.e., 5 mg by slow intravenous push at 1 mg/min, repeated if needed in 10 minutes) is actually suggested for the treatment of acute myocardial infarction. However, this dose may also be suitable for the treatment of hypertension in the patient with closed head injury.

Some practitioners advocate treatment of any sustained blood pressure above 160 mmHg. A sedative such as morphine, given alone, may provide blood pressure control. Small doses, 2.5 to 15 mg IV, given frequently (e.g., every 4 hours), may block stimuli that cause excitement. If sedation does not control blood pressure, intravenous trimethaphan or hydralazine should be used in preference to sodium nitroprusside owing to the deleterious effect of the latter on cerebral perfusion. The dose of trimethaphan is 0.5 to 1.0 mg/min IV until the desired systolic blood pressure is achieved, which should not be less than 100 mmHg, as discussed earlier. It is also recommended to drop blood pressure to less than two-thirds of the initial level (Ropper, 1994). The hydralazine dosage for hypertensive emergencies is 10 to 20 mg IV, repeated as necessary, and the dose can be increased within this range. The drug is metabolized to its inactive but hepatoxic metabolites, hydrazine and acetylhydrazine, by acetylation. Rapid acetylators generally require higher doses than slow acetylators. This is a potential problem primarily in whites and blacks, approximately 50 percent of whom are slow acetylators versus only about 12 percent of Japanese-Americans (Relling and Evans 1992). Cerebrovascular dilation occurs following sodium nitroprusside administration, probably secondary to a direct effect on cerebral vasculature (Marshall and Bowers 1982). It has been demonstrated that intracranial hypertension can occur even in the presence of falling blood pressure following administration of sodium nitroprusside (Cottrell et al., 1978). However, if the patient fails to respond to trimethaphan or hydralazine, sodium nitroprusside may be tried if the patient is hypocarbic and hyperoxic. The drug should be infused slowly and the ICP closely monitored. If ICP monitoring is not available, the use of sodium nitroprusside can be very dangerous (Marshall and Bowers 1982).

Fever

Fever will increase tissue metabolic rate by 13 percent for each Celsius degree rise in temperature. The increased metabolic demand may not be able to be met by the already traumatized brain (Marshall 1988). Fever must be treated with antipyretics—aspirin or preferably acetaminophen—or a cooling blanket, and the source should be identified (Marshall 1988). Infections such as aspiration pneumonia and meningitis are most common, but drug allergies may also occur. Hypothalamic damage in severe TBI patients is a rare cause of fever. Any of the treatments for fever can cause chills and sweating due to the body's temperature fluctuations. Acetaminophen is preferred over aspirin because of its lack of effect on platelet adhesiveness. The dose of either drug is 325 to 650 mg PO every 3 to 4 hours. If the patient is comatose, the use of cooling techniques is indicated. In surface cooling advantage is taken of evaporation and convection heat loss principles by wetting the skin and blowing air across the body with fans. Direct cooling is employed by packing the body in ice. However, these patients are at risk for sudden cardiovascular collapse. Central cooling uses peritoneal, gastric, or bladder lavage with sodium chloride refrigerated to 9° to 20°C. However, fluid shifts may be significant, and electrolyte status must be continually monitored.

The neuroleptic chlorpromazine has been advocated as a pharmacologic adjunct to surface cooling and direct cooling in the treatment of hyperthermia. Neuroleptics act centrally as depressants to the hypothalamus to inhibit shivering thermogenesis. The use of chlorpromazine does present a significant problem to closed head injury patients since the drug lowers the seizure threshold. Once the temperature has fallen below 39°C, cooling procedures are discontinued (Matz 1986).

Seizures

Post-traumatic seizures can be classified into two groups, early and late. Early seizures occur within 1 week of injury, and late seizures occur after 1 week. Early seizures are further divided into immediate seizures, which occur within 24 hours of the injury, and delayed early seizures, which occur between 24 hours and 1 week of injury. Post-traumatic epilepsy consists of late recurrent seizures (Dalmady-Israil and Zasler 1993), which are not a usual consequence of mild closed head injury (Ch. 11).

Seizures increase energy requirements and cause a rise in cerebral blood flow up to 400 percent, which will worsen any increase in the ICP already present. Intravascular volume should be cautiously maintained by using salt solutions without dextrose. In experimental animals, hyperglycemia exacerbates ischemic brain injury (Marshall, 1988). When phenytoin is given within the first 7 days after a serious head injury, the incidence of post-traumatic epilepsy is reduced (Temkin et al., 1990). The efficacy of phenytoin 1 week or more following the injury is equivocal. Long-term prophylaxis has not been shown to be effective in preventing post-traumatic epilepsy. However, those patients with severe head injuries in whom the effects of seizures would further complicate management should receive preventive phenytoin therapy (Willmore, 1992). The preventive phenytoin dose is a loading dose of 18 mg/kg and then 5 mg/kg/day. The plasma phenytoin concentrations are then monitored and maintained between 10 to 20 μg/ml. The patient is then maintained on phenytoin prophylactically for the next 6 to 24 months (Willmore, 1992). However, since there are no data supporting the efficacy of long-term prophylaxis, an early taper is preferable. In patients who have had seizures, treatment and prophylaxis should be the same as in the non-head-injured population. Patients with the fewest seizures have the best prognosis. It has been observed that 50 percent of patients with posttraumatic epilepsy will be seizure-free within 15 years (Willmore, 1992). Decisions to remove patientsfrom medication should be made according to guidelines that apply to patients with idiopathic epilepsy.

Fluid and Electrolyte Therapy

The optimal fluid for a patient with closed head injury remains controversial. A patient who is hypotensive can be assumed to be hypovolemic (Tobin, 1989). Fluid levels in the body must be maintained for maximization of oxygen delivery to the brain. However, the patient must be kept from becoming fluid-overloaded to (1) minimize edema formation, (2) prevent a rise in ICP, and (3) increase perfusion of the brain. Thus, optimum fluid and electrolyte therapy strikes a balance between inadequate perfusion and fluid overload. Head trauma may induce salt retention initially, so that half-normal saline may be the most useful solution for fluid replacement and maintenance. Animal evidence suggests that crystalloid solutions (salt solutions) can cause increased ICP when used alone. Mannitol has been shown in several studies to reduce or control ICP (Feldman and Fish, 1991). The concern is that mannitol or any osmotically active agent (colloid solution) in excess of normal doses will cause or worsen hypotension.

ICP is normally between 2 and 12 mmHg, and levels between 15 and 40 mmHg can cause ischemic damage to the brain (Ropper, 1994). The damage is related to the difference between the ICP and the cerebral arterial pressure, which is termed the *cerebral perfusion pressure.* Cerebral perfusion pressure is directly related to the arterial pressure, and when it falls below 40 to 60 mmHg, it signifies an ICP that is high and detrimental to nerve cells (Ropper, 1994). Medications or physiologic changes that increase blood pressure do not necessarily increase cerebral perfusion pressure owing to the fact that increased vascular pressure can worsen brain edema in damaged areas of the brain. This will increase ICP and ultimately lower perfusion and worsen ischemia (Ropper, 1994). Dogs with a simulated epidural mass showed a lower ICP and higher cerebral perfusion pressure when treated with mannitol, while saline caused a rise in and sustained high level of the ICP (Feldman and Fish, 1991).

Administration of 20 percent mannitol, 0.25 to 1 g/kg, every 3 to 6, hours will cause hyperosmolar dehydration. A serum osmolality of 305 to 315 mOsm/L is wanted when directly measured ICP is not being used as a guide. Ventricular or subarachnoid drainage is desirable whenever possible.

Hypertonic solutions may improve overall survival in patients with closed head injury as compared with saline alone. The fluid used in the study by Feldman and Fish (1991) was 7.5 percent saline/dextran 70, which provided an optimal combination of salt and colloidal solution.

Use of Corticosteroids

Despite many controlled trials, the use of corticosteroids to reduce ICP remains controversial. Pitts (1982) found that high-dose corticosteroids did not influence survival in patients with severe head injury but that survivors who received corticosteroids had a significantly better quality of life. One possible explanation for this beneficial effect involves brain edema. As areas of contusion resolve and osmotic pressure gradients develop within the tissue of the brain, edema can occur. Dexamethasone may prevent or ameliorate foci of edema in the injured tissue. Marshall and Bowers (1982) recommend use of 80 mg/day of dexamethasone for the first 4 days followed by a taper that terminates after 10 days.

There is no conclusive evidence that corticosteroids are beneficial in the treatment of trauma-induced cerebral edema (Tobin, 1989). Corticosteroids may be useful if there is a hemorrhage, edema, or a contusion obvious on computed tomography (CT) scan. If none of these is present, corticosteroids may complicate management and should not be used (Ropper, 1994). For example, agitation is worsened by large doses of corticosteroids. Mental status changes associated with large doses of corticosteroids include mood disorders as well as delusions or hallucinations. Haloperidol, given sparingly, can be useful (Ropper, 1994). Most studies have found that high-dose steroid therapy does not help lower ICP or affect clinical outcome (Ropper, 1994). In an anecdotal report of three cases, young patients with an initial GCS score of 10 or more and an elevated ICP for 2 days or more benefited from use of high-dose dexamethasone therapy to decrease ICP (DuPlessis, 1992). All the patients, who had been treated with mannitol and hyperventilation, were kept normovolemic and received pentobarbital but still had rising ICP. High-dose dexamethasone decreased ICP within 24 hours. The doses used were 60 mg initially and then 48 mg q6h in a 15-year-old boy, 80 mg initially followed by 48 mg q6h in a 19-year-old man, and an unspecified "megadose" in a 12-year-old boy. The data suggest that this patient group may benefit from corticosteroid therapy.

Agitation

The use of intravenous haloperidol in acutely agitated medical and surgical patients has been proved to be safe and effective. It is an especially good choice in closed head injury patients within the first 72 hours because it appears to lower ICP. The initial dose should be 5 mg IV. The line should be flushed, since haloperidol can precipitate in the presence of heparin and phenytoin. Effect on agitation can be seen within 10 to 30 minutes. If the patient remains agitated, the dose should be doubled. Doses should be given 20 to 30 minutes apart, and the patient can receive up to 75 mg/h. The dose at which the patients responds should be given at the next interval. A single dose larger than 40 mg is rarely needed, although bolus doses of up to 150 mg have been used. Older patients may need as little as 0.5 mg bid. Haloperidol can also be given as a continuous infusion at 10 to 12 mg/h (Santos et al., 1992). The intravenous route bypasses the first-pass metabolism in the liver and is quick and convenient, since head injury patients will most likely have intravenous access. Adverse drug reactions commonly seen with oral haloperidol, such as dystonia and pseudoparkinsonism, are rare with intravenous haloperidol. A rare adverse reaction associated with the use of neuroleptic agents such as haloperidol is neuroleptic malignant syndrome, which includes the symptoms of fever, autonomic instability, muscular rigidity, and altered consciousness and can be treated with bromocriptine or dantrolene. Haloperidol has minimal effects on respiratory or cardiac function and has no anticholinergic side effects (Clinton et al., 1987). However, patients with left ventricular hypertrophy and torsades de pointes seem predisposed to developing ventricular fibrillation or tachycardia, and thus haloperidol use should be avoided in these patients (Metzger and Friedman, 1993).

If the patient remains agitated after a total dose of 20 to 40 mg of haloperidol, a benzodiazepine such as lorazepam at a dose of 4 mg can be added. The combination has been shown to be more effective than either drug alone (Garza-Trevino et al., 1989). The combination of intramuscular bolus doses of lorazepam 4 mg and haloperidol 5 mg was found to be more effective than either drug alone to sedate agitated patients, particularly within the first 30 to 60 minutes (Menza et al., 1988). The safety of the lorazepam/haloperidol combination treatment was demonstrated in a group of critically ill, delirious cancer patients. Total intravenous doses of lorzepam 36 to 480 mg and haloperidol 100 to 480 mg were used successfully in 24 of 25 patients without medical complications (Adams et al., 1986).

MANAGEMENT OF CHRONIC PHASE CLOSED HEAD INJURY

The type of problems and the management of problems in the chronic phase of a head injury differ dramatically from those outlined in the previous section. Here we concentrate on aspects of pharmacotherapy in two chronic conditions, namely headache and affective disorder. More comprehensive coverage of these and other chronic effects of closed head injury are given in other chapters in this book.

Headache

Headache is a common complaint in head injury patients, even those with closed head injury (Wilkinson and Gilchrist, 1980). The problem is usually self-limited, but it may persist and require treatment (see Ch. 8).

Amitriptyline has been widely used for post-traumatic contraction headaches in doses of 25 to 50 mg (Tyler et al., 1980). Additionally, nortriptyline, doxepin, and maprotiline have been shown to be effective, but fluoxetine and imipramine were found to be less effective. These data were obtained only by incidental use of these drugs, although a study comparing amitriptyline with maprotiline found equal efficacy but fewer adverse reactions with maprotiline (Label, 1991). Maprotiline, however, is not advocated for use in patients with closed head injury because of the high incidence of seizures at therapeutic doses. Nonsteroidal anti-inflammatory drugs (NSAIDs) such as aspirin and ibuprofen may also be beneficial for the treatment of muscle contraction headaches.

Occipital neuralgia may respond to nerve blockade with a local anesthetic alone or with an injectable corticosteroid if the anesthetic alone is not effective (Sjaastad, 1990). Paroxysms of shooting pain may respond to carbamazepine; NSAIDs or transcutaneous electrical nerve stimulation (TENS) units may also be helpful (Evans, 1992).

Migraines may respond to the usual migraine headache medications. The ergotamines are the most effective abortive medication. It is important not to exceed the recommended ergotamine dose of 6 mg per attack or 10 mg per week, or else extreme vasoconstriction could result, possibly leading to gangrene. Naproxen can be tried at doses of 250 to 550 mg stat, then repeated every 8 hours as needed, and ibuprofen can be tried at 400 to 600 mg stat, then repeated every 6 hours. Isometheptane with dichloralphenazone and acetaminophen (Midrin) is effective in only 50 percent of patients and should only be used when the ergotamines are contradicted or not tolerated. The barbiturates should be used only on a low-frequency basis to avoid dependence. Sumatriptan is an injectable drug that is used for abortive purposes only. Only one 6-mg injection is generally needed, since not much benefit is obtained by adding the second 6-mg injection that is available in the kit. Not more than 12 mg should be used in a 24-hour period. It should not be given in uncontrolled hypertension or to people receiving ergotamines, and the first dose should be given under supervision in case the patient has unrecognized coronary disease. Simple analgesics such as aspirin or acetaminophen tend not to be effective for aborting migraines.

Prophylaxis of migraine involves the β-blockers, antidepressants, NSAIDs, calcium channel blockers, and valproic acid (Evans 1992). Prophylaxis should begin if the patient is having more than two migraines per month or one per week. A 70 percent response to amitriptyline or propranolol alone or in combination has been reported (Weiss et al., 1991). Propranolol is approved by the Food and Drug Administration for the use in migraines and is effective in 80 percent of cases of non-head-injured patients. Doses are low, usually 40 to 80 mg/day initially, ranging up to 320 mg/day, although doses over 160 mg are uncommon. It takes 3 to 6 months to see a beneficial effect. The heart rate should be maintained above 60 beats per minute. Amitriptyline can be tried if protriptyline is ineffective, at a dose of 75 to 100 mg/day not to exceed 200 mg/day. The calcium channel blockers are the next line of therapy. They have a delay of onset of 2 to 8 weeks, and tolerance may develop after several months. Doses used in migraine are nifedipine 10 mg tid up to 60 mg/day and nimodipine 60 to 120 mg/day. Diltiazem and verapamil may also be tried. Cyproheptadine is only 40 to 50 percent effective in non-head-injured adults even though it is the drug of choice for prophylaxis in children. The adult dose is 4 mg tid not to exceed 24 mg/day. Methysergide is effective in 60 to 70 percent of non-head-injured patients, but a drug holiday is needed for 1 month out of every 6 months owing to the risk of pulmonary fibrosis and retroperitoneal fibrosis, thereby limiting the drug's desirability. The dose is 2 mg tid not to exceed 8 mg/day.

Cluster headaches, rare following closed head injury (Evans, 1992), can be aborted with ergotamine, oxygen, prednisone, or lithium. Lithium is usually thought of as the drug of choice for acute treatment or prophylaxis of cluster headaches, with 75 percent effectiveness. It is given in doses of 300 mg two to four times daily. The plasma lithium levels should not exceed 1.2 mEq/L. Signs of toxicity, which include slurred speech, confusion, and lethargy, need to be monitored. Ergotamine has the same dose as in migraines. Also effective is 100 percent oxygen at 8 to 10 L/min for 10 to 15 minutes, which can be used up to five times daily. Prednisone 40 to 60 mg may be used acutely to treat the cluster headaches and is effective in 40 to 75 percent of patients. Prednisone is a second-line prophylactic therapy and is effective in 50 to 75 percent of patients. However, it is only effective for a short time and rebound of headaches may occur if the drug is discontinued. Prednisone at doses of 40 to 60 mg/day with a 21-day taper are recommended. The ergotamines can be used if the attacks occur regularly, and the dose should be 2 mg given 2 hours before the attack, up to 10 mg/week. Methysergide is effective but should be avoided because of adverse reactions, of which retroperitoneal fibrosis is the most serious. Drugs that are not as effective in cluster headache include β-blockers, antihistamines, carbamazepine, tricyclic antidepressants, acetaminophen, and NSAIDs. It should be kept in mind that all therapies discussed are for non-brain-injured patients. Therapy for brain-injured patients has not been well delineated (Marshall, 1988).

Affective Disorders

Depression

Approximately 27 percent of closed head injury patients suffer from depression after the injury (Fedoroff et al., 1992). The cause is not necessarily a brain injury (see Ch. 15).

Unfortunately, the literature on treatment is dominated by case studies, and no double-blind treatment trials and few open treatment studies have been reported. In one study 10 patients with closed head injury and depression were treated with amitriptyline or phenelzine (Saran, 1988). Curiously, none of the head-injured patients responded, while all 12 patients with primary depression did. A more recent study by Dinan and Mobayed (1992) compared 13 closed head injury patients with depression (diagnosed by DSM-III [Diagnostic and Statistical Manual of Mental Disorders, 3rd ed.] and Hamilton Depression Rating Scale criteria) with 13 "functional depressives." Only 4 of the 13 head-injured patients responded, while 11 of the 13 "functional depresives" responded after 6 weeks of amitriptyline therapy. Two of the head-injured patients still failed to improve after electroconvulsive therapy. Six others had lithium augmentation of the amitriptyline; of those, two improved, while four remained depressed. The authors also reported treating five patients not in the study with maximally tolerated doses of phenelzine for 4 to 6 weeks with no reponse, which is similar to the report of Saran (1988).

Perhaps depression following closed head injury is pathophysiologically different from primary depression. In this vein, few closed head injury patients were nonsuppressors on the dexamethasone suppression test, in contrast to patients with primary depression (Saran, 1985). The test is performed by administering dexamethasone 0.5, 1, or 2 mg PO at 11 P.M. and drawing a plasma cortisol level the next day at either 8 A.M., 4 P.M., or 8 P.M. An abnormal result (elevated cortisol $> 5\ \mu g/dl$) is observed in approximately 40 percent of depressed patients (Andreasen and Black, 1991). A study of 55 male patients with mild head injury, 8 of whom were depressed, found a significantly blunted prolactin response to buspirone in the depressed head injury patients as compared with 10 healthy controls (Mobayed and Dinan, 1990).

Mania

Jorge et al. (1993) evaluated 66 consecutive closed head injury patients for mania at 3, 6, and 12 months after injury. They used a structured psychiatric interview and DSM-III-R criteria (Jorge et al., 1993). Six patients (9 percent) met the criteria for mania at some point. This 9 percent incidence is higher than that seen in other brain injuries such as stroke. Frontal lobe trauma may be a factor, unfortunately. There are no reports of controlled drug trials in patients with mania after closed head injury. Anecdotal reports have indicated that some patients respond to lithium treatment while others are resistant and respond better to carbamazepine (Shukla et al., 1987; Starkstein et al., 1991).

EFFICACY OF INDIVIDUAL DRUG TREATMENTS

As indicated earlier in this chapter, numerous drugs have been used in the pharmacotherapeutic management of the closed head injury patient. Importantly, the effects of these drugs must be clearly understood to avoid potential adverse reactions in both the acute and chronic settings. These drugs include the barbiturates, CNS stimulants, tricyclic antidepressants, levodopa/carbidopa, lithium, clozapine, β-blockers, calcium channel blockers, clonidine, cytidine diphosphorylcholine, and N-acetylcysteine.

Barbiturates

If ICP remains elevated in acute, severe cases, high-dose barbiturates may be added. Barbiturartes may cause a reduction in both ICP and blood pressure, which overall does not improve cerebral perfusion. The beneficial effects of barbiturates are sedative and anticonvulsive, but other benefits have not been established. The routine use of barbiturates in acutely ill closed head injury patients is not recommended, especially considering that they can cause severe hypotension. Pressor agents required to support barbiturate use provide little increase in the cerebral perfusion pressure. In general, high-dose barbiturate therapy should only be an adjuvant therapy and should only be used when standard treatments have failed.

Pentobarbital, 5 to 10 mg/kg administered over several minutes, is the initial recommended dose (Marshall and Bowers 1982). If the patient is hypovolemic, lower doses should be used. Pentobarbital can be administered until the ICP is reduced to 20 mmHg and preferably to below 15 mmHg. The target pentobarbital serum concentration is approximately 30 mg/L. There is no further reduction in ICP with levels above 50 mg/L. It is important to note that a pentobarbital level of 40 mg/L almost always causes respiratory arrest and an isoelectric electroencephalogram; thus this ought to be the upper limit for pentobarbital dosing. Other barbiturates, specifically thiopental and phenobarbital, have the same doses and target concentrations. Phenobarbital at this serum level only causes drowsiness.

It is unknown if any barbiturate is more effective than pentobarbital (Marshall and Bowers, 1982). Sodium thiopental has the theoretical advantage of free-radical scavenging, but there is little evidence that free radical formation contributes to the pathogenesis of brain injury. Sodium thiopental also has to be given much more frequently, and serum sodium levels may rise owing to the large amount of drug that is required.

Stimulants

Stimulant medications have been used in patients with closed head injury to treat chronic behavioral disturbances, such as impaired arousal, attention, vigilance, initiation, memory and emotional control. Case reports suggest that dextroamphetamine and methylphenidate may improve functioning as measured by tests of concentration or behavior (Evans et al. 1987; Lipper and Tuchman 1976; Parmalee and O'Shanick 1987; Stern, 1978). One controlled investigation examined the efficacy of methylphenidate, 0.15 mg/kg twice daily (9 patients) or 0.30 mg/kg twice daily (6 patients), in a group of 15 closed head injury patients well past the initial recovery stage (47 ± 41 months post injury) in a double-blind, placebo-controlled, crossover design (Gualtieri and Evans 1988). Of these patients 14 were said to be subjective responders according to self-rating scales filled out by the patients and a co-informant, and 10 showed evidence of subjective and objective response (psychometric test battery). However, there was no characteristic behavior that was improved in all patients, and there was no pattern to the stimulant effects. This resulted in no statistically significant results. Moreover, long-term efficacy was questionable, and there was strong evidence of a placebo effect.

Another study evaluated the effectiveness of methylphenidate (0.3 mg/kg twice daily) in 12 chronic closed head injury patients using a double-blind, placebo-controlled, randomized, crossover design (Speech et al., 1993). Methylphenidate treatment was instituted 14 to 108 months postinjury. Outcome measures were cognitive tests of attention, learning, and cognitive processing speed, and a rating scale that was completed by a close friend or relative. No significant differences were found between methylphenidate and placebo on any of these measures. To summarize, only case reports have found any benefit with stimulant medications in closed head injury patients.

Antidepressants

Protriptyline is a nonsedating tricyclic antidepressant. A series of case reports in brain-injured patients with suspected depression, anergia, withdrawn affect, and cognitive problems showed good responses at doses of 5 to 30 mg daily within a few days (Wroblewski et al., 1993). A usual therapeutic trial of protriptyline would be 30 to 60 mg/day administered for 3 to 4 weeks. Interestingly, however, the patients may have responded to the early activating or stimulating noradrenergic agonist effect of the drug, not the antidepressant effect. Two patients developed tolerance to the drug. Anticholinergic side effects, such as urinary retention, constipation, blurred vision, memory impairment, and confusion were noted. The anticholinergic delirium associated with the tricyclic antidepressants makes their use especially problematic in acute or chronic closed head injury patients. Thus, if a patient with closed head injury becomes depressed, it is perhaps advisable to treat the patient with a nonanticholinergic antidepressant such as one of the selective serotonin reuptake inhibitors (fluoxetine, sertraline, or paroxetine) or bupropion. The efficacy of the latter medication in closed head injury remains to be determined.

Levodopa/Carbidopa

The effectiveness of Sinemet (levodopa/carbidopa) was evaluated in 12 patients aged 17 to 54 with brain injuries due to anoxia, diving and driving accidents, gunshot wounds, and blunt trauma (Lal et al., 1988). Patients were treated at times that varied from 3.7 to 52 months after their injury. All patients had physical, cognitive, communicative, emotional, and behavioral defects and had reached a plateau in their rehabilitation programs for at least 2 weeks before Sinemet was initiated. The drug was initiated at a dose of 10 to 100 mg three times daily or 25 to 250 mg four times daily. Doses were increased for the following reasons: (1) no change in status was observed for 1 week on current dose, (2) change was observed but dose was changed to see if a higher dose would provide a more rapid or different response, or (3) the initial improvement had reached a plateau. The dose was decreased if the patient deteriorated or developed unwanted effects. Improvement was noted as early as 48 hours after initiation of therapy. All patients were withdrawn from the drug after 2 to 24 months except for two who deteriorated when withdrawal was attempted. Curiously, functional improvement was retained after Sinemet was discontinued in all patients. The most impaired patients reportedly showed the most improvement. Treatment begun within 18 months of the injury was better than later. Adverse drug reactions that deserve monitoring with Sinemet include anorexia, nausea, vomiting, reversible dykinesias, mental status changes, depression, dementia, palpitations, or orthostatic hypotensive episodes. The role of Sinemet in closed head injury remains unsettled.

Lithium

Lithium carbonate has been used successfully to treat aggressive behavior in non-brain-injured and mentally retarded individuals (Glenn and Joseph, 1987; Smith and Perry, 1992). Additionally, a case series found lithium useful in the control of aggression in brain-injured patients. Glenn et al. (1989) treated 10 brain-injured patients with severe cognitive impairment and unremitting aggressive, combative, or self-destructive behavior. There was no systematized method for evaluating behavioral and cognitive changes. However, the authors reported that five patients had a dramatic response, which significantly improved their participation in rehabilitation. Another experienced a moderate response. Of these six responding patients, attempts to withdraw resulted in behavioral regression in four, but reinstitution of lithium treatment resulted in decreased aggression in three of these four patients. Of the four nonresponding patients, one improved initially but regressed in spite of continued lithium levels in the high therapeutic range. Another experienced neurotoxic drug reactions. The remaining two patients developed polyuria and polydipsia.

Lithium must always be used with caution. Neurotoxicity is a potential drawback if the plasma concentration exceeds 1.5 mEq/L, especially of the patient is already receiving an antipsychotic medication. Side effects include distractibility, poor memory, disorientation, incoherence, poor concentration, impaired judgment, involuntary movements, ataxia, dysarthia, delirium, nystagmus, and potentially, coma. Lithium is also toxic to the kidney and should not be used in patients with renal dysfunction. Other adverse reactions to lithium include nausea, vomiting, diarrhea, nephrogenic diabetes insipidus, polyuria and polydipsia, T-wave depression, teratogenicity, thyrotoxicosis, tremor, weakness, and weight gain. Monitoring parameters should include baseline blood counts, electrolyte levels, blood urea nitrogen (BUN), serum creatinine, thyroid function tests, and an electrocardiogram if clinically indicated. Lithium levels should be checked monthly for 3 months and then every 3 months and should be between 0.9 and 1.4 mEq/L (Perry et al., 1991).

Clozapine

Clozapine is a neuroleptic drug used to treat refractory schizophrenia or psychotic disorder. Clozapine has relative selectivity for D_1 and D_4 receptors as compared with the D_2 dopamine site, where typical antipsychotics mainly exert their effect. Thus it could be beneficial to patients with CNS trauma for the treatment of associated symptoms of delusions, hallucinations, suspiciousness, aggression with psychotic features, rage, and aggression refractory to other medications.

Clozapine was used by Michals et al. (1993) to treat nine patients with brain injury who displayed psychotic symptoms or outbursts of rage and aggression refractory to other medications. Evidence of cognitive impairment was based on a retrospective review of the patients' records, including hospital progress notes. Doses ranged from 300 to 750 mg daily, with the average dose being approximately 400 mg daily for 3 weeks to 5 months. One patient had dramatic decrease in bizarre speech, and two patients had marked decrease in verbal and physical aggression. Three patients had mild improvement in agitation and frequency of auditory hallucinations. Length of treatment was inadequate in three patients, although one of these was receiving amoxapine, which confounded the response. Common adverse drug reactions included drowsiness, dizziness, headache, excess salivation, vomiting, and weight gain. Two patients experienced "seizures," one of whom was already receiving valproic acid while the other was also receiving amoxapine, which, like clozapine, may lower the seizure threshold. Treatment of clozapine-induced seizures includes discontinuation of the drug, dosage reduction, or addition of anticonvulsant medication. Double-blind controlled studies are needed to determine the efficacy of clozapine versus haldol in treating psychotic and behavioral sequelae of brain injury. One potential advantage of clozapine is the reduced incidence of tardive dyskinesia. Michals et al. suggest reserving clozapine for brain-injured patients with psychosis or aggression refractory to β-blockers, lithium, and anticonvulsants. Limiting the maximal dose to 600 mg daily or adding anticonvulsant medication may help to reduce the risk of seizures.

β-Blockers

β-Adrenergic antagonists, or β-blockers, may have many uses and may even help control disruptive or violent behavior in patients with "organic brain syndromes" (Horn, 1987; Smith and Perry, 1992). Propranolol in doses of 60 to 240 mg/day has been used. The response tends to be rapid but can take as long as several days or weeks. It appears that in many cases efforts to taper the drug result in reappearance of symptoms of behavioral disturbance. There are no specific symptoms, electroencephalographic findings, injury locations, or temporal relationships indicating that a particular patient will respond to β-blockers. Some side effects include dizziness, lethargy, depression, and ataxia. The patients should be monitored for bradycardia and hypotension. Contraindications to therapy are chronic obstructive pulmonary disease, asthma, brittle diabetes, congestive heart failure, bradycardia, and hypotension. Selective β-blockers such as atenolol and metoprolol may be safer, but their efficacy is unknown as compared with the nonselective agent propranolol. Pindolol is the β-blocker of choice since, unlike propranolol, it did not cause significant bradycardia or hypotension in agitated demented patients at the recommended dose of 40 to 60 mg/day (Smith and Perry, 1992).

Greendyke et al. (1980) used propranolol, titrated to 520 mg/day over 11 weeks, in nine treatment-refractory assaultive patients. Head trauma was the etiology of the organicity in four of the patients; the others had alcoholism, brain tumor, encephalitis, or Huntington's disease. The patients with head injury became assaultive and combative only following their injury. Overall, propranolol was more effective than placebo in reducing assaultive behavior. Five patients showed marked improvement, two moderate, and two little or no improvement. The etiology of the organic brain disease apparently did not affect the response to treatment.

Clonidine

Clonidine is an α_2-adrenergic agonist which is used in hypertension and opiate withdrawal. Clonidine reportedly has produced beneficial effects on memory in children with attention-deficit hyperactivity disorder. Two patients with post-traumatic memory deficits were treated with clonidine in an attempt to improve their memory (McIntyre and Gasquoine, 1989). The two patients received the drug titrated to doses of 0.1 every morning and 0.4 mg at bedtime in one patient and to 0.2 mg four times daily in the other. Two weeks after initiation of clonidine, the patients showed no objective improvement.

Nimodipine

Calcium channel blockers have been found to be effective in experimental models of cerebral ischemia and also in the prevention of ischemic brain damage in acute treatment of patients who suffered a subarachnoid hemorrhage (Pickard et al., 1989). Nimodipine is a calcium channel blocker that is structurally similar to nifedipine. A randomized prospective double-blind trial was conducted to determine the effect of nimodipine on the outcome of head-injured patients (Bailey et al., 1991). The subjects were not obeying commands at entry to the study, which was within 24 hours of injury. Nimodipine was given to 175 patients at a dose of 2 mg/h IV for up to 7 days, while 176 patients received placebo. After 6 months, 53 percent of the nimodipine group had moderate or good recovery as compared with 49 percent of the control group, which was not significant. Mortality was initially lower in the nimodipine group, but more late deaths in vegetative or severely disabled patients caused the 6-month mortality rates to be equal. The means of diastolic and systolic blood pressure and ICP did not differ between groups. No subgroup was identified that could benefit from the drug. Nimodipine was well tolerated. It was concluded that there were no data supporting the use nimodipine following head injury.

Amantadine

Amantadine acts presynaptically to enhance the release of dopamine or to inhibit dopamine reuptake. Gualtieri et al. (1989) treated 30 brain injury patients with amantadine during the rehabilitation phase of therapy. Treatment lasted up to 12 months and began 2 to 144 months after injury. All patients were stable and receiving no other psychotropic medications. Indications for treatment were agitation, assaultiveness, distractibility, and mood swings or the need to increase the amount of responsiveness and arousal. Initial doses were 50 to 100 mg, raised gradually by 50 to 100 mg weekly until response or adverse effects occurred. The mean dose was 288.3 ± 87.3 mg/day. If no benefit was noted in 6 weeks, therapy was discontinued. The only evaluation performed to define a positive response was consensus agreement among the treatment team, patient, and the family of the patient experiencing clinical improvement. Fourteen patients were unequivocal responders and five more responded but developed unacceptable side effects. The optimal dose was 50 to 400 mg/day. Side effects noted were irritability, rigidity, depression, lethargy, edema, seizures, hyperactivity, ataxia, dyskinesia, and nausea. (The occurrence of seizures in two of the 30 patients is a disturbing finding.) Amantadine appears to be a reasonable alternative therapy for the treatment of behavioral or arousal problems in head injury patients.

Cytidine Diphosphoryl Choline

Cytidine diphosphoryl choline (CDP choline) was evaluated in a randomized, placebo-controlled study of 14 patients (Levin 1991). The patients were tested for memory, fluency, and attention, as well as being interviewed about postconcussive problems with headache, fatigue, dizziness, sleep, memory, depression, anxiety, appetite, thinking, and concentration. Entry criteria were mild to moderate head injury and hospitalization, with resolution of post-traumatic amnesia. More patients in the cytidine diphosphoryl choline group had improvement in memory than in the placebo group, 100 versus 29 percent, $P<.02$. Memory was measured by a verbal recall test, a spatial memory test, and a recognition test. The 100 percent memory increase reflects recalling or recognizing twice as many words, patterns, or objects, depending on the test. This improvement was reflected in subjective symptoms but not in cognitive tests. Fluency and attention was unaffected by the treatment. The patients in the placebo group complained more of the postconcussive symptoms of headaches, dizziness, and tinnitus. The cytidine diphosphoryl choline group complained more of gastrointestinal distress, probably secondary to the drug. The author suggested that further studies need to be done.

DRUG INTERACTIONS

The Appendix consists of abridged lists of drug interactions involving those drugs commonly used in the treatment of the closed head injury patient. The lists are partial, and drug interaction comments are not duplicated. Thus, for a given pair of drugs, both tables must be consulted to determine if a significant potential drug interaction exists. For example the calcium channel blocker (Table 17-2) / lithium (Table 17-9) interaction is only listed in Table 17-2. A list of individual drugs or drug classes in alphabetical order is also presented (Table 17-16). More complete and detailed compendia are available in the two standard drug interactions texts, *Drug Interactions and Updates* by Hansten and Horn (1994) and *Drug Interaction Facts,* by Tatro (1994).

REFERENCES

Adams F, Fernandez F, Anderson BS: Emergency pharmacotherapy of delirium in the critically ill cancer patient. Psychosomatics, suppl. 1, 27:33, 1986

Andreasen NC, Black DW: Laboratory tests. p. 94. Introductory Textbook of Psychiatry. American Psychiatric Press, Washington, 1991

Bailey I, Bell A, Gray J et al: A trial of the effect of nimodipine on outcome after head injury. Acta Neurochir (Wien) 110:97, 1991

Clinton JE, Sterner S, Stelmachers Z, Ruiz E: Haloperidol for sedation of disruptive emergency patients. Ann Emerg Med 16:319, 1987

Cottrell JE, Patel K, Turndorf H, Ransohoff J: Intracranial pressure changes induced by sodium nitroprusside in patients with intracranial mass lesions. J Neurosurg 48:329, 1978

Dalmady-Israel C, Zasler ND: Post-traumatic seizures: a critical review. Brain Inj 7:263, 1993

Damasio A: The frontal lobes. p. 360–412. In Heilman KM, Valenstein E (eds): Clinical Neuropsychology. Oxford University Press, New York, 1979

Dinan TG, Mobayed M: Treatment resistance of depression after head injury: a preliminary study of amitriptyline response. Acta Psychiatr Scand 85:292, 1992

DuPlessis JJ: High-dose dexamthasone therapy in head injury: a patient group that may benefit from therapy. Br J Neurosurg 6:145, 1992

Evans RW: The postconcussion syndrome and the sequelae of mild head injury. Neurol Clin 10:815, 1992

Evans RW, Gualtieri CT, and Patterson D: Treatment of chronic closed head injury with psychostimulant drugs: a controlled case study and an appropriate evaluation procedure. J Nerv Ment Dis 175:106, 1987

Federoff JP, Starkstein SE, Forrester AW et al: Depression in patients with acute traumatic brain injury. Am J Psychiatry 149:918, 1992

Feldman JA, Fish S: Resuscitation fluid for a patient with head injury and hypovolemic shock. J Emerg Med 9:465, 1991

Garza-Trevino ES, Hollister LE, Overall JE, Alexander WF: Efficacy of combinations in intramuscular antipsychotics and sedative-hypnotics for control of psychotic agitation. Am J Psychiatry 146:1598, 1989

Glenn MB, Joseph AB: The use of lithium for behavioral and affective disorders after traumatic brain injury. J Head Trauma Rehabil 2:68, 1987

Glenn MB, Wroblewski B, Parziale J et al: Lithium carbonate for aggressive behavior or affective instability in ten brain injured patients. Am J Phys Med Rehabil 6:221, 1989

Greendyke RM, Kanter DR, Schuster DB et al: Propranolol treatment of assaultive patients with organic brain disease: a double-blind crossover, placebo-controlled study. J Nerv Ment Dis 174:290, 1986

Gualtieri T, Chandler M, Coons TB, Brown LT: Amantadine: a new clinical profile for traumatic brain injury. Clin Neuropharmacol 12:258–270, 1989

Gualtieri CT, Evans RW: Stimulant treatment for the neurobehavioral sequelae of traumatic brain injury. Brain Inj 2:273, 1988

Hansten PD, Horn JR: Drug Interactions and Updates. Applied Therapeutics, Vancouver, WA, 1994

Horn LJ: "Atypical" medications for the treatment of disruptive, aggressive behavior in the brain-injured patient. J Head Trauma Rehabil 2:18, 1987

Jorge RE, Robinson RG, Starkstein SE et al: Secondary mania following traumatic brain injury. Am J Psychiatry 150:916, 1993

Label LS: Treatment of post-traumatic headaches: maprotiline or amitriptyline? Neurology suppl. 1, 41:247, 1991

Labi MLC, Horn LJ: Hypertension in traumatic brain injury. Brain Inj 4:365, 1990

Lal S, Merbtiz CP, Grip C: Modification of function in head-injured patients with Sinemet. Brain Inj 2:225, 1988

Levin HS: Treatment of postconcussional symptoms with CDP choline. J Neurol Sci 103:S39, 1991

Lipper S, Tuchman MM: Treatment of chronic post-traumatic organic brain syndrome with dextroamphetamine: first reported case. J Nerv Ment Dis 162:366, 1976

Marshall LF: Injury to the head and spinal cord. p. 2224. In Wyngaarden JB (ed): Cecil Textbook of Medicine. 19th Ed. WB Saunders, Philadelphia, 1988

Marshall LF, Bowers SA: Medical management of intracranial pressure. p. 129. In Cooper PR (ed): Head Injury. Williams & Wilkins, Baltimore, 1982

Matz R: Hypothermia: mechanisms and countermeasures. Hosp Pract 1:45, 1986

McIntyre FL, Gasquoine P: Effect of clonidine on post-traumatic memory defects. Brain Inj 4:209, 1990

Menza MA, Murray GB, Holmes VF, Rafuls WA: Controlled study of extrapyramidal reactions in the management of delirious, medically ill patients: intravenous haloperidol versus intravenous haloperidol plus benzodiazepines. Heart Lung 17:238, 1988

Metzger E, Friedman R: Prolongation of the corrected QT and torsades de pointes cardiac arrhythmia associated with IV haloperidol in the medically ill. J Clin Psychopharmacol 13:128–132, 1993

Michals ML, Crimson ML, Roberts S, Childs A: Clozapine response and adverse effects in nine brain-injured patients. J Clin Psychopharmacol 13:198, 1993

Mobayed M, Dinan TG: Buspirone/prolactin response in post head injury depression. J Affective Disord 19:237, 1990

Parmelee DX, O'Shanick GJ: Neuropsychiatric interventions with head injured children and adolescents. Brain Inj 1:41, 1987

Perry PJ, Alexander B, Liskow BI: Antimanic agents. pp. 93–125. In Psychotropic Drug Handbook. 6th Ed. Whitney Publications, Cincinnati, 1991

Pickard JD, Murray GD, Illingworth R et al: Effect of oral nimodipine on the incidence of cerebral infarction and outcome at three months following subarachnoid hemorrhage: British Aneurysm Nimodipine Trial (BRANT). Br Med J 298:636, 1989

Pitts LH: Medical complications of head injury. pp. 327–342. In Cooper PR (ed): Head Injury. Williams & Wilkins, Baltimore, 1982

Relling MV, Evans WE: Genetic polymorphisms of drug metabolism. p. 7–1. In Evans WE, Schentag JJ, Jusko WJ (eds): Applied Pharmacokinetics: Principles of Therapeutic Drug Monitoring. 3rd Ed. Applied Therapeutics, Vancouver, WA, 1992

Robinson RG, Boston JD, Starkstein SE, Price TR: Comparison of mania with depression following brain injury: causal factors. Am J Psychiatry 145:172, 1988

Robinson RG, Starr LP, Kubos KL, Price TR: A 2-year longitudinal study of post-stroke mood disorders: findings during the initial evaluation. Stroke 14:736, 1983

Ropper AH: Trauma of the head and spine. p. 2320. In Isselbacher KJ (ed): Harrison's Principles of Internal Medicine. 13th Ed. McGraw-Hill, New York, 1994

Santos AB, Wohlreich MM, Pinosky ST: Managing agitation in the critical care setting. J S C Med Assoc 88:386, 1982

Saran A: Antidepressants not effective in headache associated with minor closed head injury. Int J Psychiatry Med 18:75, 1988

Saran AS: Depression after minor closed head injury: role of dexamethasone suppression test and antidepressants. J Clin Psychiatry 46:335, 1985

Shukla S, Cook BL, Mukherjee S, Godwin C, Miller MG: Mania following head trauma. Am J Psychiatry 144:93, 1987

Sjaastad O: The headache of challenge in our time: cervicogenic headache. Funct Neurol 5:155, 1990

Smith DA, Perry PJ: Nonneuroleptic treatment of disruptive behavior in organic mental syndromes. Ann Pharmacother 26:1400, 1992

Speech TJ, Rao SM, Osmon DC, Sperry LT: A double-blind controlled study of methylphenidate treatment in closed head injury. Brain Inj 7:333, 1993

Starkstein SE, Federoff P, Bertheir ML, Robinson RG: Manic-depressive and pure manic states after brain lesions. Biol Psychiatry 29:149, 1991

Stern JM. Cranio-cerebral injured patients: a psychiatric clinical description. Scand J Rehabil Med 10:7, 1978

Tatro DS: Drug Interaction Facts. Facts and Comparisons, St. Louis, 1994

Teich S, Chernow B: Specific cardiovascular drugs utilized in the critically ill. Crit Care Clin 1:491, 1985

Temkin NR, Dickmen SS, Wilensky AJ et al: A randomized double-blind study of phenytoin for the prevention of post-traumatic seizures. N Engl J Med 323:497, 1990

Tobin MJ: Neurologic disorders. p. 463. In: Essentials of Critical Care Medicine. Churchill Livingstone, New York, 1989

Tyler GS, McNeely HE, Dick ML: Treatment of post-traumatic headache with amitriptyline. Headache 20:213, 1980

Weiss HD, Stern BJ, Goldberg J: Post-traumatic migraine: chronic migraine precipitated by minor head or neck trauma. Headache 31:451, 1991

Wilkinson MN, Gilchrist E: Post-traumatic headache. Ups J Med Sci Suppl 31:48, 1980

Willmore LJ: Posttraumatic epilepsy. Neurol Clin 10:869, 1992

Wroblewski B, Glenn MB, Cornblatt R et al: Protriptyline as an alternative stimulant medication in patients with brain injury: a series of case reports. Brain Inj 7:353, 1993

APPENDIX
Common Drug Interactions

TABLE 17-1. Common Drug Interactions of Acetaminophen

Drug	Mechanism
Barbiturates	Enhance hepatotoxic potential of acetaminophen overdose by increasing rate of formation of toxic metabolites
Cholestyramine	Inhibits gastrointestinal absorption of acetaminophen
Ethanol	Acute use of ethanol protects against acetaminophen toxicity while chronic use increases toxicity because of inducing acetaminophen metabolism

TABLE 17-2. Common Drug Interactions of Calcium Channel Blockers (e.g., Amlodipine, Diltiazem, Nifedipine, Nimodipine, Verapamil)

Drug	Mechanism
Barbiturates	Increased metabolism
β-Blockers	Inhibition of β-blocker metabolism, additive negative inotropic effect
Carbamazepine	Inhibits metabolism
Cimetidine/ranitidine	Increases oral absorption, blocks metabolism of cimetidine
Lithium	Enhances neurotoxicity
Neuromuscular blocking agents	Prolongs neuromuscular blockade
Quinidine	Inhibits metabolism

TABLE 17-3. Common Drug Interactions of β-Blocking Agents

Drug	Mechanism
Barbiturates	Stimulate hepatic metabolism of metoprolol and propranolol
Calcium channel blockers	May increase serum concentrations of some β-blockers
Cimetidine	Inhibits metabolism of propranolol
Clonidine	Abrupt withdrawal of clonidine may produce exaggerated hypertensive rebound for patients receiving propranolol, timolol, nadolol, and pindolol
Disopyramide	Additive inotropic effect
Epinephrine	Enhances pressor activity of epinephrine when combined with noncardioselective β-blockers (e.g., propranolol)
NSAIDs	Reduce hypotensive effects of β-blockers
Isoproterenol	May reduce effectiveness of isoproterenol in the treatment of asthma
Methyldopa	Produces increased pressor response
Neuroleptics (chlorpromazine, thioridazine, thiothixene)	Competitive metabolic inhibition, thereby increasing pharmacologic activity of both classes of drugs
Prazocin	Additive effect can produce acute postural hypotension
Propafenone	Inhibits metabolic clearance of propranolol and metoprolol
Propoxyphene	Inhibits metabolism of propranolol and metoprolol
Quinidine	Inhibits metabolism of propranolol, timolol, and metoprolol
Rifampin	Enhances metabolism of propranolol and metoprolol
Theophylline	β-Blockers inhibit xanthine metabolism and antagonism bronchodilation

TABLE 17-4. Common Drug Interactions of Clozapine

Drug	Mechanism
Anticholinergics	Additive anticholinergic effects
Carbamazepine	Additive bone marrow suppression
Phenytoin	Stimuates metabolism

TABLE 17-5. Common Drug Interactions of Corticosteroids (e.g., Dexamethasone)

Drug	Mechanism
Barbiturates	Enhancement of corticosteroid metabolism
Oral hypoglycemics	Corticosteroids increase blood glucose concentrations
Carbamazepine	Enhancement of corticosteroid metabolism
Estrogens and oral contraceptives	May enhance pharmacologic effects of corticosteroids
Isoniazid	Enhancement of hepatic metabolism and renal excretion of isoniazid with a net decrease in isoniazid serum concentrations
Rifampin	Enhancement of corticosteroid metabolism
Salicylates	Enhancement of salicylate metabolism

TABLE 17-6. Common Drug Interactions of Haloperidol

Drug	Mechanism
Barbiturates	Increased haloperidol metabolism
Lithium	Enhanced neurotoxicity risk
β-Blockers	Severe hypotensive episodes
Carbamazepine	Increased haloperidol metabolism
Fluoxetine	Combination associated with severe extrapyramidal adverse drug reactions
Guanethidine	Combination associated with increase in blood pressure

TABLE 17-7. Common Drug Interactions of Hydralazine

Drug	Mechanism
Diazoxide	Severe additive hypotensive effects
NSAIDs	Inhibit antihypertensive response of hydralazine

TABLE 17-8 Common Drug Interactions of Neuromuscular Blocking Agents (Pancuronium and Succinylcholine)

Drug	Mechanism
Verapamil and other calcium channel blockers	Prolong neuromuscular blockade by interfering with presynaptic release of neurotransmitters (i.e., pancuronium)
Aminoglycosides	Potential additive neuromuscular blocking effect may prolong respiratory depression associated with succinylcholine
Amphotericin B	Hypokalemia associated with amphotericin may prolong muscle relaxation
Cyclophosphamide	Prolongs neuromuscular blockade by inhibiting pseudocholinesterase
Monoamine oxidase inhibitors (phenelzine)	Prolong neuromuscular blockade by inhibiting pseudocholinesterase
Quinidine	Enhances effects of neuromuscular blocking agents

TABLE 17-9. Common Drug Interactions of Lithium

Drug	Mechanism
ACE inhibitors	Possible increased lithium toxicity risk
Carbamazepine	Possible increased risk of lithium-induced neurotoxicity
Chlorpromazine	Reduced serum concentrations of both drugs
NSAIDs	Indomethacin reduces lithium clearance to increase serum concentrations
Thiazides	Reduced lithium clearance with transiently increased serum concentrations
Benzodiazepines	Hyperthermia with the combination
Iodized salts	Additive in precipitating hypothyroidism
Methyldopa	Increased lithium neurotoxicity risk

TABLE 17-10. Common Drug Interactions of Lorazepam

Drug	Mechanism
Cimetidine	Inhibits metabolism of lorazepam
Ethanol	Enhances psychomotor retardation

TABLE 17-11. Common Drug Interactions of NSAIDs

Drug	Mechanism
ACE inhibitors	Indomethacin may inhibit the antihypertensive response to ACE inhibitors
Cyclosporin	Increased risk of cyclosporin-induced nephrotoxicity
Furosemide	Indomethacin reduces antihypertensive and diuretic effect
Potassium sparing diuretics	Indomethacin-induced acute renal failure with the combination
Salicylates	Reduced NSAID serum concentrations
Osmotic diuretics (mannitol)	Increased lithium clearance
Theophylline	Decreased serum lithium concentration due to increased clearance
Carbonic anhydrase inhibitors	Transient (24 hours) increase in lithium clearance
Sympathomimetics	Decreased pressor effect to direct-acting but not indirect-acting sympathomimetics

TABLE 17-12. Common Drug Interactions of Phenytoin

Drug	Mechanism
Antineoplastics	Increased phenytoin metabolism and reduced metabolism of cisplatin, vinblastin, bleomycin, doxorubicin, methotrexate, and carmustine
Aspirin	Decreased total levels of phenytoin but not free phenytoin due to protein binding displacement
Chloramphenicol	Blocking of phenytoin metabolism
Cimetidine	Blocking of phenytoin metabolism
Oral contraceptives	Enhanced oral contraceptive metabolism
Corticosteroids	Enhanced corticosteroid metabolism
Cyclosporin	Enhanced cyclosporin metabolism
Diazoxide	Enhanced phenytoin metabolism
Digitalis glycosides	Enhanced digoxin metabolism
Disulfiram	Phenytoin metabolism inhibited
Doxycycline	Enhanced metabolism of doxycycline but not other tetracyclines
Felbamate	Phenytoin metabolism inhibited and felbamate metabolism stimulated
Fluconazole	Phenytoin metabolism inhibited
Folic acid	Increased phenytoin metabolism
Furosemide	Gastrointestinal absorption of furosemide inhibited

(*Continued*)

TABLE 17-12. (*Continued*) Common Drug Interactions of Phenytoin

Drug	Mechanism
Isoniazid	Phenytoin metabolism inhibited
Levodopa	Antiparkinsonian activity of levodopa inhibited
Mebendazole	Enhanced mebendazole metabolism
Methadone	Enhanced methadone metabolism
Mexiletine	Enhanced mexiletine metabolism
Omeprazole	Phenytoin metabolism inhibited
Primidone	Enhanced metabolism of primidone to phenobarbital
Quinidine	Enhanced quinidine metabolism
Rifampin	Enhanced phenytoin metabolism
Sulfonamides	Phenytoin metabolism inhibited and phenytoin displaced by sulfisoxazole from protein binding sites
Theophylline	Enhanced theophylline metabolism
Thyroid hormones	Enhanced thyroid hormone metabolism
Valproic acid	Enhanced, decreased, or had no effect on phenytoin metabolism but phenytoin may have decreased valproic acid concentrations
Warfarin	Transient hypoprothrombinemia; after two weeks inhibition of hypoprothrombinemic response occured

TABLE 17-13. Common Drug Interactions of Pressor Agents (Dopamine)

Drug	Mechanism
Ergot alkaloids (ergonavine)	May result in excessive peripheral vasoconstriction

TABLE 17-14. Common Drug Interactions of the Selective Serotonin Re-uptake Inhibitors (e.g., Fluoxetine, Fluvoxamine, Paroxetine, Sertraline)

Drug	Mechanism
Tricyclic antidepressants	Inhibition of metabolism
Carbamazepine	Inhibition of metabolism
Monoamine oxide inhibitors	Potentially fatal serotonin syndrome
l-Tryptophan	Potentially fatal serotonin syndrome

TABLE 17-15. Common Drug Interactions of the Tricyclic Antidepressants (e.g., Amitriptyline, Nortriptyline, Imipramine, Desipramine, Protriptyline, Clomipramine, Trimipramine)

Drug	Mechanism
Alcohol	Additive impairment of motor skills
Amphetamine	Theoretical increase in amphetamine effect
Anticholinergics	Additive anticholinergic effects
Barbiturates	Stimulate metabolism
Bethanidine	Inhibits antihypertensive effect
Carbamazepine	Induces hepatic metabolism
Chlorpromazine	Inhibits metabolism
Cimetidine	Blocks metabolism
Clonidine/phenylephrine	Impairs hepatic metabolism
Fluoxetine	Increases pressor response two- to fourfold
Guanethidine	Possible metabolism inhibition
Labetalol	Inhibit antihypertensive response
Methylphenidate	Reduces metabolism
Monoamine oxidase inhibitors	Inhibit metabolism
Neuroleptics (antipsychotics)	Excessive sympathetic response, mania, impair metabolism
Phenytoin	Increases tricyclic antidepressant plasma concentrations
Quinidine	Impairs phenytoin metabolism
	Impairs cytochrome P450 metabolism

TABLE 17-16. Trade Names of Drugs Commonly Used to Treat Closed Head Injuries

Generic Name	Trade Name
Amitriptyline	Elavil
Amphotericin B	Fungisone
Alprazolam	Xanax
Bupropion	Wellbutrin
Buspirone	Buspar
Carbamazepine	Tegretol
Chlorpromazine	Thorazine
Cimetidine	Tagamet
Clomipramine	Anafranil
Clonidine	Catapres
Desipramine	Norpramin
Fluvoxamine	Luvox
Fluoxetine	Prozac
Furosemide	Lasix
Guanethidine	Ismelin
Haloperidol	Haldol
Imipramine	Tofranil
Isoniazid	INH
Labetalol	Normodyne
Lorazepam	Ativan
Mebendazole	Vermox
Methadone	Dolophine
Methylphenidate	Ritalin
Mexiletine	Mexitil
Nortriptyline	Pamelor
Omeprazole	Prilosec
Phenytoin	Dilantin
Paroxetine	Paxil
Primidone	Mysoline
Protriptyline	Vivactil
Quinidine	Quinaglute
Ranitidine	Zantac
Rifampin	Rifadin
Sertraline	Zoloft
Theophylline	Theo-Dur
Thioridazine	Mellaril
Thiothixene	Navane
Trimipramine	Surmontil
Valproic acid	Depakene, Depakote
Verapamil	Calan, Isoptin

Neurologic Impairment and Disability Evaluation

18

Nathan D. Zasler

The area of impairment and disability evaluation is probably one of the more confounding and misunderstood areas of health care-related work as it applies to caring for persons with injury residua and/or functional limitations due to disease. Traditionally, impairment and disability evaluation has not been taught as part of the medical school curriculum, nor is it typically included in any neuroscience-related residency training program.

The task of making determinations regarding impairment and disability in persons with postconcussive syndrome is fraught with potential obstacles and confounding issues. This is due to the subtle yet complex nature of the deficits involved, as well as the lack of formal "rating systems" for postconcussive-type deficits. The boundaries remain unclear between different medical disciplines—neurology, physiatry, neurosurgery, and other specialty areas—involved with the ongoing care of this patient population relative to impairment and disability evaluation as well as care in general.

This chapter attempts to provide a physiatrically based review of the issues germane to evaluating both impairment and disability of persons with postconcussive syndrome, who compose one of the more challenging patient populations seen by neuromedical specialists. Physiatry is a medical specialty concerned with the optimal functional restoration of patients with disabilities, including physical treatment of neuromuscular impairments and the use of electrodiagnostic studies, such as electromyography and evoked potentials. Its focus also extends to helping disabled individuals adapt psychosocially to their physical or cognitive impairment.

NOMENCLATURE ISSUES

Within the field of neurorehabilitation and disability, a historic problem relating to a lack of a common language existed prior to the World Health Organization (WHO)'s publication in 1980 of a system for classifying consequences of disease. WHO developed this taxonomy, known as the International Classification of Impairments, Disabilities, and Handicaps (ICIDH), to assist with structuring of a comprehensive model of illness. Probably the most important concept introduced by this model is that any illness can be represented at four levels: pathology, impairment, disability, and handicap. The term *illness* is generally used to refer to all the consequences of any disease as well as its social implications. On the other hand, the term *disease* is more restrictive and refers to a specific diagnosis or pathology.

Understanding this terminology is important in the sense that health care interventions, including rehabilitation, may affect one level and not another. For example, a person with short-term memory deficits following a mild traumatic brain injury may be able to learn compensatory strategies utilizing memory aides and may show no impairments on neuropsychological tests of short-term memory. It is also critical not to "bundle" terms, as often happens in the real world, for example when a physician performs a *whole person impairment rating* using the American Medical Association's (1993) Guidelines for Evaluation of Permanent Impairment (GEPI) and claims in the report to have done a *disability* evaluation. Appropriate distinctions must be made between the aforementioned WHO classification categories for clinical, research, and disability administrative purposes.

Pathology refers to the perturbation in function occurring within an organ or organ system in the body. Pathology has traditionally been the focus of medical care in our society both from a clinical and an administrative perspective. The International Classification of Diseases (ICD), for example, focuses primarily on pathologies, not impairments, disabilities, or handicap. As it applies to postconcussive syndromes, a pathologic diagnosis is important in order to optimize effective management and make statements regarding prognosis and natural history.

Impairments are the direct and indirect neuroanatomic and neurophysiologic consequences of the underlying pathology. The types of impairments germane to assessing persons with postconcussive syndromes include diplopia, hearing loss, olfactory dysfunction, balance dysfunction, and cognitive deficits. Psychological aberrations would also be classified as impairments in line with the ICIDH definition. Importantly, certain pathologic entities, including trauma, multiple sclerosis, and stroke, may produce no measurable impairment. In contrast, some entities such as conversion disorders, factitious disorders, and other "nonorganic" conditions (Ruff et al., 1993) produce functional difficulties despite the absence of any anatomic lesion. Finally, impairment evaluation does not take into account a person's vocational, avocational, sociocultural, or educational background.

Disability can be thought of as the functional loss that the individual suffers and how the said loss interacts with the environment as a result of the impairment. This disability can be viewed as a behavioral manifestation of the disease under a specific set of circumstances. In postconcussive syndrome as in other conditions, this may be reflected in a decreased ability to work, drive, and/or pursue hobbies. Psychological issues and the local milieu impact significantly on the manner in which a disability is manifested relative to severity and nature.

Handicap is the expression of the impact of a given pathology, impairment, or disability on an individual's specific social roles and activities. In this situation, normality is defined relative to the patient's own social context. Variables that may dictate what is "normal" for an individual include age, sex, and social and cultural factors. Importantly, there may arise situations in which the degree of handicap correlates poorly with the degree of functional disability; handicap is shaped by environmental factors such as social expectations, legal stipulations, family network, financial solvency and community physical barriers, whereas disability is not. The term *social disadvantage* is a valuable near synonym for handicap (National Institutes of Health, 1993).

PRACTICAL CONSEQUENCES OF THE ICIDH MODEL

The focus of clinical intervention should evolve over time from concentration on making a pathologic diagnosis to diagnosing and treating the resultant disability in order to reduce handicap. In practical terms, this requires the clinician to spend adequate time in inquiring as to the functional difficulties. Consequently, the examiner must also include assessment of functional abilities during the physical examination as opposed to purely "clinical" signs. Our evolving health care system, driven by health care reform, has not given adequate consideration to the aforementioned aspects of clinical care with models such as diagnostic-related groups. This has led to little or no consideration of such factors when considering hospital use trends. Additionally, our general model of health care has historically been curative, not ameliorative. In other words, we tend to focus, as a health care system, on management of acute illness, which is viewed to be self-limiting and to occur within a social vacuum without much heed being given to potential resultant functional disability or handicap. Finally, multidisciplinary medical management allows for the most effective methodologies to be instituted for treating the breadth of neurologic disease from pathology to handicap (Ragnersson et al., 1993).

In sum, impairments need to be measured to understand and prescribe appropriate treatment. Impairment measures allow the examiner to determine whether the outcome is due to neurologic recovery processes, environmental alterations, or compensatory adaptations. Measures of clinical disability or functional limitations can tell us whether function is improving in a manner that will be meaningful for the person. Real world disability measures give information regarding whether the skill was in fact utilized by the individual. Handicap measures tell us if the interventions as a whole correlate with outcomes valued by most of society (Johnston et al., 1993).

MEASUREMENT ISSUES IN NEUROLOGIC ASSESSMENT

It is critical for clinicians, and in particular those who formally evaluate impairment and disability, to be familiar with currently available measurement techniques applicable to neurologic conditions such as traumatic brain injury (TBI). Quantification of an observation in an objective fashion is essential if such evaluations are to serve as the basis for administrative decisions regarding disability determination. Practitioners should become familiar with standardized measures of cognition, behavior, and when available, the array of postconcussive somatic conditions such as hearing loss, vertigo, and tinnitus. Reasons for using objective measurement tools include establishment of diagnosis, prognosis, severity, and outcome. Clinicians should also be aware of whether or not the measure is generalizable from one population to another; specifically, a measure of affective status used in stroke populations may not be transferable to a person with depression following concussion. Additionally, it is critical to remain aware of both the false negative and false positive rates with any particular measure for the population in question.

One must also be familiar with the variety of levels of measurement, including nominal, ordinal, interval, and ratio (Wade, 1992). There are significant differences between these levels of measurement, which affect the utility of the data generated and how they are interpreted. Finally, measure construction can be of three types. The simplest involves mere description, of which multi-item indices such as the Barthel ADL Index are one example. True ratio measurements probably give the most absolute data, such as measuring the gait speed or stride length.

There is significant consensus in medical rehabilitation that functional assessment needs to be improved and standardized. Recent publications have espoused specific criteria to guide selection of rehabilitation-related standards (Johnston et al., 1992). Practical criteria for assessment of persons with brain injury can be extracted from these standards. Issues regarding validity, both predictive and construct, and reliability must be analyzed carefully. Ceiling and floor limitations of existing functional measures must be kept in mind. This is particularly germane to the mild TBI group with respect to ceiling effects of most measures. Most of the functional assessment measures used in the field of medical rehabilitation require clinician training and "following by the book" the assessment methodology. The aforementioned approach is in contradistinction to the more traditional methods used by physicians in the evaluation of impairment and disability, such as the GEPI (American Medical Association, 1993). It is my opinion that the GEPI is suboptimal for the evaluation of impairment following TBI, particularly in cases of mild neural insult, such as results in postconcussive syndromes. There are no scientific studies establishing the predictive validity of the guidelines for its common use, nor are there any correlation and/or scientific data demonstrating a link between level of impairment and potential for the injured person to return to work, school, or other activities, including independent living. There are no published data in the GEPI or elsewhere for that matter, that demonstrate reliability of the recommended impairment ratings.

We know that human work performance is a multifaceted interaction of strengths as well as weaknesses, which are determined by many factors aside from impairments per se. These factors include community barriers, job demands, and willingness of the employer to work together with the person to facilitate job reentry. Clinicians *and* administrators are generally not in a position to judge adequately the summation of these factors relative to traditional methodologies used to determine impairment and disability as affecting work reentry potential. If we are to provide responsible opinions on disability status, we are obliged to evaluate not only impairment but also the resultant disability and handicap. Evaluation of disability and handicap is a time-consuming process because it requires lengthy inquiries regarding the functional implications, if any, of the impairments and a thorough understanding of the patient's environment both at work and in the community. Community-based issues that need to be clarified include availability of transportation, mobility barriers in the community and workplace, accessibility issues, and need for workplace modifications (whether for cognitive, behavioral or physical sequelae of brain injury) (Wehman and Kreutzer, 1990).

THE GUIDES TO EVALUATION OF PERMANENT IMPAIRMENT

First published in 1971, the AMA Guides provide information to assist clinicians in rating *permanent* impairment. The GEPI is presently in its fourth edition. Comprehensive rating systems are provided for all types of impairments and organ systems except for those germane to psychologic and psychiatric disease. The GEPI is divided into four main sections: (1) concepts of impairment evaluation; (2) records and reports; (3) definitive protocols for evaluation of a particular body part, function, or system; and (4) reference tables keyed to evaluation protocols. The examiner must describe the specific clinical findings related to each impairment noted, as well as document any absent data or inability to obtain specific relevant data. Each impairment rated should be referenced to the appropriate section of the GEPI with an explanation of the percent rating assigned. All impairment ratings should be subsequently listed in summary fashion prior to determining a whole-person impairment rating.

As per the GEPI, the evaluating clinician should include a narrative history; results of the most recent clinical evaluation; assessment of current clinical status; plans for future treatment, including rehabilitation and reevaluation; diagnosis and clinical impressions; and an estimate of time for full or partial recovery. The clinician must also analyze the findings relative to the impact of the medical condition(s) on life activities, static or stabilized nature of the medical condition, or chance of sudden or subtle incapacitation as a result of the medical condition. The risk of injury, harm, or further impairment with activity needed to meet personal, social, or occupational demands must also be addressed. The clinician should also elaborate on any restrictions or accommodations regarding required activities to meet life demands. The medical condition in question must be stable before permanency can be established and/or rated.

The GEPI lists four criteria that must be met before a medical condition may be considered stable: (1) the clinical condition is stabilized and not likely to improve with surgical intervention or active medical treatment, and thus medical maintenance care only is warranted; (2} the degree of impairment is not likely to change by more than 3 percent within the next year; (3) employability is not likely to improve with surgical intervention or active medical treatment; and (4) the patient is not likely to suffer sudden or subtle incapacitation. If the aforementioned conditions are not met, impairment evaluation should be deferred.

There continues to be controversy over the duration of both neurologic and functional plateaus following TBI, including postconcussive syndrome. It should also be realized that the concept and/or definition of permanency may differ between the GEPI and other disability determination systems or programs. Additionally, examiners should be fully aware of the fact that the GEPI was developed in an attempt to produce a system that enabled clinicians to predict disability level by evaluating simple physical organ system impairments. The basic flaw in this tenet is that it mistakenly analogizes the task of impairment rating with determination of disability status. This not only is a grave mistake but it is potentially a significant disservice to the disabled person, society, and the administrative disability determination system.

When a patient presents with multisystem trauma, there may be impairments involving several parts of the body as well as several parts of the nervous system (e.g., the brain, spinal cord, and/or peripheral nerves). Individual impairments should be separately calculated and their whole-person values combined by using the Combined Values Chart in the GEPI. In general, only the medical condition causing the greatest impairment should be evaluated. This presents a problem in a patient with postconcussive deficits concurrent with more significant bodily impairments such as loss of a limb. When assessing central nervous system (CNS) impairment, one can assign five categories based on functional neuroanatomy, relative to

1. Impairments involving structures of the cerebrum
2. Impairments involving structures of the midbrain
3. Impairments involving structures of the pons
4. Impairments involving structures of the medulla
5. Impairments involving the spinal cord

There are multiple disorders of the cerebrum that need to be considered, including disturbances of consciousness and awareness, aphasia or other communication disorders, mental status abnormalities, behavioral disturbances, and special types of preoccupation/obsession. The most severe of the aforementioned cerebral deficits should be used to represent the cerebral impairment. Other secondary cerebral impairments include major motor or sensory abnormalities, movement disorders, episodic neurologic disorders, and sleep and arousal problems. Any of these last four categories may be combined with the most severe of the first five categories by means of the combined values chart, and the result would represent the estimate of the total cerebral impairment.

According to the GEPI, the evaluation of sensory and motor impairments due to cerebral disorders should be based on the examinee's ability to perform activities of daily living (which again brings up the concern of analogizing impairment and disability rating in the process of what should otherwise be only an impairment rating system). Sensory disturbances may be related to thalamic pain, phantom limb pain, causalgia, disorders of stereognosis, and disturbances of two-point and position sense. Motor disturbances may occur with or without associated weakness. Nonparetic motor deficits may include movement disorders, tonal aberrations, restrictions in expression of motor behavior, as in bradykinesia, and ataxia.

Impairments due to aphasia or dysphasia are based on gradations of impairment severity and on the results of specific language/communication-based testing. Some of the objective assessment strategies include naming objects by sight or describing them after reading about them, repeating speech, following oral and written commands, reading and comprehending, writing, spelling, and demonstrating the use of an object (a test for aphrasia). As with other impairments, the combined values chart should be used to calculate the whole-person impairment.

Mental status and integrative functions are determined of the basis of bedside assessment (see Ch. 19). Ten "traditional" measures of cognitive function are used:

1. Orientation to time, person, and place
2. Recent recall
3. Ability to remember and repeat a series of digits and repeat them in reverse order
4. Ability to perform serial subtraction of 7s from 100 or 3s from 20
5. Ability to perform other simple calculations
6. Ability to repeat three unrelated words
7. Ability to spell a word forward and backward
8. Ability to repeat a short paragraph
9. Ability to understand and explain proverbs or abstract thought
10. Judgment

The aforementioned tests of cognitive function can only be performed in the absence of significant aphasia. In the presence of a significant communication disturbance and a disturbance of mental status, the greater of the two impairments should be used as the impairment estimate. The methodology for bedside mental status testing may underestimate the extent of more subtle albeit functionally significant cognitive deficits in patients following mild TBI. Once again, the GEPI requires the examiner to grade mental status impairment based on ability to carry out activities of daily living, thereby confounding impairment and disability assessment procedures.

Emotional and behavioral disturbance ratings are again based on the relative degree of impairment in "daily functions," ranging from mild to severe. The disorders that may fall under this category of impairments include depression, emotional lability, mania, pathologic laughing or crying, psychosis, disinhibited behavior, and others. As with many other impairment measures, there is a significant degree of subjectivity within each category of impairment relative to the percent impairment assigned.

Disturbances in the level of consciousness and awareness are rated on the basis of patients' ability to care for themselves relative to the overall level of altered consciousness, with persistent vegetative state or irreversible coma correlating with a 50 to 90 percent impairment rating. Brief repetitive or persisting alteration in state of consciousness that limits ability to perform usual activities correlates with an impairment rating of 0 to 14 percent. The impairment criteria for disturbances in consciousness and awareness do *not* apply to seizure disorders, syncope (neurogenic or cardiogenic), or sleep/wake cycle disturbances.

Episodic neurologic disorders include three main subcategories: syncope with alteration in awareness, convulsive disorders, and sleep and arousal disorders. As these disorders may relate to other organ systems outside the CNS, the impairments should be combined. If a disorder is expected to change to a moderate or greater degree within the next year, the impairment should not be rated, as it is not permanent. This class of disorders should be described relative to onset, duration, associated symptoms, and impact on daily function. Even in the worst case scenario, the highest level of whole-person impairment would be 70 percent for this class of disorders.

The forebrain assessment should also include cranial nerves I and II. All too often, examiners neglect to assess cranial nerve I, which is responsible for olfactory function. Taste may be perceived by the examinee to be altered when in fact only the sense of smell has been perturbed. Olfactory impairment may be partial or complete (see Ch. 21). Additionally, dysosmia may occur in the form of parosmias or cacosmias, which need to be taken into consideration in the impairment rating. The maximum impairment rating for loss of smell is 5 percent of the whole person. Optic nerve impairments related to decreased visual acuity should be combined with any other visual system impairment. The GEPI provides a table to assist in rating impairment due to visual field loss.

Of the remaining CNS structures, namely midbrain, pons, medulla, and spinal cord, most are not relevant to evaluation of impairment following mild TBI. Exceptions are provided by the following correlations of specific impairments with CNS dysfunction. Midbrain injury that results in extra-ocular muscle dysfunction related to cranial nerves III, IV, and VI may produce diplopia. The extent of diplopia in the various directions of gaze is determined in an arc perimeter at 33 cm or with a bowl perimeter. Pontine dysfunction may result in vestibulocochlear nerve aberrations. Tinnitus in the presence of unilateral hearing loss may impair speech discrimination and adversely influence the patient's ability to conduct daily activities. Up to 5 percent may be added because of tinnitus to an impairment estimate for severe unilateral hearing loss. Vestibular dysfunction may be unilateral or bilateral (see Ch. 9). Vertigo is rated as a single entity without reference to its many potential associated symptoms. Impairment ratings range from 1 to 70 percent of the whole person. Disorders of station and gait may result from a variety of conditions involving the central as well as the peripheral nervous system. Whole-person impairments for gait disturbance range from 1 to 60 percent. Altered libido, a common postconcussive complaint, can be rated under sexual impairment criteria and receives a whole-person impairment rating of 1 to 9 percent.

The foregoing information on the GEPI provides at best a brief introduction to its utility, as well as limitations, for rating permanent impairments in persons with mild TBI. Clinicians should remember, however, that such injuries often occur in conjunction with both cranial adnexal and musculoligamentous injuries, such as occur following cervical whiplash injury, which requires rating of these sequelae and combined whole-person impairments (American Medical Association, 1993).

POSTCONCUSSION SYNDROME AND DSM-IV

Appendix B of the DSM-IV contains a "Criteria Sets and Axes Provided for Further Study" (American Psychiatric Association, 1994). Included in this appendix is a listing for "post-concussional disorder." This diagnostic category and others were excluded as official categories or axes owing to a presumption of insufficient research-based information. As defined in DSM-IV, a diagnosis of mild neurocognitive disorder, also listed as a "further study" item, should not be used in the presence of a history of TBI, concussive or otherwise.

The proposed research criteria for postconcussional disorder include a history of "head trauma" that has caused significant cerebral concussion, with quantified cognitive assessment demonstrating attention or memory deficits. *Suggested* threshold criteria for postconcussive syndrome include two of the following: (1) a period of unconsciousness lasting longer than 5 minutes, (2) a period of post-traumatic amnesia lasting more than 12 hours, or (3) a new-onset seizure disorder (or marked worsening of a preinjury seizure disorder) that occurs within the first 6 months after injury. It is my opinion that the first two of these threshold criteria potentially exclude patients with true organicity following mild TBI, in that mild TBI without associated loss of consciousness and/or significant amnesia occurs quite regularly (Dalmady-Israel and Zasler, 1993). Seizures are, in fact, fairly much a nonissue for this patient population and should in my opinion *not* be used as a threshold criterion (Horn and Zasler, 1992). Three of the following symptoms must occur shortly after the trauma (time frame unspecified) and last at least 3 months: easy fatigability; disordered sleep; headache; vertigo/dizziness; irritability and/or aggression (with little or no provocation); behavioral changes, including anxiety, depression, or affective lability; personality changes; and/or apathy. The cognitive, behavioral, and somatic symptoms must have their onset following the concussion and/or must represent a substantial (not defined) worsening of a preexisting symptom. According to the proposed research criteria, the disturbance must cause significant impairment in social or occupational functioning and represent a significant decline from a prior level of functioning, including a decline in academic performance that was temporally correlated with the injury in question.

The presenting symptoms following concussion must be differentiated from dementia due to brain injury and other mental disorders. Concurrent unrelated as well as related psychiatric diagnoses must be considered even in the presence of a clear injury and resultant concussion. Clinical psychological and psychiatric conditions such as depression, pain disorder, and less frequently, post-traumatic stress disorder need to be considered in both litigating as well as nonlitigating patients. Less commonly, clinicians may encounter examinees with somatoform disorders, factitious disorders, and malingering, which must all be considered in the differential diagnosis of the individual after mild TBI, particularly in cases that involve readily apparent secondary gain, as with litigation, avoidance of work, and/or financial gain (Zasler, 1993).

Memory impairments following concussion would fall under the category of "amnestic disorder due to traumatic brain injury" (American Psychiatric Association, 1994). The diagnostic criteria for amnestic disorder include memory impairment manifested by difficulties in ability to learn new information or by the inability to recall previously learned information. By definition, the impairment must produce disability relative to social and/or occupational functioning and represent a significant decline in prior level of functioning. There must also be evidence of a direct pathophysiologic link between the condition (mild TBI) and the amnestic disorder.

DISABILITY EVALUATION UNDER WORKERS' COMPENSATION

Workers' compensation laws typically define three categories of payments for persons unable to work owing to injury or illness (American Medical Association, 1993). Financial compensation may be for (1) lost wages due to temporary total disability; (2) payment for medical bills; or (3) permanent disability, partial or total. The criteria for temporary total disability, as defined by most workers' compensation boards, are met when a claimant is unable to earn wages, return to work is expected, and the medical condition has not yet stabilized. On the other hand, temporary partial disability implies that the claimant has returned to work but is earning a lower wage than previously. Regarding permanent disability, worker's compensation awards are normallly independent of work capacity; rather, financial remuneration is dependent upon the associated economic loss associated with the permanent medical impairment. Benefits are normally paid based on an average weekly wage with a capped payment schedule. A rating of partial permanent disability as necessary when the loss of use or loss of the body part, function, or system is less than total. No formulas exist that combine physician-determined impairment ratings with other factors to determine the percentage by which the industrial use of the employee's body is impaired (American Medical Association, 1993). The final determination regarding work capacity status is made by an agency representative based on available medical and nonmedical information on the claimant's ability to meet personal, social, or occupational demands or to meet statutory or regulatory requirements (LaForge and Harrison, 1987).

DISABILITY EVALUATION UNDER SOCIAL SECURITY

According to the Social Security Administration (1992), disability is defined as the "inability to engage in *any* substantial gainful activity by reason of a medically determinable physical or mental impairment which can be expected to result in death or has lasted or can last for a continued period of not less than 12 months." The latest disability evaluation guidelines published by the Social Security Administration in early 1994 do not affect in any significant manner the assessment of neurologic impairment and/or disability. There are two sections, one for adults and one for children, each divided into thirteen subsections. Adults are classified on the basis of chronological age older than 18 years. If an applicant's impairment is consistent with his or her symptoms, signs, or laboratory findings, a presumption is made in the absence of work that the applicant meets Social Security requirements for disability.

Social Security presently has two programs for disability, Title II, the Social Security Disability Insurance (SSDI) program and Title XVI, the Supplemental Security Income (SSI) program, respectively. The definitions for disability are essentially the same under both programs—specifically, an individual must have a "medically determinable impairment." This translates to an impairment with medically demonstrable anatomic, physiologic, or psychological abnormalities. Such abnormalities are medically determinable if they manifest themselves as signs or laboratory findings apart from symptoms. Abnormalities that manifest only as symptoms are not medically determinable.

The Title II program is provided through a trust fund into which workers contribute through FICA tax on their earnings. There are three basic categories under Title II. Title XVI provides supplemental income to individuals who meet specific financial criteria, are 65 years of age or older, or are blind. There are four basic categories to Section XVI. There are four sections in the SSDI booklet, including general information, confidentiality of Social Security records, program information, and medical evaluation criteria. According to SSDI criteria, the examiner must stipulate both degree and duration modifiers. Specifically, degree of impairment modifiers include "partial" and "total" whereas duration modifiers include "temporary" and "permanent." This is in contrast to the GEPI, which only is used for assessment of permanent impairment. Examiners should also be aware of "presumptive disability" determinations, which allow a person with a disability to receive benefits prior to the required normal duration stipulated by the Social Security Administration if they are expected to persist with a level of disability that is severe enough and anticipated to last at least 1 year from the date of disability onset (Olsheski and Growick, 1994).

The most relevant section for evaluation of impairment associated with any level of TBI is Section 11.18 (cerebral trauma). Other potentially relevant sections include 11.02 (epilepsy, major motor seizures), 11.03 (epilepsy, minor motor seizures), 11.04 (central nervous system vascular accident), and 12.02 (organic mental disorders) (Social Security Administration, 1992). The impairment criteria as set forth by the Social Security Administration are inadequate for assessment of deficits associated with postconcussive syndromes.

EMPLOYABILITY: MANAGEMENT AND ADMINISTRATIVE CONSIDERATIONS

One of the major issues relative to the administrative determination of claimant's work capability of a claimant is whether the claimant can work with or without accommodation. Employability determinations are dependent on several variables, including capacity to travel to and from work, ability to perform assigned tasks and duties at work and/or related to work, and ability to be at work (Cailliet, 1969). Employability determination is also dependent on ongoing reassessment of work performance through monitoring of attendance, work quality, and conduct. From a medical standpoint the initial burden of proof typically lies with the claimant. The medical evaluation protocol relative to any employment determination should remain independent of the person's motivation to work. Medical determination of employability should include developing an understanding of the job specifics, assessing available medical documentation, and demonstrating a causal relationship between the medical condition and the employment deficiency. Inquiries should be made regarding job specifics, including performance, physical activity requirements, reliability, availability, productivity, and "useful service life" (Koppenhoefer, 1988).

GLOBAL DISABILITY MEASURES IN TRAUMATIC BRAIN INJURY

The Glasgow Outcome Scale (GOS) is probably the most commonly used global assessment measure in the brain injury research literature (Jennett et al., 1976). It provides an ordinal rating using five outcome points: dead, vegetative, severe disability, moderate disability, and good recovery. GOS ratings strongly correlate with measures of TBI severity, including the Glasgow Coma Scale. Disability evaluators should be familiar, however, with the limitations of a "gross" outcome measure such as the GOS for a condition in which measurement of impairment and functional disability is relatively subtle. Specifically, persons with mild TBI may have significant functional disability and yet have a "good outcome" by the GOS based on its rather broad outcome criteria.

The Disability Rating Scale (DRS) is probably the best overall global methodology for functional status following TBI (Rappaport et al., 1970). The DRS actually combines both impairment and disability determination in the final formulation of the numerical score, which ranges from 0 to 30. The DRS has been well studied and has been found to be a reliable and valid measure. Once again, however, the DRS, like the GOS but to a lesser extent, tends to be insensitive to the types of functional deficits that are seen in the postconcussive population.

There are also multiple measures of activity of daily living status that are used to measure disability level in persons with TBI. Some of the more commonly used measures are the Functional Independence Measure, Functional Assessment Measure, Program Evaluation Conference System, Glasgow Assessment Scale, and Sickness Impact Profile (Hall, 1992; Hall et al., 1993). Because of the general significant reliance that these measures have on gross physical capabilities, as well as their lack of adequately sensitive cognitive, behavioral, and psychosocial parameters, these measures are relatively insensitive to functional disability issues in patient status following mild TBI (Hall, 1992).

The multidimensionality of dysfunction following mild TBI, as well as its tendency to be subtle, makes the presently available and commonly used global outcome and assessment measures insufficiently sensitive for clinical management or rehabilitation planning. Further research directed at development of multidimensional outcome assessment instruments for postconcussive patients is needed within the field of neurorehabilitation and neurologic care (Johnston et al., 1991). Table 18-1 lists recommended general functional measures for TBI, with the caveat that the majority will be too general and insensitive to accurately rate functional performance in persons with mild TBI.

PAIN ISSUES IN IMPAIRMENT AND DISABILITY EVALUATION

Two of the most difficult postconcussive complaints to assess relative to impairment and disability are headache and chronic pain. The examiner should attempt to quantify any pain complaint, including that of headache, and its impact on functional skills as part of the evaluation.

The GEPI contains an entire section on impairment evaluation of pain, including headache. The need is crucial to assess the "eight Ds": duration, dramatization, diagnostic dilemma, and drugs, dependence, depression, disuse, dysfunction. If the pain condition is to be rated, it must be stable and unlikely to change in the future despite therapy. Pain intensity (minimal, slight, moderate, and marked) as well as pain frequency (intermittent, occasional, frequent, constant) must be documented. Headache impairment is estimated by using the general pain impairment guidelines in the GEPI. A pain intensity-frequency grid is used to describe the degree of impairment resulting from any pain disorder (American Medical Association, 1993).

Multiple methodologies are available for providing some level of pain quantification beyond gross subjective reporting by the examinee. Measurement of overt motor behaviors, cognitive verbal responses, and physiologic variables comprise the three major approaches to pain quantification.

Methods for measurement of overt motor behaviors include direct behavioral observations; automated measurement devices such as "uptime" recorders; self-monitored observations such as daily diaries; and self-reports of functional disability using such standardized methods as the Sickness Impact Profile (Bergner et al., 1981; Bradley et al., 1989). Although measurement of overt motor behaviors is a very practical approach to assessment of the impact of pain on physical functioning, it is limited by patient initiation of behavior change due to the assessment procedure itself, as well as by the lack of information provided to the examiner regarding affective and sensory components of the pain experience. Examiners should understand that in patients with cognitive impairment following mild TBI, self-monitored ob-

TABLE 18-1. Functional Measures in Traumatic Brain Injury

Scale	Reliable	Valid	No. of Items	Time (min)	Phone	Self-Report
Disability Rating Scale	Yes	Yes	8	10	Yes	No
Glasgow Outcome Scale	Yes	Yes	1	<5	Yes	No
Modified Barthel index	Yes	Yes	15	15	Yes	No
Functional Inventory Measure	Yes	Yes	18	<30	Yes(?)	No
Functional Assessment Measure	Yes	?	30	<40	Yes(?)	No
Rancho Los Amigos Scale	Yes(?)	Yes(?)	1	<5	Yes	No
Adapted pulses	Yes	Yes	6	10	Yes	No

(Adapted from M Hall, 1992, with permission.)

servations must be taken with a "grain of salt" and probably should not be used as the *only* assessment strategy.

The area of pain assessment that has received the most attention by far is measurement of affective responses to pain. The earliest affective responses to pain typically are driven by the autonomic nervous system and produce symptoms of anxiety. Chronic pain, on the other hand, tends to produce vegetative signs of depression and hypochondriasis. Multiple psychometric measures have been used to evaluate "chronic pain behavior" and associated affective status. These include the Minnesota Multiphasic Personality Inventory (MMPI), Illness Behavior Questionnaire, pain drawing, Symptom Checklist-90, and Million Behavioral Health Inventory (Bradley et al., 1989). The examiner must be aware of the limitations of such testing and the anticipated "deviations from the norm" when testing persons with mild TBI (e.g., MMPI profile elevations typically occur on scales 1, 2, 3, 7, and 8 in persons with mild TBI as opposed to the population at large. Interestingly, such MMPI scale elevations are fairly parallel to those seen in chronic pain patients.

Several methods of assessing cognitive distortions and coping strategies related to pain have been developed. There are several questionnaires that measure cognitive distortions concerning general life experiences and pain-related problems. Several pain assessment techniques have been developed that rely on subjective judgments, including category scales, visual analog scales, the McGill Pain Questionnaire, and ratio scales of verbal pain descriptors. The examiner should also establish how pain has affected spousal relationships and family interactions where this consideration is applicable (Bradley et al., 1989).

Although not commonly used for "objectification" of pain complaints, measurement of physiologic variables may provide additional information regarding subjective pain complaints. Some of the methods used include electromyographic techniques, particularly with surface electrodes; use of pressure algometers or "dolorimeters" to assess myofascial trigger point sensitivity; measurement of galvanic skin response; and measurement of skin surface temperature (including thermographic evaluation). The last remains the most controversial (Bradley et al., 1989).

Given the frequency of pain complaints following concussion, examiners should be aware of the aforementioned assessment techniques as well as the GEPI section on pain impairment evaluation (see Ch. 15 in DSM-IV [American Psychiatric Association, 1994]). Obviously, pain issues need to be integrated, when present, with the other observed impairments, and overall disability determinations should only be made once this is accomplished.

PRACTICAL CONSEQUENCES OF CURRENT ASSESSMENT METHODOLOGIES

Tradition has dictated that disability determination remain within the administrative purview. I have always been faced with an ethical dilemma relative to leaving "disability determination" to administrative personnel, given their lack of medical and disability training. Presently, most administrative bodies making such decisions do so according to general criteria relative to ability to perform prior duties based on education, training, and experience and on ability to perform *any* competitive employment (McBride, 1963).

Administrative personnel make such decisions based on available medical and paramedical documentation, including impairment ratings, insurance company impairment forms, and "functional capacity" evaluation forms, which are all typically completed by the treating physician. In most cases, however, there is only an estimation of functional capabilities and no true functional assessment is completed. This practice is in my opinion irresponsible. Either physicians should have a functional capacity evaluation performed or should document that the forms cannot be filled out owing to lack of objective, standardized information. Bedside assessment of impairment may not necessarily correlate particularly well with a person's general level of functional disability and handicap, particularly following mild TBI. To an even greater extent, there are concerns regarding how such impairment ratings correlate with a specific set of job responsibilities and/or with the work environment.

RECOMMENDATIONS FOR IMPAIRMENT AND DISABILITY EVALUATION IN MILD TBI

The following section delineates a proposed methodology for impairment and disability evaluation of the postconcussive claimant. Since adequate valid and reliable impairment measures for this population are lacking, the following approach is suggested relative to one potential systematic alternative.

Given the importance of neuropsychological testing in the assessment of cognitive impairment in this patient population, any clinician working in this area should develop a relatively sophisticated appreciation of the sensitivity, specificity, validity, and reliability of the measures used. The following ten caveats should be assessed when reviewing the quality of neuropsychological testing (Zasler, 1994):

1. Has preinjury intellectual function been adequately estimated? Look for review of educational and/or military records. It is critical that assessment be made relative to standardized scores, and if these are not available, data should be corrected for patient age, education, and demographics (i.e., by using Heaton norms, the Barona regression equation, etc.).
2. Were unbiased collateral informants interviewed who could testify to pre- and/or postinjury status?
3. Was adequate acknowledgment of preinjury medical and psychological history, including prior TBI, taken into consideration?
4. Were other factors potentially affecting test performance adequately taken into consideration and acknowledged as potentially contributing to the profile generated (e.g., psychoemotional issues, pain, vestibular symptoms)?
5. Were actuarial cutoff scores and norm-referenced actuarial judgment methods used to support the diagnosis of organic brain dysfunction? Was the degree of impairment quantified via use of T scores, average impairment units, or percentile ranks?
6. Were measures of validity, simulation, and/or dissimulation included in the evaluation (e.g., validity measures on MMPI such as the F-K score, subtle versus obvious scores, "malingering tests" such as forced choice testing, and the Rey 15 item memory test)?
7. Was adequate consideration given to the initial degree of neurologic insult relative to GCS score, duration of post-traumatic amnesia, altered level of consciousness, etc., and was this correlated with symptom severity and onset to determine consistency with degree and temporal onset of impairment?
8. Was the pattern of change (if serial testing was performed) analyzed for consistency with anticipated recovery curves following central neurologic insult?
9. Was the impact (both positive and negative effects) of medication on test performance noted in the report?
10. Was the pattern of symptoms reported and the temporal onset of symptoms correlated with anticipated complaints after injuries of equal magnitude *and* with the neuropsychological testing results?

The examiner should consider using a DSM-IV axis-type grid to define any particular examinee's overall clinical status. Specifically, the clinician should delineate any and all associated primary and secondary psychological and psychiatric conditions in addition to the medical diagnoses at hand. The diagnosis of mild TBI should be based on patient and chart history; temporal relationship of symptoms to injury in question; nature of postconcussive complaints and "fit" with expected symptomatology; corroboration by others, including "noninvested" individuals; and degree to which symptom improvement matches expected natural history of neurologic recovery. Adequate consideration must be given to alternative explanations for each subjective impairment reported by the claimant. In a parallel fashion, the examiner must address each subjective impairment with appropriate bedside assessment maneuvers and, as necessary, further diagnostic testing or at least recommendations for such testing.

I would recommend that examiners minimize the initial use of the word "mild" in their diagnostic codes and simply document that the person has had a "traumatic brain injury." As part of the defining elements, the initial severity of neurologic injury should be defined via as many parameters as are available, including initial GCS score, the presence and duration of post-traumatic amnesia (retrograde and anterograde), and alteration or loss of consciousness. The clinician should then delineate each and every "postconcussive" impairment, noting where data are subjective or objective (e.g., the patient may complain of tinnitus, yet there is no way to objectively confirm the presumptive diagnosis). Symptom descriptors used as "diagnoses," such as "post-traumatic headache," "post-traumatic tinnitus," and "post-traumatic dizziness," are not only incomplete but provide no pathoetiologic information that can translate to appropriate diagnostic and treatment strategies. Each condition should be listed with a presumptive pathoetiology; for example, "post-traumatic headache" might be "post-traumatic headache secondary to right greater occipital neuralgia, right-sided referred cervical myofascial pain, and right frontotemporal migraine without aura." Prognostic statements should be made about each and every listed impairment. Functional implications of each impairment should be discussed based on patient and corroboratory witness reports and anticipated norms. Examining clinicians should remember that the best way to assess a particular functional capability is to have the examinee perform that specific activity, not some simulation of the activity that only approximates the behavior in question.

Neuropsychological testing often falls short of predicting real world performance, particularly in patients with executive function deficits related to frontal lobe insult. This shortfall of neuropsychological testing must be kept in mind. Bedside assessments are at best of limited utility in assessing higher-level cognitive, behavioral, linguistic, and social function in the case of a person with postconcussive complaints. The limitation of the bedside assessment relative to functional disability needs to be acknowledged up front by the examining clinician (Dalmady-Israel and Zasler, 1993).

A good "independent medical evaluation" assessing impairment and disability should include, along with appropriate assessment and assignments, the following key areas: history of medical condition; present complaints and current treatment; past medical history; work status; job description; physical examination including maneuvers to assess for nonorganic presentations; diagnostic studies; review of records; and medical summary and diagnostic impressions. Issues regarding causation, impairment, functional disability, permanent work preclusions, recommendations for further testing/treatment, maximum medical improvement opinions, apportionment, vocational rehabilitation, and future medical care should all be included in the report as appropriate.

Causation technically refers to the relationship of an incident, accident, or biologic factor to any physical, physiologic, or psychological disruption or alteration that may initiate the abnormality or aggravate a preexisting condition. The examiner must also differentiate spontaneously appearing conditions from preexisting pathology. *Apportionment* is the act of estimating how much of an impairment is related to a specific incident when more than one causative factor is involved. Maximum medical improvement defines the point at which further time and/or treatment is unlikely to produce significant improvement. This criterion is used to mark the termination of curative effort, initiate return to work, initiate vocational training, and/or establish a degree of permanent impairment. Employment determinations are made based on the ability of the claimant to work, with or without accommodation, with an impairment and to meet job demands and other conditions of employment, including travel to and from work (Kessler, 1970; Ziporyn, 1983). Appendix 1 presents an example of an Independent Medical Evaluation on a patient with a presumptive history of mild TBI.

CONCLUSIONS

Impairment and disability evaluation is by no means a simple undertaking for any clinician regardless of specialty affiliation. Clinicians must take the time to familiarize themselves with the variety of disability and impairment evaluation protocols and must understand their limitations relative to the specific clinical condition being assessed. Presently, there is no ideal system for rating impairment and disability following mild TBI relative to the claimant or patient with postconcussive residua (Hinnant and Tollison, 1994). A thorough understanding of the underlying disease process as well as associated injuries is paramount for optimal evaluation and reliable neurologic and vocational reentry prognosis.

REFERENCES

American Medical Association: Guides to Evaluation of Permanent Impairment. 4th Ed. Chicago, 1993

American Psychiatric Association: Diagnostic and Statistical Manual of Mental Disorders. 4th Ed. Washington, 1994, pp. 704–706

Bergner M, Bobbitt RA, Carter WB, Gibson BS: The Sickness Impact Profile: development and final revision of a health status measure. Med Care 19:787–805, 1981

Bradley LA, Anderson KO, Yound LD, Williams T: Psychological testing. In Tollison CD (ed): Handbook of Chronic Pain. Williams & Wilkins, Baltimore, 1989

Cailliet R: Disability evaluation: a physiatric method. South Med J 62:1380–1382, 1969

Dalmady-Israel C, Zasler ND: Post-traumatic seizures: a critical review. Brain Inj 7:263–273, 1993

Hall KM: Overview of functional assessment scales in brain injury rehabilitation. Neuro Rehabil 2:98–113, 1992

Hall KM, Hamilton B, Gordon WA, Zasler ND: Characteristics and comparisons of functional assessment indices: Disability Rating Scale, Functional Independence Measure and Functional Assessment Measure. J Head Trauma Rehabil 8(2):60–74, 1993

Hinnant D, Tollison CD: Impairment and disability associated with mild head injury: medical and legal aspects. Semin Neurol 14:84–89, 1994

Horn LJ, Zasler ND (eds): Rehabilitation of Post-Concussive Disorders. Hanley & Belfus, Philadelphia, 1992

Jennett B, Teasdale G, Braakman R et al: Prediction of outcomes in individual patients after severe head injury. Lancet 1:1031–1035, 1976

Johnston MV, Findley TW, DeLuca J, Katz RT: Research in physical medicine and rehabilitation XII: Measurement tools with application to brain injury. Am J Phys Med Rehabil 70:40–56, 1991

Johnston MV, Keith RA, Hinderer S: Measurement standards for interdisciplinary medical rehabilitation. Arch Phys Med Rehabil suppl. 73(12):S6–S23, 1992

Johnston MV, Wilkerson DL, Maney M: Evaluation of the quality and outcomes of medical rehabilitation programs. In DeLisa J et al (eds): Rehabilitation Medicine: Principles and Practice. JB Lippincott, Philadelphia, 1993

Kessler H: Disability Determination Evaluation. Lea & Febiger, Philadelphia, 1970

Koppenhoefer RM: In DeLisa JA (ed): Disability Evaluation in Rehabilitation Medicine: Principles and Practice. JB Lippincott, Philadelphia, 1988

LaForge J, Harrison D: Limited and unlimited Workers' Compensation wage replacement benefits and rehabilitation outcomes. Journal of Applied Rehabil Counseling 18(2):3–5, 1987

McBride ED: Disability Evaluation and Principles of Treatment of Compensable Injuries. JB Lippincott, Philadelphia, 1963

National Institutes of Health, National Institute of Child Health and Human Development: Research Plan for the National Center for Medical Rehabilitation Research. NIH Publication No. 93-3509. National Institutes of Health, Rockville, MD, 1993

Olsheski JA, Growick B: The Social Security disability system and rehabilitation in review. NARPPS J 8(4):143–156, 1994

Ragnarsson KT, Thomas JP, Zasler ND: Model system of care for individuals with traumatic brain injury. J Head Trauma Rehabil 8(2):1–11, 1993

Rappaport M, Hall KM, Hopkins HK et al: Disability Rating Scale for severe head trauma: coma to community. Arch Phys Med Rehabil 51:118–123, 1970

Rogers R (ed): Clinical Assessment of Malingering and Deception. Guilford Press, New York, 1988

Ruff RM, Wylie T, Tennant W: Malingering and malingering-like aspects of mild closed head injury. J Head Trauma Rehabil 8(3):60–73, 1993

Social Security Administration: Disability Evaluation Under Social Security: A Handbook for Physicians. Social Security Administration, 1992

Wade DT: Measurement in Neurological Rehabilitation. Oxford University Press, New York, 1992

Wehman P, Kreutzer JS (eds): Vocational Rehabilitation for Persons with Traumatic Brain Injury. Aspen Publishers, Rockville, MD, 1990

World Health Organization: International Classification of Impairments, Disabilities and Handicaps. World Health Organization, Geneva, 1980

Zasler ND: Mild traumatic brain injury: medical assessment and intervention. J Head Trauma Rehabil 8(3):13–29, 1993

Zasler ND: Ten Point Checklist for Neuropsychological Assessment. National NeuroRehabilitation Consortium, Inc. Richmond, 1994

Ziporyn T: Disability evaluation a fledgling science. JAMA 190:873–874, 1983

APPENDIX
Sample Independent Medical Evaluation

NAME: Mr. X
DATE OF BIRTH: 7/23/60
CHRONOLOGICAL AGE: 33

REFERRED BY:

Janet W, RN, BS, CCM
Richmond, Virginia 23294
Telephone Number: 804-555-1234
FAX: 804-555-2345
On behalf of Ms. V.K., Aetna Life and Casualty, P.O. Box 10137, Fairfax, VA 22030
DATE OF INJURY: 7/17/91
SOCIAL SECURITY NUMBER: 000-000-000
HANDEDNESS: Right

REASON FOR REFERRAL:

Neurophysiatric assessment of presumptive residua from accident of 7/17/91

BASIS OF REPORT

Records provided through Ms. W in addition to records provided through C.C.G., Esq. (the patient's attorney), history and physical exam of 12/13/93, and results of the Concussion Care Center of Virginia questionnaire. It should be noted that there are separate packets of medical records for the chiropractor's reports and the psychologist's reports. No emergency medical service records are available for review.

HISTORY OF PRESENT ILLNESS (as per report)

Mr. P is a 30-year-old right-handed, married white male who, based on available history, fell approximately 14 feet from a scaffold while working on a roof in Charlottesville. The accident was apparently on the job. He lost consciousness based on available information, although there are no documented eyewitness reports. The patient apparently fell such that he struck the right side of his torso/back, his right knee, and the right side of his head and had a "knot" in the right parieto-occipital area. He also acknowledged that he had a whiplash injury to the best of his recollection. The exact duration of loss of consciousness was unclear based on the medical records. It should be noted that in the emergency room note from the University of Virginia, Charlottesville, it is documented that the patient regained consciousness en route to the hospital. The patient stated initially on the Concussion Care Center of Virginia questionnaire that the duration of loss of consciousness was unknown, and when asked specifically to try to give an estimate he said 6 to 8 hours. The last thing he remembers is falling backward, and the first thing he remembers is waking up somewhere in Charlottesville. He was apparently sent home from the hospital after spending several hours (more than five) in the emergency room. Based on emergency room records his neurologic exam was nonfocal although he was oriented only times 2 in that he did not know what time it was. Neck exam was incomplete, and all that the emergency room record documented was that the neck was "currently immobilized." There was no obvious head trauma noted by the emergency room physician.

Note: For brevity the remainder of the history of present illness has been deleted.

PATIENT'S BACKGROUND

Allergies

No known drug allergies.

Developmental History

Full-term pregnancy with vaginal delivery. Milestones are normal based on patient report.

Past Medical History

1. Right knee surgery 1989, secondary to motor vehicle crash.
2. Vasectomy 1989.
3. Eye surgery at the age of approximately 14 after a penetrating injury to the right cornea.
4. Motor vehicle crash 1988. No loss of consciousness by history. It should be noted, that the patient's prior medical records were available for review (unclear whether these are all his records). However, the patient had been seen following his 1988 accident (based on the 9/21/89 note) for physical therapy at "KDH" for treatment to his back and neck but recently had been to the University of Virginia and Medical College of Virginia (MCV) for extensive workup and had had surgery on the right elbow for an entrapment syndrome. He also, apparently, had complaints at that time of left lower extremity pain. He was encouraged at that time to consider retraining for something other than his previous work as a carpenter since it appeared doubtful that he was going to be able to return to work any time soon. He apparently was also having sacroiliac joint discomfort and hip pain bilaterally, based on the 9/21/89 note. The patient was apparently seen in early 1991 by Dr. Mark Leadbetter, an expert in orthopedic reconstructive surgery, for problems with his knee.
5. Prior surgical repair of right lateral epicondylitis and testicular hydrocele repair.
6. Testicular torsion injury secondary to 1989 MCV report (unclear based on his history).

Present Medications

1. Sertaline 150 mg daily
2. Alprazolam (dose not known)
3. Clonazepam 5 mg bid
4. Amitriptyline 25 mg in the morning, 50 mg at night
5. Phenytoin 100 mg, bid
6. Lioresal 10 mg qid
7. Tylox prn

Family History

Patient denies any significant family history of psychiatric, neurologic, or other disease in his immediate family.

Psychosocial History

Patient states a positive history of tobacco use, which began at the age of 14. Generally he averages about 1 pack per day. He denies drinking alcohol now or in the past; however, this is in contradiction to other aspects of his medical records, which endorse a positive history of alcohol use, specifically beer consumption. It is interesting to note that in several places in his record there is a disparity in the reports regarding alcohol consumption. As noted, he denied any past or present consumption when I questioned him. In Dr. Kreutzer's report, the patient apparently reported that he had 1 to 3 drinks 2 to 3 times per month and was now (i.e., since the accident) abstinent from alcohol; yet elsewhere in his medical documentation there is a report of his drinking 3 to 4 beers per week. The patient denies illicit drug use. He endorses caffeine use, 1 to 2 cups of coffee a day and 1 to 2 caffeinated sodas a day. He is presently in his third marriage and has four children. The couple's 4-year-old son lives with them. Presently he spends much of his time watching TV and visiting doctors. The patient reports that one of his hobbies includes working on small engines.

Educational History

Patient states that he dropped out of school in the tenth grade. He has not received a GED. The reason he stated this happened was the fact that he needed to go to work; however, in Dr. Kreutzer's report the rationale for this was that "my father and I fell out, and I moved away." The patient denied ever being held back in school or labeled as learning disabled. He reported that he got Cs and Ds in school.

Vocational History

Patient apparently had just begun work 2 weeks prior to his accident as a carpenter with a construction company in Charlottesville. He had previously worked in chimney sweeping as well as carpentry. He has not been competitively employed since his accident nor has he tried to return to work at any level since his accident. He denies ever being on disability prior to his injury. He states that his job was very physically demanding, frequently requiring him to lift more than 100 lb. From a mental/cognitive standpoint he reported that his job was also very demanding. His work status at the time of injury by his report was full-time. He presently thinks he is capable of limited light duty. He stated that if his condition got completely better during the next few weeks he thought his employer would let him return to the job he was doing before his injury. He feels that his employer has treated him fairly. He denies having anyone in his family who has been on disability.

Legal Issues

The patient endorsed that he has had prior legal problems and/or suits. Presently an attorney is assisting him with his Workers' Compensation-related claim.

General Coping

On a scale of 0 to 10, 0 being none and 10 being maximal, the patient noted that his anxiety was at a level of 8 since his injury, depression at a level of 9, and irritability at a level of 8.

General Health Information

The patient endorsed that Dr. Kline was his primary care physician. Phone number is 703-555-4115.

SYMPTOMS, TREATMENT, AND NON-NEUROLOGIC EXAMS

Review of Symptoms

The patient endorsed that during the past year he has had the following symptoms: unexplained fevers at night, night sweats, excessive fatigue, probable depression, difficulty sleeping, chest pain or tightness, persistent or unusual cough, and trouble breathing with exercise. When asked to illustrate areas that were bothering him relative to pain, the patient marked off the neck and left shoulder girdle area as having an ache-type sensation. He also noted that his left arm hurt him around the area of the elbow. Finally, he noted a pins-and-needles sensation in the left lower extremity.

On a symptom checklist the patient endorsed the following symptoms as occurring always since his injury: difficulty lifting heavy objects; ringing/buzzing in ears (patient stated that this was only in the left ear and it began right after he fell); trouble falling asleep; trouble hearing; and trouble staying asleep. He reported the following symptoms as recurring often since his injury: difficulty in smelling things, headaches, muscle aches, muscle numbness, tiredness, weakness, can't get mind off of certain thoughts, difficulty performing chores; concentration is poor; confused; forgets people's names; forgets phone numbers; learns slowly; makes mistakes doing arithmetic; misplaces things; reads slowly; thinks slowly; trouble making decisions; trouble following instructions; loses train of thought; bored; hard getting started on things; impatient; excessive fatigue; problems with motivation; difficulty thinking of the right word; difficulty pronouncing words; writes more slowly; and writing is more difficult to read.

The patient reports that his headaches tend to occur mainly in the left occipital region with referral to the parietotemporal region. The character of the pain is throbbing in nature. Headaches can last up to 2 to 3 days. Onset tends to be sudden. Headache is exacerbated by loud sounds and movement. It is relieved by manipulation and medication, specifically Tylox. On the average his headache is reported on a scale of 0 to 10 (where 0 is no pain and 10 is maximal pain) to be 8. When it is at its worst it is a 10 and at its best it is a 0. The patient also reports that in his opinion his top three physical problems in order (most important first) buzzing in left ear (tinnitus), headache, and low back pain. The patient attributes his low back pain to sacroiliac joint dysfunction. The patient also reports "panic attacks" when he is at heights, with sweating, palpitations, and generalized fear response.

Treatment Issues

The following is a list of the treatments that the patient endorsed having received since his injury and the comments he made on whether or not the treatments were beneficial. The following treatments were all considered to have helped his condition . . . ultrasound, icing, massage, electrical stimulation, TENS, and chiropractic treatment. The patient also listed epidural injections, narcotics, muscle relaxants, and antidepressants but did not mark off whether these were helpful or not.

Diagnostic Testing Since Injury

The patient reports that he has had regular spine X-rays, CT scan of the brain, MRI scan of the brain, bone scan, EMG, nerve block, EEG, and neuropsychological testing.

Physical Exam (Focused)

Vital signs: Afebrile and stable.

General: Well nourished, slightly overweight, large-boned, white man who appears somewhat older than his stated age of 32. He did appear somewhat guarded and suspicious when first introduced to me, however, this seemed to decline during the remainder of our time together.

Head, eyes, ears, nose, throat: Atraumatic normocephalic. ENT Ear, nose, and throat grossly intact. Nose somewhat "stuffy." Fundi benign. Visual fields full to confrontation. Pupils equally round and reactive to light and accommodation.

Neck: No jugular vein distension, lymphadenopathy, or thyromegaly. Please refer to musculoskeletal exam for other findings.

Lungs: Clear to auscultation and percussion.

Cardiac exam: Regular rate and rhythm without audible murmur, gallop, or rub.

Abdomen: Deferred.

Extremities: No clubbing, cyanosis or edema. Right knee in brace. Scar over right lateral epicondyle. Negative Tinel's sign at the elbow and wrist bilaterally.

NEUROLOGIC EXAM

Cranial nerves I through XII: Grossly intact except for decreased smell on testing of cranial nerve I by the motor conduction velocity (MCV) olfactory screening test (unclear if this is due to the patient's "stuffy" nose). Patient had a negative head shaking test and Nilen-Barany test. Weber was nonlateralized. Visual acuity 20/40 in the right and 20/30 in the left. The patient had a positive "water test"; specifically, when he put his ear near running tap water his tinnitus was modulated downward in intensity.

Deep tendon reflexes: Symmetric, normoreflexic, without associated pathologic reflexes. Plantar responses, flexors bilaterally.

Sensory exam: No gross sensory deficit revealed. There were no dermatomal abnormalities noted on assessment of cervical roots C1 through C7. There was no hemi-inattention or extinction of double simultaneous stimulation. Parietal sensory function was deemed intact by testing of graphesthesia or tactile gnosis. The patient also had a sensory deficit in a rather circumscribed area in the left lateral thigh.

Cerebellar exam: Without evidence of nystagmus, dysmetria, or ataxia. There was no check or rebound noted. Romberg and sharpened Romberg were within normal limits. Gait was within normal limits.

Motor exam: No focal motor weakness revealed. There was no pronator drift. Frontal motor sequencing tasks were well within normal limits, as was bilateral Mandrake maneuver.

Mental status exam: Patient revealed to be alert and oriented × 3. On bedside testing of short-term memory, the patient performed three for three items immediately, three for three at 15 seconds, and three for three at 5 minutes. When asked to repeat the alphabet, skipping every other letter, the patient had multiple errors the first time; however, on the second attempt he did fine. He was able to spell words forward and backward. He was able to repeat six numbers forward and four numbers backward. Affect was full. Mood was a bit frustrated at times. There was no obvious thought disorder. The patient did endorse several neurovegetative symptoms, as delineated in review of systems section. He denied suicidal or homicidal ideation. There was no evidence of dysprosody, dysphasia, or dysarthria.

Musculoskeletal exam: On both active and passive examination of cervical range of motion, the patient demonstrated decreased right cervical rotation as well as decreased extension. There was right lateral cervical muscular myodystonia noted on palpation. Temporomandibular joint function was less than two fingerbreadths jaw range of motion using the nondominant three-finger rule. A left "click" was noted. Patient had a negative compression test and a negative Spurling's maneuver. The patient showed no evidence of sacroiliac dysfunction on either the left or the right side. He had some very mild thoracic vertebral segmental dysfunction at the T2-T3 level.

Tests for Dissimulation

The patient was given three tests to assess for dissimulation at the bedside. The first, the Rey 15 Item Memory Test, was performed with 100 percent accuracy. The Rey Dot Counting Test was also performed. The patient did not make any errors on dot counting, and his items all were in line with the number of dots, suggesting no attempt to appear worse than he actually was. The Hiscock Forced Choice Testing was also done (revised version, 36 items) . . . the patient performed at 100 percent level on this testing, thereby strongly suggesting that there was no attempt at dissimulation (purposeful attempt to perform/ appear badly).

Impressions/Recommendations

Status Post-Traumatic Brain Injury on 7/17/91

Based on all available *documented* information the patient incurred a mild TBI. Of some interest is the fact that there is unclear documentation regarding the exact mechanism of injury, which would have some implication for the overall magnitude of the neural insult; specifically, if the patient fell directly 14–16 feet and hit his head, one would anticipate a more severe insult to the brain than if he fell 6 feet, broke his fall somewhat, and subsequently fell an additional 8 feet, as is documented in the nursing assessment sheet from the ER in Charlottesville. Additionally, there is quite a bit of disparity in reports regarding the duration of loss of concsciousness. Apparently, the job site that he was working on is right adjacent to the UVA Medical Center which implies that the duration of unconsciousness is probably much less than the number of hours reported by both patient and his wife, given that the patient regained consciousness on the way to the hospital. Further clarification of this fact based on eyewitness reports would be helpful. Based on the CT and MRI reports there is no evidence whatsoever of any *significant* brain pathology resulting from his injury. Given the suspected magnitude of the patient's brain injury, one would anticipate that in all likelihood he should have a good neurologic and functional recovery. Although the extent of his cognitive impairment could potentially be related to a mild TBI, I consider that there are too many other variables present to state that his present deficits are solely a result of cerebral dysfunction secondary to trauma (see below).

Cognitive Deficits as per Neuropsychological Testing on 4/13/93

Although I fully agree with the rationale of ordering neuropsychological testing, I believe that Dr. Kreutzer has not adequately analyzed the "abnormal neuropsychological profile produced by the patient." (By history this man didn't even complete the tenth grade and received Cs and Ds while he was in school. My anticipation is that many of the areas of functional skills that were rated as impaired relative to preinjury status probably are no different than they were preinjury, i.e. it would not surprise me if this man was performing at a borderline impaired to impaired range in a number of intellectual spheres prior to his injury. Some of his areas of deficit might even be consistent with a learning disability. Second, this patient is on an extremely inappropriate medical regimen for somebody with a mild TBI. There is no attribution *at all* to the potential effects of the medications that he is taking on cognitive performance, particularly relative to tasks of attention, concentration, auditory memory, and motor performance. Issues regarding the effects of drugs on cognitive performance are particularly germane to the fact that he is taking two different types of benzodiazepines, specifically alprazolam and clonazepam, in addition to phenytoin and baclofen. All these medications are centrally acting with sedative properties, and all are known to potentially have an adverse effect on cognitive function. Finally, the patient's affective status, which in my opinion has been poorly documented and defined, needs to be taken into consideration as it is germane to his cognitive performance, specifically as it relates to both historical and clinical evidence of depressive symptomatology. It is well known that major depression can contaminate neuropsychological performance following mild TBI. Specifically, patients with major depression are known to exhibit deficits in attention, sustained vigilance, abstraction, fluency, memory, visual spatial skills, and motor skills. They are also likelier to have deficits in visual, spatial, motor and memory skills than in verbal skills. However, verbal tasks that require sustained attention may also be impaired in depression. Therefore, it is not always possible to make a clear diagnostic distinction between depression and other factors on the basis of neuropsychological test data alone. What is required is for a distinction to be made on clinical grounds over time by clinicians familiar with the patient's condition. The mere fact that this patient produces a Beck Depression Inventory score in the mid 20s strongly suggests that his depression has been inadequately addressed in terms of his lack of a more adequate clinical response to what has been, in my opinion, long-term treatment, apparently from both a psychological and psychiatric perspective.

Post-Traumatic Headache

Based on the available history, symptom profile, and exam findings, the patient most likely is experiencing cervicogenically mediated headache. Although there is some objective evidence of myofascial dysfunction on his neck exam, his symptoms appear to be more severe than one would expect given his exam findings. Obviously, pain, being a subjective phenomenon, is difficult to quantify in an objective fashion. It remains unclear as to what role, if any, the patient's C3-C4 herniated disc is playing in his chronic pain. The congenital vertebral anomaly at C1-C2 is an unlikely source of the patient's pain. What is probably of greater importance in terms of the patient's clinical history is that this is a man with a *chronic* history of neck and head pain predating his accident of July 1991. Based on available records and patient reports, there is seemingly an attribution of his present symptoms solely to the fall incurred in July 1991. Based on available medical records this is, indeed, not the case; however, it is impossible to say how much, if any, of his present condition is truly a result of his fall. There is no question, however, that he has pathology presently related to a persistent, albeit possibly clinically insignificant, C3-C4 herniation and associated cervical segmental dysfunction as well as chronic myofascial pain. The exact causal relationship, if any, with his July 1991 accident cannot be definitely concluded based on available records. Even though there may be a temporal relationship between these clinical findings and his accident, it does not negate the possibility that all these problems were present prior to his fall. The fact that the patient's myofascial findings are right-sided and that his limitations in cervical range of motion are to the right, with cervical rotation and in extension, are consistent with the patient's documented right C3-C4 posterolateral disc extrusion. My recommendation, as a nonsurgeon, would be that given the clinical findings this disc may indeed by symptomatic and responsible for the promulgation of the patient's pain and mysofascial dysfunction. A second neurosurgical opinion might, therefore, be beneficial. Additionally, a discogram might also help in further clarifying whether or not his symptoms are related to this disc extrusion.

Auditory Problems

Subjective complaints of tinnitus with evidence of bilateral sensorineural hearing loss, which is of a greater magnitude in the left ear than the right but also of higher frequency in the left than the right (i.e., 6,000 versus 4,000 Hz). It should be noted that tinnitus is a symptom, not a disease entity, and its etiology is not well defined. Theoretically, it is believed to be due to an electrophysiologic derangement in the cochlea, 8th cranial nerve, or deeper within the central nervous system. Further audiologic testing, including otoacoustic emissions and brainstem auditory evoked responses, may be beneficial in documenting objective pathology; however, even if these tests are abnormal, they in no way demonstrate a causal relationship with the patient's injury. If, indeed, the tinnitus only became a problem many months after the injury, it is less likely to be causally related to the injury; however, given the fact that the patient did not seek *specialized* care, it is quite possible that the symptom was there, but since no one ever asked him about it he never reported it. The patient states on my interview that he has had tinnitus since the time of his accident. It should be noted, however, that tinnitus may be caused by other phenomena aside from brain injury, including cervical pathology as well as temporomandibular joint dysfunction. The patient definitely has evidence of both these aforementioned conditions. Tinnitus may also be exacerbated by stress, anxiety, and other affective disturbances, and therefore appropriate treatment to rule out peripheral causes and/or promulgating factors needs to be addressed more aggressively. Adjuvant treatment should include mechanisms of decreasing stress and anxiety through biofeedback, avoidance of stimulants, including caffeine (patient endorses positive caffeine use), proper sleep hygiene, and potential use of anxiolytic and antidepressant medication. There is no FDA-approved drug presently for the treatment of tinnitus; however, recent literature suggests that alprazolam (which the patient is already taking) may be beneficial. In addition, there has been a smaller amount of literature on the use of oral tocainide and gingko biloba for this condition (regardless of its etiology). If further evaluation is indicated, I would recommend that the patient be referred to the group Atlantic Coast Ear Specialists in Virginia Beach and that the patient be seen by Drs. Prass and Gutnick. Given the patient's positive response to the tap water test (i.e., his tinnitus diminished when his ear was close to the running tap water) I do think that he is an appropriate candidate for consideration for a tinnitus masker. This does not per se improve the concurrent high-frequency sensorineural hearing loss; however, it would optimize hearing by diminishing the interference from the tinnitus.

Bilateral High-Frequency Sensorineural Hearing Loss

High-frequency sensorineural hearing loss is more profound in left ear than right ear and at higher frequency in left ear than right ear (6,000 versus 4,000 Hz). It is difficult to say, based on the patient's occupation and history of gun use, that this is indeed a post-traumatic phenomenon without having preinjury audiologic assessments for comparison. The patient states, however, that he did not have any hearing problems prior to his accident. A 6,000 Hz loss, however, is probably outside the "functional hearing range," and the patient has excellent speech discrimination, which is what is important from a functional standpoint. There is no indication per se for use of a hearing aid to treat from a functional standpoint the patient's high-frequency sensorineural hearing loss. On a speculative note, since he is right-handed, he will shoot his gun off from his right shoulder, thereby exposing the right ear to a significantly greater potential for noise-induced high frequency hearing loss even with the use of earplugs. The fact that his hearing loss is of higher frequency and greater amplitude in the left ear does not go along with this history; however, one should also note that the impact to his head was on the right rather than the left side, which would be against a left ear as opposed to a right ear concussive injury.

Neurobehavioral/Affective Status

At the present time the patient reports subjective complaints consistent with a phobia of heights (acrophobia). I was unable to evaluate this in an objective fashion in the clinic. Based on available objective documentation there is only evidence for depression. At present I do not believe the patient meets criteria for post-traumatic stress disorder (PTSD). Additionally, given his loss of consciousness and associated retrograde and anterograde amnesia, it would be unlikely, based on the understanding of the mechanisms by which PTSD is generated, that the patient ever actually experienced this clinical psychiatric phenomenon. Admittedly, he does have some PTSD-like symptoms, but this is quite common in the postconcussive population. It is my opinion that at present his depression is not being treated adequately, based solely on his continued subjective report and his recent Beck Depression Inventory score. I also have *significant* concerns that some of the medication he is taking may actually be promulgating depressive symptomatology, specifically, benzodiazepines in the form of alprazolam and clonazepam. These drugs should be weaned if at all possible. The patient may also be an excellent candidate for referral to a psychologist specialized in postconcussive disorders, particularly as it is germane to adjustment issues.

Left Lateral Femoral Cutaneous Nerve Syndrome

This is most likely a consequence of the patient's weight gain and compression of the lateral femoral cutaneous nerve as it passes over the anterior superior iliac spine. It can be treated with local blocks, but primarily the treatment should be weight loss. This nerve is solely a sensory nerve, and therefore the patient should not have any major functional impairment as a result of this problem. It is unlikely that it is post-traumatic in etiology given the fact that the patient fell on his right, not on his left, side.

Current Psychological/Psychiatric Needs

As a specialist in physical medicine and rehabilitation, I have concerns about the documentation provided from Dr. Carter (as previously noted). No documentation has been provided by Dr. Dort to permit understanding of what the treatment or plan has been from a psychiatric perspective. My feeling is that his behavioral care has been suboptimal, based on the available documentation, his present medication regimen, and his present affective status. It would be my recommendation, as noted above, to have the patient referred to a clinician who can broach his behavioral problems from a holistic standpoint and work along with a psychologist experienced in dealing with TBI and chronic pain issues. Any treating clinician should have a list of goals, specific treatment plans, and specific end points for the therapy. My concern with Dr. Carter's treatment is that I see none of these things elucidated in the medical record. If I have not seen the complete medical record, obviously this opinion is open for modification.

Rehabilitation Needs

At the present time it is my opinion that there are a number of medical issues that need to be clarified before any further rehabilitation efforts are made. One of my major concerns with this case is that there does not seem to be a "captain of the ship," and the care being rendered seems to be splintered and noncoordinated. After the aforementioned medical issues are addressed, I believe that the patient, should he persist with cognitive, behavioral, linguistic, and/or physical problems, would be a good candidate for entry into a high-level TBI program, one that also had the capability of dealing with his musculoskeletal chronic pain issues. By centralizing this man's care it would also lessen the overall "sickness role" that he seems to have taken on even though he states that he is motivated to return to work. He also does not seem to have been encouraged by treating clinicians to resume any type of active structured schedule, which will be important for community, avocational, and vocational reentry. Once his medical condition is addressed as I have recommended above, I believe reevaluation for rehabilitation needs should occur. He may be quite appropriate for high-level occupational and speech/language pathology referrals, as well as referral to an experienced physical therapist who is comfortable dealing with chronic myofascial pain and dysfunction.

Vocational Status

At present it is my impression that the patient is not employable based on the aforementioned issues. It is my opinion, however, that he has good potential for vocational re-entry once the aforementioned issues have been aggressively pursued. I would envision that with appropriate direction to his care and referral to appropriate specialized clinicians, and potentially with the aid of a vocational rehabilitation specialist this man should be competitively employable at least on a part-time basis within 6 months.

Maximal Medical Improvement

It is my opinion that until my recommendations are put in place, it is difficult to say whether Mr. P has reached maximum medical improvement (MMI) given all the confounding variables. It is my opinion that his current functional status is masked by several issues, as discussed above. While I do not believe that Mr. P is making a conscious effort at appearing to be worse than he is, there obviously are some secondary gain issues that must be taken into consideration. These are most likely occurring at a subconscious level, although it is impossible for the examiner to totally rule out dissimulation or at least a component thereof. Based on my bedside evaluation there was no indication that the examinee was making a conscious effort to appear bad on cognitive and/or musculoskeletal testing. The results seem to be consistent across different maneuvers to elicit deficits in given areas, whether cognitive, behavioral, or physical.

Apportionment Issues

At present, it is my opinion that the examinee has evidence of injury-related impairments and disability related to a multiplicity of factors, in addition to secondary psychoemotional factors affecting physical health. Given the aforementioned maximum medical improvement issues, it is my opinion that brain injury sequelae per se are the least of this examinee's problems (less than or equal to 25 percent); however, the brain injury residua are causally related to his injury of 7/17/91. There is good to very good clinical evidence for the majority of the patient's complaints in the absence of any likely (> 50 percent) chance of dissimulation; however, the latter cannot obviously be ruled out with certainty.

NOTE ABOUT THE REPORT

This independent medical evaluation is based on the subjective complaints, the history given by the examinee, the objective medical records, and the tests provided to me as well as the physical findings of the examinee at the time of my assessment. Recommendations regarding work are given totally independently of the requesting agents. The opinions are based upon reasonable medical probability. Medicine is both an art and a science, and although the patient may be fit for return to duty, there is no guarantee that the patient will not be reinjured or suffer additional injury once he returns. If further information is required, please contact the undersigned.

The opinions rendered in this case are the opinions of this evaluator. This evaluation has been conducted on the basis of the medical examination, and documentation was provided with the assumption that the material is true and correct. If more information becomes available at a later date, opinions are subject to change. The opinions expressed herein do not constitute per se a recommendation for specific claims or administrative functions to be made or enforced.

Should there be additional questions, please feel free to cal me at NNRC, Inc.: 1-800-914-NNRC or by fax at 804-346-1956.

Sincerely,

Nathan D. Zasler, MD, FAAPM&R, FAADEP, BCFE
Fellow American Academy of Disability Evaluating Physicians
Board Certified Forensic Examiner
CEO & Executive Medical Director, National NeuroRehabilitation Consortium, Inc.
Director, Concussion Care Centers of America, Inc.

Neuropsychological Assessment of Patients with Traumatic Brain Injury: The Iowa-Benton Approach

19

R. D. Jones

This chapter reviews the approach to neuropsychological assessment that has come to be known as the "Iowa-Benton approach." Other approaches will also be considered, to facilitate comparison with the Iowa-Benton approach. The interested reader is referred to Reitan (1986), Reitan and Wolfson (1985), Jones and Butters (1983), Golden et al. (1985), Milberg et al. (1986), and McKenna and Warrington (1986) for more detailed information regarding other major schools of neuropsychological assessment.

In practice, few clinical neuropsychologists are dogmatic or rigid in their approach to assessment. For example, although the Halstead-Reitan Neuropsychological Battery (HRNB) (Reitan and Wolfson, 1985) remains an important force in the field, its use in isolation is less common than in the past. By the same token, it is common for a psychologist trained in the "Iowa-Benton" or "Boston" schools to use tests from the Halstead-Reitan Battery or items from the Luria Nebraska Neuropsychological Battery (Golden et al., 1985). As a general statement, practitioners in the field of clinical neuropsychology have recognized the importance of using the best features of several different approaches.

CURRENT SCHOOLS OF NEUROPSYCHOLOGICAL ASSESSMENT: FIXED BATTERY VERSUS FLEXIBLE BATTERY

An important conceptual distinction exists in clinical neuropsychology between the so-called fixed battery and flexible battery approaches to assessment (Jones and Butters, 1983). In the fixed battery approach, the clinician administers a predetermined set of tests, typically with known sensitivity and specificity in the detection of brain dysfunction. Perhaps the best-known example is the HRNB (Reitan and Wolfson, 1985).

There are several advantages to the fixed battery approach. First, every patient is administered a relatively comprehensive set of probes; thus the clinician is less likely to miss an impairment that may not have been evident before testing. Second, given the fixed format, the psychometric properties of the battery as a whole can be determined. Third, because test selection is not idiosyncratic depending on the patient and the laboratory, communication between clinicians may be enhanced. Finally, case selection for retrospective research is relatively easy with the fixed battery approach, because all patients have been administered a standard set of measures.

However, there are disadvantages to this approach. The fixed battery method has been criticized for being potentially unresponsive to the specific clinical situation (Benton, 1992). For example, in a patient with a relatively pure syndrome such as aphasia from a single left perisylvian lesion or amnesia from bilateral temporal lobe dysfunction, it can be argued that the clinical examination should focus on the relevant syndrome rather than unrelated or uninformative constructs (e.g., motor skills). A related criticism has been that fixed battery approaches can be inefficient. Four or more hours of testing is not uncommon with some current fixed batteries. In addition to this already lengthy battery, further specific measures that probe functions that are not well tapped in the standard battery are often administered (e.g., a verbal memory test in addition to the HRNB) (Reitan, 1986; Reitan and Wolfson, 1985). The sheer length of such an examination can be beyond the capacity of many patients with traumatic brain injuries (TBI), particularly in the acute recovery period.

The fixed battery is typically contrasted to either the flexible approach to assessment or to the "process approach" (Benton, 1992; Jones and Butters, 1983; McKenna and Warrington, 1986). The essential benefits of the flexible approach are that it is viewed as more efficient and more responsive to the clinical situation, as compared with the fixed battery. It typically includes a series of tests tailored to the patient's clinical condition, the referral question, and questions that may have arisen in the initial interview with the patient and the results of earlier testing. In the process approach, there is great emphasis on how the patient came to his or her answer, as opposed to simply whether the answer was correct. That is, in this approach there is less emphasis on comparing a patient's scores with empirically derived normative data and greater emphasis on the process of the patient's problem-solving method. The Iowa-Benton approach does not abandon entirely qualitative observations related to the process of the patient's problem solving but does have a strong emphasis on the use of empirical normative data.

Flexible batteries and the process approach have been cited as being more efficient, more responsive to the clinical situation, and more directly related to the referral question than fixed battery approaches. Retrospective research is often hindered, however, because there is no guarantee that patients have received the same tests in all instances. Also, these approaches have been criticized for not being comprehensive and thus not appreciating the complexity of brain-behavior relationships. Finally, communication between clinicians may be hindered by the flexible battery approach, because there are likely to be idiosyncrasies associated with individual patients or practitioners.

THE IOWA-BENTON APPROACH

In this section, the Iowa-Benton approach to neuropsychological assessment of TBI is described. This approach is inextricably tied to Arthur Benton, whose work has influenced the field of clinical neuropsychology for five decades (see Hamsher, 1985; Tranel, in press).

Benton developed a flexible, hypothesis-driven approach to assessment. Flexibility in this context imparts the belief that the clinician should have the opportunity to explore diagnostic possibilities with a variety of measures rather than a fixed set of assessment tools for every patient. The selection of measures depends on multiple factors such as patient condition and complaints, the results of earlier tests, the referral question, known brain pathology (e.g., the site of the lesion), and the history of the patient.

However, this flexibility is built on a brief relatively standard set of tests, or "core battery." The core battery provides the clinician with a broad sampling of the patient's behavior, using tests that are informative in a general sense rather than specific to a given lesion or condition. In part, the core battery is intended to serve as a screening tool for unsuspected impairments (e.g., memory impairments that were not apparent in another context). Further, the core battery is used to establish a preliminary baseline in critical areas of cognition (e.g., memory, attention, language, intellect, orientation, praxis, executive control).

This rationale for this approach to assessment has been set forth in several papers by Benton and students (Benton, 1985, 1992, 1994; Tranel, in press). As Benton (1985) has stated, neuropsychological assessment is viewed "in the same way as we view the physical or neurological examination, i.e., as a logical, sequential decision making process rather than simply the administration of a fixed battery of tests" (p. 15).

Features of the Iowa-Benton Approach

Hypothesis Testing

The approach to assessment is hypothesis-driven. The core battery, which takes 40 to 60 minutes, is administered, and based on the patient's performance on this brief battery, he or she may be given more tests of a particular type. For example, if a patient performs poorly on a test of visuoconstruction in the core battery (e.g., the Block Design subtest from the Wechsler Adult Intelligence Scale-Revised [WAIS-R]) (Wechsler, 1981), he or she may be given a variety of other tests to delineate the defect more clearly, for example, the Facial Recognition Test (Benton et al., 1994b) to assess the extent to which visual perception contributes to the defect or the Judgment of Line Orientation Test (Benton et al., 1994b) to assess the extent to which spatial judgment may be contributing to the defect.

Similarly, selection of follow-up tests is guided by the patient's condition and other factors noted above, such as the patient's complaints, the referral question, and known brain pathology. Patients with TBI will invariably be given tests of anterograde verbal and visual memory, because such defects are common in the condition. Similarly, brain trauma that results in contusions of the orbital frontal lobes that are confirmed by neuroimaging will be given additional tests of executive control, because such impairments are commonly associated with such lesions (Damasio and Anderson, 1993). Patients who are involved in medicolegal disputes after TBI will be given a broader range of tests than those patients referred simply for documentation of current defects, because the questions posed in legal referrals often require unusually precise characterization of acquired impairments (Matarazzo, 1990).

The essence of this feature of the approach is that the psychologist must consider the *meaning* of the defects presented by any given patient. The assessment is veiwed as an active, hypothesis-testing, logical procedure, in which the patient is both a subject and a collaborator who provides valuable information to help guide the examination.

Empirical Data

A cornerstone of the approach is reliance on normative empirical data. Performances on tests are adjusted for age, education, and other factors found to be relevant to performance. Scores are compared with normative values of subjects without known brain damage or cognitive dysfunction, and the results are interpreted in the setting of the individual patient. This reliance on empirically derived normative data can be seen in the many tests that have been developed at the Benton Laboratory (e.g., Benton et al., 1994a; Sivan, 1992; Spreen and Benton, 1985).

The Referral Question

Along with several other factors outlined in this section, the referral question drives test selection. When the referring agent is concerned about a given patient's memory after closed head injury, for example, the psychologist will place greater emphasis on tests of memory in an attempt to document more fully a patient's strengths and weaknesses in that area. For example, any (or all) of the following memory tests may be given: tests of anterograde verbal list learning, recall, and recognition such as the Auditory Verbal Learning Test (AVLT) (Lezak, 1983; Wiens et al., 1988), tests of anterograde verbal story learning and recall such as the Logical Memory section of the Wechsler Memory Scale-Revised (WMS-R) (Wechsler, 1987), tests of short-term visual memory such as the Visual Retention Test (Sivan, 1992), tests of delayed visual memory such as recall of the Complex Figure Test (Lezak, 1985), tests of retrograde autobiographic memory such as the Iowa Autobiographical Memory Questionnaire (Jones et al., 1993), tests of retrograde visual memory for faces such as the Boston Famous Faces (Albert et al., 1979) or the Iowa Famous Faces (Benton Neuropsychology Laboratory, 1995), or tests of procedural memory such as the Rotor Pursuit or Mirror Tracing test (Benton Neuropsychology Laboratory, 1995).

Patient Condition and Patient Complaints

Test selection is also driven by a patient's complaints. In all cases, the patient is interviewed regarding his or her perception of their own cognitive functioning, and complaints are investigated either through further clarification by interview or formal assessment procedures. For example, if a patient is referred for a memory problem after closed head injury and appears to be depressed during the initial interview, the psychologist will assess the possibility of depression in depth by, for example, administration of the Beck Depression Inventory (Beck et al., 1961) and/or Minnesota Multiphasic Personality Inventory-2 (MMPI-2) (Hathaway et al., 1989). Similarly, if a patient is referred for depression and is also complaining of memory defects, the memory defect will be assessed in greater depth.

In nearly all cases of TBI, we interview collateral sources regarding the cognitive functioning of the patient. Similar to patient complaints, collateral observations that bear on the neuropsychological characterization of the patient are explored through formal assessment (e.g., by the Iowa Rating Scales for Personality Change) (Benton Neuropsychology Laboratory, 1995), further interview, or both.

Results of Other Tests

Results of other tests are regarded as important ancillary data to the final analysis of the case. Since the advent of modern neuroimaging in the mid-1970s, there has been substantially less emphasis on lesion localization in our approach and greater emphasis on defining and describing performances in various areas of cognition affected (e.g., language, visuoperceptual skills, memory).

The results of the neuropsychological assessment are never interpreted in isolation from other sources of data. For example, in addition to the results of other medical tests, the neuropsychologist considers factors such as the patient's sociocultural background, information from collateral sources, and features of the event that is hypothesized to have caused the neuropsychological dysfunction. Particularly in cases of mild TBI when the acquired impairments may be subtle, it may be necessary to have access to extensive information to arrive at a final diagnosis. Such information would include, for example, the medical history; findings of electroencephalographic (EEG) and neuroimaging studies; results of the neurologic examination; Glasgow Coma Scale (GCS) score on admission to the hospital; the duration of retrograde amnesia, post-traumatic amnesia, and loss of consciousness; the observations of witnesses to the trauma; police reports; ambulance attendant's and paramedic's notes; and emergency room records. One does not observe impaired test performances and attempt to interpret them post-hoc; rather, one works "forward" from the facts of the injury. This approach to building an impression of the patient's condition reflects the fact that poor neuropsychological test performances can derive from many possible etiologies other than brain dysfunction from trauma (e.g., depression and other psychiatric disease, poor effort, malingering, and fatigue).

Implications of the Iowa-Benton Approach

Patient Care

Benton (1992) has noted the importance of recognizing the effects of nonneurologic factors in patient performances. Thus he expressed the opinion that

> **too many neuropsychologists are not sufficiently sensitive to the physical condition and affective status of their patients. They are seemingly unaware that the performances which they are eliciting are also determined by a variety of nonneurological factors of a physical, emotional, and motivational nature. (p. 414)**

The approach to assessment is solidly grounded in concern for patients. There is great emphasis placed on efficiency, relevance, and consideration of the above-noted nonneurologic factors such as age, fatigue, depression, and motivation. Such factors may be particularly salient in patients with TBI, because the condition itself is broadly disabling. Further, in the case of traumatic injury, the issues of limited motivation, fatigue, and depression must be addressed with care, because such conditions can be "organic" as well as nonneurologic features of the condition.

Clinical Research

The core battery is administered in most cases; thus retrospective research can be accomlished using the measures in this battery (e.g., Jones et al., 1992). However, the follow-up tests are less predictable; thus retrospective research is often hindered with these measures. Specific projects must be initiated prospectively, rather than by using existing clinical files. Historically, the approach to research in the Benton Neuropsychology Laboratory has been largely prospective testing of a specific test or hypothesis that arose in the clinical setting. This can be seen in the many studies of the individual tests that have been produced in the Benton Laboratory. For example, research interest in the Gerstmann syndrome resulted in clinical tests of finger localization and right-left disorientation, whereas interest in hemispheric dominance led to the development of tests of visuoperception, visuospatial judgment, and constructional praxis (Benton et al., 1994b) and interest in aphasia led to the development of many tests of language (Benton et al., 1994a; Spreen and Benton, 1985).

Training

In its current form, the approach to training in the Benton Laboratory conforms to the American Psychological Association (APA) Division 40 guidelines for training of postdoctoral fellows in clinical neuropsychology (APA Division 40 Task Force on Education, Accreditation, and Credentialing, 1987). Postdoctoral trainees typically have backgrounds in clinical psychology according to APA criteria and have obtained additional training at the graduate level in neuroanatomy and basic neuroscience. The period of training is typically 2 years, of which the first year is devoted largely to clinical practice and coursework. The second postdoctoral year integrates a research component, and at the end of this period, trainees are expected to have demonstrated accomplishment in research through publication or presentation at a regional or national meeting.

In addition to postdoctoral training, there is opportunity for graduate level training in the Benton Laboratory. Several graduate students per year train at our site, usually with a focus on clinical practice and didactic courses. This emphasis on training at both the graduate and postgraduate levels carries on the tradition of training established by Benton at the inception of the Iowa Laboratory (see Tranel, in press).

ASSESSMENT INSTRUMENTS: A SAMPLING

This section provides an overview of the tests commonly used in the Benton Neuropsychology Laboratory, many of which were developed at this site. Table 19-1 presents the tests most commonly used and the core battery, and Table 19-2 presents the commonly used follow-up tests.

The Core Battery

The core battery in the Iowa-Benton approach to neuropsychological assessment is intended to be a brief, broad, sensitive, and generally informative screening tool from which the examiner proceeds to build a profile customized to the patient. The core battery typically takes 40 to 60 minutes of patient time. The component tests have changed gradually over the years. Currently, the typical core battery consists of the tests listed (in italics) in Table 19-1.

TABLE 19-1. Current Battery: Benton Neuropsychology Laboratory[a]

1. Visual acuity screen
2. Auditory acuity screen
3. *Orientation to personal information, time, and place*
4. *Recall of recent presidents*
5. *WAIS-R Information*
6. *Complex Figure Test-Copy administration (with 30-minute) recall administration at appropriate time)*
7. *Rey Auditory Verbal Learning Test (with 30-minute recall and recognition at appropriate time)*
8. Draw a clock
9. WAIS-R Arithmetic
10. *WAIS-R Block Design*
11. WAIS-R Digit Span
12. WAIS-R Similarities
13. Trailmaking Test—Parts A and B
14. WAIS-R Digit Symbol
15. *Controlled Oral Word Association*
16. *Benton Visual Retention Test*
17. Facial Recognition Test
18. WAIS-R Picture Arrangement

[a] The most common "core battery" tests are in italics.
(Adapted from Appendix A, Benton Neuropsychology Laboratory, 1994, with permission.)

TABLE 19-2. Tests Commonly Used in the Benton Neuropsychology Laboratory

- Orientation
  - Time
  - Personal information
  - Place
  - Recent presidents
  - Recent news events
- Intellect/academic achievement
  - WAIS-R
    - Information
    - Digit Span
    - Vocabulary
    - Arithmetic
    - Comprehension
    - Similarities
    - Picture Completion
    - Picture Arrangement
    - Block Design
    - Object Assembly
    - Digit Symbol
  - Wide-Range Achievement Test
    - Reading
    - Spelling
    - Arithmetic
  - National Adult Reading Test-Revised
  - Stanford Binet
- Memory
  - AVLT
    - Trials 1–5
    - Delayed Recall
    - Delayed Recognition
  - Complex Figure Test
    - Copy
    - Recall
  - Benton Visual Retention Test
    - Copy of design #E10
    - # Correct
    - # Errors
  - WMS-R
    - Verbal
    - Visual
    - General
    - Attention/concentration
    - Delayed recall
  - Warrington Recognition Memory Test
    - Words
    - Faces
  - Forced Choice Memory Assessment
  - Iowa Autobiographical Memory Questionnaire
  - Iowa Famous Faces
  - Boston Remote Memory Battery
- Speech and language
  - Fluency
  - Paraphasias
  - Articulation
  - Prosody
  - Comprehension
  - Writing

TABLE 19-2 (*Continued*) Tests Commonly Used in the Benton Neuropsychology Laboratory

    - Copy
    - Dictation
    - Spont
  - Gestural Praxis
  - MAE
    - COWA
    - Visual Naming
    - Sentence Repetition
    - Token Test
    - Reading Comprehension of Word & Phrases
    - Aural Comprehension of Words & Phrases
    - Spelling: oral, written
  - Boston Naming Test
  - Boston Diagnostic Aphasia Exam
    - Automatized Sequences
    - Complex Ideational Material
    - Reading Sentence & Paragraphs
    - Repeating Phrases: high and low probability
    - Responsive Naming
    - Verbal Agility
  - Chapman Speed of Reading
  - Action Naming Test
- Visual perception/construction/motor
  - Facial Discrimination
  - Judgment of Line Orientation
  - Line Cancellation
    - Left
    - Center
    - Right
  - Hooper VOT
  - Drawing
    - Clock ("20 to 4")
    - House
    - Bicycle
  - 3-Dimensional Block Construction
  - Mirror Tracing (Triangle)
  - Grooved Pegboard Test
- Executive functions
  - Trailmaking Test
  - Wisconsin Card Sorting Test
  - Design Fluency
  - Booklet Category Test
- Mood/personality
  - Beck Depression Inventory
  - Beck Anxiety Inventory
  - MMPI
  - Iowa Rating Scales of Personality Change
  - Rorschach
- Miscellaneous
  - Dementia ratings
  - Right-left discrimination
    - Self
    - Confrontation
  - Finger Localization
  - Paced Auditory Serial Addition Test (attention)
  - Starry Night (attention)
  - Dichotic listening

(References for these tests can be found in Spreen and Strauss [1991], Lezak [1983], Benton Neuropsychology Laboratory [1994], and Wechsler [1981].)

Orientation

Orientation is measured by the Temporal Orientation Questionnaire (Benton et al., 1994b) and a series of specific questions related to personal information and knowledge of current surroundings. The Temporal Orientation Questionnaire is typical of the tests used in the Benton Laboratory in several ways; thus its development and method of administration will be described in some detail.

The test was developed by Benton and colleagues in response to their observation that assessment of temporal orientation in the context of the usual clinical interview could be misleading. Specifically, they found that a moderate degree of temporal disorientation was often overlooked. In response to this, their goal was to provide normative data that would help to define a defective performance empirically, based on observation in normals. Normative observations from a combination of three studies, comprising more than 400 subjects, are presented in Benton et al. (1994b) and are contrasted to the performances of nonaphasic brain-damaged patients in two studies of more than 100 subjects.

The Temporal Orientation Questionnaire is reproduced in Figure 19-1. The patient is asked to provide precise information regarding the date, month, year, day of week, and time of day (see "Patient Response" column of Fig. 19-1). Specific error scores are assigned if a response is incorrect (see "Correct Answer" column of Fig. 19-1), and a total error score is derived from the sum of the error scores ("Score" column, Fig. 19-1). This total score is then compared with normative data, and defects in temporal orientation are defined qualitatively by descriptors assigned to percentile ranks (e.g., a "borderline" performance is equal to −3 or the 5th percentile, a "low normal" performance is equal to −2 or the 8th percentile, and a "severely defective" performance is equal to −6 or less, or the .7th percentile or less). The test has been found to be useful in a screening examination for dementia (Eslinger et al., 1985) and is one of a few tests that are of benefit in the early differential diagnosis of dementia and so-called pseudodementia (Jones et al., 1992).

Attention

Measures of attention commonly used in the Benton Neuropsychology Laboratory include the Digit Span and Digit Symbol subtests of the WAIS-R (in the core battery) (Wechsler, 1981), the attention-concentration index of the WMS-R (Wechsler, 1987), the Paced Auditory Serial Addition Test (Gronwall, 1977), and the "Starry Night" procedure (Rizzo and Robin, 1990). We view performances on these measures as critical to the interpretation of other measures, because many higher-level abilities measured in neuropsychological assessment depend on intact or at least adequate attentional capacity. In the context of TBI, the assessment of attention becomes critical, given the substantial research literature documenting attentional impairments in such individuals (Gentilini et al., 1989; Gronwall, 1977).

Intellect

Specific intellectual skills are usually assessed with subtests of the WAIS-R (Wechsler, 1981). The specific subtests and number of subtests used have varied over the years. Currently, four subtests are most commonly used. These include (1) the Information subtest, which is often used as an index of premorbid intellect, (2) The Arithmetic subtest, which is viewed as a measure of not only verbal arithmetic skills but also as a test of problem solving and attention, (3) the Block Design subtest, which provides a measure of spatial problem solving, praxis, and motor speed, and (4) the Digit Symbol subtest, which provides an index of speeded visual-motor processing and attention.

With few exceptions, we are not particularly interested in the IQ score per se, and seldom do we report them in numerical form because such composite scores can be misleading or can obscure specific strengths or weaknesses of interest (Lezak, 1988). Particularly in the case of acquired brain damage due to trauma, we are more interested in the information provided by specific subtests, the relation between the subtests, and at times, the qualitative features of performance on these well-standardized measures (Kaplan et al., 1991; Lezak, 1993; Matarazzo, 1972). When intellectual performances are characterized, they are done so in the context of *ranges* and in relation to *expectations based on estimates of premorbid functioning* (e.g., "in the low average range, below expectations based on the patient's occupational and educational history").

Memory

Memory complaints are extremely common in patients with TBI. Memory tests can be broken down into several domains. Anterograde verbal memory is often measured by the AVLT with delayed recall, the

EXAMINER QUESTION	PATIENT RESPONSE	CORRECT ANSWER	SCORE
WHAT IS TODAY'S DATE?			
MONTH -5 for each month up to -30 maximum. Full credit if within 15 days of correct date.	________	________	____
DATE -1 for each day up to -15 maximum.	________	________	____
YEAR -10 for each year up to -60 maximum. Full credit if within 15 days of correct date.	________	________	____
WHAT DAY OF THE WEEK IS IT TODAY? -1 for each day up to -3 maximum.	________	________	____
WHAT TIME IS IT NOW? -1 for each 30 minutes up to -5 maximum	________	________	____
	TOTAL ERROR SCORE		____

Normative Data

Error Score	Percentile	Interpretation
-0	69+	Intact
-1	37	Normal
-2	8	Low Normal
-3	5	Borderline
-4	3	Moderate Defect
-5	1	Moderate Defect
-6	.1	Severe Defect

Fig. 19-1. Temporal Orientation Questionnaire (From Benton et al., 1994, with permission.)

Wechsler Memory Scale, and the Wechsler Memory Scale-Revised (WMS-R) (Lezak, 1988; Wechsler, 1987; Wiens et al., 1988). Anterograde visual memory is measured by the Benton Visual Retention Test (Sivan, 1992), recall of the Complex Figure Test (Lezak, 1988), and the visual memory index of the WMS-R (Wechsler, 1987). Retrograde memory is assessed by the Iowa Autobiographical Memory Questionnaire (Jones et al., 1993), the Iowa Famous Faces Test (Benton Neuropsychology Laboratory, 1994), and the Boston Remote Memory Battery (Albert et al., 1979). Procedural memory is assessed by the Rotor Pursuit test (Benton Neuropsychology Laboratory, 1994).

Language

A wide variety of tests of speech and language is used in the Benton Laboratory. The most widely known language measures associated with the Iowa-Benton approach are those tests that comprise the Multilingual Aphasia Examination (MAE) (Benton et al., 1994a). The MAE is composed of eight tests, of which six are most commonly used: Controlled Oral Word Association (COWA), Token Test, Aural Comprehension, Reading Comprehension, Sentence Repetition, Visual Naming (see Table 19-2). These tests, both individually and as a battery, have been shown to be sensitive to the presence of aphasia (Benton et al., 1994a; Jones and Benton, 1994).

Of the MAE tests, only the COWA is part of the core battery, based on the view that only tests that are most broadly informative belong in the battery. COWA has been shown to be sensitive to many language disorders (Benton et al., 1994a; Jones and Benton, 1994), discrimination of demented versus normal elderly (Eslinger et al., 1985), and dementia associated with human immunodeficiency virus (Jones and Tranel, 1991). It has also been viewed as a test of executive control and frontal lobe functioning (Tranel et al., 1994). The sensitivity of this test makes it especially useful in the core battery, particularly in cases of TBI when the clinical presentation can be quite varied.

Visual Perception, Construction, Judgment

Visual perception is typically assessed by the Facial Recognition Test (Benton et al., 1994b), which has been shown to be particularly sensitive to the presence of posterior right-hemisphere lesions. Visuoconstruction is measured by the Three-Dimensional Block Construction test (Benton et al., 1983) and the copy administration of the Complex Figure Test (Lezak, 1988). Spatial judgment is assessed by the Judgment of Line Orientation Test (Benton et al., 1978).

Personality, Mood, and Executive Control

Changes in personality, mood, and executive control are among the most common sequelae of brain injury due to trauma. Frequently used tests of personality include the MMPI-2 (Hathaway et al., 1989), the Beck Depression Inventory (Beck et al., 1961), and the Beck Anxiety Inventory (Beck and Steer, 1990). Less often, the Iowa Rating Scales for Personality Change (Benton Neuropsychology Laboratory, 1995) and the Rorschach may be used. The results of these tests in cases of known or suspected brain trauma can be enlightening in several respects. For example, the MMPI and MMPI-2 can be valuable in the determination of the extent to which psychiatric factors (e.g., depression, somatization disorder) may be contributing to a patient's clinical presentation, the assessment of malingering, or the extent to which response biases contribute to a patient's complaints (Berry et al., 1991; Greene, 1991). Although there is no single "organic profile" on the MMPI, there are certain scales and code types that are more likely to be elevated in patients with neurologic damage (Graham, 1977; Greene, 1991; Lachar, 1974). Further, the development of "organic" subscales derived from the MMPI has received some empirical validation in the detection and classification of patients with known neurologic conditions (Graham, 1977; Wiggins, 1969).

However, the results of such tests are always interpreted in the context of a clinical interview and the history of the patient, because it is believed by our group that the results of such probes must be understood as they pertain to the specific clinical situation. For example, a profile of depression as confirmed by the MMPI-2 and the Rorschach may represent a long-standing and stable dysthymic disorder, a "reactive" depression attributable to physical disability or cognitive impairment due to brain injury, or an "organic" depression associated with and directly attributable to brain damage. In this context, the observations of collateral sources (e.g., a spouse, parent, child, or caretaker) are sought in an effort to understand the phenomenology and etiology of the findings suggested by personality measures.

A similar approach is taken in the assessment of executive control dysfunction. Several tests are used to evaluate for such dysfunction, for example, the Wisconsin Card Sorting Test (Heaton, 1981), Category Test (Reitan and Wolfson, 1985), COWA (Benton et al., 1994a), Stroop Color Word Test (Golden, 1978), and the Trailmaking Test (Reitan and Wolfson, 1985). Several more experimental procedures can be illustrative in certain cases of suspected executive control defects, for example, the Tinkertoy Test and the Design Fluency Test (Jones-Gottmen and Milner, 1977; Lezak, 1983). However, use of such tests is typically restricted to experimental rather than clinical application (see also Tranel et al., 1994).

The results of tests of executive function must be interpreted in the context of the clinical situation. In the case of executive control defects after TBI, the observations of collateral sources become particularly critical, because many patients with rather dramatic defects in social judgment and other aspects of executive control are unaware of their disability and can even perform normally on the screening tests for such dysfunction (Anderson et al., 1991). The selection of a collateral is made in consultation with the patient. However, in litigated cases, at times it may be desirable to designate a collateral who is not immediately connected to the litigation. For example, rather than a spouse, in cases involving litigation it may be beneficial to speak with co-workers or neighbors, because such sources are distant from the litigation, and in this sense, their objectivity is less open to question.

ASSESSMENT OF TBI: CASE EXAMPLES

In this final section, a series of cases is presented that is intended to provide examples of the Iowa-Benton approach to neuropsychological assessment in the context of TBI. The cases were selected from our clinical files to represent the breadth of assessment in the Iowa-Benton model and the flexibility with which the model is applied.

Mild TBI

A 32-year-old female student was seen for neuropsychological assessment 1 month after a sports-related TBI. According to hospital records, she was admitted with a GCS score of 14 and had experienced an approximate 5-minute loss of consciousness according to observers. Acute computed tomography (CT) raised the question of a small left temporal-parietal contusion, but subsequent neuroimaging studies (CT and magnetic resonance imaging [MRI]) were normal, as was the EEG. She had virtually no retrograde amnesia and approximately 25 minutes of post-traumatic amnesia. At the time of the first neuropsychological assessment, she was taking anticonvulsant medication (Dilantin) as a prophylactic measure. In the initial interview, she complained of feeling "not as sharp" as before the accident and of problems with memory and word finding. She denied changes in mood vision, hearing, comprehension, and orientation. She stated that her grades were largely "A"s in the past.

She was evaluated on three occasions. The results of the first and the final assessments are depicted in Table 19-3. Our impression after the initial examination was that she had defects in visual perception (Facial Recognition Test) and speeded visuomotor sequencing (WAIS-R Digit Symbol and Trailmaking Test Part A) that were consistent with a mild post-TBI syndrome.

By the time of our final examination, approximately 1 year after the initial injury, her performances were within expectations based on her background. At that point, the patient was considering legal action, thus the examination was more detailed than our initial assessment. Further, as a result of this contingency, in addition to the neuropsychological data the psychologist examined pre- and post-trauma school records (which demonstrated no change in grades) and interviewed several collateral sources (husband, academic advisor, sibling), all of whom believed that she had made a full recovery. The impression of the examining neuropsychologist at the time of the last assessment was that she had recovered from her initial mild cognitive impairments but that, based on the interview with the patient and the MMPI, she continued to harbor concerns regarding her medical condition. This concern, as expressed by the patient, was related to her decision to terminate her participation in sports, given the possibility of a second and more severe brain injury. Psychotherapy for this concern was recommended. She did not pursue legal action in this case, and at the time of follow-up, she had completed psychotherapy and was successfully completing her graduate studies.

TABLE 19-3. Case Example: Mild Traumatic Brain Injury

Patient: right-handed 32-year-old female graduate student (with excellent school performances)
Features of the trauma: loss of consciousness = 5 minutes, no retrograde amnesia, approximately 25 minutes post-traumatic amnesia, admission GCS score = 14

Test	1 Month	1 Year
Orientation	Normal	Normal
Intellect		
Information	13	14
Digit Span	12	14
Vocabulary		14
Arithmetic	11	16
Comprehension		15
Similarities	14	13
Picture Completion		10
Picture Arrangement	14	16
Block Design	9	12
Object Assembly		12
Digit Symbol	7	12
Memory		
AVLT		
1	10	12
2	11	14
3	14	14
4	14	14
5	14	15
RECALL	14	15
RECOGNITION	Normal	Normal
Complex Figure Test		
Copy	35	35
Recall	19.5	25.5
Visual Retention Test		
Correct	8	7
Errors	2	3
Speech/language		
Fluency	Normal	Normal
Articulation	Normal	Normal
Prosody	Normal	Normal
Comprehension	Normal	Normal
Paraphasias	Absent	Absent
COWA	52	55
MAE Sentence repetition		14
Boston Naming Test		58
Chapman Reading		25
Category Fluency		62
Visual perception/spatial judgment		
Facial Recognition Test	39	41
Judgment of Line Orientation		25
Executive control		
Wisconsin Card Sorting Test		Normal
Booklet Category Test		16 errors
Trailmaking Test		
Part A	41	24
Part B	65	47
Personality/mood		
Beck Depression Inventory	13	17
Beck Anxiety Inventory		11
MMPI		2-1-3 profile

This case demonstrates a clinical situation that is borne out in the literature clearly—patients with mild brain traumas often, but not always, recover fully from their initial neuropsychological impairments (Dikmen et al., 1994; Ruff et al., 1989). In this case, the patient was young and highly intelligent and had a relatively minor trauma with limited loss of consciousness and post-traumatic amnesia. All these factors are associated with good recovery.

This case further demonstrates the extent to which the Iowa-Benton approach is customized to the contingencies of the clinical situation. In this case, the possibility of legal action prompted the neuropsychologist to complete a much more extensive examination than might have otherwise been completed. This stands in contrast to a strictly fixed battery approach, wherein the same tests would have been administered regardless of the question being posed.

Moderate TBI

The patient was a right-handed 45-year-old male truck driver with 12 years of education and with reportedly average school performances. He was a pedestrian involved in a motor vehicle crash wherein he sustained a left temporal depressed skull fracture. GCS score in the local emergency department was 9, and loss of consciousness was estimated to 45 minutes. Retrograde amnesia, established in the chronic examination, was estimated to be 4 to 5 hours, and anterograde amnesia was estimated to be 2 weeks. Acute CT and an MRI 1 week after the event showed a left temporal subdural hematoma (see Figure 19-2). During our first assessment, approximately 2 weeks after the injury, he was characterized as mildly agitated and aphasic, with fluent, paraphasic, and perseverative speech and severe defects in oral comprehension. The formal data from the first examination, as well as an assessment completed approximately 1 year later, are depicted in Table 19-4.

It is noteworthy that in the initial examination it was thought that the patient had memory defects in addition to aphasia. This is a somewhat unusual impression. We are typically disinclined to diagnose a verbal memory defect in the setting of aphasia, because there may be no meaningful method of assessing memory in such patients. In this case, however, it was thought by the examiner that the memory defects were beyond what could be explained by the aphasia. In sum, the findings were believed to be consistent with multiple areas of brain dysfunction. Compromises were seen clearly in language but also in memory.

The second column of Table 19-4 shows the findings of our assessment 1 year after the trauma. As can be seen, his initial language defects had largely resolved, but he was left with residual impairments in naming (MAE Visual Naming), word finding (COWA), constructional praxis (Complex Figure Test-Copy), visual perception (Facial Recognition Test), and memory (AVLT, Complex Figure Test-Recall, Visual Retention Test). It was the impression of the examining neuropsychologist that he would be unable to function in his formal job as a truck driver, and he was referred to vocational rehabilitation for assessment of occupational interests and possible skills. Further, the patient and his family were referred to a local TBI support group for information and psychological support pertaining to his condition and to neuropsychological rehabilitation for assessment of his appropriateness for further rehabilitation services (e.g., psychotherapy, couples counseling, cognitive rehabilitation). The final diagnosis was chronic post-TBI syndrome of moderate severity.

This case demonstrates some of the flexibility of the Iowa-Benton approach. Given the known left temporal hemorrhage (demonstrated on neuroimaging) and the particular language defects, the initial assessment was aimed at cognitive/linguistic abilities that were clearly compromised and that were likely to be impaired in the chronic epoch (memory, language). Of further interest in this case is a comparison of the sheer amount of data collected at the different time epochs. During the acute stages of the patient's recovery, it would have been inappropriate to give the patient an extended battery of tests. However, based on the initial examination, the psychologist was able to provide a meaningful impression to the referral source regarding the patient's cognitive and linguistic functioning and established a baseline against which to compare later assessments. This patient was not considered "untestable" during the acute stages; he was, in fact, able to provide a meaningful neuropsychological profile even in the acute epoch.

A Medicolegal Problem

The final case to be presented exemplifies a medicolegal case of alleged post-TBI. The patient was a right-handed 40-year-old mechanic with a high school education and 2 years of technical training.

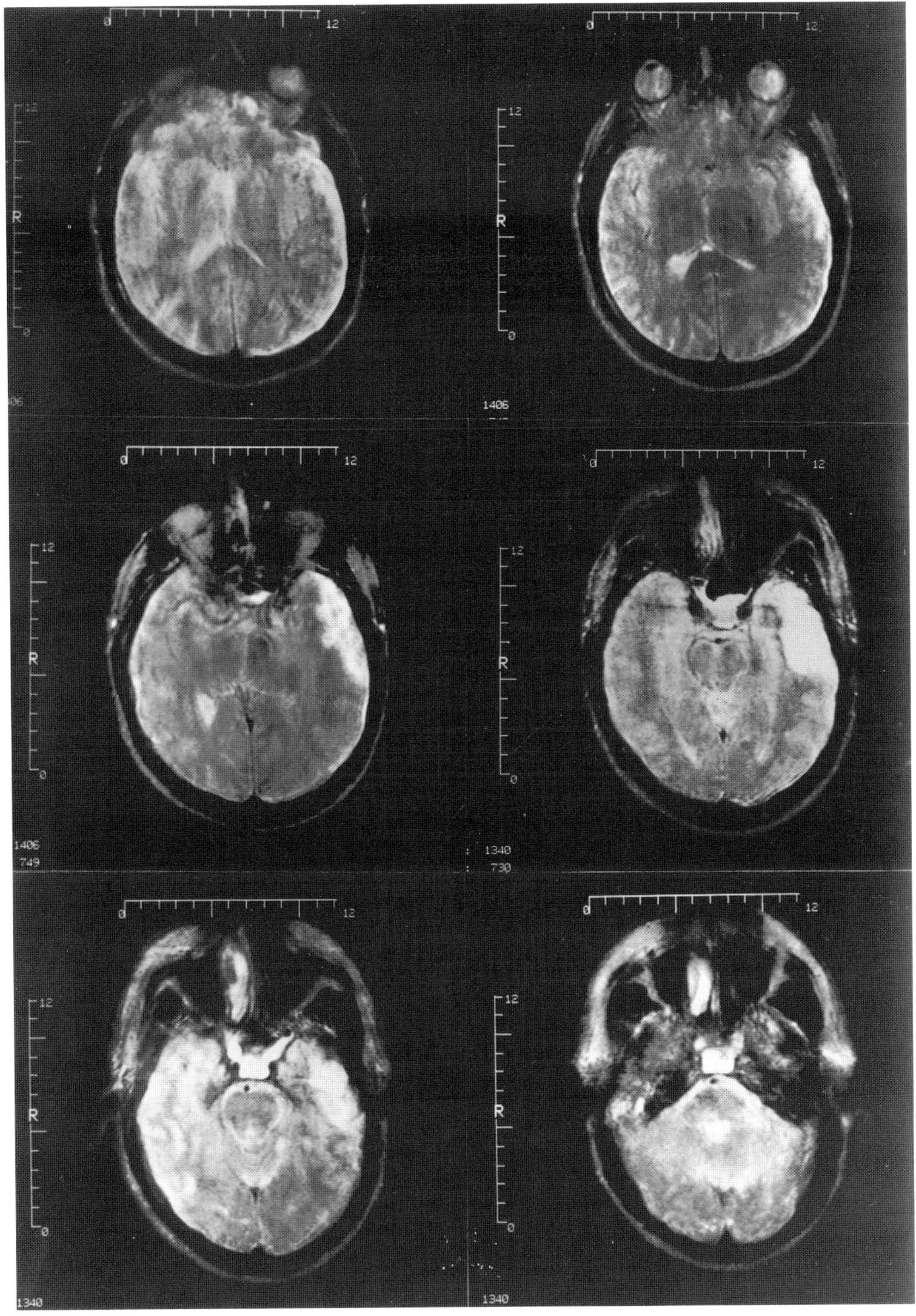

Fig. 19-2. Axial MRI slices obtained 2 weeks after a trauma, in standard radiographic orientation (left = right). Note the large left temporal hematoma, visible despite motion artifact secondary to agitation.

TABLE 19-4. Case Example: Moderate Traumatic Brain Injury

Patient: right-handed 45-year-old male truck driver with a high school education (with reportedly average school performances)
Features of the trauma: loss of consciousness = 45 minutes, 4 to 5 hours retrograde amnesia, 2 weeks post-traumatic amnesia, admission GCS score = 9, depressed skull fracture

Test	2 Weeks	1 Year
Orientation	Defective	Normal
Intellect		
Information		11
Digit Span		7
Block Design		8
Digit Symbol		6
Memory		
AVLT		
1		3
2		4
3		6
4		4
5		5
RECALL		2
RECOGNITION		Defective
Complex Figure Test		
Copy		25
Recall		6
Visual Retention Test		
Correct		3
Errors		13
Speech/language		
Fluency	Mildly dysfluent	Normal
Articulation	Normal	Normal
Prosody	Impaired	Normal
Comprehension	Impaired	Normal
Paraphasias	Perseverative, paraphasic	Normal
COWA	7	21
MAE Sentence Repetition		8
MAE Visual Naming		38
MAE Aural Comprehension	12	17
MAE Reading Comprehension	7	17
Visual perception/spatial judgment		
Facial Recognition Test		37
Draw a clock	Defective	Normal

While driving a large truck, he ran across a tire in the road and immediately thereafter stopped to check the condition of his truck. His log book indicated that he drove for several hours after this event and that he drove a normal 8-hour shift for the following 3 days. Several days after the accident, he began to experience spells of dizziness and nausea and sought medical attention. His medical assessment was negative. Several months later, he began to complain of episodic memory gaps, irritability, and word finding problems. He was referred for neuropsychological assessment, the results of which were interpreted to indicate a post-TBI syndrome as a result of the jolt he sustained when he ran over the tire in the road several months earlier. The outside neuropsychologist who had evaluated him indicated that the patient was permanently disabled due to the alleged brain trauma. It was in this context that he was referred to the Benton Neuropsychology Laboratory by the attorney for the insurance company for whom he was driving at the time of the event..

The neuropsychological data from our assessment are presented in Table 19-5. As can be seen, from a technical perspective there are several cognitive impairments, including aspects of intellect, attention, memory, and visuospatial skills. However, features of the profile appeared incongruent. For example, he generated a superb performance on the Wisconsin Card Sorting Test, which was somewhat surprising given the other deficits he demonstrated and the difficulty of this test. Also, he had a normal performance on the Complex Figure Test-Recall, whereas performances on other visual memory tests were severely defective (e.g., the Visual Retention Test, Recognition Memory Test-Faces). Also, he performed normally on Recognition Memory Test-Words but generated a severely defective performance on another verbal memory test (AVLT). Finally, although not presented here, the data showed several marked discrepancies relative to the other neuropsychological assessments (e.g., the WAIS-R Information subtest score on the other examination was 14, AVLT recall score was 9, and the Complex Figure Test-Recall score was 26).

There was no evidence of malingering on the Symptom Validity Test and a two-alternative forced choice test (Binder, 1993, Lezak, 1983). The MMPI suggested extreme somatic concern, with a clinical profile that is associated with many vague physical complaints and is suggestive of a somatoform disorder.

In our interview with this patient, he was forthcoming, pleasant, and articulate. He denied loss of conciousness, retrograde amnesia, and post-traumatic amnesia associated with the presumed brain trauma. We consider the determination of this information to be critical in cases of brain trauma, because it relates directly to the diagnosis (Brown et al., 1994). Such information in medicolegal cases can typically be obtained from both the patient and from medical records (e.g., paramedic or emergency department reports). In this case, he had vivid recall of the entire event. He expressed genuine concern that he had sustained a brain trauma, that he would be disabled for life, and that he would be unable to provide for his family. In our interview with his wife, she agreed fully with her husband's self-perceptions of impairments in memory and word finding and increased moodiness since the event. Both she and her husband stated that these impairments had become progressively worse over time and that they had not even noticed any problems with mood or cognition until several months after the event. In an extensive interview, both the patient and his wife denied the possibility of other etiologies for his complaints (e.g., toxic exposure, medication effects).

Background records reviewed in this case were extensive. In addition to the raw neuropsychological data from the prior examination, these records included a complete medical history, school records including performances on standardized achievement tests, and occupational records. Also, a second collateral was interviewed, the driving partner of the patient, who was in the truck at the time of the alleged brain trauma.

The records revealed that for several years before the alleged trauma the patient had had a series of medical complaints that had not been confirmed by diagnostic tests and in some cases were considered to be anatomically impossible (e.g., "glove anaesthesia"). On at least six occasions before the alleged brain trauma, he had complained of progressive problems with dizziness, word finding, memory, and mood changes. The records revealed that he had undergone assessment for a seizure disorder based on these complaints several years before the alleged trauma and had been diagnosed with "pseudoseizures" at that time based on 24-hour EEG studies. Several of the physicians he had consulted noted a suspicion of psychiatric disease, specifically a somatoform disorder, but the patient was never referred for psychological or psychiatric assessment. He had been an average student in high school and technical school. His partner who was riding in the truck at the time of the accident specifically denied that the patient demonstrated any behavioral change immediately after the event or for the next several days or that the patient had any complaints during the period immediately after the event.

The impression of the examining neuropsychologist was that the patient did not have a TBI but rather a long-standing psychiatric disorder. He was referred to a psychiatrist for assessment (blind to the neuropsychologist's opinion), and the patient was subsequently diagnosed with somatoform disorder. Treatment in the setting of group psychotherapy was recommended. At follow-up, the patient had returned

TABLE 19-5. Case Example: Medicolegal Problem

Patient: right-handed 40-year-old male mechanic, 14 years of education (average school performances)
Features of the trauma: loss of consciousness = none, no retrograde amnesia, no post-traumatic amnesia, admission GCS score never rated (no hospital admission)

Test	3 Years
Orientation	−1
Intellect	
Information	10
Digit Span	7
Arithmetic	8
Comprehension	13
Similarities	13
Picture Completion	9
Picture Arrangement	11
Block Design	9
Digit Symbol	6
Attention	
WMS-R Attention-Concentration	88
Memory	
WMS-R Logical Memory	
Immediate	26 %ile
30-minute delay	55 %ile
AVLT	
1	6
2	6
3	6
4	7
5	6
RECALL	2
RECOGNITION	12/30 (below chance)
Complex Figure Test	
Copy	32
Recall	19.5
Visual Retention Test	
Correct	4
Errors	10
Recognition Memory Test	
Faces	26/50
Words	45/50
Speech/language	
Fluency	Normal
Articulation	Normal
Prosody	Normal
Comprehension	Normal
Paraphasias	Normal
COWA	40
MAE Visual Naming	52 + 2
Visual perception/spatial judgment	
Facial Recognition Test	45
Judgment of Line Orientation	18
Executive control	
Wisconsin Card Sorting Test	
8 Errors	
6 Perseverative errors	
6 Categories	

(*continued*)

TABLE 19-5 (*Continued*) **Case Example: Medicolegal Problem**

Booklet Category Test	
Trailmaking Test	
Part A	44
Part B	88
Personality/mood	
Beck Depression Inventory	34
MMPI	Spike 1 (T = 100)
Motivation	
Symptom Validity Test	Normal (15/15 × 5 trials)
Two Alternative Forced Choice	Normal (70/72)

to work as a mechanic and reportedly no longer expressed concerns regarding TBI.

This case illustrates several points. First, it is important to recognize that this patient had a legitimate problem, albeit not a TBI. It is not uncommon for neuropsychologists to see patients with sincere concerns regarding their cognitive functioning, and subsequent assessment suggests that these concerns are most likely related to psychiatric disturbance. In this case, the patient very likely had some form of somatoform disorder, as was eventually diagnosed. He was not a malingerer.

Second, this case illustrates the extent to which relevant information must be reviewed to come to an opinion "within a reasonable degree of neuropsychological certainty" in medicolegal cases (Matarazzo, 1990). In such cases, we do not rely solely on the outcome of neuropsychological testing and then attempt to tie observed substandard performances to an event or presumed etiology. Rather, we view it as important to work forward from the event, in this case alleged TBI, and attempt to determine if there is a neuropsychological profile that fits with the facts of the case. Such an approach often involves extensive review of records.

Similar to the first case, this patient received an extensive evaluation. The detail of this assessment arose in response to the referral question, which demanded precise characterization of his neuropsychological profile, the patient's complaints, which were broad and somewhat vague, and the results of tests from the core battery, which in many cases were below expectations.

CONCLUSION

The Iowa-Benton approach to neuropsychological assessment of patients with TBI is hypothesis-driven and logically sequential, and it relies on empirically derived normative data. Test selection depends on multiple factors that are given different degrees of importance in any given examination: the referral question, the patient's condition, known or suspected brain pathology, the patient's complaints, and the results of earlier tests are some of the more salient factors that drive test selection. The method is operationalized by administration of a brief (40- to 60-minute) set of "core" tests that are intended to be *generally* informative and follow-up tests selected from a rich armamentarium of specific measures. The dual aim of the method is to provide a meaningful, reliable characterization of the patient's neuropsychological functioning (cognitive, affective, and behavioral) while simultaneously respecting the patient's clinical situation. The method is not seen as a "solution" to the problem of how to combine the best of the "fixed" and "flexible" battery approaches to assessment but rather a "reasonable response" to the problem (see Benton, 1992, p. 414–415).

By definition, the Iowa-Benton approach to assessment is subject to change in accordance with advances in basic knowledge. That is, although the general method of a hypothesis-testing approach in the setting of a core battery has remained in place for more than 40 years, the specific tests both in the core battery and in the follow-up tests have evolved over time. This evolution has taken place in response to new knowledge in cognitive neuroscience, clinical experience, and the development of new tests. It can be anticipated that this evolution will continue.

ACKNOWLEDGMENT

I am grateful to Arthur Benton for his comments on an earlier draft of this chapter, and for his consistently wise guidance during the time I have spent in the Benton Laboratory at Iowa.

REFERENCES

Albert ML, Butters N, Levin J: Temporal gradients in the retrograde amnesia of patients with alcoholic Korsakoff's disease. Arch Neurol 36:211–216, 1979

Anderson SW, Damasio H, Jones RD, Tranel D: Wisconsin Card Sorting Test as a measure of frontal lobe damage. J Clin Exp Neuropsychol 13:909–922, 1991

APA Division 40: Report of the Task Force on Education, Accreditation, and Credentialing. Clin Neuropsychol 1:29–34, 1987

Beck AT, Steer RA: Beck Anxiety Inventory Manual. The Psychological Corporation, San Antonio, TX, 1990

Beck AT, Ward CH, Mendelson M et al: An inventory for measuring depression. Arch Gen Psychiatry 4:561–571, 1961

Benton AL: Some problems associated with neuropsychological assessment. Bull Clin Neurosci 50:11–15, 1985

Benton AL: Basic approaches to neuropsychological assessment. In Steinhauer SR, Gruzelier JH, Zubin J. (eds): Handbook of Schizophrenia. Vol. 5. Elsevier, Amsterdam, 1991

Benton AL: Clinical neuropsychology: 1960–1990. J Clin Exp Neuropsychol 14:407–417, 1992

Benton AL: Neuropsychological assessment. Annu Rev Psychol 45:1–23, 1994

Benton AL, Hamsher K, Sivan AB: Multilingual Aphasia Examination. 3rd Ed. AJA Associates, Iowa City, IA, 1994a

Benton AL, Sivan AB, Hamsher K et al: Contributions to Neuropsychological Assessment. 2nd Ed. Oxford, New York, 1994b

Benton Neuropsychology Laboratory: Manual of Operations. Department of Neurology, University of Iowa, Iowa City, IA, 1995

Berry DTR, Baer RA, Harris MJ: Detection of malingering on the MMPI: a meta-analysis. Clin Psychol Rev 11:585–598, 1991

Binder LM: Assessment of malingering after mild head trauma with the Portland Digit Recognition Test. J Clin Exp Neuropsychol 15:170–182, 1993

Brown SJ, Fann JR, Grant I: Postconcussional disorder: time to acknowledge a common source of neurobehavioral morbidity. J Neuropsychiatry 6:15–22, 1994

Damasio AR, Anderson SW: The frontal lobes. In Heilman KM, Valenstein E (eds): Clinical Neuropsychology. 3rd Ed. Oxford, New York, 1993

Dikmen SS, Temkin NR, Machaner JE et al: Employment following traumatic brain injury. Arch Neurol 51:177–186, 1994

Eslinger PJ, Damasio AR, Benton AL, Van Allen M: Neuropsychological detection of abnormal mental decline in older persons. JAMA 253:670–674, 1985

Gentilini M, Nichelli P, Schonhuber R: Assessment of attention in mild head injury. In Levin HS, Eisenberg HM, Benton AL (eds): Mild Head Injury. Oxford, New York, 1989

Golden CJ: Stroop Color and Word Test Manual. Stoelting Company, Chicago, 1978

Golden CJ, Purisch AD, Hammeke TA: Luria Nebraska Neuropsychological Battery: Forms I and II Manual. Western Psychological Services, Los Angeles, 1985

Graham JR: The MMPI: A Practical Guide. Oxford, New York, 1977

Greene RL: MMPI-2/MMPI: An Interpretive Manual. Allyn and Bacon, Boston, 1991

Gronwall D: Paced auditory serial addition task: a measure of recovery from concussion. Percept Mot Skills 44:367–373, 1977

Hamsher K: The Iowa group. Int J Neurosci 25:295–305, 1985

Hathaway SR, McKinley JC, Butcher JN et al: Minnesota Multiphasic Personality Inventory-2. Regents of the University of Minnesota, Minneapolis, 1989

Heaton RK: A Manual for the Wisconsin Card Sorting Test. Psychological Assessment Resources, Odessa, FL, 1981

Jones BP, Butters N: Neuropsychological assessment. In Hersen M, Kazdin AE, Bellack AS (eds): The Clinical Psychology Handbook. Pergammon Press, New York, 1983

Jones RD, Benton AL: Use of the multilingual aphasia examination in the detection of language disorders. INS Prog Abstr, 1994

Jones RD, Tranel DT: Development of a screening battery for the detection of HIV-related cognitive deficits. Arch Clin Neuropsychol 6:198, 1991

Jones RD, Tranel D, Benton AL, Paulsen J: Differentiating dementia from "pseudodementia" early in the clinical course: utility of neuropsychological tests. Neuropsychology 6:13–21, 1992

Jones RD, Tranel D, Walljasper C: Disruption of autobiographical memory in patients with focal brain lesions. Clin Neuropsychol 7:340, 1993

Jones-Gottman M, Milner B: Design fluency: the invention of nonsense drawings after focal cortical lesions. Neuropsychologia 15:653–674, 1977

Kaplan E, Fein D, Morris R, Delis DC: The Wechsler Adult Intelligence Scale-Revised as a Neuropsychological Instrument. The Psychological Corporation, San Antonio, TX, 1991

Lachar D: The MMPI: Clinical Assessment and Automated Interpretation. Western Psychological Services, Los Angeles, 1974

Lezak MD: Neuropsychological Assessment. 2nd Ed. Oxford University Press, New York, 1983

Lezak MD: IQ: R.I.P. J Clin Exp Neuropsychol 10:351–361, 1988

Matarazzo J: Psychological assessment versus psychological testing: validation from Binet to the school, clinic, and courtroom. Am Psychol 45:999–1017, 1990

Matarazzo JD: Wechsler's Measurement and Appraisal of Adult Intelligence. 5th Ed. Oxford, New York, 1972

McKenna P, Warrington EK: The analytical approach to neuropsychological assessment. In Grant I, Adams K (eds): Neuropsychological Assessment of Neuropsychiatric Disorders. Oxford, New York, 1986

Reitan RM: Theoretical and methodological bases of the Halstead-Reitan Neuropsychological Test Battery. In Grant I, Adams K (eds): Neuropsychological Assessment of Neuropsychiatric Disorders. Oxford, New York, 1986

Reitan RM, Wolfson D: The Halstead-Reitan Neuropsychological Test Battery: Theory and Clinical Interpretation. Neuropsychology Press, Tucson, AZ, 1985

Rizzo M, Robin DA: Simultanagnosia: a defect of sustained attention yields insights on visual information processing. Neurology 40:447–455, 1990

Sivan AB: Benton Visual Retention Test. 5th Ed. The Psychological Corporation, New York, 1992

Spreen O, Benton AL: Neurosensory Center Comprehensive Examination for Aphasia (NCCEA). Experimental Ed. University of Iowa, Department of Neurology, Iowa City, 1985

Spreen O, Strauss E: A Compendium, of Neuropsychological Tests: Administration, Norms, and Commentary. Oxford University Press, New York, 1991

Tranel D: The Iowa-Benton school of neuropsychological assessment. In Grant I, Adams K (eds): Neuropsychological Assessment of Neuropsychiatric Disorders. 2nd Ed. Oxford, New York, in press

Tranel D, Anderson SW, Benton A: Development of the concept of "executive function" and its relationship to the frontal lobes. In Boller F, Grafman J (eds): Handbook of Neuropsychology. Vol. 9. Elsevier, New York, 1994

Wechsler D: Manual for the Wechsler Adult Intelligence Scale-Revised. Psychological Corporation, New York, 1981

Wechsler D: Wechsler Memory Scale-Revised. Psychological Corporation, New York, 1987

Wiens AN, McMinn MR, Crossen JR: Rey Auditory Verbal Learning Test: development of norms for healthy young adults. Clin Neuropsychol 2:67–87, 1988

Wiggins JS: Content dimensions in the MMPI. In Butcher JN (ed): MMPI: Research Developments and Clinical Application. McGraw-Hill, New York, 1969

Neuropsychological Sequelae of Traumatic Brain Injury

20

R. D. Jones
S. W. Anderson
T. Cole
J. Hathaway-Nepple

The cognitive, affective, and behavioral sequelae of brain damage due to head trauma are frequently the most salient features of the condition. In fact, the diagnosis of brain damage related to head trauma often primarily or entirely rests on the determination of the presence and severity of such sequelae. The precise measurement and characterization of these features of the condition are the explicit area of study in the clinical neuropsychology of traumatic brain injury (TBI). This chapter provides an overview of some of the types of neuropsychological deficits that are associated with TBI.

Diagnosis and management of patients with TBI typically occur in a multidisciplinary setting. In addition to clinical neuropsychology, specialties such as neurology, psychiatry, social work, occupational/vocational rehabilitation, cognitive rehabilitation, speech pathology, and family therapy are often asked to coordinate services. Clinical neuropsychological assessment is important in this context for several reasons. For diagnostic purposes, many patients with mild TBI have otherwise normal medical tests (e.g., neurologic examination, neuroimaging, electroencephalography [EEG]), and neuropsychological assessment is necessary to confirm the diagnosis. In cases of more severe TBI, neuropsychological assessment becomes less critical for establishing the presence of brain dysfunction, because behavioral manifestations of the injury are often clear and ancillary diagnostic tests are often positive. However, even in cases of severe injury, neuropsychological assessment remains of central importance for clarifying the nature and severity of cognitive and behavioral impairments, for evaluating the contribution of other factors such as psychiatric disease, dementia, or premorbid substance abuse, for assessing the course of recovery, and for documenting the efficacy of interventions. Finally, in virtually all cases of TBI such assessment can provide information relevant to management of the condition, for example, whether the patient can manage financial affairs, whether the patient needs rehabilitation, and appropriate goals for rehabilitation.

In this chapter, common neuropsychological sequelae of TBI are discussed. Although not all head trauma causes brain injury, the terms are often used interchangeably. In our use of the terms, head trauma will not necessarily imply brain trauma, and brain trauma may be due to multiple etiologies in addition to head trauma (e.g., penetrating missile wounds, sudden acceleration/deceleration without actual trauma to the head). The focus in this chapter is to characterize *behavioral, cognitive, emotional, and social characteristics that are compromised, exacerbated, or in some way modified by TBI.* In the first part of the chapter, the effects of brain trauma on neuropsychological functions are described. This section includes consideration of selected research on the effects of brain trauma on memory, attention and information processing, intellect, language, visuoperceptual and visuoconstructional functions, executive control and personality, and social/occupational functioning. A series of cases from the Benton Neuropsychology Clinic at the University of Iowa is presented that illustrates many of the points made earlier in the chapter. Finally, future research directions are considered.

MEMORY

The most prevalent complaint in patients with TBI is an impairment of memory (Arcia and Gualtieri, 1993; Levin, 1989; Tate et al., 1991; Van Zomeren and Van Denberg, 1985). A substantial body of research has documented this, although estimates of the prevalence of memory defects after TBI vary dramatically depending on factors such as the severity of the injury, associated complications (such as prior injury or psychiatric disease), and demographic characteristics of the patient (Oddy et al., 1985; Ruff et al., 1989; Schacter and Crovits, 1977).

Likely owing to the physics and resulting pathophysiology of acceleration/deceleration injuries in TBI, there is evidence in both animal and human studies of relatively specific memory defects after TBI (Hamm et al., 1992; Levin, 1989; Levin et al., 1988; Levin et al., 1990). Specifically, there is disproportionate representation of temporal and frontal abnormalities associated with brain injury due to trauma (Eisenberg and Levin, 1989; Levin et al., 1982), areas that are well known to contribute to memory (Damasio and Damasio, 1993; Squire et al., 1993; Tranel 1994).

In general, memory impairments associated with TBI can be divided into the anterograde epoch, referring to memory for events that occurred subsequent to the injury, and the retrograde epoch, referring to memory for events that occurred before the injury (Fig. 20-1). After the injury, there is typically, but not always, loss of consciousness, during which the patient by definition is unable to remember ongoing events. This is followed by a period of anterograde memory impairment of variable length. Typically, the initial period of anterograde memory defects is termed post-traumatic amnesia (see below) and is characterized by disorientation, confusion, and other manifestations of cognitive disruption.

The severity of the neurologic injury in the acute epoch can be defined more precisely than simple presence or absence of loss of consciousness. The subdivision of levels of coma is usually measured by the Glasgow Coma Scale (GCS) (Teasdale and Jennett, 1974) (Table 20-1), which has been found to be a more reliable index than simple judgments of "conscious" versus "unconscious" (Teasdale et al., 1978). The GCS assesses the patient's behavior in three modalities: minimum stimulus to produce eye opening, motor response, and verbal response. Total scores range from 3 to 15 and have been shown to be predictive of survival. The total GCS score has also served as a classification variable in recent research to provide an index of the severity of brain trauma. GCS scores on admission to a hospital are typically reported. For purposes of classification, several investigators have designated GCS scores of 13 to 15 as signifying mild injury, 9 to 12 as signifying moderate injury, and 3 to 8 as signifying severe injury (Levin et al., 1990).

Recent studies suggest that the presence or absence of loss of consciousness in and of itself and in the setting of otherwise mild trauma does not predict memory impairment in the chronic epoch (Leininger et al., 1990; Strugar et al., 1993). For example, Leininger et al. (1990) studied 53 patients with minor TBI, 31 of whom had sustained brief loss of consciousness and 22 of whom were only "dazed." Relative to control subjects, the two experimental groups performed poorly on five of eight neuropsychological tests administered, including tests of verbal and visual memory (Auditory Verbal Learning Test and Complex Figure Test-Recall, respectively) (see Lezak, 1985, for test characteristics). However, there were no differences in memory performances between those

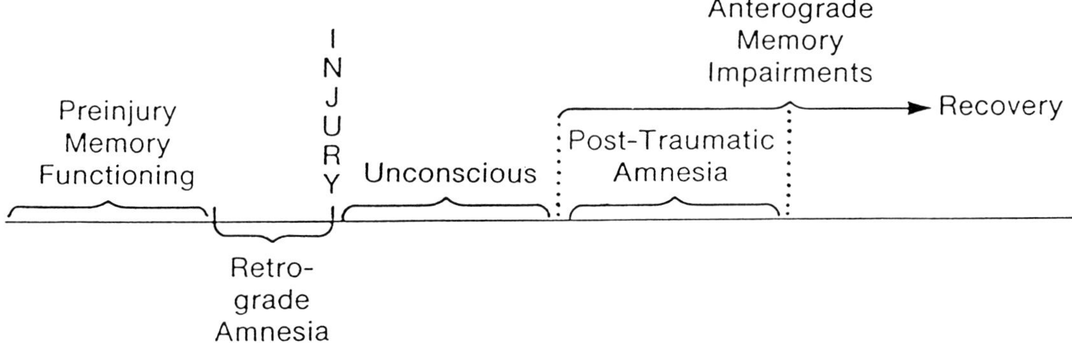

Fig. 20-1. Memory impairments from closed head injury related to time. (From Ruff et al., 1989, with permission.)

subjects who were only "dazed" and those who sustained brief loss of consciousness.

After resumption of consciousness, there may be a period of post-traumatic amnesia. This refers to the period of time after a brain injury during which ongoing events are not remembered in a continuous way. That is, the patient does not make a permanent record of ongoing events and may appear disoriented and confused. Although the measurement of post-traumatic amnesia is somewhat complicated and a matter of some debate (see Gronwall, 1989a; Levin et al., 1982), there is no question as to its practical significance in patient management in the early stages after brain trauma. One indication of post-traumatic amnesia is the degree to which a patient is oriented to his or her surroundings and ongoing events in time (i.e., orientation). Recovery of orientation after TBI has been addressed in a prospective investigation of 84 patients who had sustained mild, moderate, or severe TBI (High et al., 1990). It was reported that orientation to personal information was usually the first to recover, followed by orientation to place and time.

TABLE 20-1. Glasgow Coma Scale

Eye opening	Spontaneously	4
	To verbal command	3
	To pain	2
	No eye opening	1
Best motor response	Obeys commands	6
	Localizes pain	5
	Flexion-withdrawal	4
	Decorticate posturing	3
	Decerebrate posturing	2
	No response	1
Best verbal response	Oriented, converses	5
	Disoriented, converses	4
	Verbalizes	3
	Vocalizes	2
	No response	1
	TOTAL	

(From Teasdale and Jennett, 1974, with permission.)

It is clear that memory problems can be detected after mild TBI, and in fact, loss of consciousness is not a necessary precursor to subsequent memory impairments (Leininger et al., 1990). However, some of the methodologically strongest research to date suggests that many if not most patients with mild TBI generally recover cognitive capacities including memory (Levin et al., 1987b). For example, Ruff et al. (1989) studied 155 consecutive patients between the ages of 15 and 50 years who had GCS scores of at least 13 on hospital admission after TBI and GCS scores of 15 at 48 hours after the trauma. Loss of conciousness was limited to 20 minutes at most, and all the subjects had normal neurologic examinations. Follow-up evaluations were conducted with specific emphasis on memory functioning, and performances of TBI subjects were compared with regional controls. There were clear and significant memory problems observed in the TBI group during the baseline evaluation. At the 1-month follow-up examination, there was significant attrition, but based on 57 patients who participated in the baseline assessment and the 1-month follow-up, the authors concluded that verbal and visual memory performances in patients with mild TBI were indistinguishable from controls.

The term *retrograde amnesia* in the context of TBI refers to an inability to remember events before the trauma. Retrograde amnesia is typically briefer than post-traumatic amnesia (see Fig. 20-1). Retrograde memory defects may show a "temporal gradient" whereby events that are most temporally proximate to the injury are the most likely to be forgotten and more temporally distant memories (e.g., of childhood) are more likely to be retained (Capruso and Levin, 1992; Levin et al., 1985). Finally, retrograde memory impairments tend to recede or "shrink" over time. As patients emerge from their initial confusion and disorientation, more recent retrograde events will be recalled (Levin et al., 1985).

In sum, several basic principles can be derived from the literature: (1) it is possible that even mild TBI can result in chronic memory defects, although the likelihood of memory impairment is greater with more severe injuries, (2) the previous principle notwithstanding, most patients with mild TBI and no other risk factors recover to normal or near-normal levels of memory functioning, and (3) retrograde amnesia after TBI is brief relative to post-traumatic amnesia.

ATTENTION AND INFORMATION PROCESSING

Attention is a complex topic and a global term that can be broken down into several subcomponents. By simple sustained attention or vigilance, we mean the ability of the individual to maintain concentration on a task at hand over a specified period of time. This stands in contrast to divided attention, which refers to the ability to attend to two or more tasks simultaneously. The concept overlaps considerably with the notion of memory and, in particular, so-called working memory. Finally, *information processing* refers to the ability to synthesize and use sequential information on an ongoing basis. Attention and information processing can be affected by even mild TBI (Miller, 1970; Stuss et al., 1985; Van Zomeren, 1981). In fact, some authors argue that such abilities are selectively affected and that this selectivity can be demonstrated by specific neuropsychological methods (Gentillini et al., 1989; Gronwall, 1989b).

The measurement of attention has been undertaken in several ways. Perhaps the most common method of assessing attention is with a reaction time paradigm. There are many permutations of this paradigm, including divided-attention reaction time tasks, choice reaction time tasks, and simple reaction time tasks. For example, Hugenholtz et al., (1988) examined a group of 22 adults with mild TBI. Studies of simple and choice reaction times were completed with these subjects five times over a 3-month period and were compared with the performances of 22 normal matched controls. The results indicated that simple reaction time did not discriminate between groups but that choice reaction times, even at the 3-month follow-up, were significantly different as a function of group. Hugenholtz et al. attributed this difference to differences in the degree of "central" processing necessary in simple versus divided attention tasks and underscored the ubiquity of subtle defects in attention in even very mildly injured patients. The findings have been replicated and extended by this group in subsequent studies (see Stuss et al., 1989). A conceptually similar finding was reported by Parasuraman et al. (1991), who found that attentional performances of mildly injured patients were normal under conditions of visual "vigilance" testing but were defective when the stimulus was visually degraded. This finding was interpreted to reflect the TBI patients' inability to perform normally on tests of attention that require effortful information processing.

Information processing has been assessed extensively by the Paced Auditory Serial Addition Test (PASAT) (Gronwall, 1989b; Gronwall et al., 1977). In this task, the subject is presented with a series of digits at increasing speed and is asked to add the first to the second, the second to the third, the third to the fourth, and so on. The test has been shown to discriminate between mildly brain-injured subjects and normal controls and has been used to chart recovery curves for mildly brain-injured patients (Gronwall, 1989b). There is some suggestion that speed of information processing may be selectively impaired in patients with TBI. For example, Ponsford and Kinsella (1992) reported in a series of studies that patients with TBI were no different than controls on measures of "focused" attention or "sustained" attention but that tests of speed of information processing discriminated TBI subjects from controls. In addition to the PASAT, the neuropsychological tests that discriminated between groups included the Symbol Digit Modality Test, simple and choice reaction time tests, and the Stroop Color-Word test.

In sum, attentional and information processing defects are common after TBI, and several authors have noted that such deficits may be relatively selective. The literature suggests that the impairments can be observed, especially under conditions of divided reaction time tasks and other tests that require effortful information processing.

INTELLECT

General intellectual ability after TBI has been assessed primarily with the Wechsler Adult Intelligence Scale-Revised (WAIS-R) (Wechsler, 1981). This test consists of 11 subscales, 6 of which are designated "Verbal" and 5 of which are designated "Performance" subtests. Resultant summary scores are designated as the Verbal IQ (VIQ), the Performance IQ (PIQ), and Full-Scale IQ. VIQ is generally regarded as related more strongly to well-learned or "crystallized" information, whereas PIQ, based on nonverbal and generally novel tasks, does not rely as heavily on well-learned skills (Lezak, 1985). At the level in interpretation for the individual patient, a clinical neuropsychologist is often more interested in the pattern of results across subtests rather than the summary IQ derived from them (Kaplan et al., 1991; Lezak, 1985, 1988). Summary IQ scores, although more statistically reliable, reflect a collection of performances on multiple and disparate tasks. Much of the potentially rich information available through individual subtest analysis is lost when using only summary indices, and such indices may, in fact, be misleading regarding a patient's intellectual abilities.

However, there are clear trends in the literature regarding summary IQ indices on the WAIS-R after TBI. In general, the severity of TBI is related to the level of intellectual deficit (Barth et al., 1983; Dikmen et al., 1986a; Mandelberg and Brooks, 1975; Mayes et al., 1989; Tabaddor et al., 1979). Relative to controls, subjects with mild TBI show little if any impairments on formal tests of intellect (e.g., WAIS, WAIS-R) (Drudge et al., 1984), whereas more severely brain-injured patients do show clear defects both initially and chronically (Mandleberg and Brooks, 1975; Mayes et al., 1989; Tabaddor et al., 1984).

A second trend in the literature is that intellectual functions improve over time, from the acute stages after trauma to the chronic epoch. For example, in a longitudinal study of intellectual recovery after TBI, Mandleberg and Brooks (1975) studied 40 men who had sustained TBI of varying levels of severity, defined by the duration of post-traumatic amnesia. Performances on the WAIS were compared with performances of a control group. As might be expected, scores on most of the tests were below the scores of the control goup at the initial assessment. After 10 months, however, there was no significant difference in VIQ between the groups. Performance subscale scores of the brain-injured group showed some improvement but remained significantly lower than those of the control group until a 3-year follow-up assessment. In general, scores on the Verbal tests were not as low as scores on the Performance tests and improved to normal levels more quickly.

This latter finding reported by Mandleberg and Brooks has been reported elsewhere. That is, several studies have shown that VIQ of patients with TBI shows less initial decline and recovers more completely than PIQ (e.g., Mayes et al., 1989). This is perhaps related to the relative novelty of Performance subscale tasks, which tend to be generally more sensitive to brain dysfunction compared with Verbal subscale tasks (Jones et al., 1992; Lezak, 1983). However, this finding is not universally supported in the literature (see Tabaddor et al., 1984); thus it is probably too early to make broad statements with certainty regarding the relationship between VIQ and PIQ after TBI.

In sum, as might be expected, patients with TBI show intellectual deficits, largely related to the severity of the trauma. Assessment of overall intellectual functioning, however, is of less interest in this population in the context of clinical neuropsychological assessment, because more meaningful data can be derived from analysis of performances on specific subscales.

LANGUAGE

That a blow to the head can result in specific language impairments has been recognized since ancient Greece, and multiple cases of traumatic aphasia had been described by the 16th century (Benton and Joynt, 1960). Although firearms and motor vehicles have largely replaced stones and spears as the instruments of neural damage, TBI resulting in language impairment has remained a topic of scientific inquiry and clinical significance. Much of the knowledge base of modern aphasiology has been derived from the study of patients with cerebrovascular disease, but these findings have direct relevance to TBI.

Virtually any form of linguistic disorder commonly associated with vascular disease also can result from traumatic injury, depending on the nature, location, and severity of the injury. The pathophysiology of closed head injury makes less likely the occurrence of tightly localized damage restricted to specific language-related structures but is associated with a relatively high probability of dysfunction within the left perisylvian region. As such, language impairments are not uncommon after TBI. For example, Sarno (1980) examined 56 cases admitted to a rehabilitation unit after TBI sufficient to result in at least brief (10 to 15 minutes) loss of consciousness and found that all these subjects had some degree of language defect.

Given that impairments of word retrieval (i.e., naming and word finding) are almost universal in aphasia, it is not surprising that these are the most common language defects after TBI (e.g., Heilman et al., 1971; Levin et al., 1976, 1981). When present, paraphasias, circumlocutions, alexia, and agraphia typically are quite obvious and generally will be described by the patient or family. Impaired aural comprehension, however, may be subtle and may underlie complaints of confusion or uncooperativeness. Given that aural comprehension defects are common (e.g., occurring in one-third of the sample of Levin et al., 1976) and can influence performances on most neuropsychological tests, formal assessment of comprehension with an instrument such as the Token Test should be considered carefully in cases of TBI.

Contracoup injuries may produce aphasia even when the trauma is right-sided. However, it is uncommon for aphasia to appear in isolation after closed head injury. Most TBI patients with aphasia also have significant defects in nonlinguistic aspects of cognition, and the severity of impairment of other cognitive abilities is greater in aphasic than in nonaphasic TBI patients (Levin et al., 1976). Sarno (1980) found that most patients with subcortical or brainstem lesions resulting in dysarthria also had subtle linguistic defects evident on testing.

Fluent aphasias are relatively more common than nonfluent aphasias (Basso and Scarpa, 1990; Heilman et al., 1971). Global aphasia is rare and usually transient and is associated with severe generalized cognitive defects and with older age at the time of trauma (Levin et al., 1981; Luria, 1970; Sarno, 1980). Even when most aspects of language are well preserved, TBI patients may have significant impairments in discourse and pragmatic use of language, such as indirect requests or hints (McDonald and van Sommers, 1993).

As a general rule, recovery of language defects tends to be quite good after nonpenetrating TBI. For example, Loury (1970) found that 75 percent of patients with left-hemisphere injuries had aphasic signs in the acute period, but only 37.5 percent had persisting language defects. Along similar lines, the findings of the Traumatic Coma Data Bank (Levin et al., 1990) indicated that language recovery after 1 year surpassed recovery of memory and other cognitive abilities.

VISUAL FUNCTIONS

TBI can result in damage to components of the visual system from the retina to high-order visual and polymodal association cortices. Some form of visual dysfunction may occur in more than 50 percent of TBI patients (Gianutsos et al., 1988; Schlageter et al., 1993), and impaired vision has been found to be among the most commonly reported long-term symptoms of TBI (Carlsson et al., 1987). However, these impairments usually are at early or peripheral levels of the visual system (e.g., optic neuropathy, ocular motor palsy) and are not typically within the purview of neuropsychology. A neuro-ophthalmologic evaluation should be performed on TBI patients with visual difficulties before consideration of diagnoses of higher-order visuoperceptual disorders (see Ch. 10). Furthermore, testing of near visual acuity should be virtually routine, given the detrimental effect of visual impairment on neuropsychological test performances (Kempen et al., 1994).

As noted earlier, patients with mild TBI show impairments on measures of complex visual attention (Parasuraman et al., 1991). Heinze et al. (1992) found that a group of TBI patients tested 2 to 18 years after injury showed defects on parallel and serial visual search tasks and that these impairments were related to abnormalities of early and intermediate event-related potentials.

There has been limited investigation of higher-order visuoperceptual defects after TBI, although some studies have indicated generally good recovery of perceptual abilities. For example, Levin et al. (1977, 1990) have shown that most patients recovering from TBI have normal visuoperceptual and visuoconstructional abilities.

It is, of course, possible for the full range of cortically based visual perceptual defects to result from TBI if the tissue damage is localized to primary or association visual areas. However, this is not common, and when cortically based defects do occur (e.g., visual field defects and visual spatial impairments), it usually is in the context of widespread cognitive dysfunction. The relative preservation of visual perceptual abilities in TBI is consistent with the concentration of tissue destruction in inferior temporal and frontal cortices, away from the posterior brain regions primarily involved in visual perception.

EXECUTIVE FUNCTIONS AND PERSONALITY

The term *executive functions* has been used to describe a broad range of supraordinate cognitive abilities involved in judgment, decision making, social conduct, and the initiation, planning, regulation, and organization of behavior (Tranel et al., 1994). Executive functions are interwoven with other, subordinate cognitive abilities such as attention, perception, memory, and language. On the one hand, executive functions are dependent on these subordinate abilities, but also, the ability to apply the subordinate abilities to solve real-world problems is dependent on an intact executive function system.

It is in interaction with the real world that the presence and significance of executive function defects often become apparent. Impairments of executive functions can be difficult to assess and quantify, and much of this difficulty stems from the frequent dissociation between severely impaired behavior in real-world settings and normal performances on clinical and laboratory neuropsychological measures (e.g., Damasio and Anderson, 1993; Eslinger and Damasio, 1985). It is possible for brain damage to result in impairments of judgment, decision making, and social conduct of sufficient severity to preclude independent living, yet allow the patient to perform normally on a broad range of standardized tests of cognition, including those generally associated with executive functions. Even tasks requiring the analysis of social situations and the generation of social response options may be performed normally when presented verbally and requiring a verbal response, despite severe defects in real-world social decision making (Saver and Damasio, 1992).

The relationship between impairments of executive function and frontal lobe damage has been apparent at least since the description of Harlow's famous patient Phinias Gage (Damasio et al., 1994; Harlow, 1868; see Benton, 1991, for an historical review of early frontal lobe studies). That this relationship is not a simple one also is apparent. Consider the ability of patients with focal frontal lobe lesions to perform the Wisconsin Card Sorting Test (Heaton, 1981), which is perhaps the most widely used neuropsychological measure of executive function. Some patients with damage restricted to the frontal lobes are severely impaired in their ability to detect the relevant sorting principles and alter their response patterns contingent on feedback. However, other patients with comparable lesions have no difficulty on the task and perform within normal limits (Anderson et al., 1991). It is safe to say that, despite general acceptance of a relationship between frontal lobe damage and executive function defects, no standardized measure of executive function has been identified that is universally sensitive to frontal lobe damage.

One finding that has emerged with some consistency is that damage to the orbital surface of the frontal lobes can cause severe impairments of social conduct, rational judgment, and planning (e.g., Damasio, 1994; Damasio and Anderson, 1993; Eslinger and Damasio, 1985). This is especially relevant in the current context, because the frontal lobes, and particularly the orbital surfaces, are susceptible to damage in TBI (e.g., Adams et al., 1980; Levin et al., 1987a). It is thus not surprising that executive function defects are among the most frequent and important consequences of TBI.

Several studies have documented and helped delineate various impairments of executive functions that can result from TBI. For example, patients with TBI have been found to have impairments of anticipatory behavior on a shuttlebox analog avoidance task (Freedman et al., 1987). Relative to a control group with cerebrovascular disease, subjects with TBI were impaired in the ability to use a conditioned stimulus cue to initiate avoidance of a noxious stimulus, despite performing as well as or better than the control group on several standardized measures of cognitive and motoric abilities. These findings were interpreted as suggesting that the brain-injured patients are likely to have specific difficulty in situations in which current behavior must be guided on the basis of expected future consequences. This is consistent with recent findings regarding the cognitive impairments of patients with focal prefrontal lobe damage (Bechara et al., 1994; Bechara et al., in press).

Further evidence of an impairment after brain injury of the ability to regulate behavior when not directly guided by immediately salient stimulus conditions was provided by a set of experiments by Shallice and Burgess (1991). Three patients with TBI involving the frontal lobes (but retaining good intellectual abilities) had severe difficulties on tests that required them to prioritize, order, and carry out several simple open-ended tasks. The subjects were inefficient, poorly organized, and spent too long on individual tasks.

Self-awareness has been described as the highest cognitive attribute of the frontal lobes (Stuss and Benson, 1987), and awareness of acquired impairments has been found to be among the best predictors of rehabilitation outcome and return to employment after brain injury (Diller, 1994; Ezrachi et al., 1991). Unfortunately, patients with TBI often are unaware of their acquired cognitive impairments (Anderson and Tranel, 1989). In some cases with substantial right-hemisphere damage resulting in left hemiparesis, the unawareness may also encompass the motor defect.

To the degree that the executive function defects after brain injury include alterations of awareness, judgment, social conduct, behavior initiation and control, and emotion, it frequently is noted that the patient's "personality" has changed. Perhaps even more so than other aspects of executive function, personality changes are difficult to define and quantify, and there is little clinically useful overlap between models of personality and what is known about brain function. Among the most common personality changes after brain injury are disinhibition, irritability, low frustration tolerance, and lack of motivation. Premorbid personality characteristics will, in virtually all cases, help shape postinjury abilities and impairments in the realm of social conduct, emotion, and behavioral control (e.g., Dunlop et al., 1991). In addition to premorbid factors and expected reactions to the consequences of an injury (often including loss of employment, physical impairments, and some degree of loss of independence), personality may be affected by damage to the frontal lobes and limbic structures, among other brain areas.

A tendency to think in concrete terms or an inability to think abstractly has long been recognized as a central component of the executive function defects that result from brain injury (e.g., Goldstein and Scheerer, 1941). Abstract thinking includes abilities such as extracting and comparing the essential features of stimuli or situations, whole-part comparisons, categorization, adopting alternative perspectives, and transcending the most immediately salient aspects of a situation. These defects can be seen most clearly in brain-injured patients when they are forced to go beyond their initial response to an abstraction task. For example, brain-injured patients' performances may be normal on the WAIS-R Similarities subtest, which calls for determination of how two stimuli are alike. However, if they are then asked to generate a second response to the same items (i.e., to think flexibly or reconceptualize the information), their performances deteriorate (Grattan et al., 1994; Scherzer et al., 1993).

This finding also bears similarity to the literature on measures of "fluency," or the ability to generate multiple responses to a given cue. Impairments of controlled verbal fluency (the ability to generate words in reponse to a first-letter cue) have been found in patients with closed TBI (Levin et al., 1976; Sarno, 1980). Benton (1968) has shown that defects of controlled verbal fluency are associated with anterior left-hemisphere damage, and Levin et al. (1991) found that TBI patients with frontal lobe lesions tended to make more perseverative errors on a controlled word finding task than did patients with nonfrontal lesions. Levin et al. (1991) also found that TBI, particularly when the frontal lobes were involved, resulted in impairments on a test of design fluency (i.e., the ability to generate original unique designs). Similar to the verbal fluency task, perseverative errors tended to be common in patients with frontal lobe damage.

In sum, a growing body of experimental evidence has supported the commonly held notion that TBI often results in significant executive function defects. One of the major challenges facing neuropsychologists working with TBI patients is to refine these experimental procedures into efficacious clinical assessment tools and to better define the relationships between these measures of executive function and behavior difficulties in the real world.

SOCIAL OUTCOME

Social outcome is commonly conceptualized as including, at least, family and marital relationships, social activities and competencies, and vocational outcome. There is substantial empirical support for the notion that these functions are affected adversely by TBI. However, several important research questions remain, and several important methodologic issues have been addressed only rarely.

Perhaps most closely studied have been the effects of TBI on the marital relationship. In general, this literature suggests that the spouses of TBI patients are at increased risk for emotional disorder and reports high rates of marital breakdown relative to controls (Kreutzer et al., 1992; O'Carroll et al., 1991; Peters et al., 1990). For example, Peters et al. (1990) evaluated spouses' ratings of marital adjustment. Subjects included 55 male patients with documented TBI, of which 10 were classified as mild, 25 were classified as moderate, and 20 were classified as severe, based on GCS scores. Based on wives' responses, the Dyadic Adjustment Scale (DAS) (Spanier, 1976), Peters et al. reported that the severely injured group was more likely to have complaints as reflected on the total DAS score, the "Dyadic Consensus" subscale, and the "Affectional Expression" subscale. Similar results were reported in a subsequent study by this group, in which patients with spinal cord injuries served as controls (Peters et al., 1992). Such marital dysfunction may underlie the reported increased likelihood of divorce after TBI (Kreutzer et al., 1992; Panting and Merry, 1972; Thomsen, 1984). Further, there is some evidence of increased sexual dysfunction and dissatisfaction after TBI (O' Carrol et al., 1991), but this area has received relatively little empirical attention.

An interesting area of research has emerged in the past several years in relation to social deficits after TBI. In response to the often-noted social deficits of such patients, which have been described as some of the most "subtle and yet most handicapping" features of the condition (Lezak, 1989, p. 113), several researchers have begun to examine the precise behavioral components of the social interactional style of patients after TBI (Grattan et al., 1994; Marsh and Knight, 1991; Newton and Johnson, 1985). For example, Marsh and Knight (1991) studied 18 patients with a history of severe TBI (defined as post-traumatic amnesia greater than 7 days) and compared social interaction behavior in specific laboratory situations with a closely matched control group. The authors reported that speech characteristics significantly differentiated the two groups and that these speech characteristics in the brain-injured group may account, at least in part, for their social interaction deficits. The authors suggest that such findings may help to direct rehabilitation efforts after TBI.

In sum, the available literature indicates clearly that social interactional style and social relationships are impaired in patients with TBI. However, there are notable limitations to the currently available research in this area. For example, there is relatively little available research on the social outcome of patients with *mild* TBI—rather researchers have focused on patients with severe brain injuries. Also, modifying factors such as injuries to other systems (e.g., orthopaedic injuries) have not been studied extensively (for an exception to both of these generalizations, see Dikmen et al., 1986). Such research considerations are becoming increasingly important as researchers and clinicians recognize the importance of the quality of social relationships and its relationship to overall disability after TBI.

Return to Work

One area of social outcome after TBI that has received substantial attention is return to work. Given the costs of disability and lost income after TBI, researchers have shown interest in particular in the predictors of return to work. This literature reveals several factors about patients, neurologic status, and specific cognitive impairments that have been associated with return to work.

Regarding pretrauma characteristics of the individual, several studies have noted that age at time of injury is related to return to work, with younger patients generally more likely to resume employment (Crepeau and Scherzer, 1993; Dikmen et al., 1994). Similarly, employment status and level of employment (e.g., skilled versus semiskilled) have been related to likelihood of return to work, with more skilled workers with longer work histories more likely to resume work after TBI (Brooks et al., 1987; Dikmen et al., 1994). Gender has generally not been associated with return to work after TBI (Crepeau and Scherzer, 1993).

Most studies have supported the expected conclusion that severity of brain trauma is inversely related to likelihood to return to work. That is, the more severe the trauma, whether measured by GCS score, duration of post-traumatic amnesia, or length of hospitalization, the less likely an individual is to return to work (Fraser et al., 1988; Rao et al., 1990). Further, as might be expected, positive radiologic evidence of brain abnormality (e.g., contusion, hematoma) is related to decreased likelihood of employment after TBI (Eide and Tysnes, 1992).

Neuropsychological deficits associated with return to work after TBI have been varied. In a recent meta-analysis of variables predictive of return to work, Crepeau and Scherzer (1993) indicated that performances on tests that are generally considered to assess executive functions are those that are most reliably associated with post-trauma employment status. Related to this, emotional disturbance was reported by these investigatiors to be closely related to return to work. Other investigators have reported many cognitive impairments associated with lack of employment, including memory, attention, visuospatial impairments, and language defects (Brooks et al., 1987; Fraser et al., 1988; Schwab et al., 1993).

Two recent studies represent an important trend in the research literature on return to work. Schwab et al. (1993) and Dikmen et al. (1994) represent two large-scale studies (n = 520 and 366 patients respectively) that have used multivariate models in an attempt to predict return to work. This approach has obvious advantages, because those variables that are found to be most closely related to employment can be selectively addressed in rehabilitation. In the case of Dikmen et al., the authors provide a multivariate model using weighted variables that were predictive of employment in their sample (e.g., GCS score, preinjury job stability, injury to other systems such as orthopaedic injuries, and neuropsychological performance on the Halstead-Reitan Neuropsychological Battery). Similarly, in the Schwab et al. (1993) study, the authors provide a means to calculate a "disability score" based on seven neurologic, neuropsychological, and social/emotional variables. These studies represent a trend in the literature that is likely to continue. That is, researchers are recognizing the importance of multivariate models in the prediction of employment status after TBI and are incorporating multiple variables into research designs.

In sum, employment after TBI has been a focus of interest to researchers. There is clear risk of employment problems after TBI (with estimates of unemployment varying from 50 to 99 percent) (Crepeau and Scherzer, 1993). Recent research shows marked conceptual and methodologic improvements relative to earlier work. In particular, these recent studies have adequate sample sizes to permit generalization of the findings. Perhaps more important, these studies have incorporated multivariate models in the prediction of employment after TBI. Such models include variables related to the severity of the injury, associated neurologic sequelae (e.g., seizures or motor defects), and demographic characteristics of the injured individual, in addition to neuropsychological defects as measured after the injury. Multivariate prediction models are likely to be explored more fully in this area of research in the future.

THE IOWA SERIES

In this final section, a description is provided of a series of cases of TBI referred to the Benton Neuropsychology Laboratory at the University of Iowa. The cases were drawn from clinical files of more than 300 cases of TBI seen in our clinic between 1990 and 1994 and are intended to provide an idea of the range of types of cases, the outcome of such cases and types of deficits observed, and the range of tests administered.

Forty cases are described. Inclusion criteria for this series were that the patient (1) had to be admitted to the University of Iowa Hospitals and Clinics for initial management of the TBI, (2) had to have a confirmed trauma, as defined by observed loss of consciousness, hematoma, or other objective evidence, (3) had to be assessed neuropsychologically in the acute epoch, defined as less than 3 months after the injury, (4) follow-up neuropsychological data from the chronic epoch, defined as more than 3 months after the injury, had to be available, and (5) patients did not have a history of mental retardation or learning disability.

Demographic information are presented in Table 20-2. Patients were seen initially an average of 3 weeks after the trauma (SD, 2 weeks; range, 1 day to 10 weeks). Follow-up neuropsychological assessments were completed an average of 8.7 months after the trauma (SD, 7.6 months; range, 3.2 to 46 months). Average GCS score on admission was 10.3 (SD, 4.1; range, 3 to 15) and average GCS score 24 hours after admission was 11.5 (SD, 3.6; range, 6 to 15). The series included 31 males and 9 females. Thirty-four patients were right-handed. Average education was 12.1 years (SD, 1.9 years; range, 9 to 19 years). Estimated premorbid IQ according to the Barona et al. (1984) equation was 97.7 (SD, 6.4; range, 86 to 116). All patients had confirmed loss of consciousness, 24 of whom experienced this for greater than 15 minutes. In 28 cases, the cause of the trauma was a motor vehicle crash. Four had a history of prior TBI,

TABLE 20-2. Characteristics of the Iowa Sample of Head Trauma Cases ($n = 40$)

Characteristic	Mean	SD
Age	28.2	8.5
Education	12.1	1.9
Estimated premorbid IQ (from Barona et al., 1984)	97.7	6.4
Admission GCS score	10.3	4.1
24-Hour GCS score	11.5	3.6
Characteristic	***N***	
Gender		
Males	31	
Females	9	
Handedness		
Right	34	
Left	6	
Time one number employed	31	
Time two number employed	11	
Time one occupation (from Barona et al., 1984)		
Unskilled labor	11	
Semiskilled labor	17	
Not in labor force	9	
Skilled labor	1	
Manager/administration/clerical/sales	1	
Professional/technical	1	
Time two occupation		
Unskilled labor	2	
Semiskilled labor	6	
Not in labor force	29	
Skilled labor	2	
Manager/administration/clerical/sales	0	
Professional/technical	1	

and two had a prior psychiatric history. Thirty-one were employed at the time of the initial assessment, whereas 11 were employed at the time of the follow-up examination. Fourteen were in litigation related to their injury at the time of the second examination.

Inspection of Table 20-2 shows that 20 patients who had been employed at the time of the injury were not employed at the time of our follow-up examination. Put another way, only about one-third (9 of 31) of the patients who had been employed at the time of the injury had returned to work by the time they were reevaluated, an average of 8 months later.

Figure 20-2 represents several of the core tests of the Benton Neuropsychology Laboratory and how patients performed on these tests over time. Several findings and trends are of interest. For example, in a series of correlational analyses, we found no clear relationship between GCS scores and long-term neuropsychological performances. This lack of correspondence between outcome and initial clinical presentation has been reported previously (e.g., Barth et al., 1983). This was true for GCS scores both at admission and at 24 hours. However, there were several very significant correlations between GCS ratings and performances on neuropsychological tests in the acute epoch. One interpretation of this finding is that a substantial amount of the variance observed in recovery from TBI is due to factors other than the severity of the initial trauma. That is, the data are consistent with factors other than the severity of the trauma (perhaps age, premorbid intellect, or "complicating" conditions such as psychiatric disease, for example), having a substantial impact on eventual outcome.

Perhaps most clear is the fact that these patients recovered over time. Reported below each figure are the paired *t*-tests of the Time 1 to Time 2 performances for these patients. Given the multiple comparisons, a Bonferroni-corrected α values of 0.003 may be applied. As can be seen in the figures and is perhaps not surprising, patients improved over time on virtually all measures. This is a consistent theme in the literature, albeit with exceptions (Dikmen et al., 1983; Dikmen et al., 1986b; Drudge et al., 1984; McLean et al., 1983; but see Stuss et al., 1985).

Further, it is noteworthy that many of the constructs and themes discussed earlier in this chapter are largely borne out by these data. For example, relative to normative data for the tests presented, the data suggest a variety of impairments, but these impairments are perhaps most clear on tests of memory (e.g., Complex Figure Test-Recall, Visual Retention Test, Auditory Verbal Learning Test; for normative data related to the tests presented, the reader is referred to Wechsler, 1981, and Spreen and Strauss, 1991).

CONCLUSION

Neuropsychological impairments after TBI are common. Such impairments can be seen at the bedside, but is often the case that formal neuropsychological assessment laboratory procedures are necessary to delineate the defects. Virtually all domains of cognition can be affected by TBI, but some, such as

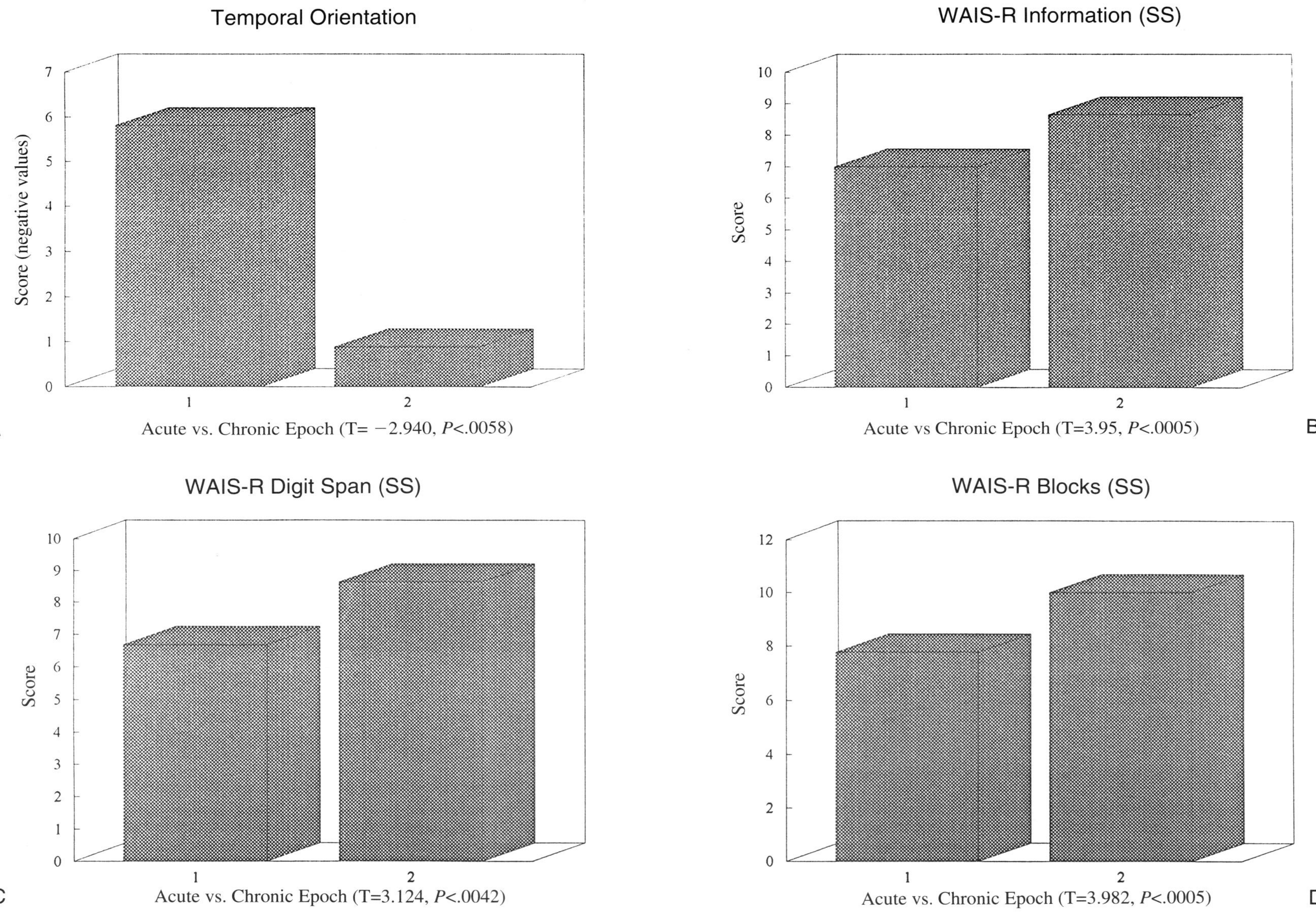

Fig. 20-2. Core neuropsychological tests conducted by the Benton Neuropsychology Laboratory and their results. **(A) Temporal Orientation; (B)** Wechsler Adult Intelligence Scale—Revised (WAIS-R) Information: SS; **(C)** WAIS-R Digit Span: SS; **(D)** WAIS-R Blocks: SS; (*Figure continues.*)

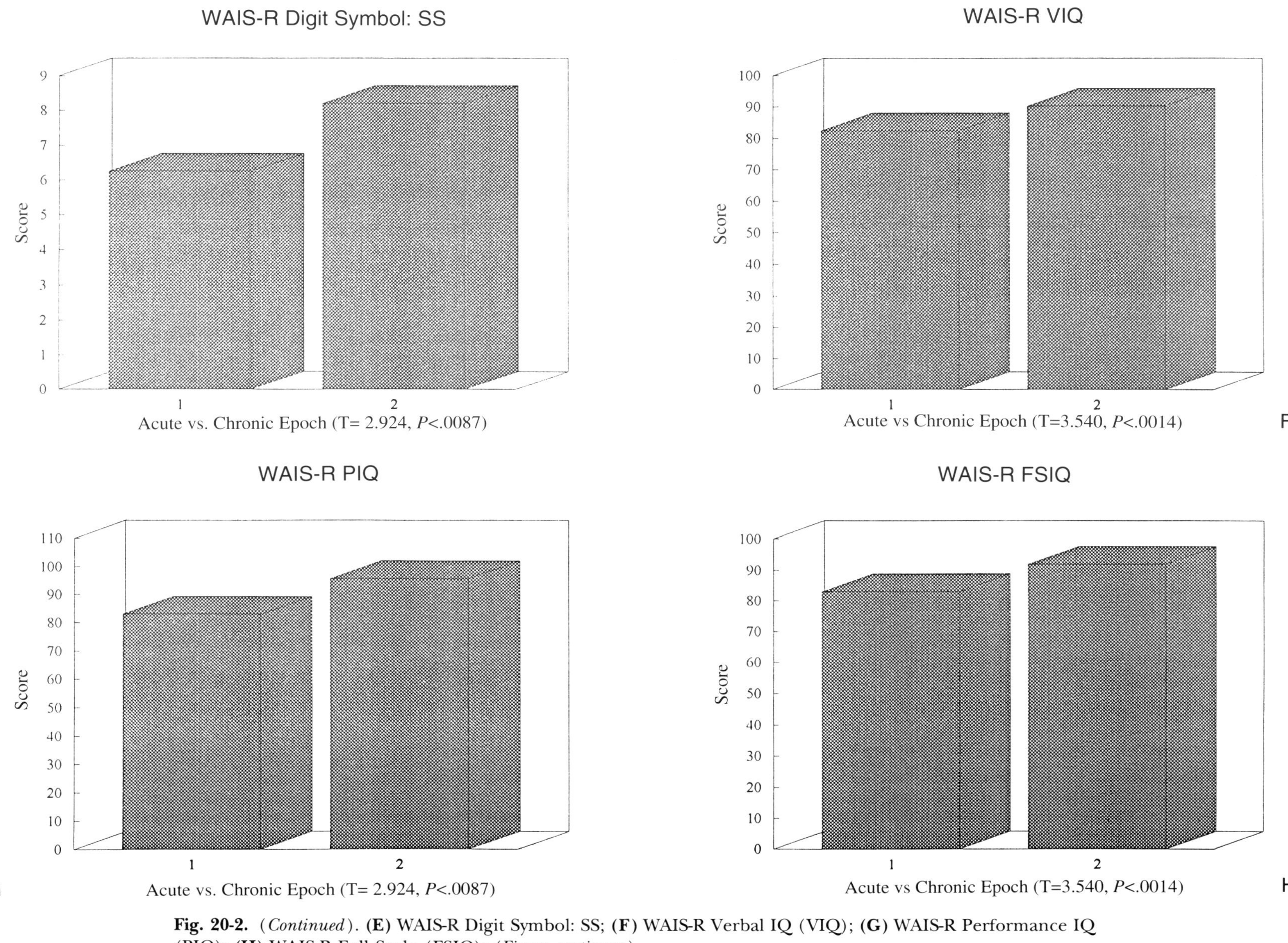

Fig. 20-2. (*Continued*). **(E)** WAIS-R Digit Symbol: SS; **(F)** WAIS-R Verbal IQ (VIQ); **(G)** WAIS-R Performance IQ (PIQ); **(H)** WAIS-R Full Scale (FSIQ); (*Figure continues.*)

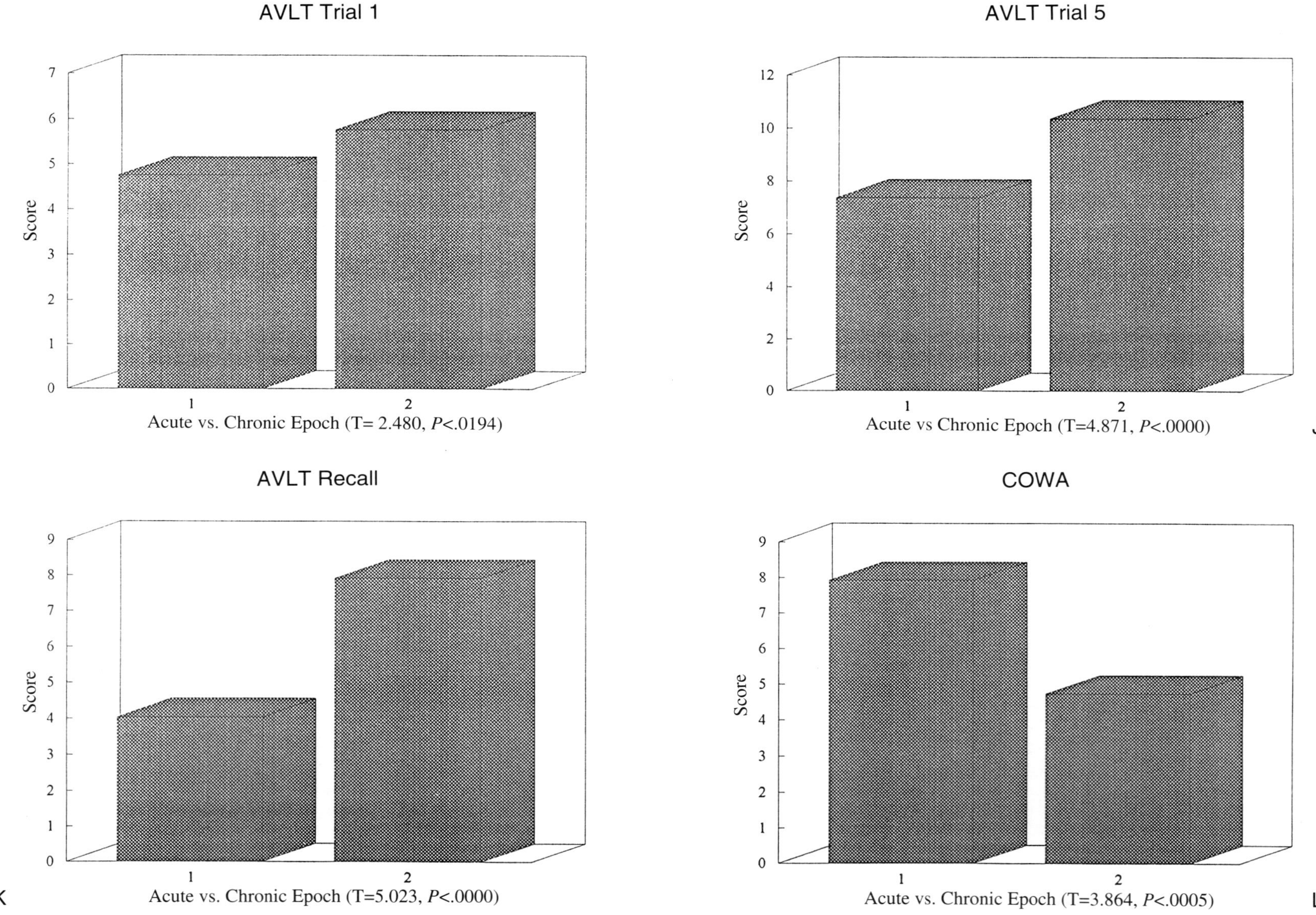

Fig. 20-2. (*Continued*). **(I)** Auditory Verbal Learning Test (AVLT) Trial 1; **(J)** AVLT Trial 5; **(K)** AVLT Recall; **(L)** Controlled Oral Word Association Test (COWA); (*Figure continues.*)

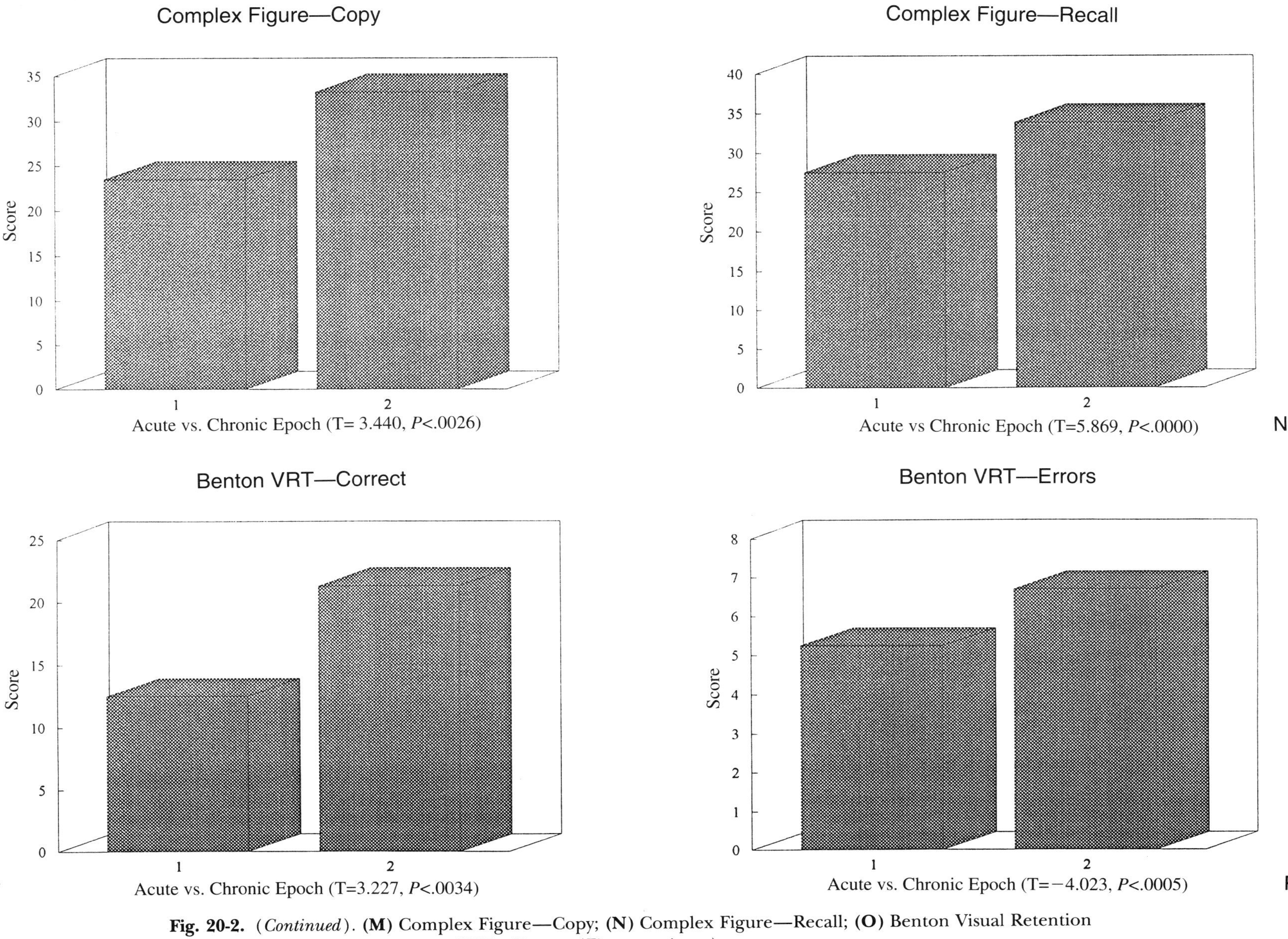

Fig. 20-2. (*Continued*). **(M)** Complex Figure—Copy; **(N)** Complex Figure—Recall; **(O)** Benton Visual Retention Test (VRT)—Correct: **(P)** Benton VRT—Errors; (*Figure continues.*)

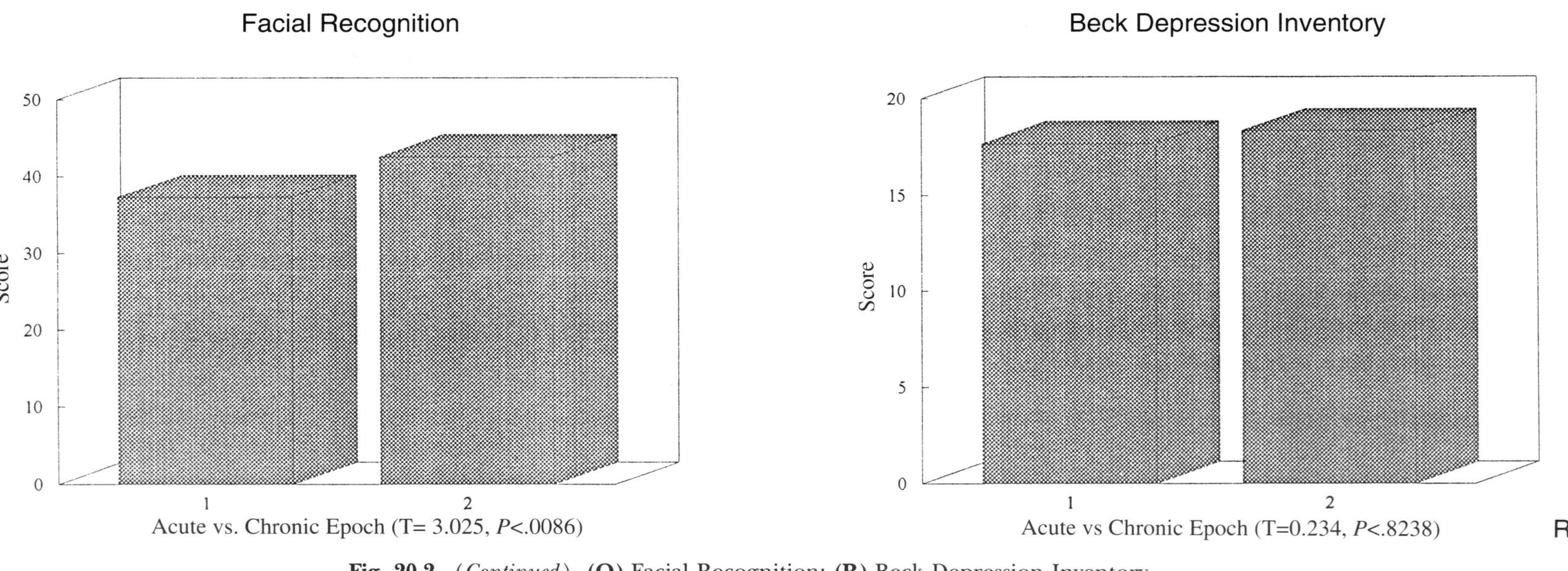

Fig. 20-2. (*Continued*). **(Q)** Facial Recognition; **(R)** Beck Depression Inventory.

attention and anterograde memory, appear to be particularly susceptible to disruption after trauma. Finally, there are characteristic profiles of deficit and recovery from TBI that have been demonstrated in group studies, and such profiles may help to guide the clinician in his or her expectations or prognosis.

Substantial knowledge has been gained regarding the pathophysiology, phenomenology, and course of TBI. However, there are still several gaps in basic knowledge surrounding the condition and several new areas of research to be explored. For example, the explication of very complex constructs such as "memory" and "attention" has been limited. Borrowing from cognitive psychology and cognitive neuroscience, research questions at this point might more profitably address what *aspects* of memory (e.g., semantic or episodic, procedural or declarative) or attention (e.g., simple or divided) are affected by TBI. This trend of delineating specific abilities subsumed under global constructs has emerged in the literature on TBI in recent years and is likely to continue.

Perhaps the most pressing research need is concerned with the extent to which laboratory-based neuropsychological procedures are related to real-world variables of interest. This construct has been termed "ecological validity" and is currently an area of vigorous research in clinical neuropsychology. For example, it is clearly of value to know that performance on a given test or set of tests is predictive of ability to drive, or amenability for rehabilitation. Efforts along these lines can be seen in some of the research related to return to work, and this attempt to relate neuropsychological performances to real-world performance is likely to continue (Crepeau and Scherzer, 1993).

However, in our view such efforts are more likely to be of value when research adopts multivariate prediction models of the real-world behavior. That is, the predictive power of any neuropsychological test in isolation is not likely to be high. For example, the impairment index from the Halstead-Reitan Battery may well have some predictive power regarding ability to return to work. But the index alone cannot address which patient will be able to return to what job and under what conditions. Also, it is clear that the predictive power of neuropsychological tests is enhanced greatly by recognition of the fact that real-world circumstances and characteristics of the individual, not just performances on tests, must be considered in predicting behavior.

ACKNOWLEDGMENT

This work was supported by NINDS Grant PO1 NS 19632

REFERENCES

Adams JH, Graham D, Scott G et al: Brain damage in fatal nonmissile head injury. J Clin Pathol 33:1132–1145, 1980

Anderson SW, Damasio H, Jones RD, Tranel D: Wisconsin Card Sorting Test performance as a measure of frontal lobe damage. J Clin Exp Neuropsychol 13:909–922, 1991

Anderson SW, Tranel D: Awareness of disease states following cerebral infarction, dementia, and head trauma: standardized assessment. Clin Neuropsychol 3:327–339, 1989

Arcia E, Gualtieri CT: Association between patient report of symptoms after mild head injury and neurobehavioural performance. Brain Inj 7:481–489, 1993

Barona A, Reynolds CR, Chastain R: A demographically based index of pre-morbid intelligence for the WAIS-R. J Consult Clin Psychol 52:885–887, 1984

Barth JT, Macciocchi SN, Giordani B et al: Neuropsychological sequelae of minor head injury. Neurosurgery 13:529–533, 1983

Basso A, Scarpa MT: Traumatic aphasia in children and adults: a comparison of clinical features and evolution. Cortex 26:501–514, 1990

Bechara A, Damasio AR, Damasio H, Anderson SW: Insensitivity to future consequences following damage to human prefrontal cortex. Cognition 50:7–15, 1994

Bechara A, Tranel D, Damasio H, Damasio AR: Failure to respond automatically to anticipated future outcomes following damage to prefrontal cortex. Cerebral Cortex, in press

Benton AL: Differential behavioral effects in frontal lobe disease. Neuropsychologia 6:53–60, 1968

Benton AL: The prefrontal region: its early history. In Levin HS, Eisenberg HM, Benton AL (eds): Frontal Lobe Function and Dysfunction. Oxford University Press, New York, 1991

Benton AL, Hamsher KD: Multilingual Aphasia Examination. University of Iowa, Iowa City, 1976

Benton AL, Joynt RJ: Early descriptions of aphasia. Arch Neurol 3:109–126, 1960

Brooks N, McKinlay W, Symington C et al: Return to work within the first seven years of severe head injury. Brain Inj 1:5–19, 1987

Capruso DX, Levin HS: Cognitive impairment following head injury. Neurol Clin 10:879–893, 1992

Carlsson GS, Svardsudd K, Welin L: Long-term effects of head injuries sustained during life in three male populations. J Neurosurgery 67:197–205, 1987

Crepeau F, Scherzer P: Predictors and indicators of work status after traumatic brain injury: a meta-analysis. Neuropsychol Rehabil 3:5–35, 1993

Damasio AR: Descartes' Error: Emotion, Reason, and the Human Brain. Grosset/Putnam, New York, 1994

Damasio AR, Anderson SW: The frontal lobes. In Heilman K, Valenstein E (eds): Clinical Neuropsychology. 3rd Ed. Oxford University Press, New York, 1993

Damasio AR, Damasio H: Cortical systems underlying knowledge retrieval: evidence from human lesion studies. In Poggio TA, Glaser DA (eds): Exploring Brain Function: Models in Neuroscience. Wiley, New York, 1993

Damasio H, Grabowski T, Frank R et al: The return of Phineas Gage: clues about the brain from the skull of a famous patient. Science 264:1102–1105, 1994

de Bruin AF, de Witte LP, Stevens F, Diederiks JPM: Sickness Impact Profile: the state of the art of a generic functional status measure. Soc Sci Med 35:1003–1014, 1992

Dikmen S, McLean A, Temkin N: Neuropsychological and psychosocial consequences of minor head injury. J Neurol Neurosurg Psychiatry 49:1227–1232, 1986a

Dikmen S, McLean A, Temkin NR, Wyler AR: Neuropsychological outcome at one month postinjury. Arch Phys Med Rehabil 67:507–513, 1986b

Dikmen S, Reitan RM, Temkin N: Neuropsychological recovery in head injury. Arch Neurol 40:333–338, 1983

Dikmen SS, Temkin NR, Machamer JE et al: Employment following traumatic head injuries. Arch Neurol 51:177–186, 1994

Drudge OW, Williams JM, Kessler M, Gomes FB: Recovery from severe head injuries: repeat testing with the Halstead-Reitan Neuropsychological Battery. J Clin Psychol 40:259–265, 1984

Dunlop TW, Udvarhelyi GB, Stedem AF et al: Comparison of patients with and without emotional/behavioral deterioration during the first year after traumatic brain injury. J Neuropsychiatry Clin Neurosci 3:150–156, 1991

Eide PK, Tysnes OB: Early and late outcome in head injury patients with radiological evidence of brain damage. Acta Neurol Scand 86:194–198, 1992

Eisenberg HM, Levin HS: Computed tomography and magnetic resonance imaging in mild to moderate head injury. In Levin HS, Eisenberg, HM, and Benton AL (eds): Mild Head Injury. Oxford, New York, 1989

Ezrachi O, Ben-Yishay Y, Kay T et al: Predicting employment in traumatic brain injury following neuropsychological rehabilitation. J Head Trauma Rehabil 6:71–84, 1991

Fraser R, Dikmen S, McLean A et al: Employability of head injury survivors: first year post-injury. Rehabil Counseling Bull 31:276–288, 1988

Freedman PE, Bleiberg J, Freedland K: Anticipatory behavior deficits in closed head injury. J Neurol Neurosurg Psychiatry 50:398–401, 1987

Gentilini M, Nichelli P, Schoenhuber R: Assessment of attention in mild head injury. In Levin HS, Eisenberg HM, Benton AL (eds): Mild Head Injury. Oxford, New York, 1989

Gianutsos R, Ramsey G, Perlin RR: Rehabilitative optometric services for survivors of acquired brain injury. Arch Phys Med Rehabil 69:573–578, 1988

Goldenberg G, Oder W, Spatt J, Podreka I: Cerebral correlates of disturbed executive function and memory in survivors of severe closed head injury: a SPECT study. J Neurol Neurosurg Psychiatry 55:362–368, 1992

Goldstein KH, Scheerer M: Abstract and concrete behaviour: an experimental study with special tests. Psychol Monogr 53, 1941

Grattan LM, Bloomer RH, Archambault FX, Eslinger PJ: Cognitive flexibility and empathy after frontal lobe lesions. Neuropsychiatry Neuropsychol Behav Neurol 7:251–259, 1994

Gronwall D: Behavioral assessment during the acute stages of traumatic brain injury. In Lezak MD (ed): Assessment of the Behavioral Consequences of Head Trauma. Alan R. Liss, New York, 1989a

Gronwall D: Cumulative and persisting effects of concussion on attention and cognition. In Levin HS, Eisenberg HM, and Benton AL (eds): Mild Head Injury. Oxford, New York, 1989b

Hamm RJ, Dixon CE, Gbadebo DM et al: Cognitive deficits following traumatic brain injury produced by controlled cortical impact. J Neurotrauma 9:11–20, 1992

Heilman KM, Safran A, Geschwind N: Closed head trauma and aphasia. J Neurol Neurosurg Psychiatry 34: 265–269, 1971

Heinze H-J, Munte TF, Gobiet et al: Parallel and serial visual search after closed head injury: electrophysiological evidence for perceptual dysfunctions. Neuropsychologia 30:495–514, 1992

High WM, Jr, Levin HS, Howard EG, Jr: Recovery of orientation following closed head injury. J Clin Exp Neuropsychol 12:703–714, 1990

Hugenholtz H, Stuss DT, Stethem LL, Richard MT: How long does it take to recover from a mild concussion. Neurosurgery 22:853–858, 1988

Jennett B, Bond M: Assessment of outcome after severe brain damage: a practical scale. Lancet I:480–487, 1975

Jones RD, Tranel D, Benton AL, Paulsen J: Differentiating dementia from "pseudodementia" early in the clinical course: utility of neuropsychological tests. Neuropsychology 6:13–21, 1992

Kaplan E, Fein D, Morris R, Delis DC: The Wechsler Adult Intelligence Scale-Revised as a Neuropsychological Instrument. The Psychological Corporation, San Antonio, TX, 1991

Kempen JH, Kritchevsky M, Feldman S: Effect of visual impairment on neuropsychological test performance. J Clin Exp Neuropsychol 16:223–231, 1994

Kreutzer JS, Marwitz JH, Kepler K: Traumatic brain injury: family response and outcome. Arch Phys Med Rehabil 73:771–778, 1992

Leininger BE, Gramling SE, Farrel AD et al: Neuropsychological deficits in symptomatic minr head injury following concussion and mild concussion. J Neurol Neurosurg Psychiatry 53:293–296, 1990

Levin HS: Memory deficit after closed head injury. J Clin Neuropsychol 12:129–153, 1989

Levin HS, Amparo E, Eisenberg HM et al: Magnetic resonance imaging and computerized tomography in relation to the neurobehavioral sequelae of mild and moderate head injuries. J Neurosurg 66:706, 1987a

Levin HS, Benton AL, Grossman RG: Neurobehavioral Consequences of Closed Head Injury. Oxford, New York, 1982

Levin HS, Gary HE, Eisenberg HM et al: Neurobehavioral outcome 1 year after severe head injury. Experience of the Traumatic Coma Data Bank. J Neurosurg 73:699–709, 1990

Levin HS, Goldstein FC, High WM, Eisenberg HM: Disproportionately severe memory deficit in relation to normal intellectual functioning after closed head injury. J Neurol Neurosurg Psychiatry 51:1294–1301, 1988

Levin HS, Goldstein FC, Williams DH, Eisenberg HM: The contribution of frontal lobe lesions to the neurobehavioral outcome of closed head injury. In Levin HS, Eisenberg HM, Benton AL (eds): Frontal Lobe Function and Dysfunction. Oxford University Press, New York, 1991

Levin HS, Grossman RG, Kelly PJ: Aphasic disorder in patients with closed head injury. J Neurol Neurosurg Psychiatry 39:1062–1070, 1976

Levin HS, Grossman RG, Kelly PJ: Impairment of facial recognition after closed head injuries of varying severity. Cortex 13:119, 1977

Levin HS, Grossman RG, Rose JE, Teasdale G: Long-term neuropsychological outcome of closed head injury. J Neurosurg 50:412–422, 1979

Levin HS, Grossman RG, Sarwar M, Meyers CA: Linguistic recovery after closed head injury. Brain Lang 12:360–374, 1981

Levin HS, High WM, Meyers et al: Impairment of remote memory after closed head injury. J Neurol Neurosurg Psychiatry 48:556–563, 1985

Levin HS, Mattis S, Ruff R et al: Neurobehavioral outcome following minor head injury: a three center study. J Neurosurg 66:234–243, 1987b

Lezak MD: Neuropsychological Assessment. 2nd Ed. Oxford University Press, New York, 1985

Lezak MD: IQ: RIP. J Clin Neuropsychol 10:351–361, 1988

Lezak MD: Assessment of psychosocial dysfunctions resulting from head trauma. In Lezak MD (ed): Assessment of the Behavioral Consequences of Head Trauma. AR Liss, New York, 1989

Loury AR: Traumatic Aphasia: Its Syndromes, Psychology and Treatment. Mouton, Paris, 1970

Mandleberg IA, Brooks DN: Cognitive recovery after severe head injury. 1. Serial testing on the Wechsler Adult Intelligence Scale. J Neurol Neurosurg Psychiatry 38: 1121–1126, 1975

Marsh NV, Knight RG: Behavioral assessment of social competence following severe head injury. J Clin Exp Neuropsychol 13:729–740, 1991

Mayes SD, Pelco LE, Campbell CJ: Relationships among pre- and post-injury intelligence, length of coma and age in individuals with severe closed-head injuries. Brain Inj 3:310–313, 1989

MacDonald S, van Sommers P: Pragmatic language skills after closed head injury: ability to negotiate requests. Cognitive Neuropsychol 10:297–315, 1993

McLean A, Temkin N, Dikmen S, Wyler AR: The behavioral sequelae of head injury. J Clin Neuropsychol 5:361–376, 1983

McLean A, Jr, Dikmen SS, Temkin NR: Psychosocial recovery after head injury. Arch Phys Med Rehabil 74:1041–1046, 1993

Miller E: Simple and choice reaction time following severe head injury. Cortex 6:121–127, 1970

Newton A, Johnson JA: Social adjustment and interaction after severe head injury. Br J Clin Psychol 24:225–234, 1985

O'Carroll RE, Woodrow J, Maroun F: Psychosexual and psychosocial sequelae of closed head injury. Brain Inj 5:303–313, 1991

Oddy M, Coughlan T, Tyerman A, Jenkins D: Social adjustment after closed head injury: a further follow-up seven years after injury. J Neurol Neurosurg Psychiatry 48:564–568, 1985

Panting A, Merry PH: The long term rehabilitation of severe head injuries with particular reference to the need for social and medical support for the patient's family. Rehabilitation 38:33–37, 1972

Parasuraman R, Mutter SA, Molloy R: Sustained attention following mild closed-head injury. J Clin Exp Neuropsychol 13:789–811, 1991

Peters LC, Stambrook M, Moore AD, Esses L: Psychosocial sequelae of closed head injury: effects on the marital relationship. Brain Inj 4:39–47, 1990

Peters LC, Stambrook M, Moore AD et al: Differential effects of spinal cord injury and head injury on marital adjustment. Brain Inj 6:461–467, 1992

Ponsford J, Kinsella G: Attentional deficits following closed head injury. J Clin Neuropsychol 14:822–838, 1992

Priddy DA, Johnson P, Lam CS: Driving after severe head injury. Brain Inj 4:267–272, 1990

Rao N, Rosenthal M, Cronin-Stubbs D et al: Return to work after rehabilitation following traumatic brain injury. Brain Inj 4:49–56, 1990

Ruff RM, Levin HS, Mattis S et al: Recovery of head injury after mild head injury. In Levin HS, Eisenberg HM, Benton AL (eds): Mild Head Injury. Oxford, New York, 1989

Russell WR: The Traumatic Amnesias. Oxford, New York, 1971

Sarno MT: The nature of verbal impairment after closed head injury. J Nerv Ment Dis 168:685–692, 1980

Saver J, Damasio AR: Preserved access and processing of social knowledge in a patient with acquired sociopathy due to ventromedial frontal damage. Neuropsychologia 29:1241–1249, 1991

Schacter DL, Crovits HF: Memory function after closed head injury: a review of the quantitative research. Cortex 13:150–176, 1977

Scherzer BP, Charbonneau S, Solomon CR, LePore F: Abstract thinking following severe traumatic brain injury. Brain Inj 7:411–423, 1993

Schlageter K, Gray B, Hall K et al: Incidence and treatment of visual dysfunction in traumatic brain injury. Brain Inj 7:439–448, 1993

Schwab K, Grafman J, Salazar AM, Kraft J: Residual impairments and work status 15 years after penetrating head injury: report from the Vietnam Head Injury Study. Neurology 43:95–103, 1993

Shallice T: Specific impairments in planning. Philos Trans R Soc Lond 298:199–209, 1982

Shallice T, Burgess PW: Deficits in strategy application following frontal lobe damage in man. Brain 114: 727–741, 1991

Spanier GB: Measuring dyadic adjustment: new scales for assessing the quality of marriage and similar dyads. J Marriage Family 38:15–28, 1976

Spreen O, Strauss E: A Compendium of Neuropsychological Tests. Oxford, New York, 1991

Squire LR, Knowlton B, Musen G: The structure and organization of memory. Annu Rev Psychol 44:453–495, 1993

Stuss DT, Benson DF: The frontal lobes and control of cognition and memory. In Pereceman E (ed): The Frontal Lobes Revisited. Lawrence Erlbaum Associates, Hillsdale, NJ, 1987

Stuss DT, Ely P, Hugenholtz H et al: Subtle neuropsychological deficits in patients with good recovery after closed head injury. Neurosurgery 17:41–47, 1985

Stuss DT, Stethem LL, Hugenholtz H et al: Reaction time after head injury: fatigue, divided and focused attention, and consistency of performance. J Neurol Neurosurg Psychiatry 52:742–748, 1989

Tabaddor M, Mattis S, Zazula T: Cognitive sequelae and recovery course after moderate and severe head injury. Neurosurgery 14:701–708, 1984

Tate RL, Fenelson B, Manning ML, Hunter M: Patterns of neuropsychological impairment after severe blunt head injury. J Nerv Ment Dis 179:117–126, 1991

Teasdale G, Jennett B: Assessment of coma and impaired consciousness. Lancet 2:81–84, 1974

Teasdale G, Knill-Jones R, Van Der Sand J: Observer variability in assessing impaired consciousness and coma. J Neurol Neurosurg Psychiatry 41:603–610, 1978

Thomsen IV: Late outcome of very severe blunt head trauma: a 10–15 year second follow-up. J Neurol Neurosurg Psychiatry 47:260–268, 1984

Thomsen IV: Late psychosocial outcome in severe blunt head trauma. Brain Inj 1:131–143, 1987

Tranel D: Memory, neural substrates. Encyclopedia Hum Behavior 3:149–163, 1994

Tranel D, Anderson SW, Benton AL: Development of the concept of executive functions in relation to the frontal lobes. In Boller F, Grafman J (eds): Handbook of Neuropsychology. Vol. 9. Elsevier, New York, 1994

Van Zomeren AH: Reaction Time and Attention after Closed Head Injury. Swets & Zeitlinger, Lisse, 1981

Van Zomeren AH, Van Denberg W: Residual complaints of patients two years after severe head injury. J Neurol Neurosurg Psychiatry 48:21–28, 1985

Wechsler D: WAIS-R Manual. Psychological Corporation, New York, 1981

Neurologic and Neuropsychologic Aspects of Frontal Lobe Impairments in Postconcussive Syndrome

21

Paul J. Eslinger
Lynn M. Grattan
Laszlo Geder

THE FRONTAL LOBE AND BEHAVIOR AFTER CONCUSSION

Studies of postconcussive syndromes have generated an increasing interest in the neurologic and neuropsychologic impairments associated with frontal lobe damage. Such interest has arisen from two lines of evidence: the high prevalence of frontal lobe damage from concussive injuries and the difficult management of the associated neurobehavioral impairments that cause disability and other negative consequences (Adams et al., 1980; Brooks, 1984; Papo et al., 1982; Prigatano, 1986). There are several mechanisms of damage that affect the frontal lobe in concussion, including white matter shearing from acceleration-deceleration and rotational forces, contusion, laceration, hemorrhagic mass lesions, edema, and other secondary pathologic effects such as in-

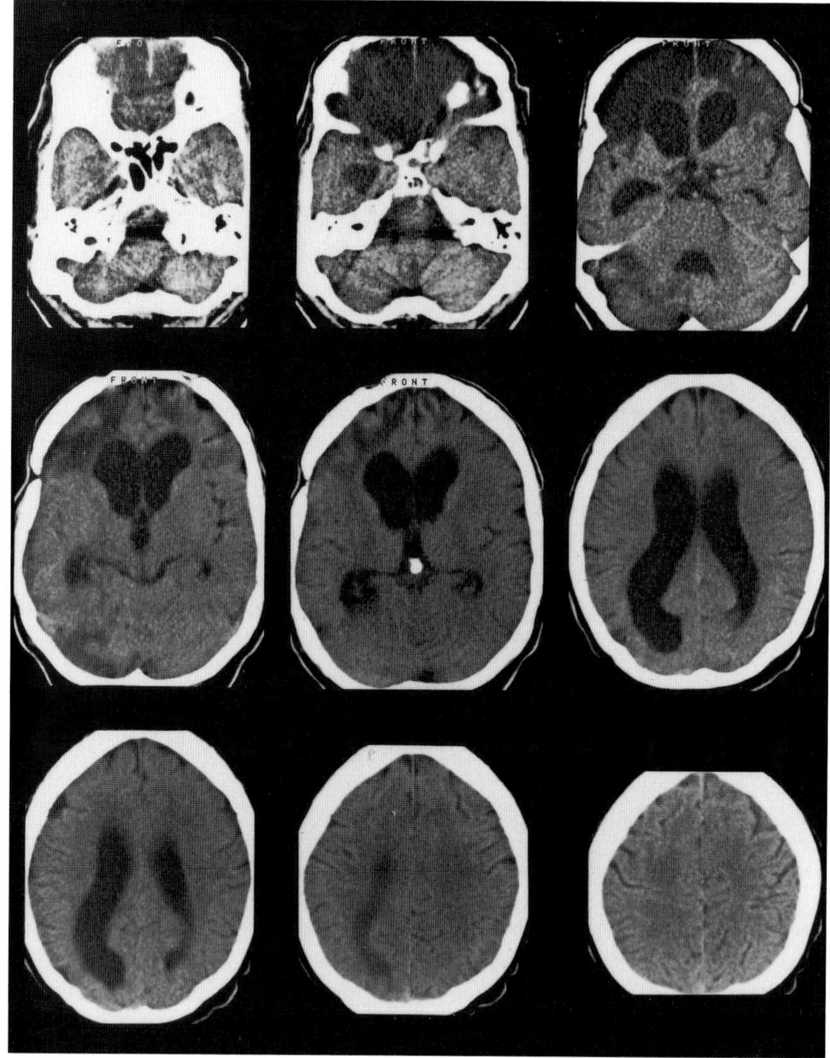

Fig. 21-1. **(A)** Chronic CT scan and **(B)** best-fitting brain templates of case 1, showing a large area of inferior and polar frontal lobe damage after head injury, which required surgical debridement of frontal skull fracture. (Fig. B adapted from Damasio and Damasio, 1989.) *(Figure continues.)*

creased intracranial pressure. The frontal lobe is particularly susceptible to direct impact and secondary pathologic injury in concussion because of its location in relation to prominent bony structures of the skull. Several studies have supported such vulnerability. In a series of 83 concussion patients with computed tomographic (CT) scan evidence of intracranial mass lesions, Papo et al. (1982) reported that 43 percent showed frontal or frontotemporal lesions. Postmortem data were also reported from 17 of their severe concussion cases with CT scan evidence of frontal lobe lesion. Damage within the frontal lobe was established to be bilateral in 65 percent of these cases and usually involved the orbital, dorsolateral, or polar regions. Although the frontal lobe lesion was often a prominent neuropathologic feature in this series, all patients had damage in other cerebral regions as well. Therefore, frontal lobe damage can be considered a common but not isolated pathologic result of concussion.

The clinical neurologic and neuropsychologic consequences of concussive injuries are numerous. Our focus in this chapter is on the cognitive, social, and neurologic alterations that are associated with frontal

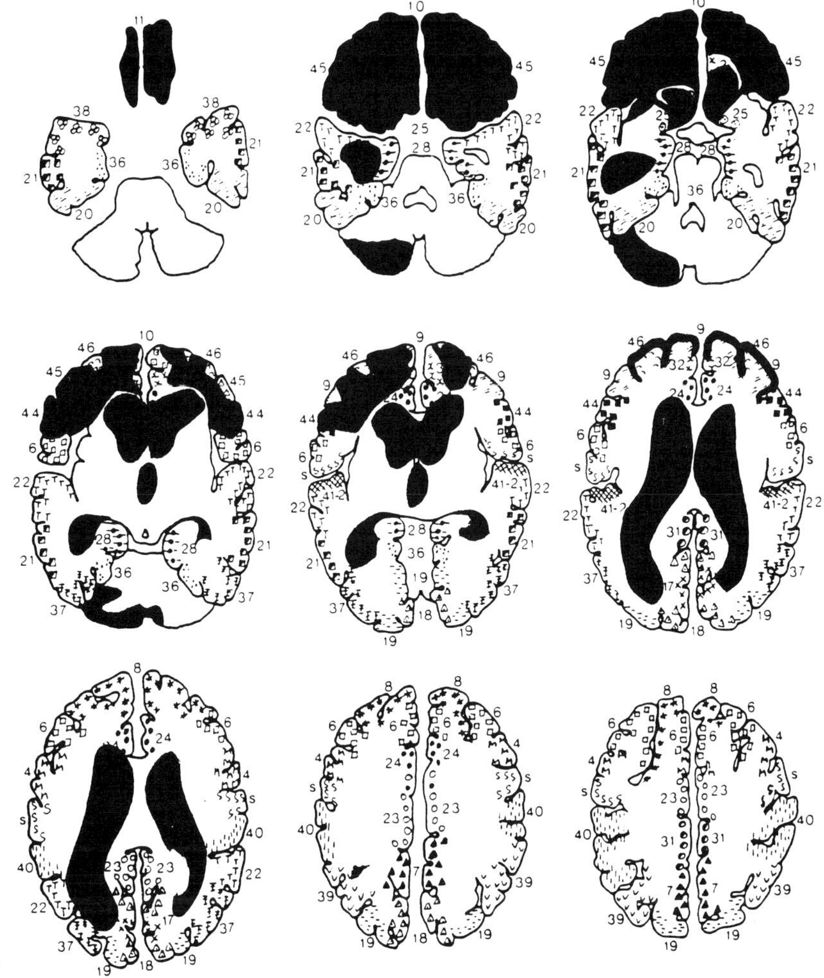

Fig. 21-1. *(Continued).*

lobe damage from concussion. Many of these alterations are commonly subsumed under the psychological construct of *executive processes* and have been identified as major contributing factors to partial and complete disability. Their effects are quite different from the discrete motor, sensory, or "modular" cognitive impairments that often characterize other regions of cortical damage, and they span several domains of cognition and behavior. The result may be compromise of a person's adaptive, independent functioning and adjustment in social, vocational, and familial endeavors.

The construct of executive functions has been delineated in a number of theoretical and research approaches, including information processing, behavioral, analytic, neuropsychological, cognitive, neurologic, and develomental (Eslinger, in press; Grattan and Eslinger, 1991). The emphasis in this chapter arises mainly from neuropsychological and neurologic approaches, although elements from other approaches are also discussed. Our definition of executive processes is that they encompass *regulatory, integrative,* and *representational* operations that are central to decisional and future-oriented mechanisms of cognition and social behavior. Neuroanatomic formulations have suggested that prefrontal cortex and interrelated cortical and subcortical structures form neural networks, which provide the crucial anatomic substrate for executive processes. The prominence of the prefrontal cortex in mediating the development and maintenance of coherence, stability, and direction in cognitive and social processes has invited the label of "executor of the brain."

The chapter first reviews and summarizes four brief case histories of concussive injuries that involved frontal lobe damage and produced different kinds of neurologic and neuropsychologic impairments. We then address the assessment and management of three categories of postconcussive impairments associated with frontal lobe damage: cognitive-executive, social-executive, and neurologic.

Case 1

Figure 21-1 is an example of extensive frontal lobe lesion after severe concussion, as observed on CT scan and localized on standardized brain templates. In this case, the 37-year-old man suffered multiple trauma when he lost control of his motorcycle while not wearing a helmet. He required surgical debridement of a frontal skull fracture and sustained bilateral damage to prefrontal structures, including the orbital frontal cortex, frontal pole, and portions of the dorsolateral frontal cortex. Diffuse ventricular enlargement can also be observed in this chronic CT scan, taken 4 years after the concussive injury because of a new right cerebellar infarct. With the exception of cerebellar-related dysmetria, the patient's motor strength and sensory examination remained normal. Anosmia was evident since the frontal lobe lesion. Even in this chronic phase of recovery, the patient showed marked executive and self-regulatory impairments. Neuropsychological examination indicated perseverative behavior, cognitive rigidity, stimulus-boundedness, distractibility, impulsivity, poor judgment for safety as well as in decision-making activities, and minimal application of learning to everyday tasks. For example, perseverative responses on the Wisconsin Card Sorting test were greater than three standard deviations above the mean, with zero categories achieved. These significant impairments encompass several important aspects of executive processes as well as the self-regulation that permits appropriate anticipation, initiation, inhibition, and shifting to alternative response strategies. In addition, social behavior was often childish, with emotional indifference toward others and little awareness of his impulsive remarks. In spite of these impairments, many basic aspects of speech, language, perception, memory, and intellect were within normal limits. For example, Block Design performance on the Wechsler Adult Intelligence Scale—Revised (WAIS-R) and recognition memory on the Rey verbal learning test were average. Clinical examination of behavior also supported the patient's need for a highly structured care setting with low stimulation parameters and frequent feedback to correct inappropriate behavior. This case is remarkable not only for prominent executive and self-regulatory impairments but also for the frontal lobe lesions that are the likely neural basis for these deficits.

Case 2

This 24-year-old man was an unrestrained passenger in a head-on motor vehicle crash, who was ejected through the front windshield and found unresponsive at the scene. He suffered a severe closed head injury and was admitted to the hospital in a coma, with a Glasgow Coma Scale (GCS) score of 5. Initial brain CT scan revealed cerebral edema. During the 12 weeks following injury, he showed very modest clinical improvement. Upon referral to our service, we observed his extreme slowness in basic sensory and cognitive processing, marked paucity of motor activity, no verbalizations, and no purposeful behavior—a clinical presentation compatible with akinesia and mutism. Review of brain CT scan taken at 1 month postconcussion (Fig. 21-2) revealed less edema but bilateral hypodense lesions, most prominently in the mid to superior regions of the mesial frontal lobe (including portions of the anterior cingulate gyrus–Brodmann's area 24, as well as areas 32 and 6). At 3 months postonset the akinesia and mutism were only slowly resolving as the patient began to orient to nearby sounds and to occasional visual stimuli as well. The marked lack of motivation and initiation severely limited his participation in physical, occupational, and other therapies and prevented evaluation of cognitive abilities. It was recommended that he be treated with a dopamine agonist in order to improve initiation and spontaneity. The rationale and results of such intervention are discussed in more detail in the section *Treatment with Bromocriptine.*

Case 3

This is an example of milder concussive injury with executive and self-regulatory impairments. CT scan in the acute phase showed intracerebral hematomas in the frontal lobe of this 19-year-old intoxicated man, who was struck by a motor vehicle and found unconscious (Fig. 21-3). In contrast to the permanent tissue

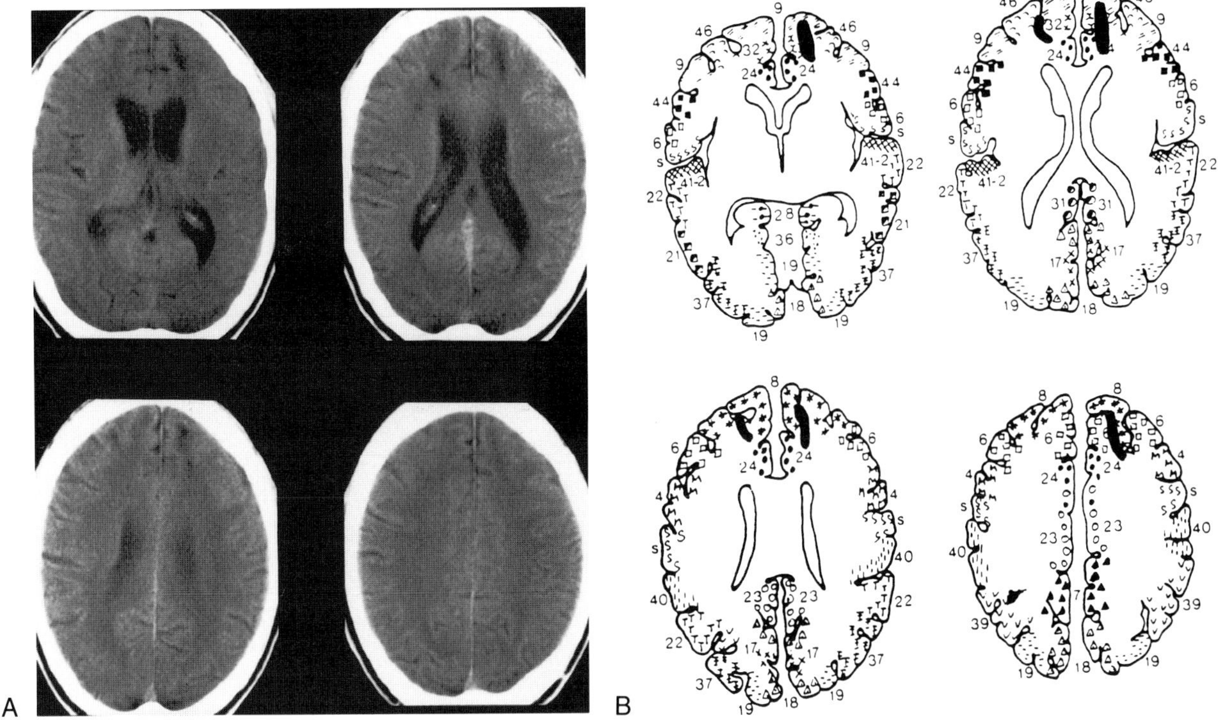

Fig. 21-2. **(A)** CT scan 1 month postinjury and **(B)** best-fitting brain templates of case 2 showing small hypodense lesions to the mesial frontal lobe (including anterior cingulate gyrus and minimally to the supplementary motor area—Brodmann's areas 24, 6, and 32) in patient with akinesia and mutism after closed head injury.

damage in cases 1 and 2, the hemorrhagic lesions and cerebral edema observed in Figure 21-3 typically show significant resolution. The GCS score of 9 improved rapidly to 12. In the emergency room he was moving all extremities, with normal reflexes, and was alert and verbalizing but confused and not following commands. Duration of post-traumatic amnesia was 2 weeks. Although he exhibited fewer cognitive and behavioral impairments than patients 1 and 2 during the inpatient rehabilitation phase, his self-regulation in social and emotional domains remained erratic and problematic. He showed marked frustration intolerance, with diminished impulse control and poor self-awareness, resulting in inappropriate outbursts of aggression and anger. These deficits were managed within the setting of a highly structured rehabilitation program with multiple therapies, all encompassing an emphasis on differential reinforcement and frequent questions and cues regarding appropriate social behaviors. Over the ensuing months, his social self-regulation and self-monitoring improved. His deficits in the chronic phase were much more subtle than in the previous cases, although formalized neuropsychological testing detected mild residual difficulties in speed of information processing, working memory, cognitive flexibility, and divided attention.

Case 4

In contrast to the previous cases, this 47-year-old electronics designer showed a postconcussive syndrome involving the frontal lobe that appeared deceptively mild. He suffered concussion from a motor vehicle accident, which killed his teenage daughter. He was briefly unconscious at the scene and was brought to the emergency room with a GCS score of 14. CT scan showed right frontal lobe hematoma, contusion, and edema (Fig. 21-4) with fractures to the right lateral orbital wall, superior orbital wall, and frontal skull (none requiring surgical treatment). He improved rapidly, with resolution of post-traumatic amnesia within 7 days and a residual retrograde amnesia of only 5 to 10 minutes. His cognition, behavior, and self-care activities were considered quite good by the medical staff. Because of the absence of such

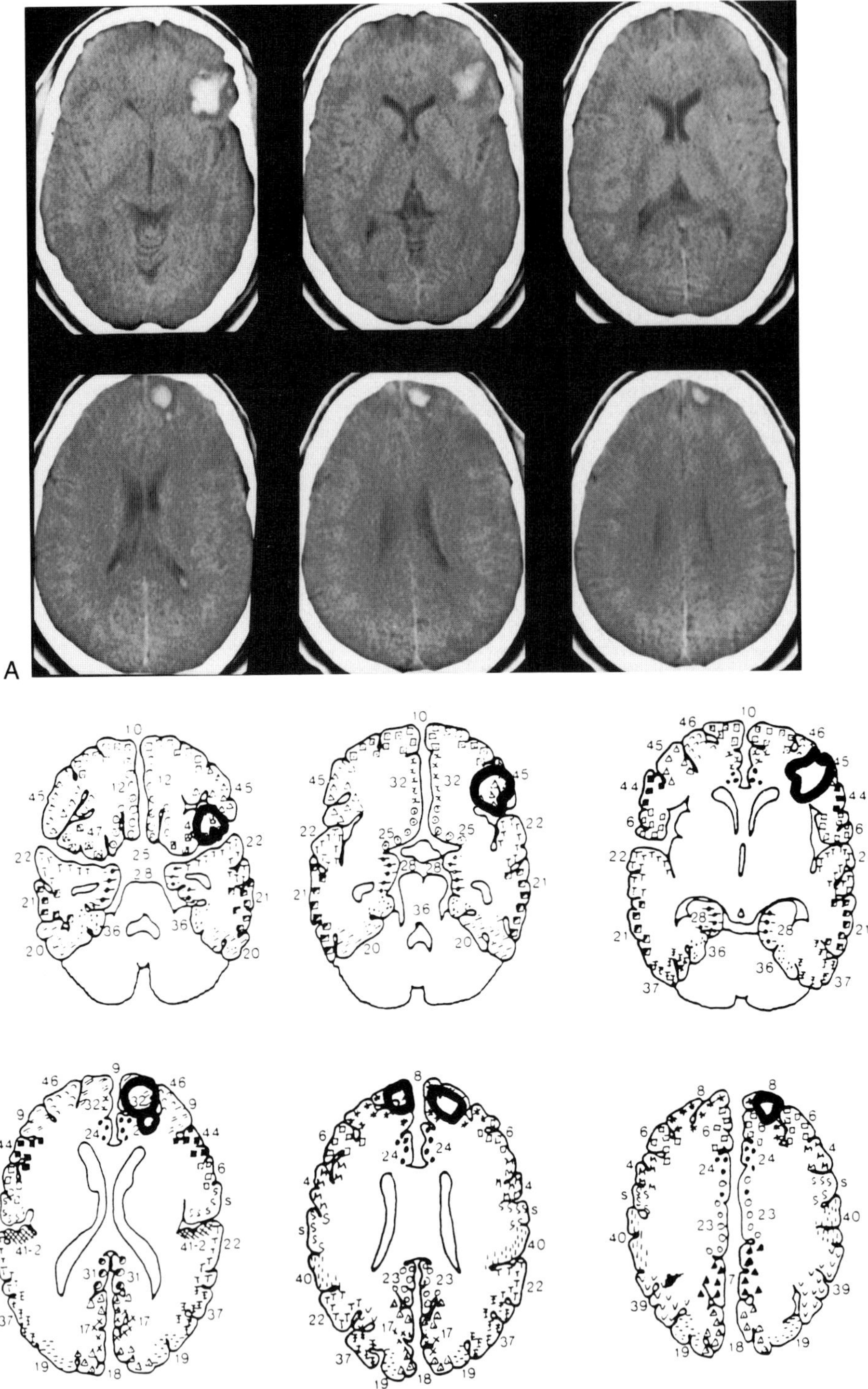

Fig. 21-3. **(A)** CT scan in the acute phase and **(B)** best-fitting brain templates of case 3 showing multiple intracerebral hematomas in the frontal lobe (indicated by open black circles) after patient was hit by a motor vehicle while intoxicated.

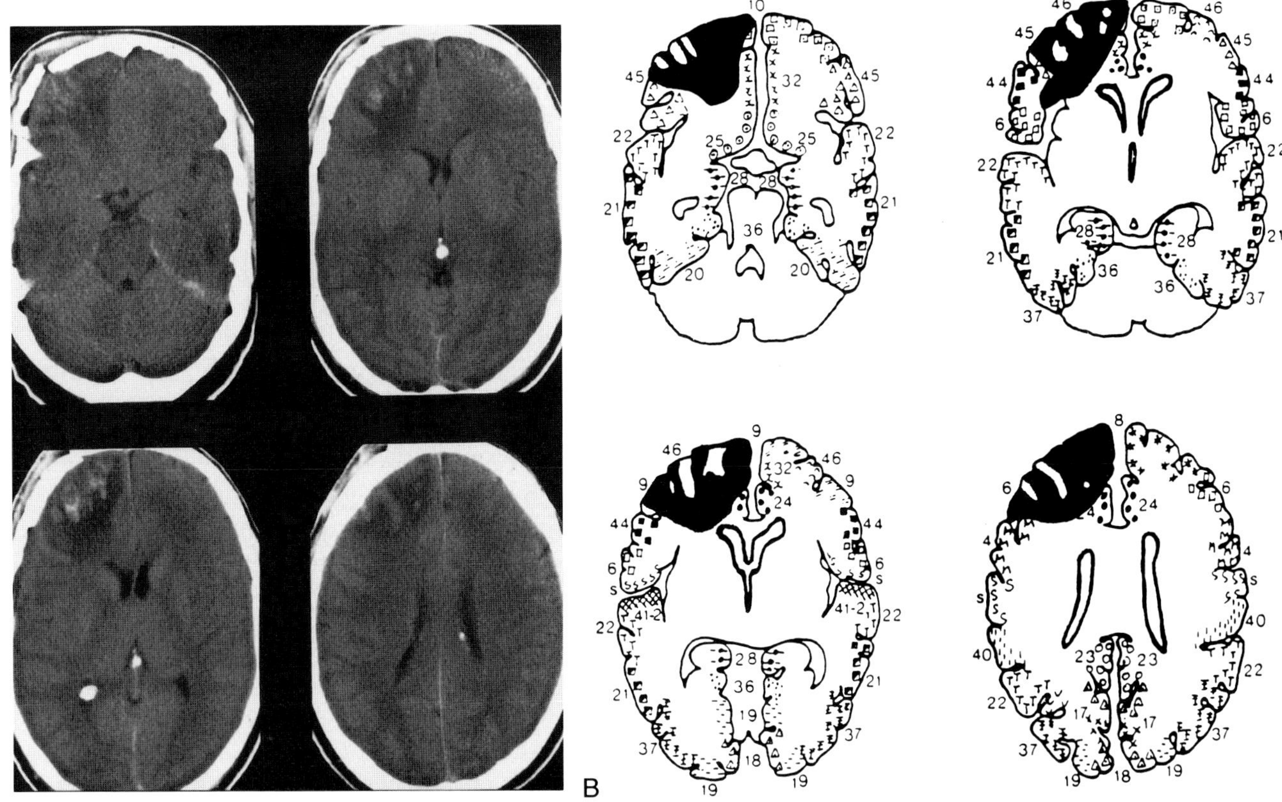

Fig. 21-4. **(A)** CT scan in the acute phase and **(B)** best-fitting brain template of case 4 showing hemorrhagic contusion to the right frontal lobe and temporal pole after a motor vehicle accident. Patient's GCS score was 14 within minutes after accident.

functional impairments, there was disagreement over his need for rehabilitation services, with the resolution being a brief evaluative inpatient admission and continuing outpatient services by the neuropsychology clinic. Bedside neuropsychological screening revealed an alert and fully oriented man who spoke in a fluent, nonparaphasic, and well articulated manner, with modest short-term memory difficulties. Formal neuropsychological testing indicated an average range of measured intellect (WAIS-R Full Scale IQ = 101, 53rd percentile), language, visual perception, and constructional praxis. Learning and memory assessment also indicated an average performance level (Wechsler Memory Scale—Revised [WMS-R] General Index = 108, 70th percentile), which was within the range expected for his educational and occupational background. Although delayed memory measures showed only a modest decline (WMS-R Delayed Index = 94, 35th percentile), a striking defect in temporal organizational aspects of learning was detected. Specifically, Digit Sequence Learning (Benton et al., 1983) performance was impaired (score 2/24, <1st percentile) and level of sequential organization imposed during word list learning trials was low (SO index .19). These temporal learning deficiencies, particularly in light of an average range of general learning and memory scores, have been specifically associated with frontal lobe damage (Eslinger and Grattan, 1994; Grattan et al., 1992), and may contribute to ongoing memory difficulties. This particular patient also showed a marked discrepancy in memory retention for the Rey and Taylor complex figures when a sequential organizational strategy was imposed by the examiner (memory retention at 80th percentile) versus the patient's self-generated figure processing (25th percentile) (Eslinger et al., 1995). Therefore, the cognitive emphasis in outpatient sessions centered on developing and applying temporal and sequential organizational algorithms in daily and vocational activities.

The other major area of cognitive impairment involved reactive and spontaneous forms of cognitive flexibility. Although the patient quickly identified and successfully achieved one category on the Wisconsin Card Sorting test (by 11 sorts), he thereafter could not achieve another category. His perseverative responses were greater than four standard deviations above the mean, with 48 percent of errors being perseverative, reflecting marked inability to react to and utilize examiner feedback. On the spontaneous flexibility measures of design fluency, the patient could not generate designs according to specific rules, despite intact constructional praxis and his background as an electronic designer.

Finally, a prominent clinical impairment was evident in emotional processing. Although he could readily acknowledge his daughter's accidental death on a verbal level, he continued to show no overt emotional reaction to this loss and no sharing of grief with his wife, who was appropriately distressed. By 2 months postconcussion, emotional reactions to his loss began percolating through his indifferent demeanor, initially in the form of agitated reactions but eventually progressing to recognized grief stages.

Discussion of Example Cases

These cases illustrate several fundamental elements of neurologic and neuropsychologic presentations in concussion, as follows:

1. The location of cerebral lesions is highly diverse across cases. This is evident not only for localization to major brain areas (e.g., brainstem, diencephalon, telencephalon), but also for specific location within those areas. In particular, the four illustrative cases showed different locations of frontal lobe damage with relatively few focal neurologic signs, and the associated impairments were most strikingly in different facets of executive and self-regulatory processes. These were not confined to one modality and affected organizational and integrative aspects of cognitive processes as well as self-regulation in behavioral, social, and emotional domains. Therefore, the neurologic and neuropsychological impairments in concussion are related to location and extent of the anatomic lesions.
2. While the pathology of concussive injuries frequently involves the frontal lobe, lesions are by no means confined there. Papo et al. (1982) succinctly stated that "In the vast majority of cases the focal lesion is nothing but the most impressive feature of diffuse brain damage . . ." Another common region of telencephalic damage, for example, is the anterior temporal lobe, particularly the temporal pole. This paralimbic cortex is anatomically interconnected with the amygdala, the orbital and polar frontal regions via the uncinate fasciculus, as well as with other limbic system, diencephalic, and cortical association areas (Markowitsch et al., 1985; Pandya and Yeterian, 1990). The interrelated processing of frontal and temporal polar areas has been linked to memory, social adjustment, primary affiliative tendencies, and emotional processes in human and nonhuman primate studies (e.g., Myers, 1972). Therefore, executive and social processing impairments after injuries that affect these interrelated areas must be viewed in terms of disrupted neural networks that subserve complex behavior (Damasio, 1985; Goldman-Rakic, 1988; Grattan et al., 1994; Nauta, 1972; Pandya and Barnes, 1987). As another example, impaired shifting of response set has been observed in patients with lesions to not only the frontal lobe, but also to posterior cortical association areas, and to the basal ganglia (specifically the region of the head of the caudate) (Anderson et al., 1991; Eslinger and Grattan, 1993; Grafman et al., 1990). Since the frontal lobe is strongly interconnected with posterior association cortices and projects powerfully to the basal ganglia, the neural network subserving response shifting may involve the frontal-cortical system (possibly for perceptual, reasoning, and working memory aspects of such tasks) and the frontal-striatal system (possibly for the motor inhibition and activation aspects of response shifting in such tasks). Although it is reasonable to focus on and extract clinical and neuropsychological data that inform us about executive functions after concussion, it is rarely the case that all such postconcussive impairments can be attributed to frontal lobe damage alone.
3. The types of lesions that occur after concussive injuries are also diverse. From the four example cases, the evident CT scan abnormalities differed between the irreversible hypodense lesions visualized in Figures 21-1 and 21-2 and the space-occupying hematomas, cerebral edema, and contusions in Figures 21-3 and 21-4, which show significant

resolution over time. Differences in lesion type (as well as location) will account, in part, for the variable patterns of recovery in executive and self-regulatory domains after concussive injuries. Other forms of pathology, in particular axonal shearing injury, constitute another source of lesion differences that could contribute to variable outcome.

4. Although the most severe social and cognitive problems tend to be observed during the early months after head trauma, their debilitating effects may become more evident during the chronic recovery phase. This was most clear in case 1 and to a lesser extent in case 4, where persistently poor adaptation and adjustment led to mounting social, financial, and familial problems. Personality changes are common after concussion and have often been attributed to damage to the frontal lobe on the basis of studies of traumatic and nontraumatic frontal lobe lesions (Ackerly and Benton, 1947; Brickner, 1934; Eslinger and Damasio, 1985; Goldstein, 1942; Harlow, 1868). Such changes may exist with or without neurologic and measurable cognitive deficits. Even when they are accompanied by neurologic or cognitive symptoms, the personality and social difficulties may present a comparatively greater barrier to successful rehabilitation, functional recovery, and return to work (Brooks et al., 1986; Lezak, 1987; Oddy, 1984). Moreover, personality and social-emotional alterations are also the primary contributors to the strain and disruption frequently reported by the family members of brain-injured patients (Brooks, 1986; Lezak, 1986).

   As the example cases illustrate, the relationship between severity of injury and subsequent social or personality changes is neither simple nor linear. The long-term result for many head-injured patients is fewer social interactions and reduced social supports. Moreover, the diversity of social and emotional alterations seems to parallel the heterogeneity in head trauma pathophysiology. Numerous factors contribute to the personality alterations associated with head trauma and deserve discussion alongside cognitive alterations. Therefore, we will address the social impairments that represent disruption of executive processes associated with frontal lobe damage in the section *Social-Executive Aspects of Postconcussive Syndrome.*

When one considers the marked variations in the neurobiologic effects of concussive injuries, it is perhaps not surprising that the neurologic and neuropsychologic consequences also vary widely and hence require intensive individual evaluation. In the following sections we discuss such evaluation of concussion from the perspectives of cognitive-executive, social-executive, and neurologic impairments.

COGNITIVE-EXECUTIVE ASPECTS OF POSTCONCUSSIVE SYNDROME

Cognitive-Executive Processes

The construct of executive processes in the neuropsychology literature emerged from important case descriptions, from clinical observations of behavior in various patient samples, and from more recent development and validation of cognitive tasks and behavioral paradigms, which are applied to neurologic as well as normal populations. Among postconcussive patients, as our example cases illustrated, many executive processing impairments can be observed. They are encountered most frequently in patients with moderate to severe injuries but can also be detected in certain mild head trauma cases.

Executive processes have been among the most difficult psychological constructs to define, model, and operationalize through behavioral measures. They differ from models of sensation, perception, language, memory, and even intelligence that have more advanced definitions and operationalized measures and yet are critically interrelated to these fundamental cognitive domains. Executive processes have sometimes been invoked to explain how nonroutine or nonautomatic situations are handled, but what demands a nonroutine response from one person may not demand such response from another person with different background and experience. Other approaches highlight the role of verbal self-regulation in executive processes, emphasizing the use of rule-based strategies to guide behavior and achieve certain goals. However, even high levels of verbal knowledge do not ensure appropriate behavioral responses, as suggested by the dissociation between "knowing" and "doing" in patients with frontal lobe damage (e.g., Eslinger and Damasio, 1985; Lhermitte, 1986; Milner, 1964).

We suggest that cognitive components of executive processes encompass representational, integrative, and regulatory features, which are central to decisional and future-oriented aspects of behavior, and have termed these *cognitive-executive processes.* Representational operations include registration of information, experience and organismic states for handling both immediate environmental-organismic demands (e.g., working memory) and longer-term assimilation of knowledge (e.g., planning, prioritization, weighing courses of action). Integrative operations necessarily span multiple modalities but are also privy to organismic states and needs. The operationalized measures of such processes, discussed in more detail below, have focused largely on complex problem-solving tasks that require cognitive flexibility, incorporation of new experiences, and identifying patterns of information. The third operation emphasizes regulatory processes that are tied to responses, internal and external, and the various effector systems associated with motor, endocrine, autonomic, and other bodily capacities influenced by central neurologic processing. The basic motor choices to initiate, sustain, inhibit, and shift are paramount examples.

The focus of these three operations is normally context-dependent, and they are organized to serve adaptation, adjustment, and appropriateness of behavior in relation to a person's goals, intentions, and participation within diverse settings.

Neuropsychological Evaluation

Neuropsychological examination encompasses several of the important approaches toward evaluating cognitive-executive processes. The initial phase of such examination is centered around establishing neurologic data about the trauma, including parameters such as duration of loss of consciousness, GCS scores, clinical neurologic examination, brain scan findings, electroencephalographic (EEG) and other neurologic test results, accompanying medical conditions, treatments, and current state of recovery as indicated by attending medical and rehabilitation staff, the patient (if possible), and family members. Interviews with the patient (if possible) and family are indicated to establish pertinent history and current neurobehavioral condition. For patients who are unable to cooperate with interview and formal neuropsychological testing, behavioral-cognitive observations and informal cognitive assessment may be possible at the bedside and during other therapies. For patients who are cooperative only for brief periods, well-focused multiple examination sessions are recommended. On inpatient units, these can range from one to five sessions per week, each 15 to 45 minutes. Early examination sessions are geared toward differential diagnosis, supported by standardized assessment of orientation, attention, memory, and basic communication and perceptual skills as well as behavioral and emotional self-regulation. For patients in a post-traumatic amnesia state, daily rechecks of orientation and memory are recommended. At this stage of neurobehavioral recovery, one of the paramount concerns is increasing patients' participation in rehabilitative therapies, usually through behavioral, pharmacologic, and structured program approaches.

For outpatients and those in the latter stages of inpatient rehabilitation, more rigorous neuropsychological examination is recommended. The emphasis in such examination is initially on formal, psychometric evaluation of basic aspects of attention, intelligence, language, perception, memory, and routine problem-solving and will involve computation of standardized IQ, and other cognitive indices. Although these composite measures are not completely devoid of influence from cognitive-executive processing, a different set of psychometric parameters generally is used to evaluate cognitive-executive processes. These parameters emphasize representational, integrative, and regulatory components, and are reflected through tests that require information storage, manipulation of information, and adaptive application of behavior. Information *storage* refers to the various classifications of knowledge in the nervous system. In the case of executive processes, these classifications are tested by the patient's assimilation of feedback as well as advanced information in problem solving tasks and by the dynamic and transient representations referred to as "working memory." *Manipulation* of information influences the rate, efficiency, and organizational structure of information retrieval and problem solving and depends on a variety of cognitive skills. *Adaptive application* of behavior refers to the insight, judgment, self-regulation, and use of knowledge that govern appropriateness of thoughts and responses in relationship to goals, intentions, and participation within diverse settings.

As can be seen in Table 21-1, there is no single modality or cognitive area that is the sole focus of cognitive-executive processing. Hence, problem solving, inferential thinking, planning, learning and memory, communication, working memory, atten-

TABLE 21-1. Cognitive-Executive Processes and Their Operationalized Measures[a]

Executive Processes	Measures
Cognitive flexibility	
Spontaneous	Fluency paradigms
Reactive	Wisconsin card sorting test
Environmental judgments	Cognitive estimation
	Frequency judgments
Planning	Tower of London Hand
	Porteus mazes
	Rey complex figure
Learning/memory	
Temporal processing	Digit sequence learning
	Recency judgments
Organization	Serial position effects
	Subjective organization
	Semantic clustering
Source-context	Time-place judgments of learning
Metamemory	Self-judgments
Encoding	Levels of processing
	Release from proactive interference
Discourse	
Organization	Narratives
Intentional states	Test of language competence
Working memory	
Verbal	Paced auditory serial addition test
Visual spatial	Delayed alternation
	Delayed responding
Attention	
Selective	Visual search
Divided	Peterson Interference Task
	Trails B
	Dichotic listening
Self-regulation/self-monitoring	
Sustained	Vigilant tasks
Paced responding	Self-ordered pacing
Response suppression-conflicting stimuli	Stroop test
Environmental independence	Utilization behavior tasks
Inhibition	Go/no go tasks

[a] See Lezak (1985)and Spreen and Strauss (1991) for details on many of these tests.

tion, and self-regulation domains must be considered, even among patients with good recovery after concussion (e.g., Barth et al., 1983; Cicerone and Wood, 1987; Glisky et al., 1986; Novoa and Ardila, 1987; Stuss et al., 1985; Stuss et al., 1989; and Van Zomeren et al., 1984).

Cognitive-Executive Impairments and Frontal Lobe Damage

The relationship between cognitive-executive impairments and frontal lobe damage has been supported by many case and group studies, most clearly in patients with focal damage to the frontal cortex. However, this correlation may not be entirely adequate to explain the consequences of concussive injuries, even when there is evidence of frontal lobe lesion from neuroimaging studies. It must also be stated that the absence of specific frontal lobe lesion after concussion cannot definitively rule out executive processing impairments. For example, Vilkki (1992) reported that closed head injury patients with nonfrontal parenchymal lesions on CT scan were as impaired on executive measures as those patients with frontal lesions patients. Furthermore, both groups scored more poorly than head injury patients without parenchymal lesions. Therefore, the presence or absence of a parenchymal lesion after concussion, rather than its anterior versus posterior location, was more predictive of executive processing impairments. As the investigator suggested, parenchymal lesion on CT scan may signal more widespread disruption of cortical-cortical and cortical-subcortical circuits. A likely mechanism for such widespread disruption is diffuse axonal injury, resulting in disconnection of the neural networks subserving executive processes. This conclusion is also supported by regional cerebral blood flow study with technetium 99m hexamethyl-propylene amineoxime (HMPAO). Goldenberg et al. (1992) reported that although significant correlations were found between executive functional test scores and reduced flow in the frontal lobe, stronger correlations were evident with reduced flow in the thalamic region. Whether the latter is a primary or secondary (e.g., deafferentation caused by cortical lesions) consequence of head injury, it may nevertheless serve as a marker of severity of diffuse injury and disruption of the neural networks that underlie executive processing abilities. These data argue for an anatomic model of executive processes that emphasizes the interrelationship of frontal lobe regions with nonfrontal brain systems that provide crucial psychological and biologic operations as well as effector mechanisms. It is our view that understanding of postconcussive executive processing impairments and their outcome requires a stronger emphasis on assessing the neural networks in which the frontal lobe is prominently involved, as neuroimaging evidence of frontal lobe lesions alone is not sufficiently predictive of consequences and outcome after concussive injuries.

With the use of standardized psychometric procedures in neuropsychological practice, it is possible to evaluate at least several aspects of executive processes. However, it is also the case that executive processes are defined in part by their independence from immediate environmental and organismic demands. In other words, developing and maintaining sets of mental representations that prolong and organize the salience of experiences and information long after their occurrence provides an important basis for human adjustment and adaptation. Examples include planning, anticipation, insight, and orderly change in goals, plans, and intentions that drive and guide behavior. These processes can be impaired by concussive injuries (e.g., Freedman et al., 1987; Grafman et al., 1993) and yet may not be fully reflected by current neuropsychological tests. Therefore, detailed clinical evaluation and interview with patients and their family members are important aspects of neuropsychological examination, which must be considered together with standardized test results. The semi-structured interview approach of the Brock Adaptive Functioning Questionnaire (Dynan, Roden, and Murphy, 1955) provides a rating based analysis of symptoms often associated with frontal lobe damage and concussion.

Management of Cognitive-Executive Impairments

Remediation and management of cognitive aspects of executive impairments is frequently required after concussive injuries, and a focused literature is continuing to emerge around this topic. Together with impairments in social behavior, cognitive-executive deficits can develop into the main class of postconcussive symptoms that impede community and vocational reintegration. This is particularly evident when other aspects of recovery (e.g., ambulation, speech, basic daily activities) are proceeding well but irregular attention is given to higher cognitive and social processes.

Executive and self-regulatory impairments in patients are among the most challenging to rehabilitation specialists. Common deficits that impede rehabilitative progress include "release" of inappropriate behaviors such as aggressive outbursts, impulsivity, distractibility, and perseveration but also include lack of motivation and slow, erratic improvement day to day. Since management of socially inappropriate behaviors and neurologic deficits (e.g., lack of initiation) are discussed later in this chapter, we here focus briefly on postconcussive cognitive deficits. As part of a neuropsychological examination, reasons for maladaptive behaviors need to be identified. These can include various forms of cognitive deficit, heightened susceptibility to environmental stimulation, stress and frustration intolerance reactions, poor self-control, and lack of self-monitoring. Increasingly, case studies have described effective behavior modification procedures, the most successful focusing on discrete, measurable behaviors (e.g., Lira et al., 1983; Whaley et al., 1986). A wide variety of behavior therapy techniques have been described and can be applied in individualized fashion to particular cases, depending on patients' cognitive-behavioral abilities and the targeted behaviors (reviewed by Mateer and Ruff, 1990; McGlynn, 1990). However, the literature pertinent to cognitive-executive impairments remains small in comparison with the domains of attention, memory, visual perception, and language. This is a result of difficulties in defining the core elements of executive processes, developing intervention strategies that address the complexity of these processes, and implementing these in a cost-effective manner.

Cognitive approaches potentially can enhance learning and alter maladaptive strategies. An example is the study of Cicerone and Wood (1987), who attempted to treat the prominent planning deficit of a young postconcussive patient some 4 years after injury. Using verbal self-regulation as a cognitive-mediational strategy, the investigators designed a self-instructional procedure for the patient. Target behaviors included reduction of off-task behaviors and problem-solving errors while training on a series of Tower of London tasks. The intervention led to marked improvement in planning performance, with evidence for transfer and maintenance of learning effects as well.

Together with behavioral modification, modeling, social learning, psychotherapeutic, and neurologic treatments, cognitive-mediation approaches can provide certain patients with enhanced skills for problem solving and adaptation. However, such research is in the early stages and requires further development and empirical validation.

SOCIAL-EXECUTIVE ASPECTS OF POSTCONCUSSIVE SYNDROME

When personality, social, and emotional difficulties are present after milder forms of head trauma, patients are most frequently described as irritable, with decreased frustration tolerance. After moderate to severe head injuries some patients have been additionally described as "childish" (e.g., giddy, demanding, or self-centered), with rapid mood changes, lack of social tact and restraint, and impulsiveness in social situations, while others display apathy, indifference, or a lack of concern for the interests and needs of others (Brooks et al., 1986; Elsass and Kinsella, 1987; Thompson, 1984).

Despite the well-documented changes in personality and social behavior after head trauma and their strong association with poor outcome, there are few taxonomies or guidelines available for diagnosing these aspects of traumatic brain injury. Some patients may meet various DSM-IV (American Psychiatric Association, 1994) criteria for personality, mood, stress, or adjustment disorders, but these are imprecise categories for the socially disruptive behaviors of postconcussive patients and do not address the synergistic effects of the cognitive, social, and emotional alterations caused by acquired brain injury. Specifically, a common difficulty for most postconcussive patients lies in prioritizing, organizing, and managing social information as well as their own emotional reactions in novel and complex social settings. This difficulty largely represents disruption of the executive system and the way in which social and interpersonal cues are utilized in the development and maintenance of adaptive social behavior. Subsequently, we are persuaded that a heuristic taxonomy of "social executors" may provide a parsimonious model for describing and classifying several types of personality and social difficulties commonly associated with postconcussive syndromes. The social executors include social self-regulation, social self-awareness, social sensitivity, and social salience (Table 21-2). These are based on the convergence of data from existing models of neuropsychologically mediated social deficits after head trauma (Brooks, 1984; Lezak, 1989; Prigatano, 1986) combined with empirical data regarding the role of the frontal lobes and interrelated cerebral regions in executive and interpersonal behavior (Grattan and Eslinger, 1991a; Grattan et al., 1994; Stuss and Benson, 1986).

TABLE 21-2. A Proposed Taxonomy of Social Impairments After Brain Injury: Types of Social-Executive Processes

Social self-regulation	Managing one's interaction with other people
Social self-awareness	Knowledge and insight about oneself in social situations
Social sensitivity (empathy)	Recognition and understanding of psychological states
Social salience	Processes that underlie the sense of meaningfulness to social situations and other people

Social Executors

Select social-emotional processes and behaviors associated with postconcussive syndromes may be subsumed under the umbrella of "executive functions." Operating as social executors, these processes serve to facilitate or impede the execution of effective and meaningful interpersonal relationships. The social executors are distinguishable from other emotional, interpersonal, and reactive processes such as depression, anxiety, or low self-esteem by virtue of their close relationship with cognitive-executive processes and their role in organizing, modifying, and integrating social perceptions, social behavior, and emotional expression within specific contexts and into stable mental models. These mental structures take into account social roles, norms, and expectations as well as what is considered "fair and just" by the culture. Although isolated impairments in each social-executive process have been found in patients with focal cerebral lesions, disruption of multiple social-executive processes is the more common pattern following moderate to severe head trauma.

The ways in which these difficulties are expressed are largely dependent upon associated cognitive deficits, the patient's premorbid personality, reactive syndromes, current environment and the adaptability of the patient's family or social system (Fig. 21-5). For instance, a person with a memory disorder may feel personally inadequate and overly dependent on others following head trauma. However, the manner in which these feelings are expressed (as genuine sadness, with efforts to be self-reliant and appreciative

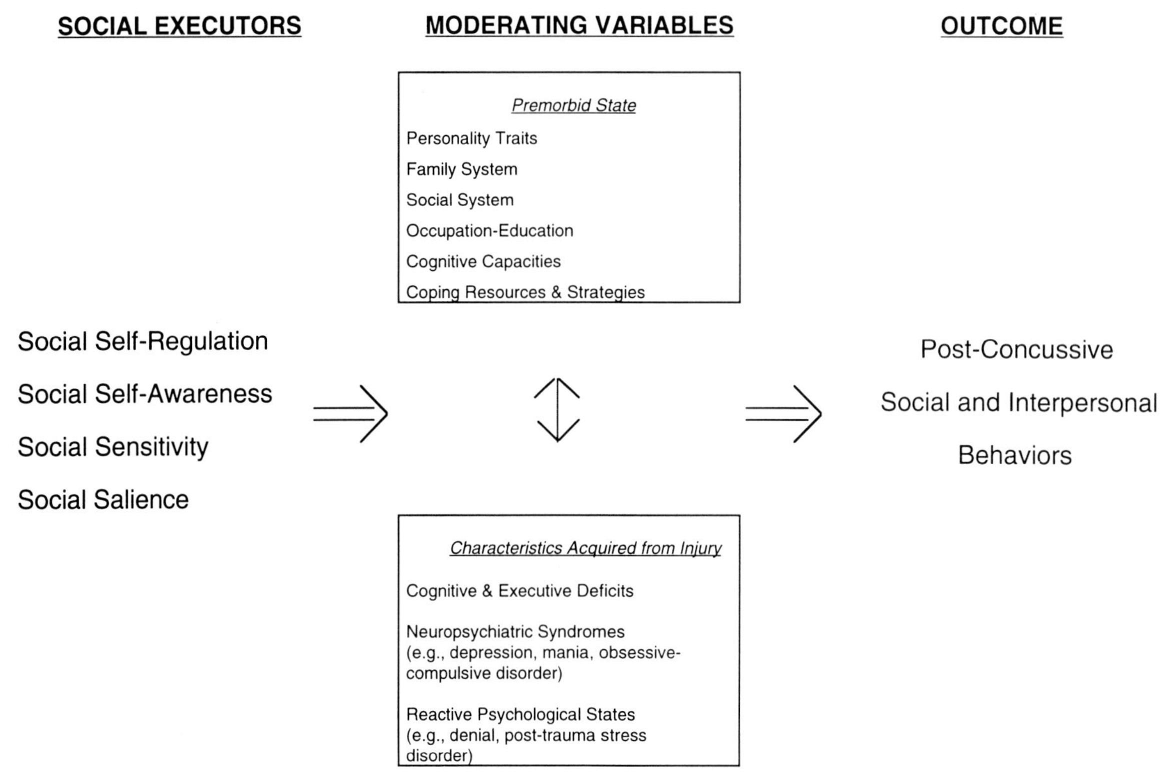

Fig. 21-5. Proposed model outlining many of the key elements of social executive processes and the moderating variables that interact to influence outcome from postconcussive injuries.

of others, as apathy and social withdrawal, or by hugging everyone the person sees and likes in any context) is largely dependent on the integrity of the social executors. The specific characteristics of the social executors are as described below.

Social Self-Regulation

Social self-regulation is the ability to effectively manage the initiation, rate, intensity, and duration of one's interaction with other persons. Difficulties with social self-regulation are common sequelae of moderate to severe head trauma and occur along a continuum, ranging from pathologic inertia to complete disinhibition (Hebb and Penfield, 1940; Lezak, 1989; Prigatano, 1986). These difficulties are most evident during acute and subacute recovery phases and may persist in milder forms as permanent features of the patient's personality. Problems with social self-regulation may be expressed in the following ways:

1. Difficulty in inhibiting impulsive responses in social contexts, resulting in frequent interruptions and bizarre or contextually inappropriate behavior.
2. Low frustration tolerance, resulting in irritable, angry, or violent over-reactions to mild inconveniences or conflicts.
3. Limited appreciation for interpersonal boundaries, resulting in inappropriate self-disclosure, overly personal questions to others, and inappropriate physical gestures such as hugging or kissing therapists and casual acquaintances.
4. A viscosity or stickiness in social situations, whereby the patient does not stop talking or leave the interpersonal situation despite clear cues that the interaction is over.
5. Reduced initiation and volition in social settings, resulting in the appearance of apathy.

Social Self-Awareness

Social self-awareness is specialized knowledge or insight about oneself in social situations (Grattan et al., 1994; Lezak, 1989; Prigatano et al., 1990; Stuss,

1991). Social self-awareness involves the accurate perception of one's own feelings, ability to manage strong emotions, the impact one has on other people, and one's general interpersonal effectiveness. Accurate social self-awareness is important for making adaptive social judgments and executing interpersonal behavior that is contextually appropriate and maintains positive relationships over time. Disruption of accurate social self-awareness may result in tactless and tasteless comments, inappropriate or bizarre behavior, and uncorrected socially malapropos remarks. Furthermore, it may decrease motivation to seek and respond to treatment for interpersonal problems. In a study of the specific knowledge deficits associated with closed head injury, Prigatano et al. (1990) demonstrated that head-injured patients disproportionately underestimated their difficulties in emotional control and social interaction as compared with cognitive and instrumental abilities. The authors hypothesized that this deficit might be associated with the extent of frontal lobe damage. A subsequent study in our laboratory supported this hypothesis and indicated that isolated deficits in social self-knowledge occurred most frequently in patients with focal frontal lobe damage (Grattan et al., 1994). Therefore, the frontal lobe may serve as an executive knowledge base and gating mechanism for accumulating and accessing specialized knowledge and insight about the self.

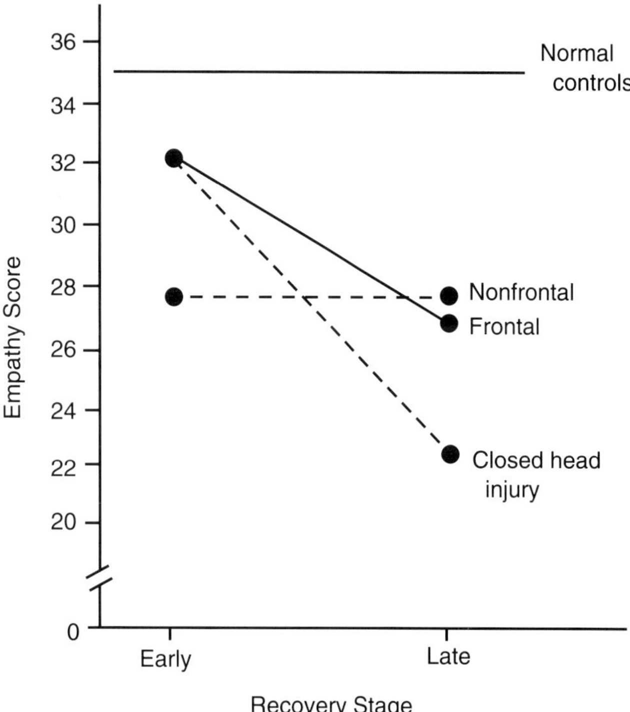

Fig. 21-6. Illustration of the different patterns of onset and change in empathy scores reported by patients with nontraumatic, focal frontal and nonfrontal lesions as well as by patients with moderate closed head injury. The empathy measure of Hogan (1969) was used with all subjects. Patients with closed head injury and nontraumatic frontal lobe lesions both showed significant reduction in cognitively based empathy between the early and late phases of recovery. According to their family member reports, they also showed lack of awareness in the social domain during early phases of recovery.

Social Sensitivity

Social sensitivity is the extent to which an individual is able to recognize and understand another's psychological state. It is generally synonymous with the construct of cognitively based empathy; that is the ability to take another person's perspective or point of view or to put oneself in another's shoes (Hogan, 1969). These perspective-taking abilities allow an individual to anticipate the behavior and reactions of others and provide a basis for satisfying and adaptive interpersonal relationships. Normal levels of cognitively based empathy have been associated with likability, social acuity, communication competence, and effective social functioning. In contrast, nonempathic individuals tend to be rigid, self-centered, and insensitive to others.

Empirical studies of cognitively based empathy have been undertaken in patients with focal cerebral lesions and head trauma (Grattan and Eslinger, 1989, 1990). The results indicated that patients report different patterns of change according to lesion location, etiology, and recovery phase. The most common alteration is a reduction in empathy score on a valid and reliable self-report inventory. In the early recovery phase (within 1 month postonset), patients with isolated nonfrontal cerebral lesions quickly reported a significant reduction in empathy, which remained stable throughout the later recovery phase (6 months postonset) (Fig. 21-6). Patients with isolated frontal lobe lesions initially reported only a modest reduction in empathy, which evolved over time to a highly significant reduction. Patients with moderate head trauma reported an even steeper reduction in empathy ($P < .01$) between early and late recovery phases, in a pattern similar to the frontal lesion sample. For both groups, it is interesting to note that family member reports on an equivalent form identified reduction in the patient's empathy levels during the early recovery phase. This supports the interpretation that the early reports by frontal lesion and head trauma patients were limited by their impaired social self-awareness but were modified as executive processes improved and social-emotional difficulties were encountered. For many patients, their reports in the late phase more closely parallel reports by family members and hence may represent improved awareness. Empirical studies have also indicated that patients who maintain normal empathy levels after frontal lobe damage have significantly better social and vocational outcome than those with reduced empathy (Grattan and Eslinger, 1991b). A similar result might be expected for head trauma patients. Moreover, the reduction in empathy after frontal lobe damage, particularly damage involving the dorsolateral sector, may be related to a specific deficit in understanding alternate perspectives when unfamiliar persons and situations are encountered (Grattan et al., 1994). Therefore, the frontal lobe provides crucial cognitive support to this social executor, permitting individuals to extricate themselves from a set perspective and consider other persons' points of view and emotional states, particularly in nonroutine situations.

Social Salience

Social salience embraces a variety of processes that contribute meaningfulness to a social situation and the individuals within it and hence distinguish among people and circumstances according to their importance. These processes have a strong biologic basis, operating at conscious and nonconscious levels, and determine an individual's level of arousal, visceral reactions, and autonomic responsiveness. They also set the emotional tone for social interactions. At a psychological level, these processes influence the allocation of attention and interest as well as mental and emotional resources in social situations. They provide important data for interpreting one's own or another's emotional state and mediate social reinforcement. Deficits in social salience carry negative social consequences and can appear as overt disregard for a person or situation, under- or over-responsiveness to the emotional experiences of others, inability to benefit from social feedback, or alterations in social anxiety.

Impaired social salience may be amenable to measurement through neurobiologic and cognitive methods. From a neurobiologic perspective, reduced autonomic responsiveness to social stimuli has been reported following nontraumatic damage to the orbital frontal region (Damasio et al., 1991), which is also a common location of damage from concussive injuries. Summarizing this work and considering its theoretical implications, Damasio et al. suggested that the somatic states associated with social reinforcers and punishments may not be evoked in patients with orbital frontal lobe lesions. As a result, they cannot learn from social experiences nor be guided by somatic cues previously acquired. Preliminary cognitive data from our laboratory, using a standardized measure of affectively based empathy, have indicated that head-injured patients in the chronic phase are rated significantly lower than normal by family members. This was interpreted as reflecting their difficulty in sharing the feelings of another at an affective level. For example, patients reported feeling too much or too little sensitivity when seeing a sad movie, visiting a sick friend, or seeing an animal in pain as compared with a normal comparison group. Although diagnostic measures are yet to be developed, we suggest that concussive injuries can be associated with inability to modulate the experience of emotion in relationship to other people and diverse social settings. The specific relationship to location and severity of head injury must also be established.

The notion of social salience embraces a diversity of physiologic processes and psychological operations, the measurable aspects of which are only beginning to emerge. Nevertheless, preliminary empirical data and theoretic formulations suggest that impairments in social salience may be a significant factor in the chain of events that produces some maladaptive social behaviors and personality characteristics. From a neurobehavioral perspective, the orbital frontal lobe and its connections with the limbic system, which are particularly prone to damage in concussive injuries, may mediate important aspects of social salience.

Assessment and Interventions

The extent to which head-injured patients can regulate their behavior in social contexts, demonstrate awareness of their impact on others, understand another's point of view, or share in another's emotional experience are important personality and social dimensions to assess. In the clinical setting, the features of social executors may be assessed through patient observation as well as by clinical interview with the patient, family members, caregivers, or treatment staff. We have also found the Patient Competency Rating Scale (Prigatano, 1986) to be a useful tool for guiding questions in the interpersonal, social, and emotional domains within the context of a more comprehensive psychological assessment. We recommend that it be administered to both the patient and a family member. There are standardized measures available for assessing both cognitively and affectively based empathy. However, these are currently more pertinent to research with brain-injured patients than to clinical diagnostic purposes. With the exception of the early recovery phase, there is generally a high agreement between patient and family member ratings on standardized inventory of cognitively based empathy. Hence, interviewing a family member can be an efficient and effective way to obtain these data.

Interventions for disturbed social-executive processes typically fall within the purview of specially trained neuropsychologists, neuropsychiatrists, or behavioral neurologists and may involve multiple treatment modalities (e.g., individual, family, or group psychotherapy), depending on the specific problem. Some of the interventions, particularly if they involve supportive counseling or behavioral interventions, may be supplemented with contacts by other treatment providers such as occupational, physical, or speech therapists. It is important to keep in mind that there is considerable diversity in the psychological character of head-injured patients, and individualized psychotherapeutic treatment plans need to be developed for each patient and that patient's family. Within this context, Table 21-3 provides a summary of some general treatment guidelines.

NEUROLOGIC ASPECTS OF POSTCONCUSSIVE SYNDROME

Neurologic Impairments

Since the impact of concussive injuries on the frontal lobe can be quite diverse, it is necessary to undertake comprehensive neurologic and neuropsychologic examinations. Neurologic evaluation encompasses motor activity, sensory, cranial nerve, reflex, and autonomic functions, as well as many clinical aspects of cognitive processes (Table 21-4).

Motor activity is mediated by a large expanse of frontal cortex. Damage to primary motor cortex results in contralateral spastic paralysis according to

TABLE 21-3. Treatment Guidelines for Disturbed Social-Executive Processes in Postconcussive Patients

1. Recognize interpersonal difficulties as an important domain for assessment and intervention.
2. Identify the source of the social difficulty with a comprehensive clinical evaluation of cognitive, executive, interpersonal, affective, and personality processes.
3. Set realistic goals, preferably multiple short-term goals, which members of the rehabilitation team can address and track.
4. Acknowledge that maintenance of acceptable social behavior is a reasonable goal.
5. Start therapy from each patient's level of interpersonal functioning. Bring the patient's attention to any inappropriate behaviors only after a positive therapeutic relationship is developed, with an emphasis on increasing self-awareness.
6. Educate the patient's family to social-emotional alterations after head trauma. This often involves confirming their observations and concerns regarding the patient's inappropriate behaviors, as well as offering support and programmatic ideas for long-term management and recovery.
7. Support the patient's strengths.
8. Reassure the patient in different ways that the troublesome behaviors may be modified.
9. Encourage a sense of optimism and hope with the patient, the family, and the rehabilitation team.
10. If group therapy is indicated, restrict group to members who are head-injured.
11. Treat the patient in a personal yet professional manner. Learn about prior interests, activities, and goals, incorporating as many aspects as possible into the patient's current self-perspective.
12. If litigation is in progress, encourage rapid resolution to reduce associated stresses.
13. When the frustration and anger of the patient or family members are directed at the treatment team, do not take it personally. This may reflect the helplessness and self-doubt of the patient and/or family. They may need assistance in expressing these anxieties more directly and productively.
14. Offer the family a "take-home" plan for how to manage residual social-emotional deficits, and provide outpatient follow-up as needed.

TABLE 21-4. Frontal Lobe Functions: Localization and Prominent Symptoms

Function	Localization	Symptom
Motor activity	Motor cortex: area 4	Contralateral spastic paralysis
	Premotor cortex: area 6	Frontal release signs, spasticity, apraxia
	area 44, 45	Nonfluent aphasia, buccofacial apraxia
Autonomic	Cingulate and medial orbital gyri	Respiratory, blood pressure, peristalsis
	Mesial frontal region	Frontal lobe incontinence
Higher cognition and behavior	Superior medial: area 24, 6	Lack of initiative, apathy, akinesia, and mutism
	Inferior medial: area 25, 32, 12 basal forebrain	Memory impairment, confabulation, disinhibition, utilization behavior
	Dorsolateral: area 8, 9, 10, 11, 43, 46, 47	Poor integration and synthesis of information, disorganization, stimulus-boundedness, concrete thinking, perseveration, poor self-monitoring and planning, neglect, semifluent aphasias
	Orbital: area 10, 11, 12, 13, 14	Personality change, poor social judgment, impulsivity, lack of sustained goal-directed behavior

the homuncular pattern of motor organization. Damage to premotor cortices induces apraxia and more spasticity than palsy, as well as sucking, groping, and grasping reflexes. These primitive reflexes, driven by the parietal lobe, can be "released" by virtue of frontal lobe damage. Injury to the inferior aspects of the premotor cortex in the left hemisphere (Broca's area) results in nonfluent aphasia and buccofacial apraxia, with transcortical motor aphasia associated with lesions rostral or deep to Broca's area. Bilateral lesions to primary motor cortex cause quadriplegia. Damage to superior mesial frontal structures, particularly the anterior cingulate gyrus (area 24) and supplementary motor area (area 6 on the mesial surface of the hemisphere) causes akinesia and mutism. This is most severe in bilateral lesion cases and is more transient with better recovery after unilateral lesions. Even after improvement, decrease of initiation, lack of concern (apathy), and emotional blunting may dominate the clinical picture. The frontal lobe also mediates important aspects of autonomic activity. The cingulate and medial orbital gyri, both closely interconnected with hypothalamic and limbic system structures, are involved in control of respiration, blood pressure, and peristalsis (e.g., Appenzeller, 1976; Brodal, 1981; Kaada, 1960). Mesial frontal damage may lead to incontinence. Olfactory impairments after concussion have been reported consistently since the early descriptions of Ogle (1870) and Legg (1873) and more recently in the studies of Sumner (1964) and Schechter and Henkin (1974). When traumatic injuries do not involve the nasal cavity or olfactory epithelium, such impairments arise from damage to the olfactory nerve or central olfactory structures including the olfactory bulbs, tract, and frontotemporal prepiriform cortex. The delicate position of the olfactory nerve as it projects from epithelial receptors through the cribriform plate of the ethmoid bone makes it particularly vulnerable to shear injury. Central olfactory structures are also highly susceptible to shear injury and contusion because of their locations along bony surfaces encasing orbital frontal and anterior temporal lobes. The complete (anosmia) or partial (microsomia) loss of olfactory sensation is most common (occurring in up to 50 percent of reported series), while a smaller percentage of patients demonstrate altered odor perception, usually in the form of distortions of smells (parosmia or dysosmia). Because of the role of olfaction in flavor appreciation, patients may also complain of changes in taste.

Clinical olfactory examination involves testing the patient's detection and recognition accuracies. Standardized psychometric tests are available such as the Smell Identification Test (Doty, 1983), which involves scratching microencapsulated crystals to release odors (i.e., scratch and sniff) and then identifying the odorant from among four word choices. These as well as other procedures have emphasized the importance of employing relatively pure odorants (e.g., musk, floral, fruit flavors) to assess olfaction, in contrast to harsher odorants that irritate the nasal mucosa and cause trigeminal nerve stimulation. In fact, clinicians may purposefully use such irritants to check the accuracy of patient responses and complaints of olfactory loss. With anosmia and dysosmia from damage to olfactory structures, detection of trigeminal nerve stimulants remains unaffected. Finally, since olfaction can be affected by upper respiratory conditions, structural defects of the nasal cavity, and environmental exposures, it is important for the clinician to inquire about and rule out such confounding afflictions.

Higher cognitive-executive impairments after concussive injuries can range from mild to severe. The strongest model for evaluating such impairments is based on study of focal lesion cases, where there is converging evidence for specialized sectors of the frontal lobe (e.g., Cummings, 1985; Damasio, 1985; Eslinger and Damasio, 1985; Grattan and Eslinger, 1991a). Several of the common clinical characteristics associated with damage to these sectors are summarized in Table 21-4. As noted above, damage to the superior mesial aspects of the frontal lobe is associated with akinesia, mutism, and less severe forms of apathy, emotional blunting, aspontaneity, and lack of initiative. Consequences of inferior mesial frontal damage involving the basal forebrain region may include memory impairment, confabulations, disinhibition, and in certain cases the environmental dependency syndrome characterized as utilization behavior. Dorsolateral frontal lesions cause a variety of impairments in higher cognition, including perseveration, poor integration and synthesis of information, disorganization in thinking, learning and responding, concrete thinking, stimulus-boundedness, distractiblity, poor self-monitoring, and inability to plan. Damage in the left dorsolateral frontal region disrupts verbal mediation of cognition despite the absence of aphasia, whereas right dorsolateral frontal lesion can cause left hemispatial neglect and spatial disorganization. Orbital frontal damage, in contrast, is associated with subtler but nonetheless disabling changes in personality, social judgment, motivation, and sustained goal-directed behavior. Emotional outbursts, lessening of the constructive and integrative forces of personality, inappropriate joking (Witzelsucht), and loss of empathy are also characteristic of damage to this frontal region, which is closely interconnected with temporal polar and other limbic system structures.

Neurologic Evaluation

The neurologic evaluation of the head-injured patient is completed by clinical examination, brain imaging procedures such as CT and magnetic resonance imaging (MRI), and neurophysiologic tests (EEG, evoked potentials). In some centers, measures of regional cerebral blood flow, cerebral metabolic activity (positron emission tomography [PET]) and functional MRI may be available. In addition to the neurologic deficits in motor activity, autonomic functions, olfaction, and higher cognition that are characteristic of frontal lobe damage, neuroimaging procedures can be extremely useful in patient evaluation. For example, Becker et al. (1977) demonstrated that 41 percent of patients who are unable to follow simple commands after head injury had mass lesions on CT scan.

Concussion patients can be classified into three groups based on brain CT findings: (1) diffuse injury with generalized contusions, intracerebral hematomas, and edema; (2) localized extracerebral or intracerebral mass lesions, particularly in the frontal and temporal lobes; and (3) normal scan. Intracerebral hematomas may be present on the initial CT scan or may appear hours to days after a head injury, representing hemorrhage into a primary injury site. Subdural, epidural, and intracerebral hemorrhages represent the localized extra- and intracerebral masses in the head-injured population.

The advantage of MRI over CT scan is the high level of anatomic definition and specificity, pathologic sensitivity, and imaging according to multiple parameters and planes. MRI scan has more value later in the course of head injury management than in the early phase. MRI detects a number of posttraumatic lesions that are not shown on the CT scan (e.g., diffuse axonal injury, contusions, primary brainstem injury and secondary injuries, tentorial arterial infarction, cerebral herniations, pressure necrosis associated with intracranial hypertension) (Gentry et al., 1988b) and appears to be much more sensitive to the occurrence of frontal lobe lesions (Levin et al., 1992). MRI also has special value in assessing cases in which there is a disparity between the neurologic state of a patient and CT findings (Gentry et al., 1988a).

Imaging techniques reflecting changes in cerebral function rather than structure may have prognostic value for the recovery of the head-injured patient. As an example, PET provides data on the pathophysiology of head injury through imaging parameters of cerebral metabolism (cerebral blood flow, cerebral metabolic rates for oxygen and glucose) and blood-brain barrier function (see Ch. 6). However, its logistical constraints and expense limit routine use. Measurement of regional cerebral blood flow with single-photon emission computed tomography (SPECT) using technetium 99m HMPAO may reveal a more comprehensive picture of the distribution and extent of brain dysfunction after concussion by showing alterations in the absence of detectable structural damage on CT and MRI scan (e.g., Jacobs et al., 1994; Masdeu et al., 1994; Newton et al., 1992). The perfusion defects appear to correlate with clinical impairments not explained by CT or MRI findings, and hence SPECT may improve the clinical assessment of outcome after traumatic brain injury, particularly in regard to executive functions (e.g., Goldenberg et al., 1992; Oder et al., 1992). However, these imaging procedures are neither routine nor fully established as standardized procedures.

The EEG can be easily used in the evaluation of head injury patients with encephalopathy or coma. The EEG recording is usually nonspecific and does not give definite information on the etiology of the underlying process, but it does provide information on its severity. Burst suppression pattern in head injury-induced deep coma is a common finding. It is a test of choice when a suspected nonstructural physiologic focal disturbance such as ischemia or postictal depression, has to be evaluated. EEG is the only test for evaluation of possible seizures.

Evoked potentials are considered physiologic measures of the severity of neural injury and may be predictive of outcome after head trauma. When evoked potential data from multiple sensory modalities (somatosensory, visual, and auditory potentials) are combined, the predictive value for outcome is further enhanced. Such measures have been shown in at least one study to accurately forecast outcome in 91 percent of a severe head injury population sample (Narayan et al., 1981).

Treatment with Bromocriptine

Dopamine, a neurotransmitter in the central nervous system, has assumed a special importance since it appeared to be involved in two severe pathologic states, Parkinson's disease and schizophrenia. The discovery of decreased levels of dopamine in the basal ganglia of parkinsonism patients and the therapeutic effect of L-dopa was followed by the discovery of dopamine in the striatum (Sano et al., 1959). The antipsychotic effect of chlorpromazine (Delay and Deniker, 1957) was related to dopamine receptor blockade (Carlsson and Lindquist, 1963).

Thiery et al. (1973, 1974) demonstrated the presence of dopamine terminals in rat and cat cerebral cortex. The dopaminergic cortical innervation in rat appeared in restricted distribution. No dopaminergic projections were identified in the primary somatosensory or motor cortices, but dense terminal fields were detected in limbic areas (anterior cingulate and entorhinal cortices) and in two rostral parts of the frontal cortex, which are homologous to the prefrontal cortex of primates.

Frontal dopaminergic receptor fields attracted interest because the frontal cortex plays a major role in the activation and control of cognitive functions (e.g., Damasio, 1985; Fuster, 1985; Goldman-Rakic, 1988). Maximum numbers of dopaminergic fibers were found in frontal agranular areas 4, 6 and 24; among these, the primary motor strip and the anterior cingulate cortex possessed the densest innervation. In the agranular areas, the dopaminergic fibers invaded all layers, but mainly layer I and to a lesser extent layers V and VI. Occasional local accumulations in layers II and III were noted. Area 9 of the prefrontal cortex shows dopaminergic innervation but of a lower density and mainly in layers I and V and VI. Dopaminergic fibers are also prominent in frontal white matter, along the corticosubcortical junction.

The ascending dopaminergic projections from the midbrain have been subdivided into a nigrostriatal and mesocorticolimbic component (Albanese et al., 1986; Björklund and Lindvall, 1978; Fallon, 1988; Moore and Bloom, 1978). The neuronal cells of the nigrostriatal pathway are located in the substantia nigra and terminate in the caudate nucleus, putamen, and globus pallidus. A decrease of the dopaminergic neurotransmission in the nigrostriatal pathway results in parkinsonism, whereas hyperactivity of this system has been implicated in Huntington's chorea. The neurons of the mesocorticolimbic pathway are located in the central tegmental area. They project to the nucleus accumbens, amygdala, septal nuclei, olfactory tubercle, and certain cortical areas. The system is divided into mesoallocortical axons terminating in the phylogenetically old cortical derivatives (olfactory tubercle, amygdala, septal nuclei, and pyriform cortex) and mesoneocortical pathways terminating in all neocortical areas. The dopaminergic innervation of the neocortex in humans is expanded and shows highly differentiated laminar distribution patterns (Berger et al., 1988; Gaspar et al., 1989). The dopamine receptors in the human cerebral neocortex are mainly of the D_1 type (DeKeyser et al., 1988; Camps et al., 1989; Cortes et al., 1989; Hall et al., 1988). In rodents the activation of D_1 receptors causes self-stimulation, (Ferrer et al., 1983), grooming (Malloy and Waddington, 1984), behavioral arousal (Orgini et al., 1985), and motivation (Shippenberg and Henz, 1988). The mesoneocortical dopamine system may have a role in human cognition (Weinberger et al., 1988) and has been shown to directly influence frontal lobe-mediated behavioral functions in the monkey model (Sawaguchi and Goldman-Rakic, 1994).

Clinical studies indicate that lesions of the superior mesial part of the frontal lobe (anterior cingulate gyrus, supplementary motor area) cause akinesia, mutism, and gait apraxia. Other forms of disturbed initiation and motor programming are evident after damage to Broca's area and the frontal pole. In focal lesions of the frontal lobe, it is assumed that the mesoneocortical pathways are disrupted postsynaptically. In partial lesions, postsynaptic dopaminergic agents such as bromocriptine might be useful in improving synaptic activation within the frontal lobe. Agents such as L-dopa, which act presynaptically, and amantadine, which increases dopamine release, are not useful, as they would require not only intact receptors but also an intact area for synthesis of dopamine as well as intact pathways to transport the dopamine to the receptors (Fleet et al., 1987). Treatment with bromocriptine and recovery from unilateral neglect has been reported in monkeys with hemispatial resection of the frontal polysensory association cortex (Deuel and Collins, 1983). Apomorphine had therapeutic effect on neglect induced by unilateral dorsomedial prefrontal cortical lesions in rats (Corwin et al., 1986).

Bromocriptine, as a dopamine agonist, has been shown to improve the speaking skills of patients with chronic nonfluent aphasia and hemispatial neglect following ischemic injury to the frontoparietal operculum and the frontotemporoparietal area (Fleet et al., 1987; Gupta and McCoch, 1992). We studied the effect of bromocriptine on the recovery from traumatic frontal lobe injury in three patients (J.S., M.C., and A.C.). One patient (J.S.) had isolated frontal polar injury on brain CT scan, while the other two suffered frontal lobe lesions as part of their multifocal brain damage. Bromocriptine treatment was not introduced for patients in the period of post-traumatic agitation, when they were medicated with antidopaminergic, psychotropic agents. Since bromocriptine has a direct role in mediating prefrontal lobe activity, we do not recommend the simultaneous use of less efficacious antidepressants, including serotonin reuptake inhibitors, and these were not used in the study sample.

The goal of this study was to determine the effect of bromocriptine on recovery of several aspects of frontal lobe executive impairments; the minimum effective dose of bromocriptine for recovery; the individual responsiveness of prefrontal signs (appreciation of social nuances, goal-directed behavior) and mesial frontal lobe signs (affect, mutism, and akinesia) to treatment with bromocriptine; and the comparative response to Bromocriptine in patients with single frontal versus multiple brain lesions.

The starting dose of bromocriptine was 5 mg PO qd for 6 days, followed by 10 mg PO qd for 22 days, then 15 mg for the rest of the treatment period. The

TABLE 21-5. Bedside Evaluation Parameters for Frontal Lobe Functions

Parameter	Score
Affect	
	1 = Normal
	0 = Blunt
Mutism	
	4 = Imminent response
	3 = Hesitation with a latency period <30 s
	2 = Slow response with a latency period of 1–2 min
	1 = Very slow response with a latency period of 2–4 min
	0 = Severe apathy, no response to questions
Appreciation of Social Nuances	
	3 = Intact
	2 = Minimally impaired
	1 = Impaired
	0 = Lack of appreciation
Goal-Directed Behavior	
	3 = Intact
	2 = Outlines acceptable goals
	1 = Inappropriate goals
	0 = Lack of goal-directed behavior
Akinesia	
	4 = Complex purposeful, voluntary movements
	3 = Good voluntary movements
	2 = Slow voluntary movements
	1 = Occasional voluntary movements
	0 = Akinesia

Score Range: 0–15

medication was started at the time of admission to the University Hospital Rehabilitation Center. Changes in affect, mutism, appreciation of social nuances, goal-directed behavior, and akinesia were followed by daily bedside evaluation at morning rounds and scored as shown in Table 21-5. The degree of frontal lobe impairment in these patients was severe and precluded formal neuropsychological testing in the pretreatment period. During the treatment period, all patients were involved in cognitive, physical, occupational, speech, and recreational therapies.

The results indicated that all patients with traumatic injury involving the frontal lobe achieved some measure of functional recovery. The two patients with multifocal brain injury that also involved the frontal lobe had the same rate of recovery as the one with restricted frontal lobe damage (Table 21-6). The pretreatment scores of appreciation of social nuances and goal-directed behavior were the lowest. However, by the end of bromocriptine treatment period, every patient in the trauma group reached maximum scores for the bedside evaluation procedure. The minimal effective dose of bromocriptine for full recovery was 15 mg qd.

The temporary early discontinuation of treatment with bromocriptine for patient J.S. resulted in the decline of appreciation of social nuances (e.g., foul language) and goal-directed behavior (Table 21-7). Reinstitution of a 15-mg qd dose of bromocriptine reversed the decline.

CONCLUSION

Patients who suffer concussive injuries frequently show diverse neurologic and neuropsychologic impairments associated with the frontal lobe and the extended neural networks that subserve complex, adaptive behavior. These were examined from cognitive, social, and neurologic perspectives. Impairments in cognitive-executive processes encompass representational, integrative, and regulatory operations that disrupt organization and control of behavior, as well as cognitive functions such as flexibility, planning, working memory, and goal-directed behavior. Because of such defects, adaptation and adjustment of postconcussion patients can be effectively reduced. Cognitive aspects of these executive impairments can be assessed with a variety of standardized neuropsychological tests, supplemented by clinical observations and interviews. Remediation of executive impairments remains an important challenge, with procedures being developed and subjected to validation.

Changes in social behavior and personality after head trauma are common and present significant problems for patients and their families. Social impairments have been conceptualized here in terms of a model of social executors. The model provides a taxonomy within which to define and describe several of the social impairments caused by head trauma and includes social self-regulation, social self-awareness, social sensitivity (empathy), and social salience. Because of the diversity of social impairments, treatment plans are individualized, involve multiple modalities, and frequently require family interventions as well.

The neurologic consequences of head trauma can affect diverse frontal lobe functions, including motor, language, olfactory, autonomic, and cognitive processes. The effect of bromocriptine on recovery from mesial frontal functions (akinesia, mutism, range of affect) and prefrontal functions (appreciation of social nuances, goal-directed behavior) were examined in a preliminary trial of three patients with traumatic brain injury involving the frontal lobe. All three patients showed significant improvement during prolonged treatment with bromocriptine, although, there were individual differences in the therapeutic response to the drug. The end-of-treatment rate of improvement was identical for patients with isolated frontal versus frontal with multiple cerebral injuries. The effective dose of bromocriptine was 15 mg qd. The abnormal affect, mutism, and akinesia responded well to bromocriptine, while appreciation of social nuances and goal-directed behavior were more refractory to treatment. Discontinuation of bromocriptine after prolonged administration (6 months) did not result in clinical deterioration. Further studies appear warranted, employing a more

TABLE 21-6. Frontal Lobe Function Scores of Pre- and Post-Bromocriptine Treatment in Patients With Traumatic Brain Injury

Patient	Pretreatment Scores[a]	End of Treatment Scores[a]
J.S.	2	15
M.C.	8	15
A.C.	5	15
Mean	5	15

[a] Score range: 0 = impaired, 15 = intact.

TABLE 21-7. The Effect of Early Discontinuation of Bromocriptine Treatment on the Recurrence of Frontal Lobe Symptoms in One Patient

		Bromocriptine Treatment Scores			
Frontal Lobe Symptoms	Maximum Scores	5 mg qd 6 days	10 mg qd 14 days	15 mg qd 35 days	Discontinued
Affect	1	0	0	1	1
Mutism	4	3	4	4	4
Appreciation of social nuances	3	1	2	3	1[a]
Goal-directed behavior	3	0	1	3	2[a]
Akinesia	4	4	4	4	4

[a] Indicates clinically evident decline during period of discontinued medication.

detailed treatment protocol, with appropriate control procedures and objective neuropsychological measures.

REFERENCES

Ackerly SS, Benton AL: Report of a case of bilateral frontal lobe defect. Res Publ Assoc Res Nerv Ment Dis 27:479–504, 1947

Adams JH, Scott G, Parker LS et al: The contusion index: a quantitative approach to cerebral contusion in head injury. Neuropathol Appl Neurobiol 6:319–324, 1980

Albanese A, Altavista MC, Rossi P: Organization of central nervous system dopaminergic pathways. J Neural Transm Suppl 22:3–17, 1986

American Psychiatric Association: Diagnostic and Statistical Manual of Mental Disorders (DSMIV), 1994

Anderson SW, Damasio H, Jones RD, Tranel D: Wisconsin Card Sorting performance as a measure of frontal lobe damage. J Clin Exp Neuropsychol 13:926–939, 1991

Appenzeller O: Autonomic Nervous System: An Introduction to Basic and Clinical Concepts. 2nd Ed. North-Holland, Amsterdam, 1976

Barth JT, Macciocchi SN, Giordani B et al: Neuropsychological sequelae of minor head injury. Neurosurgery 13:529–532, 1983

Becker DP, Miller JD, Ward JD: The outcome from severe head injury with early diagnosis and intensive management. J Neurosurg 47:491–502, 1977

Berger B, Trottier S, Verney C et al: Regional and laminar distribution of the dopamine and serotonin innervation in macaque cerebral cortex. A radioautographic study. J Comp Neurol 273:99–119, 1988

Björklund A, Lindvall O: The meso-telencephalic dopamine neuron system—a review of its anatomy. In Livingston KE, Hornykiewicz O (eds): Limbic Mechanisms—The Continuing Evolution of the Limbic System Concept. Plenum Press, New York, 1978, pp. 307–331

Brickner RM: An interpretation of frontal lobe function based upon study of a case of partial bilateral lobectomy. Res Publ Assoc Res Nerv Ment Dis 13:259–331, 1934

Brodal A: Neurological Anatomy. 3rd Ed. Oxford University Press, New York

Brooks N: Closed Head Injury: Psychological, Social and Family Consequences. Oxford University Press, New York, 1984

Brooks N, Capsie L, Symington C: The five-year outcome of severe blunt head injury: a relative's view. J Neurol Neurosurg Psychiatry 49:764–770, 1986

Camps M, Cortes R, Gueye B et al: Dopamine receptors in human brain: autoradiographic distribution of the D_2 sites. Neuroscience 28:275–290, 1989

Carlsson A, Lindquist M: Effect of chlorpromazine or haloperidol on formation of 3-methoxytyramine and normetanephrine in mouse brain. Pharmacol Toxicol 20:140–144, 1963

Cicerone KD, Wood JC: Planning disorder after closed head injury: a case study. Arch Phy Med Rehabil 68:111–115, 1987

Cortes R, Gueye B, Pazos A et al: Dopamine receptors in human brain: autoradiographic distribution of the D_1 sites. Neuroscience 28:263–273, 1989

Corwin JV, Kanter S, Watson RT et al: Apomorphine has a therapeutic effect on neglect produced by unilateral dorsomedial prefrontal cortex lesions in rats. Exp Neurol 94:683–698, 1986

Cummings JL: Clinical Neuropsychiatry. Grune & Stratton, Orlando, 1985

Damasio AR: The frontal lobes. pp. 339–376. In Heilman KM, Valenstein E (eds): Clinical Neuropsychology. Oxford University Press, New York, 1985

Damasio AR, Tranel D, Damasio HC: Somatic markers and the guidance of behavior: theory and preliminary testing. In Levin HS, Eisenberg HM, Benton AL (eds): Frontal Lobe Function and Dysfunction. Oxford University Press, New York, 1991

Damasio H, Damasio AR: Lesion Analysis in Neuropsychology. Oxford University Press, New York, 1989

De Keyser J, Claeys Al, De Backer JP et al: Autoradiographic localization of the D_1 and D_2 dopamine receptors in human brain. Neurosci Lett 91:142–147, 1988

Delay J, Deniker O: Caractéristiques psychophysiologiques des médicaments neuroleptiques. pp. 485–501. In Garattini S, Ghetti V (eds): Psychotropic Drugs. Elsevier Science Publishers, Amsterdam, 1957

Deuel RK, Collins RC: Recovery from unilateral neglect. Exp Neurol 81:733–748, 1983

Doty RL: The Smell Identification Test Administration Manual. Sensonics, Inc., Philadelphia, 1983

Dywan J, Roden R, Murphy T: Orbitofrontal symptoms are predicted by mild head injury among normal adolescents. J Intl Neuropsychol Soc 1:121, 1995

Ell PJ, Cullum I, Costa DC: A regular cerebral blood flow mapping with Tc-99m labelled compound. Lancet 2:50–51, 1985

Elsass L, Kinsella G: Social interaction following severe head injury. Psychol Med 17:67–68, 1987

Eslinger PJ: Conceptualizing, describing, and measuring components of executive function: a summary. In Lyon GR, Krasnegor NA (eds): Attention, Memory, and Executive Function. Paul H. Brookes, Baltimore, 1995 (in press)

Eslinger PJ, Damasio AR: Severe disturbance of higher cognition after bilateral frontal lobe ablation. Neurology 35:1731–1741, 1985

Eslinger PJ, Damasio AR, vanHoesen GW: Olfactory dysfunction in man: anatomical and behavioral aspects. Brain Cogn 1:259–285, 1982

Eslinger PJ, Grattan LM (eds): Perspectives on the developmental consequences of early frontal lobe damage (special issue). Dev Neuropsychol 7:257–260, 1991

Eslinger PJ, Grattan LM: Frontal lobe and frontal-striatal substrates for different forms of human cognitive flexibility. Neuropsychologia 31:17–28, 1993

Eslinger PJ, Grattan LM: Altered serial position learning after frontal lobe lesion. Neuropsychologia 32:729–739, 1994

Eslinger PJ, Grattan LM, Geder L: Impact of frontal lobe lesions on rehabilitation and recovery from acute brain injury. NeuroRehabilitation 5:161–182, 1995

Fallon JH: Topographic organization of ascending dopaminergic projections. Ann N Y Acad Sci 537:1–9, 1988

Ferrer JMR, Sanguinetti AM, Vives F, Mora F: Effects of agonists and antagonists of D_1 and D_2 dopamine receptors on self-stimulation of the medial prefrontal cortex in the rat. Pharmacol Biochem Behav 19:211–217, 1983

Fleet WSH, Valenstein E, Watson RT, Heilman KM: Dopamine agonist therapy for neglect in humans. Neurology 37:1765–1770, 1987

Freedman PE, Bleiberg J, Freedland K: Anticipatory behaviour deficits in closed head injury. J Neurol Neurosurg Psychiatry 50:398–401, 1987

Fuster JM: The prefrontal cortex and temporal integration. pp. 151–178. In Peters A, Jones EG (eds): Cerebral Cortex: Vol. 4. Plenum Press, New York, 1985

Gaspar P, Berger B, Febvret A et al: Catecholamine innervation of the human cerebral cortex as revealed by comparative immunohistochemistry of tyrosine hydroxylase and dopamine-beta-hydroxylase. J Comp Neurol 279:249–271, 1989

Gentry LR, Godersky JC, Thompson B, Dunn VD: Prospective comparative study of intermediate-field MR and CT in the evaluation of closed head trauma. AM J Radiol 150:673–677, 1988a

Gentry LR, Thompson B, Godersky JC: Trauma to the corpus callosum: MR features. AJNR 9:1129–1133, 1988b

Glisky EL, Schacter DL, Tulving E: Computer learning by memory-impaired patients: acquisition and retention of complex knowledge. Neuropsychologia 24:313–328, 1986

Goldenberg G, Oder W, Spatt J, Podreka I: Cerebral correlates of disturbed executive function and memory in survivors of severe closed head injury: a SPECT study. J Neurol Neurosurg Psychiatry 55:362–368, 1992

Goldman-Rakic PS: Circuitry of primate prefrontal cortex and regulation of behavior by representational memory. pp.373–417. In Mountcastle VB (ed): Handbook of Physiology. Vol. 5. The Nervous System. American Physiological Society, Bethesda, MD

Goldstein K: After Effects of Brain Injuries in War. Grune & Stratton, Orlando, 1942

Grafman J, Jones B, Salazar A: Wisconsin Card Sorting performance based on location and size of neuroanatomic lesion in Vietnam veterans with penetrating head injury. Percept Mot Skill 74:1120–1122, 1990

Grafman J, Sirigu A, Spector L, Hendler J: Damage to the prefrontal cortex leads to decomposition of structured event complexes. J Head Trauma Rehabil 8:73–87, 1993

Grattan LM, Eslinger PJ: Higher cognition and social behavior: changes in cognitve flexibility and empathy after cerebral lesions. Neuropsychology 3:175–185, 1989

Grattan LM, Eslinger PJ: Influence of cerebral lesion site upon the onset and progression of interpersonal deficits following brain injury. J Clin Exp Neuropsychol 12:33, 1990

Grattan LM, Eslinger PJ: Frontal lobe damage in children and adults; a comparative review. Dev Neuropsychol 7:283–326, 1991a

Grattan LM, Eslinger PJ: Characteristics of favorable recovery from frontal lobe damage. Neurology suppl.1, 41:266, 1991b

Grattan LM, Bloomer RH, Archambault FX, Eslinger PJ, : Cognitive flexibility and empathy after frontal lobe lesion. Neuropsychiatry Neuropsychol Behav Neurol 7:251–259, 1994

Grattan LM, Eslinger PJ, Mattson KE et al: Altered social self-awareness: empirical evidence for frontal lobe specialization for social self-knowledge. Neurology suppl.2, 44:A292, 1994

Grattan LM, Eslinger PJ, Matson KE: Evidence for a double dissociation among learning paradigms in patients with frontal and non-frontal cerebral lesions. Soc Neurosci Abst 18:213, 1992

Gupta SR, McCoch AG: Bromocriptine treatment of nonfluent aphasia. Arch Phys Med Rehabil 73:373–376, 1992

Hall H, Farde L, Sedvall G: Human dopamine receptor subtypes—in vitro binding analysis using ^{3}H-SCH 23390 and ^{3}H-raclopride. J Neural Transm 73:7–21, 1988

Harlow JM: Recovery from passage of an iron bar through the head. Publ Mass Med Soc 2:327–347, 1868

Hebb DO, Penfield W: Human behavior after extensive bilateral removal from the frontal lobes. Arch Neurol Psychiatry 44:421–438, 1940

Hogan R: Development of an empathy scale. J Consul Clin Psychol 33:307–316, 1969

Jacobs A, Put E, Ingels M, Bossuyt A: Prospective evaluation of technetium-99m-HMPAO SPECT in mild and moderate traumatic brain injury. J Nucl Med 35:942–947, 1994

Kaada B: Cingulate, posterior orbital, anterior insular and temporal pole cortex. In Field J, Magoun HW, Hall VE (eds): Handbook of Physiology. Sect 1:Neurophysiology. Vol. 2. American Physiological Society, Washington, 1960

Legg JW: A case of anosmia following a blow. Lancet 2:659, 1873

Levin HS, Williams DH, Eisenberg HM et al: Serial MRI and neurobehavioral findings after mild to moderate closed head injury. J Neurol Neurosurg Psychiatry 55:255–262, 1992

Lezak MD: Neuropsychological Assessment. Oxford University Press, New York, 1985

Lezak MD: Psychological implications of traumatic brain damage for the patient's family. Rehabil Psychol 31:241–250, 1986

Lezak MD: Relationships between personality disorders, social disturbances and physical disability following traumatic brain injury. J Head Trauma Rehabil 2:57–69, 1987

Lezak MD: Assessment of psychosocial dysfunctions resulting from head trauma. pp. 113–143. In Lezak MD (ed): Assessment of the Behavioral Consequences of Head Trauma. Alan R Liss, New York, 1989

Lhermitte F: Human autonomy and the frontal lobes. Part II: Patient behavior in complex and social situations: the "environmental dependency" syndrome. Ann Neurol 19:335–343, 1986

Lira FT, Carne W, Masri AM: Treatment of anger and impulsivity in a brain damaged patient: a case study applying stress inoculation. Clin Neuropsychol 5:159–160, 1983

Malloy AG, Waddington JL: Dopaminergic behavior stereospecifically promoted by the D_1 agonist R-SK & F 38393 and selectively blocked by the D_1 antagonist SCH 23390. Psychopharmacology (Berlin) 82:409–410, 1984

Markowitsch HJ, Emmans D, Irle E et al: Cortical and subcortical afferent connections of the primate's temporal pole: a study of rhesus monkeys, squirrel monkeys, and marmosets. J Comp Neurol 242:425–458, 1985

Masdeu JC, van Heertum RL, Kleiman A et al: Early single-photon emission computed tomography in mild head trauma. J Neuroimaging 4:177–181, 1994

Mateer CA, Ruff RM: Effectiveness of behavior management procedures in the rehabilitation of head-injured patients. In Wood RL (ed): Neurobehavioral Sequelae of Traumatic Brain Injury. Taylor and Francis, New York, 1990

Mattson AJ, Levin HS: Frontal lobe dysfunction following closed head injury. J Nerv Ment Dis 178:282–291, 1990

McGlynn SM: Behavioral approaches to neuropsychological rehabilitation. Psychol Bull 108:420–441, 1990

Milner B: Some effects of frontal lobectomy in man. In Warren JM, Akert K (eds): The Frontal Granular Cortex and Behavior. McGraw-Hill, New York, 1964

Moore RY, Bloom FE: Central catecholamine neuron systems: anatomy and physiology of the dopamine systems. Annu Rev Neurosci 1:129–169, 1978

Myers RE: Role of prefrontal and anterior temporal cortex in social behavior and affect in monkeys. Acta Neurobiol Exp (Warsz) 32:567–579, 1972

Narayan RK, Greenberg RP, Miller JD: Improved confidence of outcome prediction in severe head injury: a comparative analysis of the clinical examination, multimodality evoked potentials, CT scanning and intracranial pressure. J Neurosurg 54:751–762, 1981

Nauta WJH: Neural associations of the frontal cortex. Acta Neurobiol Exp (Warsz) 32:125–140, 1972

Newton MR, Greenwood RJ, Britton KE et al: A study comparing SPECT with CT and MRI after closed head injury. J Neurol Neurosurg Psychiatry 55:92–94, 1992

Novoa OP, Ardila A: Linguistic abilities in patients with prefrontal damage. Brain Lang 30:206–225, 1987

Oddy M: Head injury and social adjustment. In Brooks N (ed): Closed Head Injury. Oxford University Press, New York, 1984

Oder W, Goldenberg G, Spatt J et al: Behavioral and psychosocial sequelae of severe closed head injury and regional cerebral blood flow: a SPECT study. J Neurol Neurosurg Psychiatry 55:475–480, 1992

Ogle W: Anosmia: cases illustrating the physiology and pathology of the sense of smell. Med Chir Trans 53:263–290, 1870

Orgini E, Caporali MG, Massotti M: Stimulation of dopamine D-1 receptors by SKF 38393 induces EEG desynchronisation and behavioral arousal. Life Sci 37: 2327–2333, 1985

Pandya DN, Barnes CL: Architecture and connections of the frontal lobe. pp. 41–72. In Perecman E (ed): The Frontal Lobes Revisited. IRBN Press, New York, 1987

Pandya DN, Yeterian EH: Prefrontal cortex in relation to other cortical areas in rhesus monkey: architecture and connections. Prog Brain Res 85:63–94,1990

Papo I, Caruselli G, Scarpelli M, Luongo A: Mass lesions of the frontal lobe in acute head injuries. A comparison with temporal lesions. Acta Neurochir (Wien) 62:47–72, 1982

Prigatano GP: Neuropsychological Rehabilitation After Brain Injury. Johns Hopkins University Press, Baltimore, 1986

Prigatano GP, Altman IM, O'Brien T: Behavioral limitations that traumatic-brain-injured patients tend to underestimate. Clin Neuropsychol 4:163–176, 1990

Sano I, Gamo T, Kakimoto Y et al: Distribution of catechol compounds in human brain. Biochim Biophys Acta 32:586–588, 1959

Sawaguchi T, Goldman-Rakic PS: The role of D1-dopamine receptor in working memory: local injection of dopamine antagonists into the prefrontal cortex of rhesus monkeys performing an oculomotor delayed-response task. J Neurophysiol 71:515–528, 1994

Schechter PJ, Henkin RI: Abnormalities of taste and smell after head trauma. J Neurol Neurosurg Psychiatry 37:802–810, 1974

Shippenberg TS, Henz A: Motivational effects of opioids: influence of D-1 versus D-2 receptor antagonists. Eur J Pharmacol 151:233–242, 1988

Spreen O, Strauss E: A Compendium of Neuropsychological Tests. Oxford University Press, New York, 1991

Stuss D: Disturbance of self-awareness after frontal system damage. pp. 63–83. In Prigatano GP, Schacter DL (eds): Awareness of Deficit After Brain Injury. Oxford University Press, New York, 1991

Stuss DT, Benson DF: The Frontal Lobes. Raven Press, New York, 1986

Stuss DT, Ely P, Hugenholtz H et al: Subtle neuropsychological deficits in patients with good recovery after closed head injury. Neurosurgery 17:41–47, 1985

Stuss DT, Stethem LL, Hugenholtz H et al: Reaction time after head injury: fatigue, divided and focussed attention, and consistency of performance. J Neurol Neurosurg Psychiatry 52:742–748, 1989

Sumner D: Post-traumatic anosmia. Brain 87:107–120, 1964

Thierry AM, Blanc G, Sobel A et al: Dopaminergic terminals in the rat cortex. Science 182:499–501, 1973

Thierry AM, Hirsch JC, Tassin JP et al: Presence of dopaminergic terminals and absence of dopaminergic cell bodies in the cerebral cortex of the cat. Brain Res 79:77–88, 1974

Thompson IV: Late outcome of very severe blunt head trauma: a 10 to 15 year second follow-up. J Neurol Neurosurg Psychiatry 41:611–616, 1984

Vilkki J: Cognitive flexibility and mental programming after closed head injuries and anterior or posterior cerebral excisions. Neuropsychologia 30:807–814, 1992

Weinberger DR, Berman KF, Chase TN: Mesocortical dopaminergic function and human cognition. Ann N Y Acad Sci 537:330–338, 1988

Whaley AL, Stanford CB, Pollack IW, Lehrer PM: The effects of behavior modification vs lithium therapy on frontal lobe syndrome. J Behav Ther Exp Psychiatry 17:111–115, 1986

Van Zomeren AH, Brouwer WH: Deelman BG: Attentional deficits: the riddles of selectivity, speed, and alertness. pp. 74–107. In Brooks N (ed): Closed Head Injury. Oxford University Press, New York, 1984

Neurologic and Neuropsychological Aspects of Minor Head Injury in Children

22

Jane H. Cerhan
Elsa G. Shapiro
Robert L. Kriel

Head injury is a significant public health problem, with large human and financial costs (Jaffe et al., 1993). In children, head injury occurs frequently and accounts for the largest number of children's visits to emergency rooms (Kraus et al., 1986). Because of this prevalence, most physicians and psychologists will encounter a pediatric patient with a head injury at some point in their practice.

The vast majority of pediatric head injuries are mild. In this chapter, the nature and outcome of pediatric mild closed head injuries is reviewed and an approach to neurologic and neuropsychological evaluation and management is presented.

In cases of very mild head trauma without neurologic symptoms it is not always clear whether there has been actual brain involvement. Therefore, the term *head injury* is used unless *brain injury* is dictated by the contrast (see Chapter 1).

PATHOPHYSIOLOGY

The pathophysiology of minor brain injuries in humans is not well understood, primarily because autopsy material is never available unless the patient dies from other systemic injuries. In mild brain injury it is presumed that there are transient neuronal, axonal, and glial as well as vascular injuries. Rotational accelerational forces may be largely responsible for these effects.

The nature of injury in very young children may be somewhat different from that in adults. The skull's flexibility, the softer consistency of young brains, and the relatively large head size together with poor head control seem to make very young children more vulnerable to minor injuries. Infants and toddlers have been hypothesized to develop cerebral edema more readily because of their higher metabolic rates and increased vasoreactivity (Merton and Osborne, 1983). It has also been proposed that young children are particularly vulnerable to diffuse axonal injury because of incomplete myelinization and shallower convolutions, which may result in greater sensitivity to shearing (Calder et al., 1984). After age 2 there is rapid maturation of the skull and brain, and by 8 to 10 years the skull and intracranial structures of children likely respond to trauma similarly to those of adults (Masters et al., 1987). For a more complete discussion of the pathophysiology of mild brain injury, readers are referred to the discussion by Elson and Ward (1994).

EPIDEMIOLOGY

We are not aware of any epidemiologic studies specifically examining the incidence of *mild* head injury in children. Such data are particularly difficult to collect as many mild injuries go unreported. Kraus et al. (1986) considered the number of fatal brain injuries and hospital admissions for head injury in children up to 15 years old in San Diego County, California for all of 1981. They found an incidence of 185 per 100,000 children per year. These rates were similar to the rates reported for the general population in that region over the same time period and to the incidence rates for children found in other studies (e.g., 220 per 100,000 reported by Annegers, 1983). However, only about 2 to 3 percent of children presenting to emergency rooms with trauma are admitted. In other words, for every patient admitted, 30 to 50 are treated and discharged home (Rivara, 1994; Rivara et al., 1989). Clearly, the incidence rates would be very much higher if milder head injuries were included.

Most brain injuries in children under the age of 5 years are sustained in falls. In older children most are related to recreational activities (e.g., especially with bicycles) and car accidents (often a car hitting a child pedestrian or bicyclist) (Kraus et al., 1986). The distribution of causes of minor head injuries is similar to the distribution found in the larger epidemiologic studies, but motor vehicle accident is the predominant cause of severe injury. Table 22-1 shows the causes of minor head injury in a series of 53 children ages 6 to 15 studied by Fay et al. (1994). It is estimated that child abuse accounts for about 10 percent of pediatric head injuries (Bruce and Zimmerman, 1989; Rivara, 1994) and an even higher percentage in infants (Duhaime et al., 1992). The prevalence rates for abuse are somewhat lower in many of the major studies (e.g., 6 percent in Fay et al., 1994 and <2 percent in Kraus et al., 1986), probably because many cases of abuse go unreported or are misclassified as a result of false reporting of cause by caretakers.

Risk Factors

Boys are more likely to incur head injuries than girls, especially after age 5. This is likely related to differences both in boys' behavior and exposure to risks (Rivara et al., 1982). Children from lower-income families are reported to be at greater risk of head injury (Kraus et al., 1986), although this finding has been less consistent (Goldstein and Levin, 1987). Rivara (1994) proposed that decreased supervision, less information about and less use of prevention strategies, exposure to more hazardous environments such as high-rise apartments, and residence nearer to heavy and fast-moving traffic could account for the greater risk for children from low socioeconomic status families. Hyperactivity has also been considered by many clinicians to predispose some

TABLE 22-1. Causes of Injury Among Pediatric Cases

Cause	Number	Percent[a]
Fall	23	43
Bicycle	12	23
Motor vehicle versus bicycle	4	8
Motor vehicle versus pedestrian	3	6
Assault	3	6
Motor vehicle passenger	2	4
Motor vehicle versus motorcycle	2	4
Sports	1	2
Other	3	6
Total	53	100%

[a] Percentages do not add to 100 because of rounding. (From Fay et al., 1993, with permission.)

children to head injury, although empirically results have been mixed (Davidson et al., 1992).

The relationship between age and closed head injury is complex. For example, many experts believe that a greater proportion of the head injuries incurred by younger children are mild. However, because of a lower threshold for bringing young children to medical attention, measuring numbers of emergency room visits might inflate incidence statistics. On the other hand, head injuries caused by abuse are probably under-reported and brought to the emergency room only in the most severe cases.

Deaths from brain injury are declining (Hoekelman, 1994). This can be attributed in large part to a reduction in motor vehicle crashes after enforcement of stricter speed limits, more severe penalties for drunk driving, the mandated use of seat belts and infant car seats, and improved automotive design. More advanced emergency medicine both on the scene and in emergency rooms also has contributed to decreasing mortality due to brain injury (Hoekelman, 1994).

GRADING OF INJURY SEVERITY

Grading brain injury severity provides important prognostic information because of the strong relationship between injury severity and outcome. Classifying severity is the most important first step not only in the study of head injury but also in its practical management. Severity has been determined, by using a variety of methods such as depth and duration of coma and length of post-traumatic amnesia. McDonald et al. (1994) found that all three of these methods were good predictors of children's cognitive outcome 1 year after head injury. With mild injury, imaging results, such as those obtained by magnetic resonance imaging (MRI) rarely add to the long-term predictive value of these more traditional severity measures (Levin et al., 1992).

The most widely applied measure of initial neurologic status is the Glasgow Coma Scale (GCS) (Teasdale and Jennett, 1974). It is a 15-point scale based on three variables: eye opening, best verbal response, and best response of the arm and hand (see Chs. 1 and 21). Although the GCS is used worldwide as an index of coma severity, there are problems in applying it to infants and young children. For example, the rating of verbal response is not applicable to children who have not yet learned to talk. Furthermore, young children who are capable of responding to commands will not always do so in an unfamiliar situation. Consequently, several adaptations of the GCS for use with young children have been proposed although not yet validated. Table 22-2 shows an example of one such adaptation.

Duration of unconsciousness is another index of head injury severity that is often used. In some studies duration of unconsciousness has been a better predictor of cognitive outcome than initial GCS score. However, because there are degrees of unconsciousness, precise operational definition is important. Levin et al. (1982) defined duration of impaired consciousness as the time until a GCS of 9 was achieved. McDonald et al. (1994) looked at time until achievement of GCS of 15. We have used the following functional definition of consciousness: child is able to follow commands or gestured requests, to respond socially, to discriminate animate from inanimate objects, and to spontaneously initiate adaptive motor activity according to appropriate age expectations and premorbid functional ability. Duration of unconsciousness is sometimes difficult to judge clinically, especially with milder injuries in which the child has already regained consciousness on arrival at the hospital. If an injury is not witnessed by an adult, accurate information often cannot be obtained.

The period of *post-traumatic amnesia* is the duration of time after brain injury during which the patient cannot store and recall ongoing events (Russell, 1932; Russell and Smith, 1961). Post-traumatic amnesia has been found to have good predictive value (Ruijs, 1992; Rutter, 1981). In the McDonald et al. (1994) study, duration of amnesia was superior to initial GCS and duration of unconsciousness in predicting outcome. However, as with the other indices of severity, there are drawbacks. The length of post-traumatic amnesia is more difficult and less practical to determine than duration of unconsciousness or GCS. Amnesia can extend for a much longer time than unconsciousness and therefore requires a more extended period of observation.

Another problem is that no general consensus exists on how to measure post-traumatic amnesia. In adults, length of amnesia is most often measured by retrospectively determining when a person first began storing episodic memories about ongoing events after the injury. However, this method of measuring severity is especially problematic in children, whose retrospective reporting is unreliable and who may not have a well established concept of time relationships. Objective measurement of amnesia during

TABLE 22-2. Glasgow Coma Scale[a] Modified for Pediatric Patients

Eye-Opening Response		
Score	>1 Year	<1 Year
4	Spontaneous	Spontaneous
3	To verbal command	To shout
2	To pain	To pain
1	None	None

Motor Response		
Score	>1 Year	<1 Year
6	Obeys commands	Spontaneous
5	Localizes pain	Localizes pain
4	Withdraws to pain	Withdraws to pain
3	Abnormal flexion to pain (decorticate rigidity)	Abnormal flexion to pain (decorticate rigidity)
2	Abnormal extension to pain (decerebrate rigidity)	Abnormal extension to pain (decerebrate rigidity)
1	None	None

Verbal Response			
Score	>5 Years	2 to 5 Years	0 to 23 Months
5	Oriented and converses	Appropriate words and phrases	Babbles, coos appropriately
4	Confused conversation	Inappropriate words	Cries, but is consolable
3	Inappropriate words	Persistent crying or screaming to pain	Persistent crying or screaming to pain
2	Incomprehensible sounds	Grunts or moans to pain	Grunts or moans to pain
1	None	None	None

[a] Glasgow Coma Score = sum of best eye opening, motor, and portal responses. Range = 3 to 15. Usual definitions of severity of head injury: severe, score of <9, moderate = score of 9 to 12; mild = score of 13 to 15.
(Adapted from Fay et al., 1993, with permission.)

the recovery period is obviously preferable. Ewing-Cobbs et al. (1990) introduced the Children's Orientation and Amnesia Test (COAT), which is a brief test aimed at measuring post-traumatic amnesia during the recovery period (Fig. 22-1). They found that this measure was superior to the GCS in predicting memory scores 6 and 12 months after injury.

MEDICAL MANAGEMENT

Every emergency room physician and primary care doctor will be faced with the evaluation of pediatric head injury. This requires skill in the evaluation and treatment of the anxious child and the often more anxious parent. As noted above, determining injury severity is the crucial first step in determining the course of medical management. Often pediatric head injuries are not witnessed or are witnessed only by other children, making the exact events difficult to ascertain. However to the extent feasible, once a patient has been stabilized, a thorough history must be obtained, including any information that can be gleaned about the circumstances of the injury. The mechanism of the injury can also provide important information. For example, injuries involving high velocity (e.g., motor vehicle crashes) are often more severe than low-speed injuries, and diffuse axonal shearing is more likely. To the extent possible, the child's level of consciousness immediately after the injury and up to the time of the examination should be determined. Once it has been verified that the

Children's Orientation and Amnesia Test (COAT)

General Orientation:

1. What is your name? first (2) ________ (5) ____
   last (3) ________
2. How old are you? (3) ________ When is your birthday?
   month (1) ________ day (1) ________ (5) ____
3. Where do you live? city (3) ________
   state (2) ________ (5) ____
4. What is your father's name? (5) ________
   What is your mother's name? (5) ________ (10) ____
5. What school do you go to? (3) ________
   What grade are you in? (2) ________ (5) ____
6. Where are you now? (5) ________ (5) ____
   (May rephrase question: Are you at home now?
   Are you in the hospital? If rephrased, child must
   answer both questions to receive credit.)
7. Is it daytime or night-time? (5) ________ (5) ____

General Orientation Total ____

Temporal Orientation: (administer if age 8–15)

8. What time is it now? (5) ________ (5) ____
   (correct=5; < hr. off = 4; 1hr. off = 3; >1hr. off = 2;
   2 hrs. off = 1)
9. What day of the week is it? (5) ________ (5) ____
   (correct=5; 1 off = 4; 2 off = 3; 3 off = 2; 4 off = 1)
10. What day of the month is it? (5) ________ (5) ____
    (correct=5; 1 off = 4; 2 off = 3; 3 off = 2; 4 off = 1)
11. What is the month? (10) ________ (10) ____
    (correct=10; 1 off = 7; 2 off = 4; 3 off = 1)
12. What is the year? (15) ________ (15) ____
    (correct=15; 1 off = 10; 2 off = 5; 3 off = 1)

Temporal Orientation Total ____

Memory:

13. Say these numbers after me in the same order. (Discontinue when the child fails both series of digits at any length. Score 2 points if both digit series are correctly repeated; score 1 point if only 1 is correct.)

3	5	____	35296	81493	____	
58	42	____	539418	724856	____	
643	926	____	8129365	4739128	____	(14) ____
7216	3279	____				

14. How many fingers am I holding up? Two fingers (2) ____
    three fingers (3) ____ 10 fingers (5) ____ (10) ____
15. Who is on Sesame Street? (10) ________
    (can substitute other major television show) (10) ____
16. What is my name? (10) ________ (10) ____

Memory Total ____

OVERALL TOTAL ____

Fig. 22-1. The Children's Orientation and Amnesia Test answer form. (From Ewing-Cobbs et al., 1990, with permission.)

child meets the criteria for *minor* injury, it is equally important to observe whether the child *remains* in good neurologic condition.

Sequential observation is the cornerstone of management of minor brain injuries. Several clinical series have supported the validity, and safety of this approach (Ros and Ros, 1989; Tecklenburg and Wright, 1991). This can be done either in the emergency department, in a short-stay hospital unit, or at home (if patients are reliable and have not themselves been injured and are not under extreme stress). Generally, it is best if parents can be given written instructions as to how to observe the child and when to call or return to the hospital. Written instructions should indicate that the child is to be observed carefully for the next 24 hours and should be awakened every 2 to 3 hours during the night so that responses can be assessed. One common misconception among parents is that they should not let the child fall asleep. That obviously will lead to sleep deprivation, which will only compound the problems of assessment. It is important to stress to families that symptoms such as mild irritability and fatigue are common and generally resolve within weeks. The best evidence indicates that the vast majority of children will be symptom-free a few months after mild head injury (see the section *Outcome*).

Extended outpatient observation (i.e., for a few hours) is a useful option for patients with minor brain injury who have had brief periods of unconsciousness, headache, vomiting, or amnesia but no focal deficits. During the observation period children should have sequential examinations and repeat evaluations with the GCS. Delayed deterioration has been reported after mild brain injury in children (Snoek et al., 1984), but it is extremely uncommon, especially when there is no loss of consciousness (Casey et al., 1986).

Again, clinical judgement is necessary when deciding whether neuroimaging is indicated for the individual patient. General guidelines for management of pediatric head injuries are provided in Table 22-3. Of course, clinical judgement is necessary in determining the course of intervention for the individual patient.

Imaging

Since the mid-1980s the consensus in the medical literature is that skull radiographs generally do not provide clinically useful information in the management of pediatric head injury (Bernardi et al., 1993). They are indicated only when depressed skull fractures are suspected. In contrast, a dramatic increase in the availability and use of computed tomography (CT) has occurred. In clinical practice, CT scans are more frequently obtained than MRIs in the acute evaluation of brain injuries. There are many reasons for this: CTs are more widely available, they are very useful in demonstration of lesions that require neurosurgical intervention, and they are more rapidly completed, which is especially important for children who are anxious and upset. However, neuroimaging procedures are generally not indicated for *minor* head injuries in children. Mohanty et al. (1991) studied 348 patients who met the following criteria for mild injury: initial GCS scores of 14 or 15; lack of deterioration in the first 20 minutes of observation; absence of any focal sensory or motor deficits; and absence of clinical signs of basilar skull fracture such as blood in the ears, Battle's sign, or rhinorrhea. Of these 348 adult subjects, 3.4 percent had brain scans showing acute changes such as petechiae or subarachnoid blood. Small subdural hematomas were identified in two cases, but they did not require surgical intervention. Of particular relevance is that the CT findings, even when abnormal, did not affect clinical management. Others (e.g., Jerret et al., 1993) have reported similar findings.

In 1987 the *New England Journal of Medicine* reported the findings of a multidisciplinary panel on the indications for radiographic evaluation of head injury (Masters et al., 1987). They developed clinical criteria for radiography and then applied the protocol in a large prospective study in 31 hospital emergency rooms. Their criteria define three groups of patients at high, medium, and low risk of intracranial injury (Table 22-4). No intracranial injuries were discovered in any of their low-risk patients, who were defined as those who were asymptomatic or had headache, dizziness, scalp hematoma, laceration, contusion, or abrasion. The panel recommended eliminating radiographic imaging for low-risk patients. The high-risk group consisted primarily of patients with clearly severe open or closed head injuries. These patients were candidates for emergency CT scanning, neurosurgical consultation, or both. The so-called moderate risk group was less well defined, and the panel indicated that skull radiography in this group may sometimes be appropriate.

Neuroimaging may be more frequently indicated in children under the age of 2 because they may be at greater risk of intracranial lesions (Pietrzak et al., 1991). Furthermore, many head injuries in children under 2 are due to abuse, and abuse victims have a higher incidence of abnormal scans and mass lesions (Mohanty et al., 1991). Objective documentation for legal purposes in the case of a battered child is also helpful (Masters et al., 1987).

TABLE 22-3. Observation and Management of Pediatric Head Injuries

Type of Observation	Indications	Instructions and Action
Home	No loss of consciousness, normal neurologic examination, no polytrauma, reliable caretakers	Home observation instruction sheet, return to hospital if deterioration
Extended outpatient observation for 6 hours	Brief loss of consciousness, GCS ≥13, over 2 years old, not abuse victim, no polytrauma	Sequential observations during 6 hours with repeated GCS scores. CT scan, neurosurgical consultation, and admission if GCS deteriorates
Hospital inpatient	Unconscious longer than 10 minutes, GCS < 13, suspected abuse or asult, polytrauma	Neurosurgical consultation, CT scan, inpatient admission for extended observation

TABLE 22-4. Management Strategy for Radiographic Imaging in Patients with Head Trauma[a]

Low-Risk Group	Moderate-Risk Group	High-Risk Group
Possible findings Asymptomatic Headache Dizziness Scalp hematoma Scalp laceration Scalp contusion or abrasion Absence of moderate-risk or high-risk criteria	Possible findings History of change of consciousness at the time of injury or subsequently History of progressive headache Alcohol or drug intoxication Unreliable or inadequate history of injury Age less than 2 yr (unless injury very trivial) Post-traumatic seizure Vomiting Post-traumatic amnesia Multiple trauma Serious facial injury Signs of basilar fracture[b] Possible skull penetration or depressed fracture[c] Suspected physical child abuse	Possible findings Depressed level of consciousness not clearly due to alcohol, drugs, or other cause (e.g., metabolic and seizure disorders) Focal neurologic signs Decreasing level of consciousness Penetrating skull injury or palpable depressed fracture
Recommendations Observation alone: discharge patients with head-injury information sheet (listing subdural precautions) and a second person to observe them	Recommendations Extended close observation (watch for signs of high-risk group) Consider CT examination and neurosurgical consultation Skull series may (rarely) be helpful, if positive, but do not exclude intracranial injury if normal	Recommendations Patient is a candidate for neurosurgical consultation, emergency CT examination, or both

[a] Physician assessment of the severity of injury may warrant reassignment to a higher-risk group. Any single criterion from a higher-risk group warrants assignment of the patient to the highest risk group applicable.

[b] Signs of basilar fracture include drainage from ear, drainage of cerebrospinal fluid from nose, hematotympanum, Battle's sign, and "racoon-eyes."

[c] Factors associated with open and depressed fracture include gunshot, missile, or shrapnel wounds; scalp injury from firm, pointed object (including animal teeth); penetrating injury of eyelid or globe; object struck in the head; assault (definite or suspected) with any object; leakage of cerebrospinal fluid; and sign of basilar fracture.

(From Masters et al., 1987, with permission.)

Sports Injuries

Sports injuries merit special consideration. Severe brain injury to young athletes is exceedingly rare, especially before the age of 12 (Bruce et al., 1982), but minor head injury occurs frequently—approximately 20 percent per year among high school football players, according to Gerberich et al. (1983). The potential long-term impact of minor concussions on young athletes is not known. In a prospective study of college football players, Barth et al. (1989) found neuropsychological sequelae within 24 hours of sustaining minor "dings" in play. Fortunately, there was a return to premorbid status by postseason.

Of particular concern is the so-called second impact syndrome. In this syndrome an athlete has a mild head injury, recovers uneventfully, and then, sometime within the next week, has another seemingly mild head injury but rapidly develops cerebral edema and dies within hours. Saunders and Harbaugh (1984) described a case in which a college football player died when a mild head injury occurred several days after another mild trauma. Autopsy revealed a frontal contusion from the first injury. They hypothesize that there may be a compounding effect of consecutive mild injuries because of residual mild cerebral swelling and diminished intracranial compliance caused by the initial insult. To add to the concern, some studies have found that athletes who sustain one minor head injury are at significantly (two- to fourfold) increased risk of sustaining a subsequent head injury (Albright et al., 1985; Gerberich et al., 1983). Thus, an important issue in the treatment of injured athletes is deciding when they should be allowed to return to play.

There are published guidelines in the sports medicine literature (Table 22-5), but the success of these guidelines in averting catastrophe has not been confirmed. Saunders and Harbaugh (1984) suggest that, even with mild injury, CT scanning may be indicated in any athlete who has persisting symptoms before clearance is given to resume play. Certainly, departing from published guidelines on the basis of clinical judgment may be appropriate in individual cases.

PREVENTION

Another role for the physician involved in the treatment of pediatric head injury is that of advocating prevention. Some prevention strategies have been found to be remarkably effective. For example, Rivara (1994) describes a study conducted in Seattle, which demonstrated that bicycle helmets decrease the risk of head injury by 85 percent and the risk of brain injury by 88 percent. The increased use of seatbelts and infant car seats has dramatically reduced the risk of brain injury fatalities from car crashes. Baby walkers frequently lead to falls down steps, and parents should be advised to avoid them. Rivara (1994) suggests strategies for advising patients about prevention. For example, he emphasizes that specific instructions such as "Get rid of the baby walker" are much more effective than general statements such as "Childproof your home."

CHILD ABUSE

Child abuse is a potentially preventable yet common cause of pediatric head injury. Head injury caused by abuse appears to have more devastating outcome in terms of death and long-term cognitive and motor impairment than injuries of other etiologies (Bruce and Zimmerman, 1989; Goldstein et al., 1993; Kriel et al., 1989). One reason that abuse causes particularly pernicious injuries is the high potential for repetitive insults (Brink et al., 1980; Caffey, 1974). Furthermore, very young children are rarely exposed to comparable force from accidents (Billmire and Meyers, 1985). Subdural hematoma or loss of consciousness in an infant from an alleged low-velocity event (e.g., a low fall) raises the question of possible abuse.

Children under 1 year of age often incur brain injury when they are victims of the "shaken baby syndrome." Bruce and Zimmerman (1989) have preferred to call this the "shaken impact syndrome," as acceleration/deceleration forces over 10 g (10 times the acceleration of gravity) impossible to generate just by shaking a model of an infant. However, when the model was struck against even a soft mattress, forces up to 300 g could be generated, which is more than enough force to cause significant brain injury (Duhaime et al., 1987). In these shaking injuries, acceleration/deceleration and rotational forces occur that can cause diffuse axonal shearing, subdural hematomas, and retinal hemorrhages. Retinal hemorrhages in children under 3 years of age almost always are the result of child abuse. No retinal hemorrhages were found even with dilated funduscopic examinations of 75 children with accidental injuries

TABLE 22-5. Guidelines for Return to Play After Concussion

	1st Concussion	2nd Concussion	3rd Concussion
Grade 1 (mild)	May return to play if asymptomatic[a] for 1 week	Return to play in 2 weeks if asymptomatic at that time for 1 week	Terminate season; may return to play next season if asymptomatic
Grade 2 (moderate)	Return to play after asymptomatic for 1 week	Minimum of 1 month, may return to play then if asymptomatic for 1 week; consider terminating season	Terminate season; may return to play next season if asymptomatic
Grade 3 (severe)	Minimum of 1 month; may then return to play if asymptomatic for 1 week	Terminate season; may return to play next season if asymptomatic	

[a] No headache, dizziness, or impaired orientation, concentration, or memory during rest or exertion.
(From Cantu, 1986, with permission.)

(Buys et al., 1992). In contrast, retinal hemorrhage is commonly seen in young children whose head injuries are the result of abuse (Billmire and Meyers, 1985; Buys et al., 1992). Kaufman and Dacey (1994) conclude that "Retinal hemorrhages should always raise the suspicion of abuse, and in the child with less than severe trauma, retinal hemorrhages are diagnostic of a shaking injury" (see also Buys et al., 1992).

Any case of suspected abuse must be reported to the appropriate agency for investigation. If there is doubt, it is best to err on the side of reporting. The law tends to protect the individual making a report of suspicion even if it later proves unfounded. Needless to say, protection of the child takes precedence over doubt.

OUTCOME

Age Effects

In the past it was believed that young children were less vulnerable to the long-term effects of brain injury than older children or adults. This idea originally came from animal studies reporting that cortical lesions had less severe effects on the behavior of infant monkeys than on that of adults (Kennard, 1936; Kolb, 1989). Research on humans also appeared to support this idea since children suffering focal left hemisphere cortical lesions in the first few years of life seemed to have much better language recovery than persons with aphasia acquired in adulthood (Lennenberg, 1967). This sometimes remarkable recovery has been attributed to greater flexibility or "plasticity" of the young brain in using mechanisms of reorganization or backup systems or to unrelated neural systems taking over a function.

More recent animal and human research generally fails to support the idea that young brains recover better or compensate better after injury (Goldman, 1974). Differences based on focal lesions are not consistently seen (Geschwind, 1974; Isaacson, 1975; Rutter, 1981), and younger children do not appear to recover better from severe diffuse injury (Filley et al., 1987; Kriel et al., 1989; Mahoney et al., 1983). The relationship between age and outcome of brain injury appears to be quite complex, depending on a variety of mediating factors such as the nature and timing of the injury and the environmental context (Kolb, 1989). Findings in the animal research (Kolb, 1989; Kolb and Wishaw, 1989) suggest that for some lesions a developmental window of time may occur, during which recovery of a specific function is worse than for the same lesion acquired earlier or later in life. Similarly, Ewing-Cobbs et al. (1987) suggest that skills undergoing a rapid stage of development are more vulnerable to cerebral injury than well consolidated skills. In any case, the best evidence to date suggests that the outcome of *minor* head injury is similar in adults (Dikman et al., 1986) and children (Fay et al., 1994). Few data have been collected regarding the outcome of mild head injury in infants.

Cognitive Function

It is clear that severe brain injury can have profound long-term impact on various aspects of a child's cognitive functioning (i.e., perceptual and information processing abilities). Transient sequelae are commonly observed following minor brain injuries to children, such as headache and problems with thinking and concentration (Gulbrandson, 1984). However, the clinician should be aware that with mild injury, symptoms beyond 3 months are unlikely and permanent changes are exceedingly rare (Fay et al., 1994; Levin et al., 1993).

When studying cognitive outcome after pediatric head injury, proper control groups are critical. As a group, children sustaining head injury may have more premorbid behavioral and learning problems than the general population (Bijur et al., 1986; Chadwick et al., 1981). For example, Rutter (1981) suggests that "impulsive, overactive children are more likely to engage in dangerous play activities which result in head injuries." Thus, in research a lack of proper control groups can lead to a spurious appearance of deficit following head injury, when the problems were actually premorbid. In other cases children might perform at normal levels when compared with published norms but actually demonstrate impairment when compared with well-matched controls (Fay et al., 1994).

In the most carefully controlled study to date, Fay et al. (1994) examined neuropsychological functioning in 94 children with head injury, divided into three groups: (1) mild, initial GCS of 13 to 15; (2) moderate, initial GCS score of 9 to 12 or initial score of 13 or 14 but a score of 15 not achieved within 3 days; and (3) severe, initial GCS score of 3 to 8. Subjects were individually matched on a variety of premorbid characteristics, including behavioral and school performance factors. The moderately and severely injured groups scored lower than matched controls on several measures. Impairments were identified at 1 year in intellect, problem solving, academic performance, memory, motor speed, and psychomotor abilities. In contrast, the mildly injured subjects did not significantly differ from controls one-year post injury.

Fay et al. (1994) concluded: "Results from this study suggest that mild CHI [closed head injury] produces virtually no clinically significant long-term deficits in intellectual, neuropsychological, academic, or 'real world' functioning." These findings are consistent with the results of other controlled studies of mild head injury in children (Bijur et al., 1990; Chadwick et al., 1981) and adults (Dikman et al., 1986). They are also consistent with the findings of Levin et al. (1987) that parenchymal lesions found on MRI in subjects with minor to moderate head injury tended to resolve within 1 to 3 months. The improvement on imaging was accompanied by improved neuropsychological performance. It should be noted that MRI findings had no influence on surgical management of the patients in this study.

In contrast to mild injury, moderate to severe head injury can lead to problems in a variety of cognitive domains, depending on the extent and nature of the injury. These include potential deficits in memory, attention, language, visuospatial abilities, psychomotor speed, and executive functions. (See Fletcher and Levin [1988] and Levin et al. [1982] for more thorough reviews of the research on neuropsychological sequelae of moderate and severe closed head injury.)

Behavioral Function

As with cognitive impairment, behavioral disturbance is rarely seen after mild head injury in children (Bijur et al., 1990; Brown et al 1981; Fletcher et al., 1990). Although it is possible that there will be short-term sequelae, carefully controlled studies find no lingering deficits after 3 months. This is contrary to the frequently encountered misconception among lay-persons that such changes are likely. Unfortunately, parental expectation of deficits could actually contribute to their development if the child is overprotected, held out of school for a long period, or otherwise treated differently after a mild head injury.

Behavioral disturbance can occur after more severe head injury. A wide range of difficulties have been reported, such as disinhibition, hyperactivity, impulsivity, lethargy, behavioral regression, aggressiveness, and mood disturbances. These changes are often exacerbations of premorbid behavior patterns but can also be entirely new problems (Brown et al., 1981). Premorbid family dysfunction makes behavioral disturbance more likely after both milder and more severe head injury (Casey et al., 1986). In fact, Rivara et al. (1993) found that premorbid family dysfunction was a stronger predictor of behavioral disturbance after head injury than was injury severity.

In summary, long-term cognitive or behavioral deficits resulting from mild head injury are very rare. This does not imply that such impairment never occurs; isolated cases are possible. Furthermore, sometimes a head injury will prove to have been more severe than originally thought (e.g., an unwitnessed accident). But as the data from Fay et al. (1994) and Bijur et al. (1986, 1990) have so elegantly demonstrated, most academic and behavioral problems lasting more than 3 months after minor head injury are unrelated to brain damage. When problems occur, environmental factors and the child's premorbid status often contribute to or entirely explain the current difficulties. In any case in which a child is having problems (behavioral, cognitive, or otherwise) following an injury, referral for psychological evaluation is indicated. Regardless of the etiology of the problems, the clinician's contact with a child for minor head injury may present a window of opportunity in which to refer an at-risk child who otherwise might never come to appropriate attention for services.

NEUROPSYCHOLOGICAL EVALUATION

If behavioral, emotional, or cognitive problems are observed by the clinician or mentioned by the family, referral for neuropsychological evaluation is indicated. A comprehensive neuropsychological evaluation includes assessment of mood, adjustment, cognition, and environmental factors, which all have distinct treatment implications. In other words, the evaluation focuses on the child as a whole, with an eye toward implementing appropriate interventions. With adults it is often preferable to postpone neuropsychological evaluation until several months after mild head injury, when the results will be more indicative of long-term outcome. However, with children it is often reasonable to conduct the testing earlier because even short-term effects can create a major setback for a youngster if there are impairments that disrupt ongoing learning. On the other hand, the need to identify deficits must be balanced with the need to normalize a child's experience and to emphasize the likelihood of excellent outcome.

In most cases, persistent changes occurring after minor head injury are not related to actual tissue damage. For example, the development of hyperactivity after a head injury could be a symptom of post-traumatic stress disorder if the injury was sustained under violent or otherwise terrifying circumstances. Concentration problems in school could be related to depression or anxiety. Many children who are evaluated after head injury may have had symptoms of attention deficit disorder premorbidly, perhaps not previously diagnosed. Similary, problems due to other premorbid learning, mood, or behavior disorders may come to professional attention for the first time following mild head injury.

It is often extremely difficult to determine what amount of dysfunction is directly related to the injury, is exacerbated by the injury, or preceded the injury, and a combination of these influences may be at work. Sorting out these factors can be especially difficult with very young children, who have not established a premorbid record of standardized test scores and school performances. Furthermore, if problems arise as a child enters a new developmental stage, it is often impossible to determine whether the problems would have arisen despite the head injury. Precise determination of etiology actually has limited implications for treatment planning once a problem has been accurately defined. On the other hand, mistakenly attributing a problem to brain damage can influence parental and teacher reaction to the child, encourage litigation, and be damaging to a child's self-concept.

The latter point is illustrated by the case of a 10-year-old girl who was seen for neuropsychological evaluation. Two years prior to the evaluation she was was struck by a car while riding her bicycle. She hit her head on the windshield and immediately ran home to tell her mother. She was treated in the local emergency room for a parietal scalp laceration, and a head CT scan was performed, which was negative. There was no loss of consciousness, confusion, or pre- or post-traumatic amnesia. Her mother reported that in the year following the accident she experienced irritability and school difficulty (including difficulty in following instructions and failure to complete homework). Despite a normal MRI and 24-hour electroencephalogram, a neurologist prescribed anti-seizure medication and instructed the family that she should not be allowed to participate in contact sports (prior to the accident she had been an avid soccer player).

During the neuropsychological evaluation, the patient appeared depressed, and interview confirmed depressive symptoms. When her mother described her daughter's school problems, she became tearful and upset (vomited). Throughout testing she was nervous and uncertain. Cognitive test performances in a wide variety of domains were entirely normal, with the exception of a low fund of general knowledge. Intellectual abilities were generally in the low average range. Thorough review of premorbid school records, including teacher reports, and two premorbid evaluations by the area education agency revealed a pattern of difficulty in school involving poor attention, low self-esteem, and difficulty with comprehension and following directions, which was virtually indistinguishable from the post-morbid complaints.

Premorbid intellectual abilities were in the low average range.

It was concluded that there was no evidence of cognitive impairment attributable to brain damage but rather that the child had premorbid learning problems and was depressed. Referral for counseling was provided, and it was recommended that remedial assistance in school (initiated prior to the accident) be continued. It was also strongly recommended that the restriction on sports participation be reconsidered by the physician, as sports participation had been a critical source of self-esteem prior to the accident.

Assessment Approach

The clinical interview, with both parents or guardian and the child, is the most fundamental part of the assessment of behavioral changes after mild head injury and guides the course of the examination including test selection. It is necessary to be alert to any parental tendencies to minimize or exaggerate deficits. Particular caution is warranted when there is litigation or the potential for litigation related to the accident. The best interview is thorough without invoking the power of suggestion. Interview topics should include (1) ascertainment of changes that have been observed since the accident; (2) extent of the initial injury (e.g., length of unconsciousness, if any); (3) post-traumatic confusion and amnesia observed; (4) premorbid behavior and learning; (5) psychosocial factors contributing to behavior; and (6) medical, academic, and social history prior to the accident. The interview can be supplemented with questionnaires administered to parents and teachers. Instruments such as the Personality Inventory for Children (Wirt et al., 1982) or the Child Behavior Check List (Achenbach, 1991) can be useful in understanding the behavior and psychosocial adjustment of the child in a broad context. The Vineland Adaptive Behavior Scale (Sparrow et al., 1984) has a structured interview format and can be useful when there are deficits in the performance of everyday functional skills.

The child is interviewed to elucidate his or her experience of the injury with regard to both cognitive and emotional factors. Exploration of post-traumatic stress symptoms, attention deficit, depression, anxiety, or other behavioral abnormality should be included. Self-report measures such as the Revised Children's Manifest Anxiety Scale (Reynolds and Richmond, 1985) and the Children's Depression Inventory (Kovacs, 1992) are useful to supplement interview material. Observation of the child in the testing situation, in the waiting room or play area, and in the school setting (when feasible) can provide important information about response inhibition, activity level, and other self-regulatory behaviors.

In addition to the interview, information from the school regarding premorbid functioning is essential for the neuropsychological evaluation. Having the teacher fill out a Conners Inventory (Conners, 199) or Child Behavior Checklist (Achenbach, 1991) is necessary but not sufficient for behavioral description. Having the teacher describe the child in the classroom in as much detail as possible to ascertain changes in behavioral control can be very helpful. In addition, records of previous group testing and school grades should be obtained. If the child received special services, individual educational plans and school testing will help to distinguish the effects of head injury from premorbid problems.

Regarding cognitive assessment, a flexible approach is recommended. We use a set of core tests with most patients to explore critical aspects of cognitive functioning (e.g., attention, motor function, memory). Then, other tests are added on an individual basis in response to hypotheses relating to the particular case (e.g., findings on neuroimaging, specific referral questions, parental description or observation, and findings on the core battery). This combination of the fixed and flexible approach is the one most commonly used by neuropsychologists in North America (Benton, 1994; Tranel, 1992; Tranel, 1995).

With the exception of forensic evaluation, the emphasis within the cognitive assessment is to outline abilities and identify areas of weakness for purposes of planning interventions and developing strategies for remediation. If problems are identified, any of a number of treatments may be indicated in the individual case, such as psychotherapy, cognitive rehabilitation, speech and language therapy, occupational therapy, special education placement, or educational adaptations. For example, children with head injury sometimes have trouble with behavioral inhibition and attention. In these cases parents and teachers may be given ideas about how to increase structure, minimize overstimulation, and develop organizational strategies (e.g., by using cognitive-behavioral techniques). Overemphasis on localization of impairment is a mistake, because most neuropsychological tests perform localization poorly, localization of function is more difficult in children, and although focal lesions can occur, the primary mechanism of damage in most brain injuries is diffuse.

Public law stipulates that children with head injury-related school problems are entitled to evaluation and individualized programming provided by the school district. These school-based evaluations vary in terms of thoroughness and the evaluators' familiarity with head injury. Often school-based assessments are limited to tests of intelligence and previously learned skills such as reading and spelling, which are not sensitive to the deficits seen after head injury. In such situations, the pediatric neuropsychologist can serve as a consultant to the educational team and sometimes as an advocate for special services if a child does not meet criteria based on formulas derived for children with developmental learning disabilities.

In the evaluation of cognitive functioning, non-speeded tests of verbal intellectual ability, such as the Wechsler Intelligence Scale for Children, Third Edition (WISC-III) and other measures of "crystallized" intelligence are unlikely to be sensitive to the effects of head injury, but they can provide useful clues about a child's premorbid ability level. Similarly, a child's previously acquired fund of knowledge and overlearned material, such as well established word recognition and spelling skills, are less likely to be affected by brain injury than processes that require concentration and manipulation of concepts, such as mathematical reasoning (Levin and Benton, 1986).

Since the frontal lobes are particularly vulnerable to insult in head injury, neuropsychological evaluation includes assessment of functions mediated by this complex brain region. The so-called executive functions include higher level planning, organization, and social and emotional self-monitoring (Tranel et al., 1994). We disagree with the assertion of some neuropsychologists that because of incomplete myelination of the frontal lobes, assessment of executive functions is inappropriate in the evaluation of children. Executive functions are developing throughout childhood (Welsh and Pennington, 1988), and these functions are crucial for children's behavioral adaptation and academic success.

The development of adequate clinical measures of executive functions has been elusive. Often persons with a profound deficit in a particular executive function in daily life can perform well on laboratory tests designed to measure that function and can articulate what they should do in situations in which they fail to respond appropriately in real life (Damasio and Anderson, 1993; Eslinger and Damasio, 1985). Furthermore, *executive functions* is not a unitary concept but rather encompasses a variety of higher-level operations, which may be affected differentially, or even in opposite directions, in different patients. Thus, evaluation of executive functions requires a multimodal approach including standardized tests and analysis of problems in everyday functioning.

Tests of executive functions are not specific, as they can be affected by breakdown in lower-order abilities that are required to perform the higher-order operation. A variety of brain regions and systems are likely involved. Thus, the common term "frontal lobe tests" is inappropriate (Anderson et al., 1991). Although not specific, certain tests appear to be sensitive to impairment in certain executive functions in children. These include established tests such as the Wisconsin Card Sorting Test (Chelune and Bauer, 1986; Heaton, 1981), the Traimaking test and Color Trails (Spreen and Strauss, 1991; Williams et al., in press), and the Tower of London (Levin et al., 1994; Shallice, 1982) and more experimental measures such as the 20-question task described by Levin et al. (1993). As with all measures, age-appropriate norms are essential for clinical use.

There are many variables to consider in developing rehabilitation or special education interventions, including the nature of the cognitive impairment, the family situation, the school setting, and the child's premorbid status (including age). Because of the many variables, individualized plans are preferable. For the mildly head-injured child, brief modification of school performance expectations and temporary individual help are appropriate. The school is usually able to provide all the services necessary for the mildly head-injured. For the child with moderate to severe head injury, both school services and outside rehabilitation services may be needed. In many cases the school will be able to assume most of the service after the initial period of intense intervention. Recommendations for rehabilitation usually include striking a balance between remediation efforts and teaching compensation techniques and will depend on the locus and severity of the injury.

Again, in the case of mild injury, it is important to convey to parents and teachers the expectation of full recovery. Also, a child's activities should not be unnecessarily restricted. If deficits continue to be seen, further evaluation may clarify the nature of the problem whether it relates to the head injury or another factor. The pediatric neuropsychologist should continue to follow the child until parents are reassured either that the child has recovered or that interventions are well in place.

CONCLUSIONS

The intent of this chapter was to provide important background for physicians and neuropsychologists who will encounter pediatric patients with mild head injury. A rational approach to management will help prevent physical, psychological, and academic complications, and can be used as an opportunity to refer certain at risk children for appropriate services.

ACKNOWLEDGMENTS

The authors thank Cyndi Walljasper and Ellen Steffensmeier for technical assistance and Dr. Richard Ugland for reviewing the manuscript.

REFERENCES

Achenbach T: Child Behavior Checklist (Parent Report Form and Teacher Report Form). University of Vermont, Burlington, VT, 1991

Albright JP, Mcauley E, Martin RK et al: Head and neck injuries in college football: an eight-year analysis. Am J Sports Med 13:147–152, 1985

Anderson SW, Damasio H, Jones RD, Tranel D: Wisconsin Card Sorting Test performance as a measure of frontal lobe damage. J Clin Exp Neuropsychol 13:909–922, 1991

Annegers, JF: The epidemiology of head trauma in children. pp. 1–10. In Shapiro K (ed): Pediatric Head Trauma Futura Mount Kisco, NY, 1983

Barth JT, Alves WM, Thomas VR et al: Mild head injury in sports: neuropsychological sequelae and return of function. pp. 257–275. In Levin HS, Eisenberg HM, Benton AL (eds): Mild Head Injury Oxford University Press, New York, 1989

Benton AL: Neuropsychological assessment. Annu Rev Psychol 45:1–23, 1994

Bernardi B, Zimmerman RA, Bilaniuk LT: Neuroradiologic evaluation of pediatric craniocerebral trauma. Top Magn Reson Imaging 5:161–173, 1993

Bijur PE, Haslum M, Golding J: Cognitive and behavioral sequelae of mild head injury in children. Pediatrics 86:337–344, 1990

Bijur PE, Stewart-Brown S, Butler N: Child behavior and accidental injury in 11,966 preschool children. Am J Dis Child 140:487–492, 1986

Billmire ME, Meyers PA: Serious head injury in infants: accident or abuse. Pediatrics 75:340–342, 1985

Brink JD, Imbus C, Woo-Sam J: Physical recovery after severe closed head trauma in children and adolescents. J Pediatr 97:721–727, 1980

Brown G, Chadwick O, Shaffer D et al: A prospective study of children with head injuries: III. Psychiatric sequelae. Psychol Med 11:63–78, 1981

Bruce DA, Schut L, Sutton LN: Brain and cervical spine injuries occurring during organized sports activities in children and adolescents. Clin Sports Med 1:495–514, 1982

Bruce DA, Zimmerman RA: Shaken impact syndrome. Pediatr Ann 18:482–494, 1989

Buys YM, Levin AV, Enzanauer RW et al: Retinal findings after head trauma in infants and young children. Ophthalmology 99:1718–1723, 1992

Caffey J: The whiplash shaken infant syndrome: manual shaking by the extremities with whiplash-induced intracranial and postocular bleedings, linked with residual permanent brain damage and mental retardation. Pediatrics 54:396–403, 1974

Calder IM, Hill I, Scholtz CL: Primary brain trauma in non-accidental injury. J Clin Pathol 37:1095–1100, 1984

Cantu RC: Guidelines for return to contact sports after a cerebral concussion. Physician Sports Med 14(10):75–79, 1986

Casey R, Ludwig S, McCormick MC: Morbidity following minor head trauma in children. Pediatrics 78:497–502, 1986

Chadwick O, Rutter M, Brown G et al: A prospective study of children with head injuries: II. Cognitive sequelae. Psychol Med 11:49–61, 1981

Chelune GJ, Bauer RA: Developmental norms for the Wisconsin Card Sort Test. J Clin Exper Neuropsychol 8:219–228, 1986

Connors, K: Conners' Rating Scales. Multi-Health Systems, North Tonawanda, NY, 199

Damasio AR, Anderson SW: The frontal lobes. In Heilman K, Valenstein E (eds): Clinical Neuropsychology. 3rd Ed. Oxford University Press, New York, 1993

Davidson LL et al: Hyperactivity in school-age boys and subsequent risk of injury. Pediatrics 90:697–702, 1992

Dikman S, McLean A, Temkin N: Neuropsychological and psychosocial consequences of minor head injury. J Neurol Neurosurg Psychiatry 49:1227–1232, 1986

Duhaime AC, Alario AJ, Lewander J et al: Head injury in very young children: mechanisms, injury types, and ophthalmologic findings in 100 hospitalized patients younger than 2 years of age. Pediatrics 90:179–185, 1992

Duhaime AC, Gennarelli TA, Thibault LE et al: The shaken baby syndrome: a clinical, pathological, and biomechanical study. J Neurosurg 66:409–415, 1987

Elson , Ward : Mechanisms and pathophysiology of mild head injury. Semin Neurol 14:8–18, 1994

Eslinger PJ, Damasio AR: Severe disturbance of higher cognition after bilateral frontal lobe ablation: patient EVR. Neurology 35:1731–1741, 1985

Ewing-Cobbs L, Levin HS, Eisenberg HM, Fletcher JM: Language functions following closed-head injury in children and adolescents. J Clin Exp Neuropsychol 9:575–592, 1987

Ewing-Cobbs L, Levin HS, Fletcher JM et al: The Children's Orientation and Amnesia Test: relationship to severity of acute head injury and to recovery of memory. Neurosurgery 27:683–691, 1990

Fay GC, Jaffe KM, Polissar NL et al: Mild pediatric traumatic brain injury: a cohort study. Arch Phys Med Rehabil 74:895–901, 1993

Filley CM, Cranberg LD, Alexander MP, Hart EJ: Neurobehavioral outcome after closed head injury in childhood and adolescence. Arch Neurol 44:194–198, 1987

Fletcher JM, Ewing-Cobbs L, Miner ME et al: Behavioral changes after closed head injury in children. J Consul Clin Psychol 58:93–98, 1990

Fletcher JM, Levin HS: Neurobehavioral effects of brain injury in children. pp. 258–295. In Routh DK (ed): Handbook of Pediatric Psychology. Guilford Press, New York, 1988

Gerberich SG, Priest JD, Boen JR et al: Concussion incidences and severity in secondary school varsity football players. Am J Public Health 73:1370–1375, 1983

Geschwind N: Late changes in the nervous system: an overview. In Stein DG, Rosen JJ, Butters N (eds): Plasticity and recovery of Function in the Central Nervous System. Academic Press, Orlando, 1974

Goldman PS: An alternative to developmental plasticity: heterology of CNS structures in infants and adults. pp. 149–174. In Stein DG, Rosen JJ, Butters N (eds): Plasticity and Recovery from Brain Damage. Academic Press, Orlando, 1974

Goldstein B, Kelly MM, Bruton D, Cox C: Inflicted versus accidental head injury in critically injured children. Crit Care Med 23:1328–1332, 1993

Goldstein FC, Levin HS: Epidemiology of pediatric closed head injury: incidence, clinical characteristics, and risk factors. J Learning Disabilities 20:518, 1987

Gulbrandsen GB: Neuropsychological sequelae of light head injuries in older children 6 months after trauma. J Clin Neuropsychol 6:257–268, 1984

Heaton RK: Wisconsin Card Sorting Test Manual. Psychological Assessment Resources, Odessa, Florida, 1981

Hoekelman RA: A pediatrician's view: why deaths from head injuries are on the decline. Pediatr Ann 23:8–10, 1994

Isaacson RL: The myth of recovery from early brain damage. In Ellis NE (ed): Aberrant Development in Infancy. John Wiley & Sons, London, 1975

Jaffe KM, Massagle TL, Martin KM et al: Pediatric traumatic brain injury: acute and rehabilitation costs. Arch Phys Med Rehabil 74:681–686, 1993

Jeret JS, Mandell M, Anziska B et al: Clinical predictors of abnormality disclosed by computed tomography after mild head trauma. Neurosurgery 32:9–15, 1993

Kaufman BA, Dacey RG: Acute care management of closed head injury in childhood. Pediatr Ann 23:18–27, 1994

Kennard MA: Age and other factors in motor recovery from precentral lesions in monkeys. J Neurophysiol 1:496, 1936

Kolb B: Brain development, plasticity, and behavior. Am Psychol 44:1203–1212, 1989

Kolb B, Wishaw IQ: Plasticity in the neocortex: mechanisms underlying recovery from early brain damage. Prog Neurobiol 32:235–276, 1989

Kovacs M: Children's Depression Inventory. Multi-Health Systems, North Tonawanda, NY, 1992

Kraus JF, Fife D, Cox P et al: Incidence, severity, and external causes of pediatric brain injury. Am J Dis Child 140:687–693, 1986

Kriel RL, Krach LE, Panser LA: Closed head injury: comparison of children younger and older than 6 years of age. Pediatr Neurol 5:296–300, 1989

Lennenberg E: Biological Foundations of Language. John Wiley & Sons, New York, 1967

Levin HS, Amparo E, Eisenberg HM et al: Magnetic resonance imaging and computerized tomography in relation to the neurobehavioral sequelae of mild and moderate head injuries. J Neurosurg 66:706–713, 1987

Levin HS, Benton AL, Grossman RG: Neurobehavioral Consequences of Closed Head Injury. Oxford University Press, 1982

Levin HS, Culhane KA, Mendelsohn D et al: Cognition in relation to magnetic resonance imaging in head-injured children and adolescents. Arch Neurol 50:897–905, 1993

Levin HS, Eisenberg HM, Wigg NR, Kobayashi K: Memory and intellectual ability after head injury in children and adolescents. Neurosurgery 11:668–673, 1982

Levin HS, Mendelsohn D, Lilly MA et al: Tower of London performance in relation to magnetic resonance imaging following closed head injury in children. Neuropsychology 8:171–179, 1994

Mahoney WJ, D'Souza BJ, Haller JA et al: Long-term outcome of children with severe head trauma and prolonged coma. Pediatrics 71:756–762, 1983

Masters SJ et al: Skull x-ray examinations after head trauma: recommendations by a multidisciplinary panel and validation study. N Engl J Med 316:84–91, 1987

McDonald CM, Jaffe KM, Fay GC et al: Comparison of indices of traumatic brain injury severity as predictors of neurobehavioral outcome in children. Arch Phys Med Rehabil 75:328–337, 1994

Merton DF, Osborne DRS: Craniocerebral trauma in the child abuse syndrome. Pediatr Ann 12:882–887, 1983

Mohanty SK, Thompson W, Rakower S: Are CT scans for head injury patients always necessary? J Trauma 31:801–805, 1991

Pietrzak M, Jagoda A, Brown L: Evaluation of minor head trauma in children younger than two years. Am J Emerg Med 9:153–156, 1991

Reynolds CR, Richmond BO: Revised Children's Manifest Anxiety Scale. Western Psychological Services, Los Angeles, 1985

Rivara FP: Epidemiology and prevention of pediatric traumatic brain injury. Pediatr Ann 23:12–17, 1994

Rivara FP, Bergman AB, LoGerfo J, Weiss NS: Epidemiology of childhood injuries. II: Sex differences in injury rates. Am J Dis Child 136:502–506, 1982

Rivara FP, Calogne N, Thompson RS: Population based study of unintentional injury incidence and impact during childhood. Am J Public Health 79:990–994, 1989

Rivara JB, Jaffe KM, Fay GC et al: Family functioning and injury severity as predictors of child functioning one year following traumatic brain injury. Arch Phys Med Rehabil 74:1047–1055, 1993

Ros SP, Ros MA: Should patients with normal cranial CT scans following minor head injury be hospitalized for observation? Pediatr Emerg Care 5:216–218, 1989

Ruijs MBM: Assessment of post-traumatic amnesia in young children. 1992

Russell WR: Cerebral involvement in head injury. Brain 55:549–603, 1932

Russell WR, Smith A: Post-traumatic amnesia in closed head injury. Arch Neurol 5:4–17, 1961

Rutter M: Psychological sequelae of brain damage in children. Am J Psychiatry 138:1533–1544, 1981

Saunders RL, Harbaugh RE: The second impact in catastrophic contact-sports head trauma. JAMA 252: 538–539, 1984

Shallice T: Specific impairments of planning. Philos Trans R Soc Lond [Biol] 298:199–209, 1982

Snoek JW, Minderhoud JM, Wilmink JT: Delayed deterioration following mild head injury in children. Brain 107:15–36, 1984

Sparrow SS, Balla DA, Cicchetti DV: Vineland Adaptive Behavior Scales. American Guidance Service, Circle Pines MN, 1984

Spreen O, Strauss E: A Compendium of Neuropsychological Tests. Oxford, New York, 1991

Teasdale G, Jennett B: Assessment of coma and impaired consciousness: a practical scale. Lancet 2:81–84, 1974

Tecklenburg FW, Wright MS: Minor head trauma in the pediatric patient. Pediatr Emerg Care 7:40–47, 1991

Tranel D: Neuropsychological assessment. Psychiatr Clin North Am 15:283–299, 1992

Tranel D: The Iowa-Benton School of Neuropsychological Assessment. In Neuropsychological Assessment of Neuropsychiatric Disorders. 2nd Ed. Oxford University Press, New York, 1995

Tranel D, Anderson SW, Benton AL: Development of the concept of executive functions in relation to the frontal lobes. In Boller F, Grafman J (eds): Handbook of Neuropsychology. Vol 9. Elsevier, New York, 1993

Welsh MC, Pennington BF: Assessing frontal lobe functioning in children: views from developmental psychology. Dev Neuropsychol 4:199–230, 1988

William J, Rickert V, Hogan J et al: Children's color trails. Arch Clin Neuropsychol (in press)

Wirt RD, Lachar D, Klinedinst JK, Seat PD: Personality Inventory for Children. Western Psychological Services, Los Angeles, 1982

Cognitive Rehabilitation in Closed Head Injury

23

S. W. Anderson

Cognitive and behavioral impairments are the most common sequelae of traumatic brain injury (TBI) and are the factors most likely to lead to long-term disability (e.g., Medical Disability Society, 1988; see also Ch. 20). The tendency in traditional head injury rehabilitation has been to focus on mobility and physical aspects of recovery, but the prevalence and impact of cognitive and behavioral alterations have made increasingly apparent the need for efficacious rehabilitation procedures directed at these impairments. Despite this need and the considerable recent progress of cognitive neuroscience, current treatment options for acquired cognitive and behavioral defects remain highly unsatisfactory.

Although pharmacologic interventions clearly have use in the management of some behavioral and emotional problems after brain injury (e.g., Gualtieri, 1988, see also Ch. 21), it is unlikely that neurochemical manipulations alone ever will be able to address most cognitive impairments resulting from brain injury. Another potential avenue of treatment, neural transplant techniques, holds promise for helping some brain-injured patients, but this technology awaits considerable basic research before it becomes a viable treatment option and likely never will be feasible for most TBI patients.

This state of affairs leaves the use of environmental and psychological interventions as the treatment option with the most immediate and realistic promise for the rehabilitation of cognitive and behavioral impairments after brain injury. This is the domain of neuropsychological or cognitive rehabilitation.

Cognitive rehabilitation is a relatively new therapeutic service involving the application of psychological and environmental interventions to facilitate recovery of behavioral competencies after damage to the brain. The goals of cognitive rehabilitation are explicitly tied to real-world behaviors (i.e., to allow an individual with brain damage to function optimally, to reduce the burden on his or her support system such that less assistance is needed, and to develop skills and use environmental resources to overcome residual impairments from a brain injury). This chapter focuses on treatment of nonlinguistic cognitive and behavioral defects; speech and language therapies are not reviewed.

Brain-injured patients have been a primary source of information used to guide theory development in cognitive neuroscience. It is becoming increasingly apparent that cognitive neuroscience and clinical neuropsychology have developed to a point where it now is a realistic challenge to apply these domains of knowledge to the rehabilitation of patients with brain dysfunction. Continued integration of ongoing theoretical developments in cognitive neuroscience with the practice of cognitive rehabilitation should result in increased understanding of individual neuropsychological conditions, improved neuropsychological evaluations, and more rational cognitive rehabilitation techniques.

Cognitive rehabilitation involves procedures aimed at both (1) restoration or direct retraining of defective cognitive abilities and (2) learning compensatory strategies such that tasks may be accomplished via alternate mean that circumvent impaired cognitive abilities. The restorative approach places greater faith in neuronal plasticity and redundancy of functional neural systems and is based on the assumption that systematic retraining of a basic cognitive ability will allow the patient to resume functional competence in real-life tasks that depend on that cognitive ability. The compensatory approach begins with recognition of the fact that many acquired cognitive defects are refractory to treatment and is based on the idea that patients can be trained in the use of coping strategies and external aids, such that some degree of functional competence in performing real-life tasks is maintained despite the presence of underlying cognitive impairments. One of the advantages of compensatory approaches is that they are more directly tied to performance on real-world tasks.

Consumer demand has been a powerful force in the development of cognitive rehabilitation, and the fact that clinical practice has outstripped research has contributed to controversy regarding the field. Some skepticism has occurred because cognitive rehabilitation procedures often have been developed and applied in the for-profit sector of the rehabilitation industry, raising the concerns that the field has been driven more by economic than scientific and clinical factors.

A certain amount of skepticism also arises from the common belief that a damaged biologic system such as an injured brain is impervious to psychological or environmental intervention. However, this runs counter to a wealth of animal studies that describe positive effects of enriched environment and/or training after brain damage (e.g., Finger and Stein, 1982; Will and Kelche, 1992).

The most important criticism of neuropsychological rehabilitation is that the evidence for its efficacy is weak. That this is a function of the early stage of development of the field rather than an indictment of its already realized and potential value is attested to by the accumulation of empirical support for specific procedures in recent years. Importantly, the field is evolving as a result of the incoming data. Expectations for outcome are being refined, and cognitive "muscle-building" approaches have been replaced by an emphasis on training of compensatory behaviors. Some initial guidelines have been published by the American Psychological Association Division 40 (Clinical Neuropsychology) and the American Academy of Rehabilitation Medicine (Harley et al., 1992; Mathews et al., 1991).

There is little doubt that cognitive rehabilitation will prove to be a cost-effective and standard component of brain injury rehabilitation. In addition to the demand for these services from patients and caretakers, as well as the efficacy already documented, cognitive rehabilitation is relatively inexpensive, inherently practical, and has very little risk of harming a patient. The ongoing efforts to collect data regarding the efficacy of cognitive rehabilitation will be continued and expanded.

AN APPROACH TO COGNITIVE REHABILITATION

The approach to cognitive rehabilitation in use at the University of Iowa has its roots in the flexible, hypothesis-testing, Iowa-Benton approach to neuropsychological assessment (Tranel, 1994; see also Ch. 19), as well as the pioneering efforts of the New York University Medical Center cognitive rehabilitation program (e.g., Ben-Yishay and Diller, 1993; Diller et al., 1988). In our approach, planned short-term interventions are directed at specific circumscribed goals, drawing on empirically validated procedures. Cognitive rehabilitation programs are individually tailored on the basis of the neuropsychological evaluation, patient goals, and practical considerations.

Treatment is provided by neuropsychologists, as well as by rehabilitation counselors, clinical psychology graduate students, and technicians, under the supervision of a neuropsychologist. Most patients are seen on an outpatient basis in 1- to 2-hour sessions, with the frequency of rehabilitation sessions ranging from daily to once per week. Determination of frequency of sessions is based primarily on the ability of the patient or patient-caretaker team to carry out homework assignments outside of the hospital setting.

In today's cost-conscious era, we have found it necessary to place primary emphasis on short-term efficacious interventions. At the present time, precise guidelines do not exist to determine the optimal amount or intensity of cognitive rehabilitation for an individual patient. To accommodate the spectrum of cognitive and behavioral outcomes after head injury, as well as the practical considerations of a catchment area spanning several hundred miles, we have provided a continuum of treatment plans, ranging from a single consultation session to daily rehabilitation sessions over a period of months. Most patients are seen for 12 or fewer sessions, although many are involved for a considerably longer period. We typically will contract with a patient for a program of approximately 10 rehabilitation sessions, after which follow-up measures (including both laboratory tests and indices of real-world behavior) are obtained. Rehabilitation is continued if there is reason to expect it will continue to contribute to meaningful behavioral improvement; additional follow-up evaluations are used to monitor progress and the need for additional therapy.

Virtually any patient who has sustained a TBI resulting in cognitive or behavioral impairments may be a candidate for cognitive rehabilitation. Of course, treatment goals, expectations for outcome, and intervention procedures are heavily influenced by the severity of the injury and the resultant impairments. We have found patient motivation for behavioral improvement to be a key factor in determining rehabilitation success. In the absence of such motivation (e.g., in a patient with severe unawareness), the participation of a family member or caretaker is critical. Contraindications for successful intervention include a history of significant preinjury behavioral problems or ongoing substance abuse.

Time since injury has not emerged as a critical variable in determining who will benefit from cognitive rehabilitation, although it is likely that some procedures will prove to be more or less effective in the acute or chronic epochs. On one hand, it seems desirable to implement treatment as soon as feasible to provide optimal conditions for "spontaneous" recovery to occur to the fullest extent possible. On the other hand, it may be more efficacious to wait until the patient's neuropsychological condition has stabilized to take full advantage of the individual's cognitive strengths and not to invest in the treatment of deficits that would recover without intervention.

Formulation of a patient's cognitive rehabilitation plan begins with a comprehensive neuropsychological evaluation. The evaluation serves to identify cognitive strengths and weaknesses, and it provides a source of hypotheses regarding what interventions are likely to be effective. An important challenge facing practitioners and researchers in cognitive rehabilitation and neuropsychological assessment is to bridge the gap between the cognitive abilities assessed in the neuropsychological evaluation and functional behavior in the setting of real-world demands.

After assessment, interventions are applied in a manner to test specific hypotheses regarding the patient's cognitive abilities and behavior (Gordon et al., 1989). Interventions are housed in a framework of an educational, teaching and learning encounter bearing some similarities to a classroom experience but also being individualized, collaborative, and highly participatory. The basic sequence of application of these procedures is illustrated in Figure 23-1.

The ultimate goal of any intervention must be of sufficient importance that its attainment will have a significant positive impact on the patient's life, and a critical issue for any clinical intervention is that of *generalization* to real-world situations. Unfortunately, one of the earliest findings from experimental psychology was that learning tends to be task-specific (Thorndike and Woodworth, 1901). The already limited ability of the human brain to generalize new learning from one situation or task to another is further compromised after head injury. As such, steps to facilitate generalization must be built into all interventions. This might include addressing real-world problems from the onset of treatment, use of home work assignments, activities to simulate actual work and social environments, and other in vivo experiences.

COMPONENTS OF COGNITIVE REHABILITATION

Even skeptics (e.g., Volpe and McDowell, 1990) agree that the degree of impairment suffered by persons who sustain head injury can be lessened by training in social interactions, relief of depression, education about adaptation, encouragement and support, and increased understanding on the part of family members. Given the almost universal benefits of these factors, certain elements are included in nearly

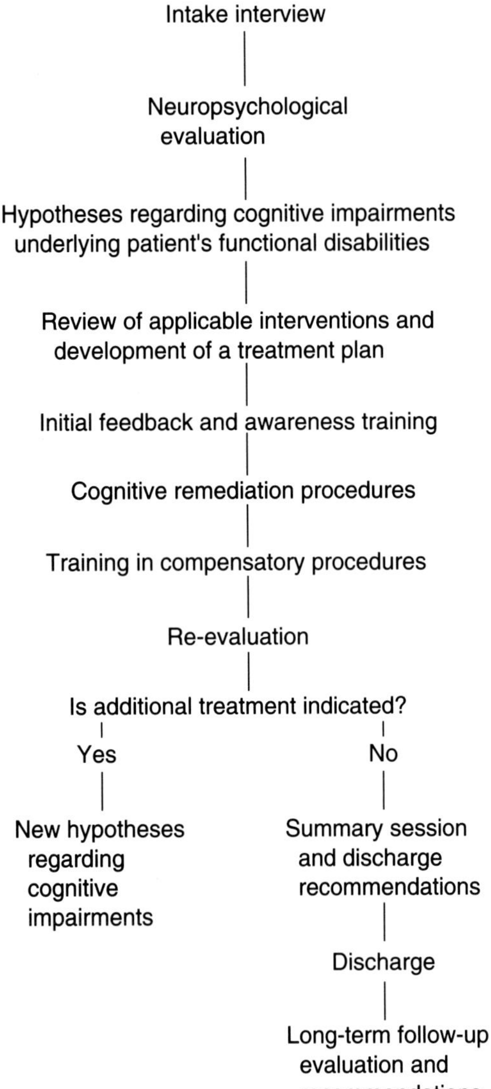

Fig. 23-1. Flow algorithm illustrating the basic sequence of procedures used in an individualized cognitive rehabilitation program.

all our individualized cognitive rehabilitation programs.

Education and Awareness Training

The pragmatic goals of cognitive rehabilitation necessitate active involvement of the patient and family from the onset of treatment. We begin most cognitive rehabilitation programs with an educational overview of brain structure and function, presented in a format that takes into consideration the individual patient's background and current level of function. This segues into a discussion of the neural and cognitive consequences of TBI and then the patient's own neuropsychological profile. For most patients, this approach provides a nonthreatening and interesting introduction to cognitive rehabilitation, as well as an opportunity to correct misconceptions regarding the patient's condition (which are common in both patients and family members).

It is critical that the patient understand why he or she is in rehabilitation and understand what is being attempted. Unawareness of acquired cognitive impairments is common after TBI, particularly when there is substantial damage to the right hemisphere; we have found that most patients with TBI underestimate the extent of their cognitive impairments (Anderson and Tranel, 1989; see also Prigatano, 1991). Furthermore, unawareness of cognitive impairments has been shown to be one of the most important predictors of rehabilitation outcome and return to employment (Diller, 1994; Ezrachi et al., 1991). Awareness of acquired cognitive impairments is particularly important when treatment plans emphasize use of compensatory procedures (i.e., the problem must be recognized before an attempt is made to compensate for it). The initial feedback session, educational sessions, and patient involvement in formulating the treatment plan provide opportunities to identify and address discrepancies between the patient's view of his condition and the impression gained from the neuropsychological assessment and report of family members.

Related to this is the importance of the patient accepting and working toward realistic goals, which are likely to be lower than preinjury expectations. Goal setting generally is a collaborative endeavor in which one of the therapist's tasks is to break down large and distant goals into a hierarchy of tangible subgoals.

Psychotherapy

As pointed out by Diller (1992), issues of awareness, motivation, and self-concept play an enormous role in the engagement of a patient in rehabilitation procedures. It follows that an element of psychotherapy is woven into virtually every neuropsychological rehabilitation program. A neuropsychologist who does not frame cognitive retraining and compensatory procedures in a context of the tools of psychotherapy (including use of motivational principles, reinforcement of adaptive behavior, empathic listening and support, exploration of emotional states, and pragmatic collaborative problem solving) is ignoring the rich literature on psychotherapy and behavior change and is doing the patient a grave disservice.

When planning the psychotherapeutic component of a rehabilitation program, there is a critical need to attend to the patient's premorbid personality characteristics. Pre-existing behavioral tendencies, modes of social interaction, and affective predispositions always contribute to a patient's personality after brain injury, and characteristics that were firmly ingrained before the injury typically are intractable to change from short-term interventions. When soliciting information regarding premorbid status, it is important to augment the patient's self-report with interviews of family members and review of available relevant records (e.g., employer evaluations, psychiatric records, academic records).

Depression, resulting from damage to the neural substrates of emotion as well as psychological reactions to the consequences of the brain injury, is a frequent target of intervention. We often combine pharmacologic treatment with psychotherapy and have found a cognitive-behavioral approach based on Beck's (1979) framework to be a useful starting point for psychotherapy. For further discussion of the role of psychotherapy in facilitating adjustment after brain injury, see Ellis (1989), Christensen and Rosenberg (1991), and Miller (1993).

Anxiety can exacerbate virtually any cognitive impairment resulting from brain damage. Our patients with TBI frequently complain of concentration problems, increased difficulty with word finding, and worsened short-term memory in anxiety-eliciting social situations. This can have devastating implications for job interviews, dating, and other interactions that help shape the patient's post-trauma life. We have found that these problems often can be addressed without resorting to anxiolytic drugs. Progressive muscle relaxation training (Bernstein and Borkovec, 1973) has proved to be an efficacious intervention for our patients with anxiety problems. This procedure involves learning to tense and relax sequentially various muscle groups throughout the body, while attending to the feelings associated with the tension and relaxation. The rationale and procedures are simple and readily mastered by most patients. Once learned, the technique can unobtrusively be applied in anxiety-eliciting situations. The fact that progressive muscle relaxation is motorically based is important for two reasons when working with brain-injured patients. First, procedural memory, including motor memory or memory for complex movement sequences, typically is preserved even when other aspects of memory are quite impaired (for reviews, see Cohen, 1984; Moscovitch, 1982; Tranel et al., 1994b). This facilitates fairly rapid learning and retention of the procedure. Second, the cognitive demands are minimal at the time of application, allowing the patient's cognitive resources to be directed to the other tasks at hand.

Drawing up therapeutic contracts that include explicit relationships between desired behaviors and reinforcement also is an effective psychotherapeutic tool across multiple situations. Contingency management or behavior modification procedures have a wide range of applicability in treating the consequences of brain injury, including such areas as overcoming behavior initiation problems, decreasing socially inappropriate behavior, and decreasing seizure frequency (reviewed by Mostofsky, 1993).

Environmental Modifications and Compensatory Devices

Use of environmental management stems from the recognition that it is difficult, and sometimes impossible, to re-establish some cognitive abilities. The patient's immediate environment, however, usually can be modified quite readily, at least to some extent. Recently, the Americans with Disabilities Act has directed increased attention to practical environmental and task modifications. Many environmental modifications take the form of increased organization (e.g., of the workplace, of records, of personal effects such as billfold and keys), which can decrease the demands on memory and executive functions, and thus benefit most brain-injured patients involved in cognitive rehabilitation. Many commercially available devices, such as wrist watches with alarms, key finders, miniature tape recorders, portable personal computers, and software with spelling and grammar corrections, can be incorporated into the compensatory training of some patients.

We encourage our patients to be innovative in finding solutions that are practical for their own unique situations. An example of this is provided by a patient of ours with right temporal lobe damage and resultant memory problems, particularly for visual and spatial information. He enjoyed working on his acreage, doing tasks such as mending fences, landscaping, and maintaining and renovating several older buildings but had a severe problem with losing his tools. He spent countless frustrating hours searching his property for missing tools and ruined some tools by leaving them outside exposed to the elements. He came on the simple and effective solution of painting the handles of all his tools bright orange. His memory defect was unchanged, but he no longer lost his tools.

SPECIFIC PROCEDURES

Attention

Attention is involved in virtually all effortful cognition, and complaints of memory and other functional difficulties often can be traced to underlying attentional defects. Because of the pervasive influence of attention and the fact that attentional impairments are common after brain injury, such defects frequently have been the target of cognitive rehabilitation programs. Unfortunately, there is much more agreement about the importance of attention and attentional defects than there is about the definition or mechanisms of attention. Given that the neuropsychological basis of attention is so poorly understood, it is not surprising that empirical findings on the efficacy of attention rehabilitation have been mixed. Several studies have reported no beneficial effects on outcome measures or a failure of improvements to generalize beyond the trained task (e.g., Gansler and McCaffrey , 1991; Niemann et al., 1990; Ponsford and Kinsella, 1988).

However, positive effects of attentional training programs also have been described in multiple studies (e.g., Gray, 1991; Gray and Robertson, 1992; Rattock et al., 1982). Sohlberg and Mateer (1987) used a single-case experimental design to evaluate the treatment of four attention-impaired patients. A series of computer-based vigilance tasks and more complex alternating and divided-attention tasks were applied over 5 to 10 weeks. Improvement was found on a measure of sustained attention, in the absence of improvement on nonattentional control tasks. Niemann et al. (1990) applied similar attention training and found greater improvement on attention and memory tasks from this approach than from training in the use of mnemonic techniques. Recently, positive findings on neuropsychological tests of attention and relatives' ratings of daily behavior were found after training on a multimodal computer system that allowed the difficulty level of training tasks to be individualized (Ruff et al., 1994).

Given the difficulties in generalizing training benefits from the specific tasks used in attention rehabilitation to other attention-demanding tasks, there is good reason to direct rehabilitation efforts to the real-world tasks for which improved performance is desired. For example, Wilson and Robertson (1992) used shaping procedures, planned breaks, and intentional controlled distraction to reduce attentional lapses while reading. This task-specific approach to attentional rehabilitation clearly warrants further investigation.

In summary, there have been sufficient positive findings to instill a sense of optimism regarding the potential benefit of attentional retraining tasks. However, it is abundantly clear that simply having a patient perform attention-demanding computer tasks does not constitute rehabilitation of attention. Task-specific attentional rehabilitation holds promise, and as pointed out by Wood (1992), repetitive practice and systematic use of reinforcement are likely to continue to emerge as practical tools of attentional rehabilitation.

Memory

Given that impairment of memory is one of the most common sequelae of brain injury, it is an unfortunate fact that memory disorder, in nearly all cases, cannot be cured or eliminated. However, this should not lead to an attitude of nihilism regarding the treatment of memory disorders. There are several avenues of intervention that can minimize the negative impact of memory problems in the daily lives of the patients and those around them.

Treatment must begin with a neuropsychological evaluation, which serves to (1) identify the severity and pattern of memory defects (e.g., the relative degree of impairment of verbal and visual memory, the possible preservation of procedural memory, or particular problems with either the acquisition or retention phases of delayed recall) and (2) characterize cognitive and behavioral factors outside of the domain of memory that either may contribute to worsening of the memory problem or, in the case of relatively preserved abilities (such as reading comprehension), be used in rehabilitation to help compensate for the memory impairment.

Memory problems after TBI can be exacerbated greatly by factors in addition to damage of the neural systems underlying memory, and often times these factors are amenable to change. For example, is the patient taking medications that may exacerbate memory problems (e.g., anticholinergic antidepressants or benzodiazepines)? Do anxiety or stress reactions contribute substantially to the patient's memory difficulties? Are the problems more in the domain of attention rather than memory? After parceling out these nonmemory factors that often contribute to memory problems, specific and circumscribed memory-related problems in the patient's daily life can be addressed.

Training in the use of compensatory strategies (e.g., increased time and deliberate attention directed toward memory tasks, use of repetition, increased organization, and external aids) has been found to be more effective than a memory drill and practice control condition, and these benefits were maintained at a 4-month follow-up (Berg et al., 1991). Likewise, Freeman et al. (1992) found that a group of subjects with TBI who underwent training in compensatory and executive strategies for memory enhancement showed better recall of paragraph-length material than did a matched control group who did not receive the treatment. The intervention consisted of approximately 15 hours of training in note-taking, rehearsal, and self-monitoring skills. Ryan and Ruff (1988) provided evidence that head-injured patients with milder impairments benefited from training in attention and memory but that patients with more severe cognitive defects did not.

Ewert et al. (1989) demonstrated that patients with severe declarative memory defects after closed head injury were able to acquire and retain procedural skills. These findings suggest that efforts directed at practical skill learning can be an efficacious approach to rehabilitation after head injury. Domain-specific learning may be a reasonable goal with patients for whom more generalized memory rehabilitation is not possible (e.g., Glisky and Schacter, 1987). Baddeley (1992) has suggested a technique by which relatively preserved procedural memory and errorless learning techniques are combined. Adequate step-by-step lists and cues are provided such that the patient is able to perform a specific behavioral routine without recourse to episodic memory and without error on the initial trial. Additional support for the use of errorless learning techniques in the rehabilitation of persons with memory impairment recently has been provided by Wilson et al. (1994).

The use of mnemonics has been associated with memory improvement since the time of ancient Greece and is fairly well known in the general public. Richardson (1992) reviewed the use of visual imagery mnemonic techniques for the rehabilitation of patients with head injury and other neurologic conditions and concluded that these techniques are of little value in helping brain-injured patients in real-life tasks. Although training in imagery mnemonic techniques can improve performance on memory tests, the benefits are primarily limited to learning lists of concrete objects (when a simple written list would suffice). Furthermore, the effective use of these procedures in the face of real-world challenges requires considerable insight and motivation, which generally are not among the strengths of persons with brain injury.

External Memory Aids

Almost everyone uses or has used external memory aids, such as taking notes during a lecture, making shopping lists, and marking events or appointments on a calendar. Given this almost universal experience, in a rehabilitation setting it usually is not difficult to explain the concept of external memory aids or to convince patients of their use. However, it can be considerably more difficult to facilitate consistent and practical use of external memory aids.

Matching the device with the specific need is a key to success. The use of any individual external memory aid will be specific to certain tasks and situations (see Herrmann and Petro, 1990), but there can be broader implications. Although much of the use of external memory aids stems from their independence from "natural" memory, it also is true that the act of using an external memory aid can facilitate memory (e.g., taking notes can aid in the encoding of information) (Kiewra, 1985).

We have found training in the use of memory books to be one of the most effective and widely applicable compensatory strategies for memory impairments. For example, a 35-year-old woman was referred to our service 1 year after a traumatic injury that damaged the inferomedial temporal lobes bilaterally. She had a severe and stable anterograde amnesia and a mild retrograde memory impairment, in the context of otherwise well-preserved cognitive abilities. With systematic training in the use of a memory notebook incorporating elements of a detailed appointment book and a personal diary, she was able to resume her role as a homemaker, including care for her two young children, and return to her secretarial job on a limited basis. Guides to overcoming initial resistance and other obstacles to successful use of a memory book are provided by Sohlberg and Mateer (1989) and Burke et al. (1994).

Visual Perception

TBI can result in damage to the visual system from the level of the retina to higher-order visual association cortices. Some form of visual dysfunction occurs in more than 50 percent of head-injured patients (Gianutsos et al., 1988; Schlageter et al., 1993), and impaired vision has been found to be among the most frequently reported long-term symptoms of head injury (Carlsson et al., 1987). Cognitive rehabilitation of higher-order visual perceptual defects must be coordinated with treatment of peripheral visual impairments, and all treatment must be based on detailed neuro-opthalmologic and neuropsychological evaluations (Anderson and Rizzo, 1995).

Visual field defects have been associated with poor outcome in a variety of daily functional activities, including driving (Grosswasser et al., 1990; Johnson and Keltner, 1983). Based on reports that monkeys with striate cortex ablations showed some reduction of visual field defects after systematic practice (Cowey, 1967; Mohler and Wurtz, 1977), patients with visual field defects have been exposed to extensive training in directing saccadic eye movements to targets in their blind visual fields. Although some positive results have been obtained (Zihl, 1981), others have failed to replicate this, suggesting the improvement in the original studies was in test-taking behavior rather than vision (Balliet et al., 1985).

Given the limited success of procedures aimed at restoration of visual fields, the future of visual field rehabilitation likely lies in training patients in scanning strategies that would allow them to compensate for visual field defects. Pommerenke and Markowitsch (1989) provided compensatory scanning instruction to patients with chronic, stable visual field defects and found that despite no change in the size of the field defect, improvement occurred in the efficiency, accuracy, and scope of visual search patterns. More recently, Kerkoff et al. (1994) provided 22 patients with hemianopias with 30-minute daily training sessions over approximately 5 weeks in a effort to improve saccadic eye movement strategies. Twelve of 22 patients (54 percent) showed partial restitution of visual fields as mapped with visual perimetry, although in 9 of the 12, the visual field increase was less than 8 degrees. The greatest improvement in visual field size was 24 degrees. Of more importance was the finding that all 22 patients showed significant increases in visual search field. The rehabilitation program included specific steps to transfer the treatment gains to daily life; improvements were found on an ecologically valid visual search test, and 20 of 22 patients returned to work. Treatment gains were maintained at a 3-month follow-up. These findings support the use of training in compensatory eye movement strategies for patients with acquired visual field defects.

Executive Functions and Interpersonal Skills

The interaction between brain and skull in TBI is such that the ventral surface of the frontal lobes is particularly vulnerable to damage. The relationships between damage to this brain area and impairments of decision making, rational judgment, planning, and interpersonal behavior are becoming increasingly apparent (Damasio, 1994; Damasio and Anderson, 1993). These so-called executive functions (Tranel et al., 1994a) are not only critical to normal dailyactivities in and of themselves but also affect and potentially thwart rehabilitation of other cognitive and physical impairments.

When such defects are severe, as is more commonly the case in early stages of recovery, contingency management procedures often can result in some degree of behavioral improvement. Somewhat paradoxically, the milder and more subtle defects of executive functions seem to be more difficult to diagnose accurately and treat. For example, occasional problems with social disinhibition, poor decision making, or amotivation may wreak havoc on the life of a person with TBI.

There has been little controlled research on the treatment of defects such as impaired problem solving or planning in the brain-injured population that would allow conclusions to be drawn regarding real-world implications, although provision of increased structure (e.g., checklists, schedules) and training in self-instruction appear to have some support. For example, Burke et al. (1991) described a series of case studies in which checklists and extensive feedback were used to improve behavior initiation and problem solving in patients with head injury, and several studies have reported positive effects of self-instructional training (e.g., Cicerone and Giacino, 1992; Cicerone and Wood, 1987; Webster and Scott, 1983).

Perhaps more so than with any other aspect of cognitive rehabilitation, treatment of executive function defects requires involvement of the patient's family. Although hardly a satisfactory solution, education of the patient and family regarding the nature of his or her executive function impairments, coupled with a partial shifting of executive reponsibilities to the non-brain-injured members of the family, constitutes one of the most pragmatic interventions available, given the present limitations of empirically supported executive function interventions and the financial climate for rehabilitation services.

Behavior modification programs, including token economies, have been successfully applied to reduce inappropriate behaviors and increase prosocial behaviors in inpatient head injury rehabilitation facilities (e.g., Hopewell et al., 1991; Peters et al., 1992; Wood, 1987), but these procedures are more problematic in the less controlled setting of outpatient rehabilitation. Executive function defects that are incompatible with independent daily functioning may occur at a low base rate and often appear only in dynamic interactions with real-world exigencies, making treatment extremely difficult.

Problems with aggression and anger control are common after TBI. Successful treatment of aggression usually depends on careful analysis of the stimulus conditions in which aggressive behavior is evoked. When the patient is in a supervised environment, positive reinforcement can be used to increase the frequency of behaviors incompatible with aggression in situations likely to elicit aggression. Extinction techniques also can be effective, particularly when the powerful reinforcing effects of social attention are recognized (see Haffey and Scibak, 1989, for a discussion of the use of behavioral techniques for treatment of aggression).

Uomoto and Brockway (1992) documented the effectiveness of a short-term anger control program that combined training the patient in self-instruction anger management skills and training the family in implementing time-out procedures and other behavior management techniques. Training in self-instruction techniques also can be used to treat behavioral dyscontrol problems other than anger, such as inappropriate verbalizations (Burgess and Alderman, 1990).

Individual outpatient psychotherapy has been applied with some success in the treatment of interpersonal behavior problems, including disinhibition and social alienation, after TBI (Becker and Vakil, 1993). Selection of circumscribed and pragmatic goals, application of exaggerated reinforcement schedules, and collaboration with external social support systems (e.g., family, workplace) were among the keys to success of such interventions. Videotape feedback is a potentially useful tool in social skills training programs. Helffenstein and Wechsler (1982) found that rehabilitation sessions involving social situation role playing by the therapist and client were more effective if the sessions were videotaped and immediately reviewed.

Group interventions for social skills training also are used in many cognitive rehabilitation programs (e.g., Ben-Yishay and Diller, 1981; Deaton, 1991). In addition to being cost-effective, group interventions provide for multiple distractions and greater unpredictability than individual sessions and thus can be more comparable to social settings outside the rehabilitation facility.

CONCLUSIONS

Cognitive rehabilitation is in an early stage of development as a scientifically based clinical discipline. The need for rational treatment of cognitive impairments after TBI is immense and not likely to diminish in the foreseeable future. The potential benefits of efficacious cognitive rehabilitation programs are considerable, in terms of improved quality of life for patients and families, reduced economic burden of brain injury, and reduced long-term drain on the health care system.

The field must become increasingly accountable. A body of research needs to be developed to address the large questions of what procedures will work for which patients and what outcomes may reasonably be expected. Refinements of current techniques and development of innovative new procedures will proceed as the link is strengthened between cognitive rehabilitation and the rapid progress in cognitive neuroscience.

Given the gaps in our understanding of the neural basis of cognition, it is not surprising that our expertise is limited when it comes to fixing the system when it is damaged. Self-awareness of one's limitations is a prerequisite to behavioral improvement, and practitioners of cognitive rehabilitation need to proceed with explicit recognition of current limitations in understanding of how a particular injury resulted in the neuropsychological profile of a given patient and how it is that a patient's brain will reorganize over time to effect recovery. In this context, what can be done is to implement learning experiences that there is empirical and theoretical reason to believe will result in improvement of brain-injured patients' ability to compensate for acquired cognitive and behavioral impairments.

REFERENCES

Anderson SW, Rizzo M: Recovery and rehabilitation of visual cortical dysfunction. Neurorehabilitation, 5:129–140, 1995

Anderson SW, Tranel D: Awareness of disease states following cerebral infarction, dementia, and head trauma: standardized assessment. Clin Neuropsychol 3:327–339, 1989

Baddeley AD: Implicit memory and errorless learning: a link between cognitive theory and neuropsychological rehabilitation? In Squire LR, Butters N (eds): Neuropsychology of Memory. 2nd Ed. Guilford Press, New York, 1992

Balliet R, Blood KMT, Bach-Y-Rita P: Visual field rehabilitation in the cortically blind? J Neurol Neurosurg Psychiatry 48:1113–1124, 1985

Beck AT: Cognitive Therapy of Depression. Guilford Press, New York, 1979

Becker ME, Vakil E: Behavioural psychotherapy of the frontal lobe injured patient in an outpatient setting. Brain Inj 7:515–523, 1993

Ben-Yishay Y, Diller L: Rehabilitation of cognitive and perceptual deficits in people with traumatic brain damage. Int J Rehabil Res 4:208–210, 1981

Ben-Yishay Y, Diller L: Cognitive remediation in traumatic brain injury: update and issues. Arch Phys Med Rehabil 74:204–213, 1993

Berg IJ, Koning-Haanstra M, Deelman BG: Long-term effects of memory rehabilitation: a controlled study. Neuropsychol Rehabil 1:97–111, 1991

Bernstein DA, Borkovec TD: Progressive Relaxation Training. Research Press, Champaign, IL, 1973

Burgess PW, Alderman N: Rehabilitation of dyscontrol syndromes following frontal lobe damage: a cognitive neuropsychological approach. pp. 183–203. In Wood RL, Fussey I (eds): Cognitive Rehabilitation in Perspective. Taylor & Francis, New York, 1990

Burke JM, Danicke JA, Bemis B, Durgin CJ: A process approach to memory book training for neurological patients. Brain Inj 8:71–81, 1994

Burke WH, Zencius AH, Weslowski MD et al: Improving executive function disorders in brain injured clients. Brain Inj 5:241–252, 1991

Carlsson GS, Svardsudd K, Welin L: Long-term effects of head injuries sustained during life in three male populations. J Neurosurg 67:197–205, 1987

Cicerone KD, Giacino JT: Remediation of executive function deficits after traumatic brain injury. Neurorehabilitation 2:12–22, 1992

Cicerone KD, Wood JC: Planning disorder after closed head injury: a case study. Arch Phys Med Rehabil 68:111–115, 1987

Cohen NJ: Preserved learning capacity in amnesia: evidence for multiple memory systems. In Squire L, Butters N (eds): Neuropsychology of Memory. Guilford Press, New York, 1984

Cowey A: Perimetric study of field defects in monkeys after cortical and retinal ablations. Q J Exp Psychol 19:232–245, 1967

Damasio AR: Descarte's Error: Emotion, Reason, and the Human Brain. Grosset/Putnam, New York, 1994

Damasio AR, Anderson SW: The frontal lobes. pp. 409–460. In Heilman K, Valenstein E (eds): Clinical Neuropsychology. 3rd Ed. Oxford University Press, New York, 1993

Deaton AV: Group interventions for cognitive rehabilitation: increasing the challenges. pp. 101–200. In Kreutzer JS, Wehman PH (eds): Cognitive Rehabilitation for Persons with Traumatic Brain Injury. Paul H. Brookes, Baltimore, 1991

Diller L: Neuropsychological rehabilitation. pp. 105–114. In Rose FD, Johnson DA (eds): Recovery from Brain Damage. Plenum Press, New York, 1992

Diller L: Neuropsychological rehabilitation: current issues for theory and practice. Workshop, Twenty-second Annual Meeting of the International Neuropsychological Society, Cincinnati, OH, 1994

Diller L, Goodgold J, Kay T: Final report to NIDRR for the Rehabilitation Research and Training Center in Head Trauma and Stroke. New York University Medical Center, 1988

Ellis DW: Neuropsychotherapy. pp. 241–269. In Ellis DW, Christensen AL (eds): Neuropsychological Treatment after Brain Injury. Kluwar Academic Publishers, Boston, 1989

Ewert J, Levin HS, Watson MG, Kalisky Z: Procedural memory during posttraumatic amnesia in survivors of severe closed head injury. Arch Neurol 46:911–916, 1989

Ezrachi O, Ben-Yishay Y, Kay T et al: Predicting employment in traumatic brain injury following neuropsychological rehabilitation. J Head Trauma Rehabil 6:71–84, 1991

Finger S, Stein DG: Environmental and experiential determinants of recovery of function. pp. 175–202. In Finger S, Stein D (eds): Brain Damage and Recovery. Academic Press, New York, 1982

Freeman MR, Mittenberg W, Dicowden M, Bat-Ami M: Executive and compensatory memory retraining in traumatic brain injury. Brain Inj 6:65–70, 1992

Gansler DA, McCaffrey RJ: Remediation of chronic attention deficits in traumatic brain-injured patients. Arch Clin Neuropsychol 6:335–353, 1991

Gianutsos R, Ramsey G, Perlin RR: Rehabilitative optometric services for survivors of acquired brain injury. Arch Phys Med Rehabil 69:573–578, 1988

Glisky E, Schacter DL: Acquisition of domain-specific knowledge in organic amnesia: training for computer-related work. Neuropsychologia 25:893–906, 1987

Gordon WA, Hibbard MR, Kreutzer J: Cognitive remediation: issues in research and practice. J Head Trauma Rehabil 4:76–84, 1989

Gray JM: The remediation of attentional disorders following brain injury of acute onset. pp. 29–47. In Wood RL, Fussey I (eds): Cognitive Rehabilitation in Perspective. Taylor & Francis, New York, 1991

Gray JM, Robertson I: Microcomputer-based attentional retraining after brain damage: a randomised group controlled trial. Neuropsychol Rehabil 2:97–115, 1992

Grosswasser Z, Cohen M, Blankstein E: Polytrauma associated with traumatic brain injury: incidence, nature and impact on rehabilitation outcome. Brain Inj 4:161–166, 1990

Gualtieri CT: Pharmacotherapy and the neurobehavioral sequelae of traumatic brain injury. Brain Inj 2:101–129, 1988

Haffey WJ, Scibak JW: Management of aggressive behavior following traumatic brain injury. pp. 317–360. In Ellis DW, Christensen AL (eds): Neuropsychological Treatment after Brain Injury. Kluwer Academic Publishers, Boston, 1989

Harley JP, Allen C, Braciszeski T, et al.: Guidelines for cognitive rehabilitation. Neurorehabilitation 2:62–67, 1992

Helffenstein DA, Wechsler FS: The use of interpersonal process recall (IPR) in the remediation of interpersonal and communication skill deficits in the newly brain-injured. Clin Neuropsychol 4:139–143, 1982

Herrmann DJ, Petro SJ: Commercial memory aids. Appl Cognitive Psychol 4:439–450, 1990

Hopewell CA, Burke WH, Weslowski M, Zawlocki R: Behavioral learning therapies for the traumatically brain-injured patient. pp. 229–245. In Wood RL, Fussey I (eds): Cognitive Rehabilitation in Perspective. Taylor & Francis, New York, 1991

Johnson CA, Keltner JL: Incidence of visual field loss in 20,000 eyes and its relationship to driving performance. Arch Opthamol 101:371–375, 1983

Kerkoff G, MunBinger U, Meier EK: Neurovisual rehabilitation in cerebral blindness. Arch Neurol 51:474–481, 1994

Kiewra KA: Investigation notetaking and review: a depth of processing alternative. Educ Psychol 20:23–32, 1985

Mathews CG, Harley JP, Malec JE: Task force report Division 40-Clinical Neuropsychology, APA. Guidelines for computer-assisted neuropsychological rehabilitation and cognitive remediation. Clin Neuropsychol 5: 3–19, 1991

Medical Disability Society: Report of the working party on the management of traumatic brain injury. Royal College of Physicians, London, 1988

Miller L: Psychotherapy of the Brain-Injured Patient. W.W. Norton & Company, New York, 1993

Mohler CW, Wurtz RH: Role of striate cortex and superior colliculus in visual guidance of saccadic eye movements in monkeys. J Neurophysiol 40:74–94, 1977

Moscovitch M: Multiple dissociations of function in amnesia. pp. 357–370. In Cermak LS (ed): Human Memory and Amnesia. Lawrence Erlbaum, Hillsdale, N.J., 1982

Mostofsky DI: Behavior modification and therapy in the management of epileptic disorders. pp. 67–81. In Mostofsky DI, Loyning Y (eds): The Neurobehavioral Treatment of Epilepsy. Lawrence Erlbaum Associates, Hillsdale, N.J., 1993

Niemann H, Ruff RM, Baser CA: Computer-assisted attention retraining in head-injured individuals: a controlled efficacy study of an outpatient program. J Consult Clin Psychol 58:811–817, 1990

Peters MD, Gluck M, McCormick M: Behaviour rehabilitation of the challenging client in less restrictive settings. Brain Inj 6:288–314, 1992

Pommerenke K, Markowitsch JH: Rehabilitation training of homonymous visual field defects in patients with postgeniculate damage of the visual system. Restorative Neurol Neurosci 1:47–63, 1989

Ponsford JL, Kinsella G: Evaluation of a remedial programme for attentional deficits following closed head injury. J Clin Exp Neuropsychol 10:693–708, 1988

Prigatano GP: Disturbances of self-awareness of deficit after traumatic brain injury. pp. 111–126. In Prigatano GP, Schacter DL (eds): Awareness of Deficit after Brain Injury. Oxford University Press, New York, 1991

Rattok J, Ben-Yishay Y, Ross B et al: A diagnostic-remedial system for basic attentional disorders in head trauma patients undergoing rehabilitation: a preliminary report. In: Working Approaches to Remediation of Cognitive Deficits in Brain Damaged Persons: Rehabilitation Monograph No. 64. New York University Medical Center, New York, 1982

Richardson JTE: Imagery mnemonics and memory remediation. Neurology 42:283–286, 1992

Ruff R, Mahaffey R, Engel J et al: Efficacy study of THINKable in the attention and memory retraining of traumatically head-injured patients. Brain Inj 8:3–14, 1994

Ryan TV, Ruff RM: The efficacy of structured memory retraining in a group comparison of head injured patients. Arch Clin Neuropsychol 3:165–179, 1988

Schlageter K, Gray B, Hall K et al: Incidence and treatment of visual dysfunction in traumatic brain injury. Brain Inj 7:439–448, 1993

Sohlberg MM, Mateer CA: Effectiveness of an attention-training program. J Clin Exp Neuropsychol 9:117–130, 1987

Sohlberg MM, Mateer CA: Training use of compensatory memory books: a three stage behavioral approach. J Clin Exp Neuropsychol 11:871–891, 1989

Thorndike EL, Woodworth RS: The influence of improvement in one mental function upon the efficiency of other functions. Psychol Rev 8:247–261, 1901

Tranel D: The Iowa-Benton school of neuropsychological assessment. In Grant I, Adams KM (eds): Neuropsychological Assessment of Neuropsychiatric Disorders. 2nd Ed. Oxford University Press, New York, 1994

Tranel D, Anderson SW, Benton AL: Development of the concept of executive functions and its relationship to the frontal lobes. In Boller F, Grafman J (eds): Handbook of Neuropsychology. Vol. 9. Elsevier, New York, 1994a

Tranel D, Damasio AR, Damasio H, Brandt JP: Sensorimotor skill learning in amnesia: additional evidence for the neural basis of nondeclarative memory. Learning Memory 1:165–179, 1994b

Uomoto J, Brockway JA: Anger management for brain injured patients and their family members. Arch Phys Med Rehabil 73:674–679, 1992

Volpe BT, McDowell FH: The efficacy of cognitive rehabilitation in patients with traumatic brain injury. Arch Neurol 47:220–222, 1990

Webster JS, Scott RR: The effects of self-instructional training of attentional deficits following head injury. Clin Neuropsychol 5:69–74, 1983

Will B, Kelche C: Environmental approaches to recovery of function from brain damage: a review of animal studies. pp. 79–103. In Rose FD, Johnson DA (eds): Recovery from Brain Damage. Plenum Press, New York, 1992

Wilson BA, Baddeley A, Evans J: Errorless learning in the rehabilitation of memory impaired people. Neuropsychol Rehabil 4:307–326, 1994

Wilson C, Robertson IH: A home-based intervention for attentional slips during reading following head injury: a single case study. Neuropsychol Rehabil 2:193–205, 1992

Wood RL: Brain Injury Rehabilitation: A Neurobehavioral Approach. Aspen Publishers, Rockville, MD, 1987

Wood RL: Disorders of attention. pp. 216–242. In Wilson BA, Moffat N (eds): Clincial Management of Memory Problems. 2nd Ed. Chapman & Hall, London, 1992

Zihl J: Recovery of visual functions in patients with cerebral blindness. Exp Brain Res 44:159–169, 1981

Forensic Issues in the Neuropsychological Assessment of Patients with Postconcussive Syndrome

24

Paul R. Lees-Haley
John T. Dunn

Postconcussive syndrome has a long and controversial history. The controversy surrounding the diagnosis of this syndrome is reflected in the latest version of the diagnostic manual of mental disorders *Diagnostic and Statistical Manual of Mental Disorders*—Fourth Edition (American Psychiatric Association, 1994), which relegates postconcussive syndrome to an appendix rather than identifying it as a standard diagnostic category. It is reported in the DSM-IV that the proposal for the diagnosis of "postconcussional disorder" underwent a careful empirical review that included wide commentary from the applicable field. However, the DSM-IV task force determined that there was insufficient information to warrant inclusion of this proposal as an official diagnosis and suggested that further research be conducted on the proposed diagnosis of postconcussive syndrome to help determine its possible use and refinement of the criteria set. Adding to the controversy regarding this syndrome, the *International Classification of Diseases*—9th Revision—*Clinical Modification* (ICD-9-CM) (Med-Index, 1991) indicates that the symptoms of postconcussive syndrome may occur in other conditions and are more common in persons who have previously suffered from neurotic or personality disorders or when there is a possibility of compensation.

Although there is no generally accepted definition, certain symptoms have come to be associated with closed head injuries, often referred to as concussions or contusions of the brain. These symptoms include complaints of headache, fatigue, insomnia, dizziness, memory loss, impaired intellectual ability, moodiness, irritability, anxiety, depression, and an increased sensitivity to noise (American Psychiatric Association, 1994).

Because the symptoms of postconcussive syndrome are unclear, ill-defined, and more common among persons with neurotic or personality disorders, the primary purpose of forensic neuropsychological assessment is to evaluate the patient's current cognitive status and compare it with a thorough and reasonable estimate of preinjury status, thus determining the nature and extent of functional losses. Assessment for the general presence of organicity or brain damage is not the primary purpose, because we all have neuropsychological limitations that can be reflected in test results. For example, an examinee who has a preexisting weakness in mathematics is likely to perform poorly on the Arithmetic subtest of the Wechsler Adult Intelligence Scale-Revised (WAIS-R) (frequently administered in neuropsychological evaluations) relative to other subtests. This relatively lower performance is not the result of suspected brain damage from a recent event, but due to an innate cognitive weakness the examinee has shown throughout schooling. The goal of the forensic neuropsychological assessment is identification of functional losses in important areas of everyday living.

Certain essential questions are addressed in most forensic neuropsychological assessments of brain injury. These include determination of whether there was an injury and, if so, its nature and extent; the cause of injury; the impact of the injury on important cognitive functions and personality; whether the deficits are treatable and, if so, through what procedures; the prognosis; and other consequences of the injury that may affect the patient's life.

More specifically, questions that often need to be addressed in forensic neuropsychological evaluations are the following: In what areas is the patient showing deficits, if any? Is the patient able to work? If so, in what capacity? Are there any disabilities from a psychological or neuropsychological perspective? Is the patient able to live independently and attend to activities of daily living? Is there a need for supervision and, if so, in what areas? Has the patient's intellectual functioning returned to premorbid levels? Answering questions such as these enables an examiner to identify a patient's functional losses in the areas of everyday living. However, neuropsychological evaluations in litigated cases pose a special challenge to examiners due to the presence of secondary gain, possible financial compensation, and response bias that develops in association with litigation. Therefore, a specific methodology is suggested to ensure that the examiner obtains the most accurate assessment of a patient's neuropsychological status.

METHODOLOGY

As indicated, forensic neuropsychological assessment is essentially a measurement of pre- and postinjury status through comparison of data gathered from sources such as history, psychological and neuropsychological testing, and mental status observations. File reviews provide a basis for opinions about the patient's past status and often contain information permitting formation of opinions about future expectations. Evaluation of the patient in person permits assessment of current mental status and application of testing procedures and provides further foundation for outcome predictions.

The patient's history may be obtained through a variety of avenues, with the most common being first-person interviews of the patient and a thorough review of appropriate records. Pre- and postinjury medical records, psychological records, educational records, and employment records are especially useful and commonly offer a more objective picture of a patient's preinjury status in litigated cases than first-person interviews. Many patients have had preinjury cognitive and aptitude testing in academic settings or have been tested in other environments such as the military, employment, or psychologists' offices. For example, a review of a patient's school records with an emphasis on the examinee's grade point average, specific class performance, achievement test results (e.g., Iowa tests), and aptitude test results (e.g., SAT) will provide a useful estimation of a patient's preinjury level of cognitive functioning.

A common error when comparing a patient's preinjury cognitive functioning with postinjury cognitive functioning is overestimating the patient's preinjury status based on speculation or unreliable self-reports. For example, as opposed to giving more weight to objective school records that may indicate a low grade point average and poor aptitude and achievement test scores, neuropsychologists sometimes will rely on the patient's subjective self-report that he or she was not interested in school or was an academic underachiever but, nonetheless, possessed superior intellectual abilities before being injured.

When assessing the premorbid intelligence of a patient, it is important not to speculate about the intellectual functioning required for preinjury occupations or level of educational attainment. A good source for objective determination of the intelligence level required for a specific preinjury occupation is the reference material associated with the *Dictionary of Occupational Titles* published by the U.S. Department of Labor. Additional data useful for estimating a patient's premorbid IQ based on occupation and level of educational attainment are found in Kaufman's *Assessing Adolescent and Adult Intelligence* (1990). Kaufman presents tables that show the mean IQs earned by different occupational groups for three broad age ranges. The mean WAIS-R full-scale IQ for the professional and technical occupational group was 112, whereas the mean full-scale IQ for skilled workers was 101. Kaufman (1990) also presents the range of full-scale IQs corresponding to different levels of educational attainment and occupational category that shows surprising results. Subjects with 16 or more years of education (i.e., having at least a 4-year degree) had full-scale IQs ranging from 87 to 148. Subjects in the highest-level occupational group (professional and technical) had IQs ranging from 81 to 148. These data underscore the caution examiners need to use when estimating a patient's premorbid level of intellectual functioning in assuming that an examinee with a college education possessed a superior IQ preinjury. An additional caveat is associated with the trend for progressively greater proportions of the population to graduate from high school and obtain some college training. To the extent that a greater proportion of the population achieves a particular level of education, that level of education is indicative of a lower IQ as characterized by standard scores for age cohorts, which is the generally accepted procedure for defining IQ. Examiners should base estimates of premorbid intelligence on objective and empirical sources such as those discussed above.

HISTORY

A thorough and accurate history is essential to a comprehensive neuropsychological evaluation. One of the most common reasons experts reach inaccurate conclusions about brain injuries is lack of a thorough and accurate history. An extraordinary number of confounding variables undermine presumptive conclusions. Speculation and conjecture do not provide a basis for opinions in valid neuropsychological assessments.

Common errors are inaccurate estimates of preinjury functioning based on reports from unreliable sources, not discovering pre-existing impairments and prior injuries, lack of awareness regarding preinjury cognitive functioning and psychosocial stressors influencing the patient's performance, missing information about pre-existing psychological problems or mental disorders, and the widespread tendency for clinicians to presume etiology based on the examinee's conclusions about etiology. Alcoholism, substance abuse, and problems secondary to personality disorders can be omissions that lead to incomplete histories and erroneous conclusions.

Collateral interviews with relatives and friends of the patient are usually helpful in clinical cases to assist in determining differences between premorbid and postinjury functioning. It has also been suggested that collateral interviews are often the best single source of data regarding a patient's condition because objective neuropsychological test results lack ecologic validity (i.e., test results do not reflect a patient's true ability to function in his or her own environment) (Sbordone, 1991). However, in litigated cases, it is difficult to locate objective observers. Family members, for example, are subject to understandable response biases and a desire to assist relatives to such an extent that their data often are unreliable for purposes of scientifically accurate measurement. Observers with marked affection or animosity toward the patient are questionable prospects when seeking sources of reliable data.

BASE RATES

Neuropsychological measures are usually norm-based measures in which an individual's performance is compared with a normative population (Franzen, 1989). In forensic neuropsychological reports and testimony, deficits or impairments are defined in several ways. For example, individuals at the lower end of the spectrum (e.g., two standard deviations below the mean) tend to be characterized as impaired, regardless of the etiology. Another definition of impairment of neuropsychological deficit is a loss from pre- to postinjury cognitive functioning. When assessing pre- and postinjury differences, it is essential to keep in mind that every individual has variable attention and concentration, imperfect memory, inconsistent motivation, and variable mood states. Thus, it is critical to consider base rates and normal functioning when determining whether an examinee is suffering impairment compared with preinjury status.

Experts such as Meehl and Ziskin have argued for many years that failure to correct for base rates may render opinions erroneous or speculative (e.g., see Faust et al., 1991; Meehl, 1954; Ziskin and Faust, 1988). Recently, there has been an increase in awareness of the importance of base rates in evaluations of personal injury claimants (e.g., see Matarazzo, 1987; Matarazzo, 1990; Matarazzo and Prifitera, 1989; Matarazzo et al., 1988).

A critical problem in knowing how to weigh the value of self-reported complaints as evidence of neuropsychological injury is that so many of these complaints are routinely reported by individuals who have not sustained a brain injury. For example, Gouvier et al. (1988) found that postconcussive symptoms are common in a normal population. Lees-Haley and Brown (1993) found that patients with no history of brain injury who were undergoing a forensic psychological evaluation reported postconcussive symptoms at a high rate compared with outpatients at a group family practice clinic. Following up on this study, Dunn et al. (1993) found that neurotoxic and neuropsychological symptoms were endorsed more frequently by personal injury litigants with no history of brain injury than by outpatients at a group family practice who had a positive history of brain injury but were not involved in litigation. Due to the high base rate of neuropsychological symptoms in forensic populations with no history of brain injury, examiners should not render diagnoses of cognitive deficits without support from correctly interpreted test results. Self-reported symptoms of postconcussion syndrome simply are not sufficiently abnormal to warrant a diagnosis in most cases because they occur so frequently in normal and forensic populations and because they are associated with many other psychological and physical conditions (Med-Index, 1991).

Also, forensic examiners need to remember that statistical significance does not equal abnormality. A frequent example of this occurs when examiners cite statistically significant differences between WAIS-R Verbal and Performance IQs as evidence of cognitive impairment. As Kaufman (1990) has cautioned, statistical significance is not enough; examiners need to determine how unusual or abnormal the difference is among the normal population. Kaufman (1990) provides base rates of Verbal and Performance IQ discrepancies that characterize normal adolescents and adults. He reports that discrepancies of 9 or more points are statistically significant at the 5 percent level, and differences of 12 or more points are significant at the 1 percent level. Nonetheless, 42.4 percent of normal subjects in the WAIS-R standardization sample had Verbal and Performance IQ discrepancies of 9 or more points, and 28.6 percent had differences of 12 or more points. Kaufman (1990) concludes that it is a common phenomenon for adolescents and adults to demonstrate statistically significant differences between WAIS-R Verbal and Performance IQ, and although differences of 9 and 12 points are statistically meaningful, they are not abnormal because they occur too frequently.

FORENSIC ISSUES OF NEUROPSYCHOLOGICAL TESTING

There are a variety of cognitive functions of special interest in neuropsychological assessment. Attention, concentration, memory, and intelligence are commonly tested. Judgment and the ability to manipulate abstract concepts are important. Personality variables usually are evaluated because emotional and interpersonal functioning are frequently affected by serious brain injuries.

There are several points of view concerning which tests should be administered in neuropsychological assessments. The fixed battery approach (e.g., the Halstead-Reitan Neuropsychological Battery or Luria-Nebraska Battery) consists of administering a standard battery of tests to permit a comparison of an examinee's test results with the normative group on each of the tests contained in that standard battery (Golden et al., 1980; Reitan and Wolfson, 1985). By contrast, the flexible battery approach consists of the administration of tests based on the unique requirements or deficits of individual examinees. For example, during the evaluation, unanticipated problems or cognitive deficits may appear. The flexible battery allows an examiner to select tests based on the unique needs of the examinee. The process approach emphasizes the style or strategy that the patient uses in responding to tests rather than using scores, norms, or pass-fail criteria (Goodglass and Kaplan, 1979). Most experts use flexible batteries composed of the tests they prefer for particular applications. The most widely used tests are those to assess intelligence, memory, attention and concentration, concept formation, and personality or emotional problems. Tests from the Halstead-Reitan battery are among the most commonly used in forensic settings.

THREATS TO VALIDITY

Valid forensic neuropsychological assessments require an examiner to cope with a variety of threats to validity. Most neuropsychological tests are subject to voluntary manipulation by a patient. Patients can readily determine how to simulate impairment through intuitively obvious means. Adults, adolescents, and children have all been demonstrated to be capable of manipulating neuropsychological assessment procedures (Faust et al., 1988a; Faust et al., 1988b; Heaton et al., 1978). Lees-Haley and Dunn (1994) found that more than 64 percent of naive subjects were able to identify correctly at least 5 of 10 symptoms associated with postconcussive syndrome, suggesting that symptom self-reporting is not difficult, at least on a symptom checklist. There are many ways to simulate impairment—for example, reporting common subjective symptoms; pretending to forget colors, words, or visual designs; working slowly; responding carelessly; producing vague answers; rendering drawings of poor quality; and random responding. These are only a sampling of the potential means of stimulating impairment through neuropsychological tests and related interviews.

Based on statements in reports and expert testimony, some examiners apparently are convinced that they are able to detect deceit reliably. The research refutes this illusion of diagnostic acumen. The most reasonable working hypothesis appears to be that we can sometimes detect deception, but we all can be fooled (Ekman, 1985). We recommend focusing on the accuracy and reasonableness of the patient's self-report and observable behavior rather than attempting to infer the patient's subjective thoughts and intentions. By attending to observable performance, examiners can recognize genuine injuries in patients who deny them and can identify normal functioning in patients who overestimate their impairment.

Neuropsychological assessment presumes that the examiner obtains the best possible performance on the part of the patient (Reitan and Wolfson, 1985). Lack of or variable motivation may invalidate the results. The examinee's level of motivation needs to be monitored closely throughout the assessment.

Most neuropsychological tests lack any validity scales or internal measures for evaluating the level of cooperation of the patient. In general, these instruments grew out of environments such as inpatient hospital settings in which patient cooperation was presumed or simply was never considered to be a substantive issue. In forensic settings, evaluation of cooperation and malingering is a normal part of a competent assessment. There is a great need for more effective procedures for assessment of these issues. Recent research has focused on forced choice techniques (Hiscock and Hiscock, 1989; Pankratz, 1983, 1988). For forensic purposes, the most promising avenues for research in the near future appear to be techniques with a combination of statistical power and face validity to the trier of fact.

CONCURRENT CONFOUNDS AND PRE-EXISTING PROBLEMS

Victims of postconcussive syndrome come to neuropsychological evaluations with a wide variety of premorbid and concurrent conditions that can confound test results. It is the responsibility of the examiner to investigate these conditions, weigh their effects carefully, and reasonably determine what, if any, effects these conditions have had on the evaluation process. Pre-existing and concurrent conditions such as learning disabilities, low academic achievement, low intelligence, attention deficit disorder, or medical conditions such as diabetes or multiple sclerosis, when unknown to or not considered by the examiner, may lead to erroneous conclusions of impairment resulting from a brain injury. Other concurrent conditions that can confound test results are physical pain; medication or drugs, particularly psychotropic medication; and emotional problems such as depression or anxiety.

Pain may interfere with neuropsychological assessment both by distracting the patient and by limiting physical performance by slowing reaction times, lessening speed of movement, and limiting range of motion. For example, an examinee suffering from arthritis may exhibit reduced performance on commonly administered psychomotor tests such as Strength of Grip, the Finger Tapping Test, the Symbol Digit Modalities Test, or the Digit Symbol subtest from the WAIS-R. An examiner who fails to inquire into the examinee's premorbid physical conditions or to consider the impact of unrelated physical conditions may erroneously interpret the test results as indicative of impaired functioning due to a brain injury.

Medications such as antidepressants, antianxiety agents, analgesics, sedatives, and soporifics all tend to lower scores on neuropsychological tests (e.g., see Spiegel and Aebi, 1981). The authors have frequently encountered situations in which an examinee is involved in a motor vehicle crash, complains of back or neck pain, and is prescribed a tricyclic antidepressant as an analgesic, often along with other analgesics as needed. A few weeks later, the examinee begins to complain of cognitive deficiencies. A referral is made to a neuropsychologist who performs an evaluation and finds normal or mildly impaired results along with the examinee's self-reported cognitive complaints. Although there is no report of a head injury, the examiner concludes that the examinee is exhibiting neuropsychological impairment, possibly due to a "whiplash" injury, without recognizing the effects of antidepressant medication on cognitive functioning, alone or in combination with other psychotropic medications.

As noted by Spiegel and Aebi (1981) and others, tricyclic antidepressants impaired performance in healthy subjects on commonly administered neuropsychological tests. For example, amitriptyline was shown to impair performance in healthy subjects on finger tapping, digit span, vigilance, reaction time, digit symbol substitution, and arithmetic. The tricyclic antidepressants are also particularly problematic for memory and other cognitive functions because of their sedative and anticholinergic effects, which block hippocampal cholinergic transmission (Deutsch, 1979). More recently, a nontricyclic, selective serotonin reuptake inhibitor fluoxetine (Prozac), which is widely prescribed, was found to impair verbal memory in nondepressed subjects (Stein et al., 1993).

Emotional problems are also a frequent source of contamination of neuropsychological test results (Breslow et al., 1980; Stromgren, 1977; Wechsler, 1987). Stromgren found significant correlations between many of the Wechsler Memory Scale scores and ratings of depression. Recovery from depression was associated with improved test performance. Wechsler (1987) reports that depressed individuals tend to score lower on the Wechsler Memory Scale. More severe psychopathology (e.g., schizophrenia) is also associated with poor performance on neuropsychological procedures (Wechsler, 1987).

The premorbid and concurrent conditions outlined above are likely to confound the results of neuropsychological tests and thus contaminate the conclusions reached in the evaluation of the cognitive effects of postconcussive syndrome. It is the responsibility of the forensic neuropsychologist to recognize these premorbid and concurrent conditions and reasonably determine their impact on the evaluation.

PERCEPTUAL AND REPORTING BIASES

Perceptual biases are beliefs, forces, or actions that influence an observer's perception of an event such that the observer's representation is inconsistent with the factual event (Dunne et al., 1990; Furnham, 1986; Lees-Haley and Brown, 1992; Roht et al., 1985). For example, after a misdiagnosis of brain injury (a false-positive), a patient may begin to pay more attention than usual to normal phenomena and conclude that these experiences confirm the presence of brain damage. Such misperceptions cohere in a confirmatory bias to induce feelings of alarm, fear, and victimization. The biased perception appears to be reality from the point of view of the patient. This "social reality based on social cognition" idea, or the phenomenon of creating individual reality based on individual perceptions, has been widely investigated by psychological researchers, with much support (Fiske and Taylor, 1991; Williams and Lees-Haley, 1993).

There is a growing consensus among researchers that how people think about their health problems is often as important for determining how they respond to health threats as are the physiologic components of disease (Skelton and Croyle, 1991; see also, e.g., Cameron et al., 1993; Cioffi, 1991; Lau et al., 1989; Leventhal et al., 1980; Pennebaker, 1980; Rodin, 1978; Swartzman and McDermid, 1993). Research findings from the cognitive approach to health perception are useful for understanding the genesis of neuropsychological symptoms that lack an objective basis.

Several aspects of events may influence individuals to form an incorrect construction of a harmless event as harmful (Alexander and Fedoruk, 1986; Dunne et al., 1990; Guidotti and Jacobs, 1993; Roht et al., 1985; Smith et al., 1978; Stahl and Lebedun, 1974). By selectively attending to base rate neuropsychological limitations and symptoms and giving them unwarranted credibility as a correlate of brain injury, the perceptual process is slanted toward the erroneous conclusion that one's brain is functioning abnormally.

Preconceived notions regarding vague labels can influence the perceptions of both genuine and illusory concussions. Laypersons may not know that "concussions" almost always resolve promptly without complications. On hearing the general term *brain damage,* many persons associate that label with permanent severe brain damage. Such notions can distort the perception of an injury, leading to false attributions of an ominous nature to a harmless event.

Unfamiliar or novel situations provide no prior experience on which to base perceptions. In such situations, preconceived ideas and stereotypical notions serve as a framework for building current perceptions. To the extent that these beliefs are accurate, such reliance serves as a valuable heuristic method for cognizing our world (Jussim, 1991). However, when these preconceived beliefs are erroneous, inaccurate perceptions result, and the consequences may be serious. For example, if a patient quits working and spends substantial periods of time in unstructured activity with few goals, based on a false opinion that he or she is disabled, it is likely that the patient will become more dysphoric than usual (Myers, 1992).

By establishing a preference or value for certain traits, experts influence the facility with which those traits will be reported (Kunda and Sanitioso, 1989). This finding is especially salient in the light of specific behaviors by physicians, scientists, and attorneys after a perceived brain injury. Frequently, attorneys ask about symptoms and clinical examiners use symptoms checklists to assess the health status of patients in forensic settings. These checklists are comprised of symptoms that would be expected to result after a brain injury and often are not scientifically validated instruments. By highlighting certain symptoms as expected, attending clinicians and attorneys influence the frequency with which these symptoms are reported. Also, symptom checklists can bias the way individuals interpret their somatic sensations (Cioffi, 1991). As Cioffi noted,

> **The use of symptoms checklists as measures of somatic perception may present a pernicious problem: Many symptom labels are already biased toward a negative or pathological interpretation . . . As measures of somatic awareness, symptom checklists may not allow persons to independently report what they feel and how they feel about it. (p. 33)**

LIMITATIONS OF THE STATE OF THE ART

The field of neuropsychological evaluation of brain injuries is a curious blend of sophisticated thinking and elementary error. Data scrutinized through highly sophisticated statistical methods and superficially rigorous scientific processes often contain simple fatal errors. For example, even the most widely used assessment instruments involve conflicting definitions and varying norms. One illustration is the definition of average intelligence: there is a 14-point difference between the definition of average intelligence as reflected in the manual for the WAIS-R and the manual for the most widely used neuropsychological norms (Heaton, 1992; Wechsler, 1981).

Two widely recognized, essentially similar tests of memory functioning use very discrepant definitions of normal levels of memory (Wechsler, 1987; Williams, 1991). Widely used neuropsychological screening instruments use different definitions of impairment and of average and below average. With one test, only 1 or 2 percent of the population may be regarded as impaired, whereas with an ostensibly similar test 10 to 20 times as many persons would be found to be suffering from neuropsychological impairment. Expert opinions also vary markedly. Some experts opine that 1 or 2 percent of the population is abnormal, and others testify that as many as one-third are outside normal limits. These broad differences of opinion make it difficult to establish meaningful standards for evaluating injuries.

Many important definitions in neuropsychological assessment lack universal definitions in the scientific community. Tests that ostensibly measure the same cognitive ability may be different in nature, varying not only in the level of difficulty but also at times measuring substantially different functions. An example is the Paced Authority Serial Addition Test (PASAT) (Gronwall, 1977; Spreen and Strauss, 1991), which is purported to be a measure of the examinee's rate of information processing. In the task, a prerecorded tape delivers a random series of 61 numbers from 1 to 9. The examinee adds pairs of numbers such that each number is added to the one immediately preceding it. For example, if the given numbers are "2,8," the answer is "10"; if the next number is

"5," this is added to the previous "8" and the answer is "13"; and so on. There are four trials on the PASAT in which the 60 numbers are presented at increasingly faster time intervals (2.4, 2.0, 1.6, and 1.2 seconds). The PASAT increases processing demands by increasing the speed of stimulus input.

Spreen and Strauss (1991) report that the PASAT is very sensitive to mild brain injury, has a correlation of 0.68 with general intelligence and numerical ability, and can be a demanding and frustrating test for normal people. Thus, the PASAT is likely to have a high false-positive rate. Nonetheless, some clinicians have reported deficits in information-processing speed based solely on poor results from the PASAT without considering an examinee's premorbid intelligence and numerical ability, the significant potential of obtaining a false-positive, and the presence or absence of corroborating results from other tests measuring the same ability.

Neuropsychological testing has experienced a rapid growth that has stretched the field beyond reasonable scientific prudence. For example, many neuropsychological tests do not meet the generally accepted standards for psychological testing (American Psychological Association, 1985). Many neuropsychological tests have no manual, have never been subjected to formal peer review or cross-validation, and have poor norms. Some have never been published at all. For example, the use of consonant trigrams (nonsense "words" composed of three letters) is often used in neuropsychological evaluations as a measure of verbal memory. However, Franzen (1989) reports that there are no reliability studies for the trigram procedure, nor are there guides for the clinical interpretation of an examinee's results on the trigram procedure. Franzen (1989) concluded that more information is needed before the trigram procedure can be recommended as an evaluation procedure.

Recently, we have seen a growing confusion and blurring between the results of objective neuropsychological measures and measures of subjective self-report. Many assessment devices are not empirically validated by external criteria; rather, they are systematic versions of a self-report interview that have been validated only by establishing correlations with other similar self-report measures. There are several symptom checklists that have been recommended for use in evaluations of patients with suspected brain injuries. O'Donnell and Reynolds (1983) developed the Neuropsychological Impairment Scale, a 95-item self-reporting measure of neuropsychological symptoms. Other symptom checklists include the 93-item Neuropsychological Symptom Checklist published by Psychological Assessment Resources and the 121-item Neurotoxicity Screening Survey (Singer, 1990). In forensic neuropsychological reports, we often see these symptom checklists included under headings of "Tests Administered" and within the list of objective measures of cognitive abilities.

The assignment of numbers, standard scores, or technical labels with graphs and profiles and the characterization of symptom checklists as objective tests can be misleading, at times amounting to little more than the examiner echoing the patient's self-report. Most symptom checklists do not inquire as to whether the endorsed symptom was experienced premorbidly. Examiners using neuropsychological symptom checklists need not only to keep in mind the high base rate of neuropsychological symptoms in normal populations but should also investigate the premorbid history of endorsed symptoms and not assume that these symptoms began post-injury.

CAUSATION

The present state of development of neuropsychological tests permits measurement of functions with essentially no definitive evidence of the causation of deficits that may be present. This is not a criticism of the tests; it is a description of their nature to help clarify their limits. Neuropsychological tests measure the nature and extent of functional limitations but not their cause. Conclusions regarding causation are derived through sources such as history and the relationship between the history and the nature and extent of the deficit. Individuals with entirely different histories and different injuries may obtain identical scores on such tests.

In terms of identifying the implications of functional losses for everyday life, the field thus far relies a great deal on a blend of common-sense inference and speculation by experts. There is a dearth of empirical data on the direct occupational consequences of brain injuries. The relationships between neuropsychological tests and the requirements of specific occupations in the competitive labor market are imperfectly understood.

LITIGATION FACTORS

Litigation, perhaps because of its adversarial qualities, seems to inspire a variety of types of unreasonable opinions. For example, dose-response relationships are often ignored in litigated cases, in which nominal and even nonexistent injuries are represented as having the impact of catastrophic events. A disturbing finding in litigated cases is patients who, after experiencing a nominal injury, are subjected to adverse iatrogenic influences by doctors and lawyers and then begin to report clinically implausible or even impossible symptoms and deterioration to the point of claiming total disability. With genuinely seriously injured patients, it sometimes appears that the best strategy for patient care is sacrificed for legal strategy.

Patients in litigation behave differently than comparable nonlitigating patient populations in several respects. Litigation is associated with higher base rates of neuropsychological symptom reporting and reporting biases in history (Lees-Haley and Brown, 1993). For example, litigating patients report lower than normal rates of preinjury trauma, lower than average stress with notoriously well-recognized psychosocial stressors, and increased presumption of disability. When the examiner is unaware that plaintiffs with no history of brain injury report postconcussive complaints at a rate higher than normal medical patients, the examiner may erroneously conclude that the symptoms are evidence of brain injury.

The Barnum effect is a potential problem in litigated cases (Lees-Haley et al., 1993). The Barnum effect, named after P.T. ("There's a sucker born every minute") Barnum refers to ambiguous characterologic statements that are applicable to most individuals. When general statements or opinions are delivered by persons in authority or expertise (e.g., mental health examiners), these statements can become personalized by examinees. Thus, examinees will tend to accept interpretations of events that sound reasonable, appear somewhat individually tailored, and are provided by an authority figure (Salovey and Turk, 1991). Experts caught up in the process of litigation may express forceful opinions that otherwise would meet with derision in a scientific meeting. These opinions may lead otherwise healthy plaintiffs to see themselves as injured.

CONCLUSION

Examiners conducting forensic neuropsychological evaluations of examinees reported to be suffering a postconcussive syndrome are confronted with a plethora of challenging problems, beginning with the current controversial nature of postconcussive syndrome as reflected in the diagnostic manuals. These challenges include estimating preinjury cognitive functioning, base rates of postconcussive symptoms, obtaining an accurate and reliable history, and the limitations of neuropsychological tests. Because of the complexity of the task and the presence of many confounds, forensic evaluations present a unique challenge to examiners. This chapter has illuminated some of the more frequently ignored confounding variables and, when possible, presented solutions so that examiners can offer the most reasonable and empirically supported opinions regarding cognitive losses from premorbid status.

The field of forensic neuropsychological assessment of brain injuries is a fascinating, burgeoning field of investigation. Although subject to many validity problems typical of a young discipline, the area is a promising one for future research. In particular, there are needs for reliable measures of functions that permit prediction of performance in activities of daily living and employment, emotional distress and life satisfaction, and outcome of treatment procedures.

REFERENCES

Alexander RW, Fedoruk MJ: Epidemic psychogenic illness in a telephone operator's building. J Occup Med 28:42–45, 1986

American Psychiatric Association: Diagnostic and Statistical Manual of Mental Disorders. 4th Ed. American Psychiatric Association, Washington DC, 1994

American Psychological Association: Standards for Educational and Psychological Testing. American Psychological Association, Washington, DC, 1985

Breslow R, Kocsis J, Belkin B: Memory deficits in depression: evidence utilizing the Wechsler Memory Scale. Percept Mot Skills 51:541–542, 1980

Cameron L, Leventhal EA, Leventhal H: Symptom representations and affect as determinants of careseeking in a community-dwelling, adult sample population. Health Psychol 12:171–179, 1993

Cioffi D: Beyond attentional strategies: a cognitive-perceptual model of somatic interpretation. Psychol Bull 109:25–41, 1991

Deutsch JA: Physiology of acetylcholing in learning and memory. p. 343. In Barbeau A, Growdon JH, Wurtman RW (eds): Nutrition and the Brain. Raven Press, New York, 1979

Dunn JT, Brown RS, Lees-Haley PR, English LT: Neurotoxic and neuropsychologic symptom base rates: a comparison of three groups. Poster presented at the 13th

Annual Conference of the National Academy of Neuropsychology, Phoenix, AZ, 1993

Dunne MP, Burnett P, Lawton J, Raphael B: The health effects of chemical waste in an urban community. Med J Aust 152:592–597, 1990

Ekman P: Telling Lies: Clues to Deceit in the Marketplace, Politics, and Marriage. W. W. Norton, 1985

Faust D, Hart K, Guilmette TJ: Pediatric malingering: the capacity of children to fake believable deficits on neuropsychological testing. J Consult Clin Psychol 56: 578–582, 1988a

Faust D, Hart K, Guilmette TJ, Arkes HR: Neuropsychologists' capacity to detect adolescent malingerers. Professional Psychol Res Pract 19:508–515, 1988b

Faust D, Ziskin J, Hiers JB Jr: Brain Damage Claims: Coping with Neuropsychological Evidence. Law and Psychology Press, Marina del Rey, CA, 1991

Fiske ST, Taylor SE: Social Cognition. Addison-Wesley, Reading, MA, 1991

Franzen MD: Critical Issues in Neuropsychology: Reliability and Validity in Neuropsychological Assessment. Plenum Press, New York, 1989

Furnham A: Response bias, social desirability and dissimulation. Personality Individual Differences 7:385–400, 1986

Golden CJ, Hammeke TA, Purisch AD: Manual for the Luria-Nebraska Neuropsychological Test Battery. Western Psychological Services, Los Angeles, 1980

Goodglass H, Kaplan E: Assessment of cognitive deficit in the brain-injured patient. In Gazzaniga MS (ed): Handbook of Behavioral Neurobiology. Vol. 2, Neuropsychology. Plenum Press, New York, 1979

Gronwall DMA: Paced auditory serial—addition task: a measure of recovery from concussion. Percept Mot Skills 44:367–373, 1977

Gouvier WD, Uddo-Crane M, Brown LM: Base rates of postconcussional symptoms. Archives of Clinical Neuropsychology, 3:273–278, 1988

Guidotti TL, Jacobs P: The implications of an epidemiological mistake: a community's response to a perceived excess cancer risk. Am J Public Health 83:233–239, 1993

Heaton RK, Igor G, Matthews CG: Comprehensive Norms for an Expanded Halstead-Reitan Battery. Psychological Assessment Resources. Odessa, FL, 1991

Heaton RK, Smith HH, Jr, Lehman RA, Vogt AT: Prospects for faking believable deficits on neuropsychological testing. J Consult Clin Psychol 46:892–900, 1978

Hiscock M, Hiscock CK: Refining the forced-choice method for detection of malingering. J Clin Exp Neuropsychol 11:967–974, 1989

Jussim L: Social perception and social reality: a reflection-construction model. Psychol Bull 98:54–73, 1991

Kaufman AS: Assessing Adolescent and Adult Intelligence. Allyn & Bacon, Needham, MA, 1990

Kunda Z, Sanitioso R: Motivated changes in the self-concept. J Exp Soc Psychol 25:272–285, 1989

Lau RR, Bernard TM, Hartman KA: Further explorations of common-sense representations of common illness. Health Psychol 8:195–219, 1989

Lees-Haley PR, Brown RS: Biases in perception and reporting following a perceived toxic exposure. Percep Mot Skills 75:531–544, 1993

Lees-Haley PR, Williams CW, Brown RS: The Barnum effect and personal injury litigation. Am J Forensic Psychol 11:21–27, 1993

Lees-Haley PR, Dunn JT: The ability of naive subjects to report symptoms of mild brain injury, post-traumatic stress disorder, major depression, and generalized anxiety disorder. J Clin Psychol 50:252–256, 1994

Leventhal H, Meyer D, Nerenz D: The common-sense representation of illness danger. p. 7. In Rachman S (ed): Contributions to Medical Psychology. Vol. 2. Pergamon, New York, 1980

Matarazzo JD: Validity of psychological assessment: from the clinic to the courtroom. Clinical Neuropsychologist, 1:307–314, 1987

Matarazzo, JD: Psychological Assessment versus psychological testing. Am Psychol 45:999–1017, 1990

Matarazzo JD, Daniel M, Prifitera A, Herman D: Intersubtest scatter in the WAIS-R standardization sample. J Clin Psychol 44:940–950, 1988

Matarazzo JD, Prifitera A: Subtest scatter and premorbid intelligence: Lessons from the WAIS-R standardization sample. Psychological Assessment: A Journal of Consulting and Clinical Psychology 1:186–191, 1989

Med-Index: International Classification of Diseases—9th Revision Clinical Modification. Med-index Publications, Salt Lake City, UT, 1991

Meehl P: Clinical Versus Statistical Prediction: A Theoretical Analysis and a Review of the Evidence. University of Minnesota Press, Minneapolis, 1954

Myers DG: The Pursuit of Happiness. Avon Books, New York, 1992

Pankratz L: A new technique for the assessment and modification of feigned memory deficit. Percept Mot Skills 57:367–372, 1983

Pankratz L: Malingering on intellectual and neuropsychological measures. In Rogers R (ed): Clinical Assessment of Malingering and Deception. Guilford Press, New York, 1988

Pennebaker JW: The Psychology of Physical Symptoms. Springer-Verlag, New York, 1980

Reitan R, Wolfson D: The Halstead-Reitan Neuropsychological Test Battery: Theory and Clinical Interpretation. Neuropsychology Press, Tucson, AZ, 1985

Rodin JA: Somatopsychics and attribution. Personality Soc Psychol Bull 4:531–540, 1978

Roht LH, Vernon SW, Weir FW et al: Community exposure to hazardous waste disposal sites: assessing reporting bias. Am J Epidemiol 122:418–433, 1985

Salovey S, Turk DC: Clinical judgment and decision making. In Snyder CR, Forsyth DR (eds): Handbook of Social & Clinical Psychology. Pergamon Press, New York, 1991

Sbordone RJ: Neuropsychology for the Attorney. Paul M. Deutsch Press, Irvine, CA, 1991

Scholmerich J, Sedlak P, Hoppe-Seyler P, Gerok W: The information needs and fears of patients with inflammatory bowel disease. Heptogastroenterology. 34: 182–185, 1987

Singer RM: Neurotoxicity Guidebook. Van Nostrand Reinhold, New York, 1990

Skelton JA, Croyle RT (eds): Mental Representation in Health and Illness. Springer-Verlag, New York, 1991

Smith MJ, Colligan MJ, Hurrell JJ: Three incidents of industrial mass psychogenic illness. J Occup Med 20:399–400, 1978

Spreen O, Strauss E: A Compendium of Neuropsychological Tests: Administration, Norms, and Commentary. Oxford University Press, New York, 1991

Speigel R, Aebi HJ: Psychopharmacology: An Introduction. John Wiley & Sons, New York, 1981

Stahl SM, Lebedun M: Mystery gas: an analysis of mass hysteria. J Health Soc Behav 15:44–50, 1974

Stein RA, Jarvik ME, Gorelick DA: Impairment of memory by fluoxetine in smokers. Exp Clin Psychopharmacol 1:188–193, 1993

Stromgren LS: The influence of depression on memory. Acta Psychiatr Scand 56:109–128, 1977

Swartzman LC, McDermid AJ: The impact of contextual cues on the interpretation of and response to physical symptoms: a vignette approach. J Behav Med 16:183–198, 1993

Wechsler D: Manual for the Wechsler Memory Scale-Revised. The Psychological Corporation, New York, 1987

Wechsler, D: Wechsler Adult Intelligence Scale—Revised, Manual. The Psychological Corporation, San Antonio, TX, 1981

Williams CW, Lees-Haley PR: Perceived toxic exposure: a review of four cognitive influences on perception of illness. J Soc Behav Personality 8:489–506, 1993

Williams MJ: Memory Assessment Scales: Professional Manual. Psychological Assessment Resources, Odessa, FL, 1991

Ziskin J, Faust D: Coping with Psychiatric and Psychological Testimony. 4th Ed. Law and Psychology Press, Marina del Rey, CA, 1988

Detection of Malingering in Postconcussive Syndrome

25

Scott R. Millis
Steven H. Putnam

Malingering has been described in the DSM-IV (Diagnostic and Statistical Manual of Mental Disorders, 4th ed.) as ". . . the intentional production of false or grossly exaggerated physical or psychological symptoms, motivated by external incentives such as avoiding military conscription or duty, avoiding work, obtaining financial compensation, evading criminal prosecution, or obtaining drugs" (American Psychiatric Association, 1994). For a number of reasons the postconcussive syndrome has stimulated a considerable amount of discussion and research regarding the malingering of a subset of psychological symptoms, viz., neuropsychological deficits. First, brain dysfunction may not be the exclusive cause of all chronic postconcussive symptoms. Psychosocial factors that reinforce symptom elaboration and maintenance appear to be important in selected postconcussive cases (Dacey and Dikmen, 1987). Second, the prevalence of malingering of neuropsychological impairment may be much higher than clinicians often presume. It has been estimated that 7.5 to as high as 64 percent of personal injury litigants and as many as 47 percent of workers' compensation claimants present with exaggerated or feigned impairments (Rogers et al., 1993; Trueblood and Schmidt, 1993). Third, neuropsychological test findings are increasingly used as the primary evidence to establish the diagnosis of mild head injury. The capacity of neuropsychological tests to differentiate malingering from genuine brain dysfunction is, of course, of great interest. Some investigators have questioned the ability of neuropsychologists to detect malingering (e.g., Faust et al., 1988b). These investigators have had their critics (e.g., Adams and Putnam, 1994; McCaffrey and Lynch, 1992) as well. Fourth, the failure to detect malingering can lead to inappropriate treatment of patients, iatrogenic initiation of illness behavior, and misallocation of expensive medical and rehabilitation resources better used for patients with bona fide needs. Fifth, the DSM-III-R and DSM-IV criteria for malingering lack sufficient empirical support at this time (Rogers, 1990). Finally, the detection of neuropsychological malingering has important legal ramifications because postconcussive disorder cases are very frequently litigated.

HISTORICAL BACKGROUND

Interest in the detection of malingered emotional and cognitive disorders has not been limited to the current decade. The 1788 publication of Samuel Farr's *Elements of Medical Jurisprudence* signaled the beginning of an extensive English literature that dealt with issues of malingering and clinical detection (Geller et al., 1990). However, eighteenth and nineteenth century writings tended to focus primarily on the malingering of psychosis, particularly manic states. Among the more unusual and disputed methods to detect malingering were flagellation, emetics, beef tea enemas, the "whirling chair," and electrical shocks to the tongue from galvanic batteries (Geller et al., 1990). These methods have, of course, fallen into disuse, but nineteenth-century investigators also emphasized the use of techniques that are currently employed, namely, extensive observation of the patient combined with a complete history.

In 1838 Ray wrote, "In simulated madness, the common error is to imagine that nothing must be remembered correctly, and that the more inconsistent and absurd the discourse, the better is the attempt at deception sustained" (Geller et al., 1990). Malingering was thought to be characterized by inconsistency in behavior and gross exaggeration of typical symptoms, concepts also considered by contemporary investigators to be hallmarks of the condition (Shapiro, 1991). In fact, Geller et al., (1990) have argued that malingering detection methods have advanced little since the nineteenth century because behavioral observation and clinical interview continue to be preferred strategies.

The capacities of observation and interview to detect malingering have been questioned because of the reliance on clinical (human) judgment in contrast to actuarial or statistical methods for diagnosis. Clinical judgment as a decision making strategy may lack sufficient sensitivity and specificity to reliably identify deception at an acceptable level of accuracy (Guilmette and Giuliano, 1991). First, errors in clinical judgment have been reported to be in the direction of underdiagnosing malingering when examiners were presented solely with patient test data summaries (Faust, 1988b). Second, confirmatory bias may significantly yet insidiously influence clinical judgment and observation, defining what is deemed important or relevant to attend to or address. For instance, the knowledge that a patient has been in a motor vehicle crash provides the opportunity to find corroborative "evidence" of the neuropsychological impairment one expects to find (Wedding and Faust, 1989). Third, clinicians are inclined to be overly confident in their abilities to detect malingering and ". . . wrongly believe that they can assess motivation and sincerity by establishing an empathetic relationship. Practiced liars merely use this as an opportunity to look sincerely into the eyes of the therapist and prevaricate" (Pankratz and Erickson, 1990). Further limitations in clinical judgment include hindsight bias, overreliance on salient data, underutilization of population base rates, and human information processing constraints to analyze symptom covariation and multiple variables with unequal weightings (Wedding and Faust, 1989). Additional strategies that supplement clinical judgment are justified and necessary.

INITIAL CONSIDERATIONS

The detection of malingering in the postconcussive syndrome case is indeed a complex diagnostic process. Accurate diagnosis is difficult in general, but the diagnosis of malingering in particular can provoke strong reactions in clinicians, which may range from denial that malingering by patients even exists to the belief that malingering is present in every case in which compensation may be obtainable. The assumptions at both extremes are antithetical to the scientist-practitioner practice model and can be marked by moralistic and judgmental stances that interfere with impartial clinical evaluation. Shapiro (1991) has noted that the awareness of malingering involves ". . . a totally different 'set' or 'cognitive map' from that in the traditional office setting where one is performing psychotherapy or psychological testing." In this regard, an adaptational model has been proposed by Rogers and Cavanaugh (Rogers, 1990), which provides a framework for investigating malingering that ". . . provides testable constructs without either moral-laden assumptions or unnecessary theorizing about traits and other characteristics of the malingerer.

Assumptions inherent in this model are threefold: (a) A person perceives the evaluation/treatment as involuntary or adversarial, (b) the person perceives that he or she has either something to lose from self-disclosure or something to gain from malingering,

and (c) the person does not perceive a more effective means to achieve his or her desired goal. (Rogers, 1990)

In the postconcussive case, the possibility of malingering may be raised first when the patient claims significant, prolonged disability, the patient obtains neuropsychological test scores that are excessively impaired or inconsistent given the initial severity of the injury event, and financial and related contextual incentives are known to be present (Binder, 1993). It is important to stress that postconcussive symptoms are, in fact, diagnostically nonspecific and commonly reported by litigants with disorders not involving the central nervous system (CNS) as well as by normal individuals (Gouvier et al., 1988; Lees-Haley and Brown, 1993; Wong et al., 1994). Moreover, the current concept of postconcussive syndrome, while widely employed, seems quite inadequate and ". . . there seems to be no place in this diagnostic construct for the vast individual differences of personal history, character formation, object relations, and socioemotional or developmental status to be played out" (Adams and Putnam, 1991). In response to the need for greater diagnostic clarity, Brown et al. (1994) proposed specific criteria for the DSM-IV and its future revisions for a "postconcussive disorder" based on a review of the mild and moderate head injury literature. The criteria proposed by Brown et al. (1994) have stimulated a great deal of debate, and the American Psychiatric Association Task Force has broadened the diagnostic criteria for the postconcussive syndrome (Tucker, 1994). Unfortunately these new criteria may include sensitive indicators of possible head injury, but nonetheless many appear to lack sufficient diagnostic specificity at this time. Likewise, the proposed criteria continue to leave unaddressed the powerful role of possible psychological factors that operate in some cases of postconcussive syndrome (Putnam and Millis, 1994).

Differential diagnosis in the postconcussive syndrome case is not limited only to brain dysfunction versus malingering but characteristically involves consideration of a range of symptomatic complaints and diagnostic possibilities. Reliance on clinical judgment alone to detect malingering is likely to result in an unacceptably high error rate, as previously noted. We will recommend a multivariate approach that involves the use of injury severity data, traumatic brain injury (TBI) neuropsychological test performance patterns, demographically adjusted neuropsychological test norms, and neuropsychological detection procedures along with the consideration of alternative medical and psychiatric diagnoses (Table 25-1). No single, quick, fool-proof "malingering test" currently exists, and such a procedure is unlikely to be forthcoming. We will propose instead that the assessment of malingering should incorporate an approach that is integrated within the context of the entire neuropsychological examination and augmented with specialized procedures of known reliability and validity.

TOWARD AN INTEGRATED APPROACH

Injury Severity and Outcome

Initial depth and duration of coma as assessed with the Glasgow Coma Scale (GCS) (Teasdale and Jennett, 1974) and duration of post-traumatic amnesia as defined by the Galveston Orientation and Amnesia Test (Levin et al., 1979) are crucial for determining the severity of the head injury and for grossly predicting the likely outcome from head injury (Katz, 1992). In addition, these variables are among the best available indicators of the *severity* of diffuse axonal injury (Katz, 1992).

There is considerable evidence that mild head injury can cause neuropathologic, neurophysiologic, and neuropsychological changes (Dikmen and Levin, 1993). At the same time, base rate data clearly suggest that outcome after mild head injury in the majority of cases is likely to be favorable (Dikmen and Levin, 1993). This is not to imply that mild head-injured patients are in all cases symptom-free, but rather that severe and chronic disability after mild head injury is uncommon without additional contributing factors. Data from the International Coma Data Bank showed that 83 percent of the subjects with post-traumatic amnesia of less than 2 weeks' duration had "good"

TABLE 25-1. Multivariate Approach to the Diagnosis of Malingering

Establish initial injury severity
Consider typical neuropsychological test pattern associated with given injury severity
Consider alternative medical and psychiatric diagnoses
Use demographically adjusted neuropsychological test norms
Use specific and general neuropsychological tests to determine presence of malingering profile

recovery and none demonstrated "severe" disability as defined by the Glasgow Outcome Scale (Jennett et al., 1979). In a more recent investigation, Dikmen et al. (1994) developed statistical algorithms to determine rates and factors predictive of return to work after head injury. For example, by applying this algorithm to a 30-year-old patient with a GCS of 15 (i.e., mild head injury), mild extremity injury, bachelor's degree, and stable preinjury job history, Dikmen et al. predict about a 92 percent chance of returning to work within 6 months.

In addition to the relationship between initial injury severity and behavioral and vocational outcome, there is an accumulating literature that describes the association between injury severity and neuropsychological test performance. In well-controlled studies of consecutive mild head injury cases, impairments in memory, attention, and information processing speed were measured within a week postinjury, but resolution of these deficits occurred within 1 to 3 months later (Dikmen et al., 1986; Levin et al., 1987). At one month following mild head injury, severe impairment on tasks of attention span, reasoning, problem solving, language, motor speed, and psychomotor integration is not typical (Dikmen et al., 1986; Levin et al., 1976). In a study by Alves et al. (1993) of 587 consecutive uncomplicated mild head injury cases, other postconcussion symptoms such as headache and dizziness were common at discharge and at 3-month follow-up, with a significant decline in reported symptomotology over 12 months. Indeed, chronic multiple postconcussive symptom patterns were rare in this large sample (1.9 to 5.8 percent). Data from the Traumatic Coma Data Bank studies (Levin et al., 1987) and Traumatic Brain Injury Model Systems of Care (Kreutzer et al., 1993) similarly provide extensive information about common neuropsychological impairment patterns after head injury, which can assist the clinician in determining the correspondence between a particular case and the known course of recovery as defined by large-group, multicenter studies.

Recommendations

Chronic, disabling impairment after mild, uncomplicated head injury is uncommon in patients without other systemic injuries, premorbid psychiatric vulnerabilities, or substance abuse involvement. Moreover, excessively poor neuropsychological test scores after mild head injury are virtually always atypical. Poor neuropsychological test performances or excessive disability does not necessarily establish proof of malingering but can provide the first indication to the clinician that motivational and psychosocial factors need to be carefully considered in the differential diagnosis. Use of injury severity and outcome data from Dikmen et al. (1994), Kruetzer et al. (1993), Levin et al. (1987), and similar investigations will assist clinicians to develop empirically based expectations of outcome and disability after head injury.

Medical, Psychiatric, and Psychosocial Factors

Before malingering becomes the primary diagnostic impression, other factors need to be considered in addition to injury severity characteristics and level of performance on neuropsychological tests (Table 25-2).

An important distinction needs to be made between complicated and uncomplicated mild head injuries. The complicated mild head injury is diagnosed on the basis of a GCS score of 13 to 15 and a computed tomography (CT) scan showing the presence of an intracranial abnormality (Dikmen and Levin, 1993). In general, this type of injury appears to have a neurobehavioral outcome more similar to a moderate head injury, i.e., GCS 9 to 12 (Dikmen and Levin, 1993). Hence, the causal factors in the symptoms of the complicated mild head injury case may be very different from those in the uncomplicated case.

The fact that an individual has sustained a mild head injury does not produce immunity from other illnesses that may exist antecedent to or subsequent to the injury. Clinicians who approach assessment in a traditional and advocating fashion may be susceptible to attributing symptoms to the accident without fully considering other etiologies. That is, they may

TABLE 25-2. Diagnostic Considerations in the Postconcussive Case

Complicated versus uncomplicated mild head injury
Endocrine, hepatic, renal, pulmonary, and cerebrovascular disorders
Alcohol and other substance abuse
Non-CNS body system injuries
Mood disorders
Anxiety disorders
Learning disabilities
Somatoform disorders
Adverse life events and chronic social difficulties

unknowingly become victims of confimatory bias. Before malingering is diagnosed in the postconcussive case, other medical disorders need to be ruled out as contributors to the disability or poor neuorpsychological test performance. Endocrine, hepatic, renal, pulmonary, cerebrovascular, and substance abuse disorders have all been associated with neuropsychological and functional impairment (Tarter et al., 1988), as has the chronic use of prescription medications such as narcotics, tranquilizers, and sedative-hypnotics (McNairy et al., 1984). Evaluation for premorbid substance abuse is important because of its high prevalence reported among some head-injured patient samples (Dikmen and Levin, 1993). Also, other body systems injuries such as orthopedic or soft tissue injuries sustained in the same accident as the mild head injury appear to be related to psychosocial difficulties. Dikmen et al. (1986) found that only 18 percent of their mild head-injured subjects with other system injuries had returned to work at 1 month postinjury, whereas 88 percent of their subjects with mild head injury alone had returned. In a more recent study, McLean et al. (1993) have stated, "Another implication of these findings is the point that not all of the problems reported after a brain injury are necessarily brain injury-related."

Psychiatric disorders also need to be considered in the differential diagnosis of the postconcussive syndrome because of the known prevalence of mental illness in the general population. The National Comorbidity Survey (Kessler et al., 1994), based on a stratified multistage area probability sample of 8,098 individuals, found that about 50 percent of the subjects reported one or more lifetime psychiatric disorder. Approximately 30 percent reported one or more 12-month disorder. Curiously, less than 40 percent of subjects with a lifetime disorder had received any formal treatment. The most prevalent psychiatric disorders found were major depression, alcohol dependence, social phobia, and simple phobia. Not only can psychiatric disorders result in social and occupational disability, but some have been associated with neuropsychological impairment as well (Winokur and Clayton, 1994). It has been well established that patients with affective disorders may demonstrate slowing in the rate of information processing, poor concentration, and memory deficits (Crosson, 1994; Johnson and Magaro, 1987). Depression has similarly been associated with a reduced ability to sustain effort in formal assessment (Cohen et al., 1982). Not surprisingly, patients with anxiety disorders also report memory inefficiencies (Noyes and Holt, 1994). Premorbid learning disabilities also deserve careful evaluation because they may be overrepresented in the mild head injury population and can be associated with preinjury neuropsychological impairment. Dicker (1992) recently reported that 50 percent of the mild head injury subjects in her sample demonstrated evidence of learning disabilities or poor academic performance premorbidly.

Somatoform disorders warrant special consideration in the postconcussive syndrome case. We have argued elsewhere (Putnam and Millis, 1994) that some cases of persisting postconcussive syndrome may be conceptualized as a type of socialized disability producing features consistent with a somatoform disorder. Somatic symptoms are part of normal experience, but the meaning and significance that individuals attribute to the symptoms vary widely and involve cultural and contextual influences perhaps not always apparent to the clinical examiner (Pennebaker, 1982). The role of psychosocial factors in the exaggeration, prolongation, and intractability of pain complaints (Fordyce, 1976; Sternbach, 1974) and illness behavior has been well established (Watson and Pennebaker, 1989). Indeed, the fundamental premise of recognizing individual differences in human behavior and response needs to be appreciated by providers evaluating and treating postconcusive disorders. For instance, individuals who are premorbidly hypervigilant to and anxious in response to somatic sensations may be at increased risk for developing persisting postconcussive symptoms. In this regard, the role of *expectancy* in the etiology of somatic complaints after mild head injury has been addressed by Mittenberg et al. (1992). These investigators found that patients who had sustained mild head injury underestimated the normal prevalence of various somatic symptoms in their retrospective accounts when compared with the base rate reported by normal controls. They suggested that ". . . patients may reattribute benign emotional, physiologic, and memory symptoms to their head injury." They have proposed a model that posits that symptoms and symptom expectations evolve shortly after the head injury, which concomitantly induces autonomic and emotional arousal. This may be followed by selective and intensified attention to one's internal and somatic state. This attentional bias then elicits additional autonomic and emotional responses, with resultant reinforcement of one's expectations. This circular reinforcement of expectations in some individuals could account for the protracted course of these symptoms, which are quite often resistant to conventional treatment interventions. Moreover, since many postconcussive symptoms are common even in the absence of bona fide disease or injury, elevated anxiety may be maintained simply because the individual perceives little improvement in symptoms over time.

Psychosocial stressors appear to play an important role in some cases of postconcussive syndrome. Fenton et al. (1993) followed a group of 45 consecutively admitted patients with mild head injury without a history of alcohol abuse. A group of control subjects matched for age, sex, and socioeconomic status was also studied. The head-injured group reported significantly more "adverse life events" (mean number, 3) in the year preceding the accident than did the control group (mean number, 1.5). Among the head-injured group at 6 weeks postinjury, the symptomatic patients had four times as many chronic social difficulties as those whose symptoms had resolved. At 6 months, chronic social difficulties were twice as common in the patients with persistent symptoms as in those whose symptoms had remitted. The implications of these findings are straightforward. As suggested by Adams and Putnam (1991), ". . . it would appear that derangement of personality also happens to many patients whose crania are untraumatized. It is simply tautological and incorrect practice to attribute reflexively any problems in personality and/or psychopathology to a patient's history of head injury *quod erat demonstrandum* [which was to be proved]."

Recommendations

Compromised performance on neuropsychological measures or social and occupational disability in the postconcussive case are not tantamount to malingering. At the same time, neither are these variables singularly diagnostic of brain dysfunction. Medical illnesses need to be considered in these complex cases, and consultation with internal medicine and neurology may be especially contributory. Unquestionably, premorbid and comorbid psychiatric vulnerabilities and psychosocial stressors can have a profound impact on how an individual adapts to a mild head trauma or injury event. As noted earlier, many individuals with a lifetime psychiatric disorder will have not received professional treatment. Hence, the absence of a documented psychiatric history does not automatically rule out a premorbid psychiatric disorder that may be associated with protracted postconcussive symptoms. Consultation with neuropsychologists and psychiatrists can assist in delineating the role of potential preinjury factors in the conceptualization of the individual case and form the basis from which individualized treatment strategies are formulated. Similarly, complete and comprehensive review of medical and school records may facilitate estimates of premorbid functioning and can alert the clinician to other medical and psychosocial factors not identified from other sources. Frequent utilization premorbidly of health care resources for relatively minor or vague complaints should prompt the clinician to assess the impact of psychosocial factors in postconcussive syndrome cases as well.

Neuropsychological Test Norms

A significant amount of the variance of some neuropsychological test scores can be accounted for by demographic factors. As an example, Heaton et al. (1991), in a sample of 553 normal adults, found that age and education together accounted for 43 percent of the variance in the Halstead Category Test performance and 55 percent of that in the composite Halstead Impairment Index. This underscores the important axiom that test scores are not self-evident: they do not interpret themselves. To underscore this point, the median number of impaired scores among the 553 *normal* adults in the Heaton et al. (1991) sample was four. The practical implication of these findings is that when a panel of neuropsychological test results is examined from solely a level-of-performance perspective, low test scores can be due to factors other than brain dysfunction. Without appropriate demographically adjusted norms, the clinician runs the risk of labeling what is, in fact, normal premorbid ability as evidence of brain impairment. Some investigators have found that human judges relying on clinical judgment misdiagnosed about one-third of normal subjects as brain-impaired (Faust et al., 1988a; Leli and Filskov, 1981). A higher rate of diagnostic accuracy (93 percent) for psychologist judges interpreting young adult test scores was reported by Nadler et al. (1994). However, the test scores given to the judges were clear and unambiguously normal. When the same judges were given normal test scores for a 74-year-old individual, 58 percent misdiagnosed the test protocol as impaired, and 23 percent of the judges diagnosed it as reflective of dementia. Limitations in human clinical judgment and nonutilization of appropriate test norms may contribute to these diagnostic errors. Appropriate interpretation of examination data incorporates, but is certainly not limited to, a level of performance methodology (Reitan and Wolfson, 1993).

Recommendations

Use of demographically corrected neuropsychological test norms is highly recommended. Particularly in cases of mild head injury, where findings can be equivocal, normal individual variation in neuropsychological functions can be falsely interpreted as reflective of brain-behavior dysfunction. As well, normal test scores without demographic corrections can appear artifactually low for some individuals and unduly arouse suspicion of malingering. Heaton et al. (1991) have developed one of the more comprehensive set of norms for an expanded Halstead-Reitan Battery. Ivnik et al. (1992) provide demographically adjusted Wechsler Adult Intelligence Scale–Revised (WAIS-R), Wechsler Memory Scale-Revised (WMS-R and Rey Auditory Verbal Learning Test norms for individuals aged 56 through 97. Williams (1991) provides age and education-based norms for the Memory Assessment Scales. Demographic corrections for other selected neuropsychological measures have been presented by Spreen and Strauss (1991).

Even with demographic adjustments, the clinician still needs to be attentive to the sensitivity (true positive rate) and specificity (true negative rate) properties of the measures used that can partially overcome the limitations of between-group comparisons. However, these statistics cannot definitively determine if a given patient has the particular disorder in question (e.g., malingering). This, of course, requires the calculation of the local base rate. In considering optimal cutoff scores for their expanded Halstead-Reitan Battery, Heaton et al. (1991) found that only 10 percent of their normal subjects had absolutely normal performance across the battery of tests with no scores in the impaired range. As indicated earlier, the group median for normal subjects was four impaired test scores. Awareness and use of diagnostic test efficiency statistics and ideally of cutoff thresholds that are adjusted to local base rates may prevent clinicians from overinterpreting the significance of an isolated abnormal neuropsychological test score. Local diagnostic base rates can be derived from medical records or epidemiologic or clinical studies of comparable patient samples.

Neuropsychological Tests and the Detection of Malingering

Demographically adjusted neuropsychological test norms, injury severity and outcome data, and consideration of alternative diagnoses are useful but are insufficient alone or in combination to detect malingering. Pankratz (1988) has described the dilemma:

> **Accurate assessment is dependent on patient cooperation because neuropsychological techniques mostly measure behaviors that can be consciously modified. That is, because a patient can report wrong information, respond slowly, act uncoordinated, and deny comprehension, his cooperation must be secured in order to evaluate his case satisfactorily.**

A need exists to develop specific tests to detect malingering and to ascertain definite malingering profiles with existing neuropsychological tests. Clinicians, judges, attorneys, and juries want to see direct and understandable evidence of malingering. Patient history, test norms, and outcome data, although helpful in the diagnostic process, may provide only indirect evidence. A number of approaches have been developed that attempt to detect malingering: simple tests that appear difficult, symptom validity testing and dichotomous forced-choice techniques, pattern analysis of conventional neuropsychological tests, the presence of many aberrant responses to personality surveys, and patient interview techniques (Table 25-3).

Simple Procedures

One approach has been to devise seemingly difficult but actually simple tests that can be completed successfully even by persons with severe cognitive impairments. The assumption is that malingerers will misjudge the level of actual difficulty of the test and perform more poorly than severely impaired patients. Alternatively, some malingerers may attempt to perform all tests as poorly as possible, which would lead to defective performances on the simple malingering procedures as well as the more difficult ones. One of the most widely used procedures of this type is Rey's 15-Item Memory Test or the Memorization of 15 Items (Lezak, 1983). It is composed of five rows with three characters each. All 15 characters are exposed to the patient for 10 seconds, but the items are highly related so that the patient actually needs to remember only three or four concepts for the successful recall of all items. Lee et al. (1992) gave

TABLE 25-3. Neuropsychological and Psychological Tests in the Detection of Malingering

- "Complex" simple procedures
  - Rey 15-Item Test
  - Dot Counting
- Forced-choice procedures
  - Symptom validity tests
  - Hiscock and Hiscock procedure
  - Portland Digit Recognition Test
  - Recognition Memory Test
  - Tests of neuropsychological malingering (Pritchard and Moses)
- Pattern analysis
  - Halstead-Reitan Neuropsychological Test Battery
  - Wechsler Memory Scale–Revised
  - Wechsler Adult Intelligence Scale–Revised
  - Rey Auditory Verbal Learning Test
  - California Verbal Learning Test
- Interview strategies
  - Structured interview of reported symptoms
  - Wiggins and Brandt personal history interview
  - Minnesota Multiphasic Personality Inventory (MMPI) and MMPI-2

the test to three groups: temporal lobe epilepsy inpatients, a nonlitigating mixed neurologic disorder outpatient group, and litigating outpatients who claimed neurologic disorders. Of the litigating patients, 37.5 percent scored at or below 7, suggesting poor sensitivity. Other investigators have also found that the 15-item test has significant limitations with regard to its sensitivity and specificity. In a study of 76 subjects coached to simulate memory impairment, none performed below the score of 9 items out of 15, or three rows recalled (Schretlen et al., 1991). In this investigation, the 15-item-test had a positive predictive value of only 21.6 percent.

Dot Counting, as developed by Rey (Lezak, 1983) is another test in this category of simple procedures. Grouped and ungrouped dots of increasing number are presented, and the patient is to count and verbally report the number of dots. Response times should increase as the number of dots increases, and grouped dots should be counted more quickly than ungrouped dots. Deviations from these patterns or response latencies greater than normative data adapted from Rey (Lezak, 1983) raise suspicion of incomplete motivation or effort. Boone et al. (1994) applied the cutoff scores derived from earlier studies to a mixed neurologic disorder sample of 212 patients. Cutoff scores of more than 180 seconds total for the ungrouped dots and more than 130 seconds total for the grouped dots resulted in extremely low levels of misclassification of brain-damaged patients as malingerers, with false positive rates of 0.9 percent with ungrouped dots cutoff and 0 percent with grouped dots cutoff. Although the dot counting task may not misclassify brain-damaged patients, at present its sensitivity to detecting malingering has not been sufficiently established.

Recommendations

At best, the 15-item test may alert the clinician to the possibility of incomplete effort and motivation, but a performance within normal limits, of course, does not rule out malingering. Like the 15-item test, Dot Counting may detect more obvious forms of malingering but should not be viewed as a comprehensive assessment of motivation. Extremely poor performance on either measure can conceivably be due to severe neuropsychological impairment, lack of cooperation, or a deliberate attempt to deceive.

Symptom Validity Testing and Forced-Choice Procedures

Forced-choice procedures, sometimes also known as symptom validity testing, have been used to assess the veracity of claims of blindness, color blindness, tunnel vision, blurred vision, deafness, anesthesias, and memory impairment (Pankratz, 1988). In the case of memory testing, the patient is given a stimulus item to remember (e.g., a word or number) and is then presented with a two-choice recognition task with the original stimulus item along with a foil. This dichotomous format provides a known level of chance performance (i.e., 50 percent correct). As performances deviate below chance, the probability that the patient is deliberately choosing the wrong answer is increased: ". . . 'motivated wrong answering' is the smoking gun of intent" (Pankratz and Erickson, 1990).

Extending the work of Pankratz et al. (1975), Hiscock and Hiscock (1989) designed a forced-choice memory test in which the patient reads a five-digit number and after a delay interval is presented with two five-digit numbers, one of which is the number presented prior to the interval. There are three blocks of 24 trials with delay intervals of 5, 10, and 15 seconds. In a validation study of 89 subjects, Guilmette et al. (1993) administered this forced-choice procedure to four groups: patients with various neurologic disorders, depressed psychiatric inpatients, nonpatients instructed to feign memory impairment (simulators), and nonpatients instructed to give their best effort. The mean percentage correct for each group was as follows: mixed neurologic disorders, 96 percent; psychiatric, 98 percent; nonpatient simulators, 60 percent; nonpatients responding honestly, 100 percent. Although a score that is significantly below chance provides statistical evidence of malingering, only 34 percent of those instructed to feign impairment obtained scores significantly below chance on the forced-choice test.

Additional validation studies of the Hiscock and Hiscock forced-choice procedure paradigm have appeared in the literature. The levels of performance on the FCP of different subject groups from these investigations are summarized in Table 25-4. The findings from three different studies are quite consistent with each other and provide evidence of convergent validity for this test. Prigatano and Amin (1993) have reported on a group of six "suspected malingerers." Malingering was suspected because of litigation, claimed disability, and complaints not "compatible with the known medical history." This suspected malingering group performed at a level similar to, albeit somewhat higher than, that of the nonpatient coached simulators in the other studies reported. Normal subjects instructed to perform with best effort completed the test essentially without error across the three studies. The brain-injured groups performed at similar levels as well. The forced-choice procedure used by Martin et al. (1993) is a computerized version. Pritchard and Moses (1992) also developed a computerized package of three forced-choice procedures assessing auditory, visual, and memory abilities. Based on a sample of 30 patients and 30 nonpatient coached simulators, at a specifity level of 96.7 percent, 66.7 percent of the simulators were correctly classified. A rather consistent finding across most studies is that the majority of malingerers do not perform significantly below chance on the forced-choice test. Nonetheless, scores on forced-choice procedures that are above chance level but lower than scores typically obtained by patients with marked brain dysfunction may still be suggestive of malingering. Interpretive guidelines are discussed at the end of this section.

The Portland Digit Recognition Test (Binder and Willis, 1991) is similar to the forced-choice procedure but uses longer delay intervals (5, 15, and 30 seconds) between stimulus presentation and response and includes an interference task of counting backward during the delay phase. Binder (1993) administered this test to 203 subjects in three groups: mild head trauma patients seeking compensation (MT-Comp), patients with documented brain dysfunction not seeking compensation (BD-NoComp), and patients with documented brain dysfunction seeking compensation (BD-Comp). BD-NoComp subjects performed best, while MT-Comp subjects obtained the lowest scores. BD-NoComp subjects averaged 84 percent, and none scored below 54 percent correct. Only 17 percent of MT-Comp subjects performed significantly below chance. In an earlier study, 15 percent of nonpatients instructed to feign memory impairment scored below chance (Binder and Willis, 1991).

The dichotomous forced-choice format has also been applied to list learning tasks. Presentation of individuals words is followed by the recognition trial, in which each target word is paired with a distractor item and the subject is required to choose one of the two words. Brandt et al. (1985) created a 20-word list procedure, and Iverson et al. (1991) devised a 21-item word list test. In both investigations, the forced-choice word lists were administered to normal controls, to simulators instructed to feign impairment, and to patient groups with a variety of neurologic conditions. All the TBI subjects in Brandt et al. (1985)

TABLE 25-4. Mean Percentage Correct on Forced-Choice Procedure

Group	Martin et al. (1993)	Prigatano and Amin (1993)	Guilmette et al. (1993)
Normal controls	99.4	99.7	100
Brain-injured patients	95.8	99.5	96
Coached simulators	38.8[a] 67.9[b]	N/A	60
Clinical malingerers	N/A	73.8	N/A

[a] "Naive" malingerers.
[b] "Sophisticated" malingerers.

and all the neurologically impaired subjects in Iverson et al. (1991) scored above chance on the recognition trials. Of the subjects instructed to feign memory impairment, 33 percent in the Brandt et al. study and 60 percent in the study of Iverson et al. samples obtained scores below chance. In a more recent study of the 21-item word list developed by Iverson et al. (1991), a cutoff score of less than 9 correct out of 21 resulted in a false positive rate of 2.4 percent in a mixed neurologic disorder sample of 212 (Boone et al., 1994).

Although not originally designed to assess motivation, the Recognition Memory Test (Warrington, 1984), which uses a forced-choice recognition format with words and photographs of faces as stimuli, has been found useful in the assessment of memory impairment after TBI (Millis and Dijkers, 1993). Subjects claiming mild head injury who were seeking financial compensation (MT-Comp) obtained significantly lower scores on both recognition memory subtests than nonlitigating subjects with moderate and severe TBI (ST group) (Millis, 1992). Of course, these findings do not imply that all patients seeking compensation for injuries sustained in an accident are malingering. Indeed, many claimants seeking compensation have genuine injuries. Rather, the base rates for malingering or symptom magnification may be higher in mild head injury cases involved in litigation. The Recognition Memory Test appears to have considerable potential to detect malingering by identifying chance levels of performance. Millis (1992) found that 30 percent of the MT-Comp group performed below chance level on the words subtest and 22 percent on the faces subtest. None of the ST group performed below chance on the words subtest, and 5 percent of this group performed below chance level on the faces subtest. A discriminant function with both subtests correctly classified 76 percent of the MT-Comp and ST subjects (Millis, 1992) and was cross-validated on a new sample of subjects with an overall correct classification rate of 83 percent (Millis and Putnam, 1994). The words subtest appears to provide better discrimination than the faces subtest of brain-injured patients from mild injury patients seeking financial compensation.

Recommendations

Development and validation of symptom validity testing and forced-choice procedures represent a major advance in the detection of malingered neuropsychological impairment. In this category of measures, the Hiscock and Hiscock Forced-Choice Procedure, the Portland Digit Recognition Test, and Warrington's Recognition Memory Test currently demonstrate the strongest empirical support as strategies to detect malingered memory impairment. Perhaps the major strength of forced-choice procedures is also their major drawback, namely, the known level of chance performance. That is, one can calculate test scores to determine objectively when a performance is statistically below chance at a given level of significance. If a score is significantly below chance (i.e., $P < .05$), there is statistical "proof" of malingering. Such evidence would appear to be quite compelling. However, the majority of coached simulators and suspected clinical malingerers tend not to obtain scores significantly below chance in most of the studies reviewed. Reliance on the criterion of significantly below chance performance on forced-choice measures is likely to result in an unacceptably high rate of false negative errors (i.e., classifying malingering profiles as valid). In cases in which malingering is suspected and above-chance performance is attained on forced-choice testing, some investigators have recommended additional cutoff scores. Guilmette et al. (1993) have suggested that fewer than 90 percent correct on the 72-trial forced-choice procedure should raise the "index of suspicion" of poor effort and that fewer than 75 percent correct is likely due to symptom exaggeration. Martin et al. (1993) have suggested that fewer than 80 percent correct on their computerized forced-choice test should raise the possibility of "feigned clinical presentation." Binder (1993) has recommended the following cutoff scores for the Portland Digit Recognition Test; 19 for the "easy" item trials (5-second and 15-second interval trials), 18 for the "hard" item trials (30-second interval trials), and 39 for the entire test. For the Recognition Memory Test, Millis (1992) provides a table of sensitivity and specificity values to assist in clinical decision making.

Pattern Analysis

Because not all malingerers are likely to perform significantly below chance on forced-choice testing, another approach to detect malingering is to use standard neuropsychological measures to determine test performance patterns and derive statistical formulas that differentiate brain-injured patients from known simulators or presumed malingerers. In one of the first investigations that examined patterns of performance on the Halstead-Reitan Neuropsychological Test Battery (HRNTB), Heaton et al. (1978) compared 16 head-injured patients with 16 control subjects instructed to feign neuropsychological impairment. The simulators performed most poorly on motor and sensory tasks, including the Finger Oscillation Test, Tactile Finger Recognition, Grip Strength, Tests for Perception of Bilateral Sensory Stimulation, and Speech-sounds Perception Test, but performed better on the more brain-sensitive measures, namely the Category Test and Tactual Performance Test. Binder and Willis (1991) found a similar pattern using clinical samples. Poorly motivated patients, as defined by scores on the Portland Digit Recognition Test, with financially compensable minor head trauma performed more poorly on the Finger Tapping Test, Grooved Pegboard, Tactile Finger Recognition, Fingertip Number Writing, and the Face-Hand Test than patients who did not show motivational impairment.

In a more recent study, Trueblood and Schmidt (1993) administered the HRNTB and other neuropsychological measures to three groups of eight subjects each: mild head-injured patients; patients defined as malingering based on below-chance performance on symptom validity testing; and patients who performed above chance on symptom validity testing but had neuropsychological test performances of questionable validity. The HRNTB tests and indicators and their respective cutoff scores that best differentiated the head injury group from the malingering and/or questionable validity groups were the General Neuropsychological Deficit Scale summary score (>44), Fingertip Number Writing (>5 errors), Digit Span (aged-corrected scaled score <7), Tactile Finger Recognition (>3 errors), Speech-Sounds Perception Test (>17 errors), Rhythm Test (>8 errors), and California Verbal Learning Test recognition hits (<13 correct). When applied to this sample, these seven cutoff scores, on the average, correctly classified 93 percent of the head injury subjects and 66 percent of the malingerers. When a cutoff of three or more of the seven indicators in the "malingering" range was used all the head-injured subjects and 87.5 percent of the malingering subjects were correctly classified in this study.

Along with the HRNTB, investigators have attempted to discern patterns of malingering by using the WMS-R and WAIS-R. Mittenberg et al. (1993a) derived a discriminant function that included eight WMS-R subtests to differentiate 39 head-injured outpatients from 39 age-matched subjects instructed to feign head injury symptoms. A correct classification rate of 91 percent was achieved, and statistical cross-validation correctly classified 87 percent of the sample. Validation of this discriminant function with clinical samples of presumed malingerers has not, to date, been reported. Using a slightly different combination of seven WMS-R measures, Bernard et al. (1993) derived a discriminant function that correctly classified 85 percent of the subjects simulating malingering and 83 percent of closed head injury patients. Cross-validation of the discriminant function on a new sample correctly classified 79 percent of the simulators and 80 percent of the patients.

The WMS-R Attention-Concentration Index (ACI) scores of TBI patients have been found to be higher than their General Memory Index (GMI) scores (Crossen and Wiens, 1988). The ACI is composed of relatively simple tasks of attention span and concentration. Mittenberg et al. (1993a) performed a discriminant analysis with the ACI and GMI difference scores to separate their TBI group from the nonpatient simulators. An overall correct classification rate of 83 percent was achieved and 82 percent with statistical cross-validation. The simulators' ACI was significantly lower than that of the TBI group. The simulators also showed the reverse ACI-GMI pattern, with ACI lower than GMI. Andrikopoulos (1994) recently replicated these findings with clinical cases. A group of eight mild head injury patients with financial incentives to give poor effort had a significantly poorer performance on the ACI than a group of patients with moderate and severe brain injuries. The financial incentive group also showed the pattern of the ACI being lower than the GMI, as contrasted with the moderate and severe injury group, who showed the opposite pattern.

This finding of excessive impairment on simple tasks of attention in cases of suspected malingering was also obtained by Trueblood and Schmidt (1993), as well as by Mittenberg et al. (1993b), who used the WAIS-R in a study comparing 67 head-injured patients with 67 nonpatients instructed to malinger. Discriminant analysis with the Vocabulary-Digit Span difference score correctly classified 71 percent of the cases. A Vocabulary-Digit Span difference of two or more scaled score points (i.e., Vocabulary greater than Digit Span) was reported to provide maximum discriminative efficiency. The larger the discrepancy with Vocabulary greater than Digit Span, the greater the likelihood of malingering. In the same study, Mittenberg et al. (1993b) also used seven WAIS-R subtests in a second discriminant analysis and achieved an overall correct classification rate of 79 percent.

Rawling and Brooks (1990) and Rawling (1992} have attempted to determine if there are qualitative differences in the types of errors made by malingerers and brain-injured patients on the WAIS-R and WMS. In a study of 16 severe TBI patients and 16 mildly injured patients seeking financial compensation, Rawling and Brooks (1990) identified 20 types of errors (additions, distortions, misplacement, confabulation) on the WAIS-R and WMS, which were summed to create a simulation index. This index was cross-validated on a new sample of 20 subjects, with only one misclassification reported. In a subsequent reliability study, Rawling (1992) found agreement rating for the individual error types to range from 83 to 100 percent with 90 to 99 percent inter-rater agreement for 11 of the 15 error types.

In addition to the WMS-R, list learning tasks such as the Rey Auditory Verbal Learning Test (RAVLT) and California Verbal Learning Test (CVLT) have been used to detect malingering. The recognition component of these tests may be particularly sensitive to feigned impairment. Binder et al. (1993) compared patients with financially compensable mild head injuries with patients with documented brain dysfunction on the recognition trial of the RAVLT. Recognition was tested by using the 50-word list read by the patient (Lezak, 1983). Using the Portland Digit Recognition Test to define a subgroup of the mild injury group as poorly motivated, Binder et al. (1993) found that this subgroup obtained significantly lower recognition scores than the group with brain dysfunction and the motivationally intact mild injury group. In agreement with this finding, Millis and Ricker (1994) found that mild head-injured patients seeking financial compensation who performed below chance on a forced-choice memory test obtained significantly lower scores on the CVLT Recognition Hits and Long Delay Cued Recall and had more false positive errors than rehabilitation inpatients with documented moderate and severe TBI. The CVLT Recognition Hits subtest provided the single best discrimination between the groups. By using a cutoff score of less than 10 correct recognition hits to indicate malingering, all the brain-injured patients and 89 percent of suspected malingerers were correctly classified. Trueblood and Schmidt (1993) found that a less stringent cutoff score of fewer than 13 CVLT Recognition Hits provided good differentiation between head-injured patients and malingerers. The head-injured patients in Trueblood and Schimdt's study (1993) tended to have less severe brain injuries than the patients reported by Millis and Ricker (1994), so that the use of a higher cutoff score could differentiate the head-injured patients from the presumed malingerers.

Recommendations

Pattern analysis is likely to be as important as forced-choice strategies in the detection of malingering. Neuropsychological methods have been able to delineate specific cognitive patterns associated with a variety of neurologic and psychiatric disorders (Grant and Adams, 1986). Determining neuropsychological patterns of malingering that are distinct from neurologic disorders appears to be an attainable goal. Challenges that confront pattern analysis include the need for larger sample sizes and cross-validation of formulas in the aforementioned studies. Many investigations are hindered by poor subject-to-variable ratios, failure to ever replicate initial findings, and misapplications of discriminant analysis procedures. Currently, the neuropsychological measures for which there are the most pattern analysis data regarding malingering detection are the HRNTB and WMS-R. Such data are accumulating for the RAVLT, CVLT, and WAIS-R.

Interview Strategies

Structured interviews may be a useful approach for evaluating the genuineness of reported symptoms. Wiggins and Brandt (1988) created the Personal History Interview, which consists of 13 simple autobiographical questions readily answered by amnesic patients. All the normal control subjects and amnesic patients correctly answered the birthdate and telephone number questions while 42 percent of the nonpatient simulators failed these questions. The Structured Interview of Reported Symptoms (Rogers et al., 1991) is a detailed and well-designed instrument to detect and evaluate deliberate distortions in the self-report of symptoms associated with psychopathology. This instrument has demonstrated efficacy in the detection of specific mental disorders and the detection of simulators who have been coached on dissimulation strategies (Rogers et al., 1992). However, it was not specifically designed to detect the feigning of neuropsychological impairment. It may be useful in assessing the psychopathologic symptoms reported by patients referred for neuropsychological examination, but this application will, of course, require validation. Nonetheless, the structured interview methodology is a much-needed advancement because postconcussive patients with protracted symptomatology report numerous somatic, emotional, and cognitive complaints that are not always easily assessed or described by standard neuropsychological measures.

Minnesota Multiphasic Personality Inventories

Administration of the Minnesota Multiphasic Personality Inventory (MMPI) or MMPI-2 is a common component in most neuropsychological (Jarvis and Barth, 1994) and forensic examinations (Pope et al., 1993). These instruments may be especially helpful in determining possible psychosocial and personality factors influencing the expression and persistence of postconcussive symptoms. Prospective investigations of consecutively admitted mild head injury patients have reported that patients frequently demonstrate emotional distress, as measured by the MMPI, soon after the injury but report decreased symptomatology at 12 and 18 months postinjury (Dikmen et al., 1986). Studies that have found elevated MMPI profiles among mild head injury patients 3 to 5 years postinjury typically have been based on samples of nonconsecutive admissions and are hence nonrepresentative of mild head injury patients in general (Dikmen et al., 1992). Thus, elevated MMPI or MMPI-2 profiles in the postconcussive case should not be attributed reflexively to the mechanisms of TBI. Instead, the profile may be reflecting premorbid psychosocial difficulties, reaction to other injuries sustained, malingering, and/or individual's response to the litigation process (Dikmen et al., 1992).

The inclusion of new validity and clinical scales in the MMPI-2 represents a significant improvement over the MMPI. These new scales have been described and reviewed elsewhere (Graham, 1993), and data on their utility have recently begun to appear in the literature. The Variable Response Inconsistency scale assesses non-content-based inconsistent or random responding, while the True Response Inconsistency scale is sensitive to acquiescent and nonacquiescent sets in the individual's responses to the test items (Graham, 1993). The MMPI-2 content scales have been modified and expanded and, owing to the face validity of the items, provide an excellent source of information regarding how the patients are attempting to present themselves. These scales also are particularly valuable in clarifying interpretive uncertainties present in the clinical scales or code type configuration. The detection of malingered or exaggerated mental illness may be facilitated by examining the MMPI-2 F and Fb scales, F-K index, the MMPI-2 version of the Dissimulation Scale-Revised, the sum of the Lachar and Wrobel Critical Items, and the T-score differences between obvious and subtle items (Bagby et al., 1994).

The Fake Bad scale developed by Lees-Haley et al., (1991) to assess personal injury litigants may show some promise in the assessment of malingering in the postconcussive case. This scale was reported to be significantly higher in a sample of mild head injury patients with persisting symptoms whose WAIS-R FSIQ scores were substantially lower in proximal retesting than in a comparable group of patients whose FSIQ scores remained stable or improved (Putnam et al., 1993). Declines in measured intelligence are, of course, inconsistent with the recovery course following mild head injury and in themselves may alert the examiner to the existence of motivational and psychosocial factors.

Recommendations

Incorporating the MMPI-2 into the neuropsychological examination is very strongly recommended in the postconcussive case. Code type analysis in addition to the consideration of subscales, research scales, and content scales may yield a plethora of information regarding patient traits, states, needs, perceptions, abiding and competing dispositions, and symptomatic complaints—information that can certainly be the basis for hypotheses regarding somatization, sociopathy, dependency, relationships, and psychosocial influences on the patient's recovery course.

USE OF AN INTEGRATED APPROACH

The detection and assessment of malingering in the postconcussive syndrome is a multiple-method process. The initial phase of the assessment involves objectively determining the severity of the head injury by way of the GCS from available medical records. If a GCS score is not indicated in the record, data from medical examination can sometimes be used retrospectively to infer a GCS or coma grade estimate. Many medical centers are now routinely administering the Galveston Orientation and Amnesia Test to head injury patients on a serial basis once they are sufficiently responsive to determine duration of post-traumatic amnesia. Once depth and duration of coma and length of post-traumatic amnesia have been established and the extent of peripheral and extracranial injuries is understood, the clinician may then refer to the outcome literature (e.g., Dikmen et al., 1994) to determine if a particular patient's presentation is consistent with known patterns of outcome and disability. If the patient presents with social and occupational disability that is in excess of reasonable clinical expectations, other medical and psychiatric disorders need to be ruled out and the issue of malingering needs to be explored.

Although postconcussive patients tend to come to the attention of clinicians later rather than sooner and often in the context of litigation, the earlier a neuropsychological assessment can be completed, the easier it may be to ascertain if psychosocial factors are significantly influencing symptom formation and persistence. Because there is no single validated test for neuropsychological malingering, comprehensive assessment is recommended. At this time, much of the research in malingering detection has centered around forced-choice measures, the HRNTB, and the WMS-R. The neuropsychologist may prefer to use these measures because of the availability of empirically derived indicators of malingering or incomplete effort. Of course, these measures offer detailed information regarding an individual's neurocognitive status as well.

If other illnesses that could be responsible for a patient's impairment have been ruled out and if the postconcussive patient performs significantly more poorly than chance on forced-choice measures, it is more likely than not that the patient is deliberately exaggerating impairment and, is thus, by definition, malingering. What if the postconcussive patient does not perform below chance on forced-choice measures? Neuropsychological test pattern analysis should be conducted to determine if the patient's profile is suggestive of malingering. Single cutoff scores for tests will not suit all diagnostic situations. Diagnostic efficiency statistics for particular tests will assist in pattern analysis (Millis, 1992; Mittenberg et al., 1993a; Mittenberg et al., 1993b; Trueblood and Schmidt, 1993). The selection of cutoff scores derived from diagnostic efficiency statistics should be influenced by the likely base rates of malingering in a given population, the relative costs of false positive and false negative errors in the specific situation, and the level of diagnostic certainty required in each case. In the postconcussive case with financial or related incentives, the diagnostic likelihood of malingering increases as the number of neuropsychological test indicators increases in the direction of malingering, as described in previous sections.

FUTURE DIRECTIONS

As the number of neuropsychological and psychological investigations into malingering has increased, cautionary notes are beginning to appear in the literature about the ethical dilemmas of publishing research on malingering. Concerns have been raised about research that investigates the effectiveness of coaching with different types of malingering strategies (Ben-Porath, 1994), as well as research that examines the capacity of specific neuropsychological tests to detect malingering (L. A. Bieliauskas, personal communication, April, 1994). It has been argued that there is a risk that this research can be misused to coach nonimpaired patients to malinger successfully and evade detection.

Requests for moratoriums on publishing certain types of research and for "restraint," however, may raise as many troubling issues as they attempt to resolve. Would proponents of publishing moratoriums argue that restraint should be exercised when publishing any research on neuropsychological characteristics of head injury? Neuropsychological investigations of head injury contain detailed descriptions of how brain-injured patients actually perform on neuropsychological tests and thus may provide the best instructions to malingerers. Such studies conceivably could be used to coach individuals on which tests to perform poorly and on which to excel. Malingering studies may actually be second-rate tools with which to coach would-be malingerers because the studies may instruct someone what not to do rather than how to present as brain-injured. Scientific advancement does not do well when free inquiry is restricted. As always, the very difficult question must be asked—who will restrain the restrainers?

On the other hand, it does appear that people can be taught how to be better malingerers. In the laboratory setting, Martin et al. (1993) found that subjects instructed in strategies to minimize detection as malingerers ("sophisticated malingerers") performed above chance level on a forced-choice procedure and obtained higher scores than subjects who did not receive instruction ("naive malingerers"). However, the sophisticated malingerers still performed significantly more poorly than the brain-injured group; 65 percent performed below the lowest patient score. It is conceivable that information presented in this article could be used to coach malingering individuals on ways to attempt to avoid detection. Is the larger good served by disseminating this research to encourage clinicians to used forced-choice methods to detect malingering and to be aware that below-chance performance is likely not necessary to arouse suspicion of poor effort? Or is the larger good served by suppressing this information so as not to provide coaching to potential malingerers? Berry et al. (1994) have suggested that "Until that time when a consensus is reached by responsible parties, producers and consumers of research on coached malingering should carefully weigh the issues and keep their ethical responsibilities well in mind as they work in this complicated arena."

The postconcussive syndrome will certainly continue to generate much debate in the world literature. Probably no disease or condition brings together so many diverse influences and is so subject to different interpretations and selective emphases. Like the blind men and the elephant, some argue it is a tree while others are certain it is a wall. Consensus will not be achieved soon, although the process to define the postconcussive syndrome more precisely is certainly underway (Brown et al. 1994). We would again emphasize the incompleteness of the postconcussive construct as it presently exists. Although the presentation of patients in the acute stage following head injury is often uniform and likely referable to a neuroanatomic substrate, the cases in which symptoms persist or increase reflect a broad range of behavioral and adaptive responses, which may only indirectly be brain-related. It is these cases in which the gain inherent in personal injury litigation looms large and in which malingering is indeed most suspect.

ACKNOWLEDGMENT

The preparation of this manuscript was supported, in part, by a grant (H133A20016) from the National Institute on Disability and Rehabilitation Research.

REFERENCES

Adams KM, Putnam SH: What's minor about mild head injury? J Clin Exp Neuropsychol 13:388–394, 1991

Adams KM, Putnam SH: Coping with professional skeptics: reply to Faust. Psychol Assessment 6:5–7, 1994

Alves W, Macciocchi SN, Barth JT: Postconcussive symptoms after uncomplicated mild head injury. J Head Trauma Rehabil 8(3):48–59, 1993

American Psychiatric Association: Diagnostic and Statistical Manual of Mental Disorders. 4th Ed. American Psychiatric Association, Washington, 1994

Andrikopoulos J: Disproportionate Attention Deficit in Malingering. Poster presentation at the meeting of the International Neuropsychological Society, Cincinnati, 1994

Bagby RM, Rogers R, Buis T, Kalemba V: Malingered and defensive response styles on the MMPI-2: an examination of validity scales. Assessment 1:31–38, 1994

Ben-Porath YS: The ethical dilemma of coached malingering research. Psychol Assessment 6:14–15, 1994

Bernard LC, McGrath MJ, Houston W: Discriminating between simulated malingering and closed head injury on the Wechsler Memory Scale–Revised. Arch Clin Neuropsychol 8:539–551, 1993

Berry DTR, Lamb DG, Wetter MW et al: Ethical considerations in research on coached malingering. Psychol Assessment 6:16–17, 1994

Binder LM: Assessment of malingering after mild head trauma with the Portland Digit Recognition Test. J Clin Exp Neuropsychol 15:170–182, 1993

Binder LM, Villanueva MR, Howieson D, Moore RT: The Rey AVT recognition memory task measures motivational impairment after mild head trauma. Arch Clin Neuropsychol 8:137–147, 1993

Binder LM, Willis SC: Assessment of motivation after financially compensable minor head injury. Psychological Assessment 3:175–181, 1991

Boone ML, Schauss SL, Franzen MD et al: Accuracy of Objective Tests Designed to Detect Malingering. Poster presentation at the meeting of the International Neuropsychological Society, Cincinnati, 1994

Brandt J, Rubinsky E, Lassen G: Uncovering malingered amnesia. Ann NY Acad Sci 44:502–503, 1985

Brown SJ, Fann JR, Grant I: Postconcussional disorder: time to acknowledge a common source of neurobehavioral morbidity. J Neuropsychiatry Clin Neurosc 6:15–22, 1994

Cohen RM, Weingartner H, Smallberg SA et al: Effort and cognition in depression. Arch Gen Psychiatry 39:593–597, 1982

Crossen JR, Wiens AN: Residual neuropsychological deficits following head injury on the Wechsler Memory Scale–Revised. Clin Neuropsychol 2:393–399, 1988

Crosson B: Application of neuropsychological assessment results. pp. 113–163. In Vanderploeg RD (ed): Clinician's Guide to Neuropsychological Assessment. Lawrence Erlbaum Associates, Hillsdale, NJ, 1994

Dacey RG, Dikmen SS: Mild head injury. pp. 125–140. In Cooper PR (ed): Head Injury. 2nd Ed. Williams & Wilkins, Baltimore, 1987

Dicker BG: Profile of those at risk for minor head injury. J Head Trauma Rehabil 7(1):83–91, 1992

Dikmen SS, Levin HS: Methodological issues in the study of mild head injury. J Head Trauma Rehabil 8(3):30–37, 1993

Dikmen SS, McLean A, Temkin N: Neuropsychological and psychosocial consequences of minor head injury. J Neurol Neurosurg Psychiatry 49:1227–1232, 1986

Dikmen SS, Reitan RM, Temkin NR, Machmer JE: Minor and severe head injury emotional sequelae. Brain Inj 6:477–478, 1992

Dikmen SS, Temkin NR, Machamer JE et al: Employment following traumatic head injuries. Arch Neurol 51:177–186, 1994

Faust D, Guilmette TJ, Hart K et al: Neuropsychologist's training, experience, and clinical judgment accuracy. Arch Clin Neuropsychol 3:145–163, 1988a

Faust D, Hart K, Guilmette TJ: Pediatric malingering: the capacity of children to fake believable deficits on neuropsychological testing. J Consult Clin Psychol 56:578–582, 1988b

Fenton G, McClelland R, Montgomery A et al: The postconcussional syndrome: social antecedents and psychological sequelae. Br J Psychiatry 162:493–497, 1993

Fordyce WE: Behavioral Methods for Chronic Pain and Illness. CV Mosby, St. Louis, 1976

Geller JL, Erlen J, Kaye NS, Fisher WH: Feigned insanity in nineteenth-century America: tactics, trials, and truth. Behav Sci Law 8:3–26, 1990

Gouvier WD, Uddo-Crane M, Brown LM: Base rates of postconcussional symptoms. Arch Clin Neuropsychol 3:273–278, 1988

Graham JR: MMPI-2: Assessing Personality and Psychopathology. 2nd Ed. Oxford University Press, New York, 1993

Grant I, Adams KM: Neuropsychological Assessment of Neuropsychiatric Disorders. Oxford University Press, New York, 1986

Guilmette TJ, Giuliano AJ: Taking the stand: issues and strategies in forensic neuropsychology. Clin Neuropsychol 5:197–219, 1991

Guilmette TJ, Hart KJ, Giuliano AJ: Malingering detection: the use of a forced-choice method in identifying organic versus simulated memory impairment. Clin Neuropsychol 7:59–69, 1993

Heaton RK, Grant I, Matthews CG: Comprehensive Norms for an Expanded Halstead-Reitan Battery. Psychological Assessment Resources, Odessa, FL, 1991

Heaton RK, Smith HH, Lehman RAW, Vogt AT: Prospects for faking believable deficits on neuropsychological testing. J Consult Clin Psychol 46:892–900, 1978

Hiscock M, Hiscock CK: Refining the forced-choice method for the detection of malingering. J Clin Exp Neuropsychol 11:967–974, 1989

Iverson GL, Franzen MD, McCracken LM: Evaluation of an objective assessment technique for the detection of malingered memory deficits. Law Hum Behav 15:667–676, 1991

Ivnik RJ, Malec JF, Smith GE et al: Mayo's older Americans normative studies. Clin Neuropsychol, suppl. 6:1–103, 1992

Jarvis PE, Barth JY: The Halstead-Reitan Neuropsychological Test Battery: A Guide to Interpretation and Clinical Applications. Psychological Assessment Resources, Odessa, FL, 1994

Jennett B, Teasdale G, Braakman R et al: Prognosis in a series of patients with severe head injury. Neurosurgery 4:283–289, 1979

Johnson MH, Magaro PA: Effects of mood and severity on memory processes in depression and mania. Psychol Bull 101:28–40, 1987

Katz DI: Neuropathology and neurobehavioral recovery from closed head injury. J Head Trauma Rehabil 7(2):1–15, 1992

Kessler RC, McGonagle KA, Zhao S et al: Lifetime and 12-month prevalence of DSM-III-R psychiatric disorders in the United States: results from the national comorbidity survey. Arch Gen Psychiatry 51:8–19, 1994

Kreutzer JS, Gordon WA, Rosenthal M, Marwitz J: Neuropsychological characteristics of patients with brain injury: preliminary findings from a multicenter investigation. J Head Trauma Rehabil 8(2):47–59, 1993

Lee GP, Loring DW, Martin RC: Rey's 15-Item Visual Memory Test for the detection of malingering: normative observations on patients with neurological disorders. Psychol Assessment 4:43–46, 1992

Lees-Haley PR, Brown RS: Neuropsychological complaint base rates of 170 personal injury claimants. Arch Clin Neuropsychol 8:203–209, 1993

Lees-Haley PR, English LT, Glenn WJ: A Fake Bad scale on the MMPI-2 for personal injury claimant. Psychol Rep 68:203–210, 1991

Leli DA, Filskov SB: Clinical-actuarial detection and description of brain impairment in the W-B Form 1. J Clin Psychol 37:623–629, 1981

Levin HS, Grossman R, Kelly P: Aphasic disorder in patients with closed head injury. J Neurol Neurosurg Psychiatry 39:1062–1070, 1976

Levin HS, Mattis S, Ruff RM et al: Neurobehavioral outcome following minor head injury: a 3-center study. J Neurosurg 66:234–243, 1987

Levin HS, O'Donnell VM, Grossman RG: The Galveston Orientation and Amnesia Test: a practical scale to assess cognition after head injury. J Nerv Ment Dis 167:675–684, 1975

Lezak MD: Neuropsychological Assessment. 2nd Ed. Oxford University Press, New York, 1983

Martin RC, Bolter JF, Todd ME et al: Effects of sophistication and motivation on the detection of malingered memory performance using a computerized forced-choice task. J Clin Exp Neuropsychol 15:867–880, 1993

McCaffrey RJ, Lynch JJ: A methodological review of "method skeptic" reports. Neuropsychol Rev 3:235–248, 1992

McLean A, Dikmen SS, Temkin N: Psychosocial recovery after head injury. Arch Phys Med Rehabil 74:1041–1046, 1993

McNairy SL, Toshihiko M, Ivnik RJ et al: Prescription medication dependence and neuropsychologic function. Pain 18:169–177, 1984

Millis SR: The Recognition Memory Test in the detection of malingered and exaggerated memory deficits. Clin Neuropsychol 6:406–414, 1992

Millis SR, Dijkers M: Use of the Recognition Memory Test in traumatic brain injury: preliminary findings. Brain Inj 7:53–58, 1993

Millis SR, Putnam SH: The Recognition Memory Test in the assessment of memory impairment after financially compensable mild head injury: a replication. Percept Mot Skill 79:384–386, 1994

Millis SR, Ricker JH: The California Verbal Learning Test in the detection of feigned memory impairment. Paper presented at the meeting of the International Neuropsychological Society, Cincinnati, 1994

Mittenberg W, Azrin R, Millsaps C, Heilbronner R: Identification of malingered head injury on the Wechsler Memory Scale-Revised. Psycholog Assessment 5:34–40, 1993a

Mittenberg W, DiGiulio DV, Perrin S, Bass AE: Symptoms following mild head injury: expectation as etiology. J Neurol Neurosurg Psychiatry 55:200–204, 1992

Mittenberg W, Zielinski RE, Fichera SM et al: Identification of malingered head injury on the Wechsler Adult Intelligence Scale-Revised. Poster presentation at the meeting of the National Academy of Neuropsychology, Phoenix, 1993b

Nadler JD, Mittenberg W, DePiano FA, Schneider BA: Effects of patient age on neuropsychological test interpretation. Prof Psychol Res Pract 25:288–295, 1994

Noyes R, Holt CS: Anxiety disorders. pp. 139–159. In Winokur G, Clayton PJ (eds): The Medical Basis of Psychiatry. 2nd Ed. WB Saunders, Philadelphia, 1994

Pankratz L: Malingering on intellectual and neuropsychological measures. pp. 169–192. In Rogers R (ed): Clinical Assessment of Malingering and Deception. Guilford Press, New York, 1988

Pankratz L, Erickson RC: Two views of malingering. Clin Neuropsychol 4:379–389, 1990

Pankratz L, Fausti SA, Peed S: A forced-choice technique to evaluate deafness in the hysterical patient. J Consult Clin Psychol 43:421–422, 1975

Pennebaker JW: The Psychology of Physical Symptoms. Springer-Verlag, New York, 1982

Pope KS, Butcher JN, Seelen J: The MMPI, MMPI-2, and MMPI-A in court: A Practical Guide for Expert Witnesses and Attorneys. American Psychological Association, Washington, 1993

Prigatano GP, Amin K: Digit Memory Test: unequivocal cerebral dysfunction and suspected malingering. J Clin Exp Neuropsychol 15:537–546, 1993

Pritchard D, Moses J: Tests of neuropsychological malingering. Forensic Rep 5:287–290, 1992

Putnam SH, Adams KM, O'Leary J: MMPI-2 correlates of unexpected cognitive deterioration in mild traumatic brain injury. Paper presented at the 28th Annual MMPI Symposium on Recent Developments in the Use of the MMPI, St. Petersburg Beach, FL, 1993

Putnam SH, Millis SR: Psychosocial factors in the development and maintenance of chronic somatic and functional symptoms following mild traumatic brain injury. Adv Med Psychother 7:1–22, 1994

Rawling PJ: The Simulation Index: A reliability study. Brain Inj 6:381–383, 1992

Rawling P, Brooks N: Simulation Index: a method for detecting factitious errors on the WAIS-R and WMS. Neuropsychology 4:223–238, 1990

Reitan RM, Wolfson D: The Halstead-Reitan Neuropsychological Test Battery: Theory and Clinical Interpretation. 2nd Ed. Neuropsychology Press, S. Tucson, AZ, 1993

Rogers R: Models of feigned illness. Prof Psychol Res Pract 21:182–188, 1990

Rogers R, Gillis JR, Dickens SE, Bagby RM: Standardized assessment of malingering: validation of the Structured Interview of Reported Symptoms. Psychol Assessment 3:89–96, 1991

Rogers R, Harrell EH, Liff CD: Feigning neuropsychological impairment: a critical review of methodological and clinical considerations. Clin Psychol Rev 13:255–274, 1993

Schretlen D, Brandt J, Krafft L, Van Gorp W: Some caveats in using the Rey 15-Item Memory Test to detect malingered amnesia. Psychol Assessment 3:667–672, 1991

Shapiro DL: Forensic Psychological Assessment: An Integrative Approach. Allyn & Bacon, Boston, 1991

Spreen O, Strauss E: A Compendium of Neuropsychological Tests. Oxford University Press, New York, 1991

Sternbach RA: Pain Patients: Traits and Treatment. Academic Press, Orlando, 1974

Tarter RC, Van Thiel DH, Edwards KL (eds): Medical Neuropsychology: The Impact of Disease on Behavior. Plenum, New York, 1988

Teasdale G, Jennett B: Assessment of coma and impaired consciousness: a practical scale. Lancet 2:81–84, 1974

Trueblood W, Schmidt M: Malingering and other validity considerations in the neuropsychological evaluation of mild head injury. J Clin Exp Neuropsychol 15:578–590, 1993

Tucker GJ: In reply [letter to the editor] J Neuropsychiatry Clin Neurosci 6:58–59, 1994

Warrington EK: Recognition Memory Test Manual. NFER-Nelson, Windsor, UK, 1984

Watson D, Pennebaker JW: Health complaints, stress, and distress: exploring the central role of negative affectivity. Psychol Rev 96:234–254, 1989

Wedding D, Faust D: Clinical judgment and decision making in neuropsychology. Arch Clin Neuropsychol 4:233–268, 1989

Wiggins EC, Brandt J: The detection of simulated amnesia. Law Hum Behav 12:57–78, 1988

Williams JM: Memory Assessment Scales: Professional Manual. Psychological Assessment Resources, Odessa, FL, 1991

Winokur G, Clayton PJ: The Medical Basis of Psychiatry. 2nd Ed. WB Saunders, Philadelphia, 1994

Wong JL, Regennitter RP, Barrios F: Base rate and simulated symptoms of mild head injury among normals. Arch Clin Neuropsychol 9:411–425, 1994

Chronic Pain, Soft-Tissue Injury, and Litigation Law 26

Michael I. Weintraub

In the past decade, the subject of chronic pain and its association with litigation has aroused considerable interest and controversy. Although nearly everyone agrees that chronic pain is a major health problem and an economic burden in America, little consensus exists about its cause, pathophysiology, precise diagnosis, and treatment. Occupational musculoskeletal injuries and vehicular crashes account for the largest source of chronic pain complaints, and traditionally, these injuries have been viewed with some skepticism due to lack of specific tissue damage. The role of financial incentives has long been thought to be the fuel for this national epidemic. With a rising skepticism about the legitimacy of complaints in litigation and the soaring number of claims for chronic pain syndrome, pain, and suffering, there is a critical need to redefine this syndrome in terms of its relationship to legal as well as medical etiologies.

The public awareness of remuneration for illness and traumatic complaints has not been forgotten and has helped to generate 18 million lawsuits in the United States per year (Margolick, 1993). Individuals are compensated for both economic and noneconomic damages. In the latter category are the subjective and intangible pain and suffering, loss of consortium, and hedonic pleasures. Despite the fact that these cannot be quantified scientifically, they are responsible for 80 percent of the current awards. The recent fraudulent trials of *Lenahan* (Lavin, 1991) and *Matos* (Crane, 1994) fooled jurors and medical personnel and were successfully detected only by active videotaped surveillance. Thus, the fundamental questions are the following: does chronic pain truly exist, and how legitimate are complaints when litigation is pending? Alternatively, how does the clinician confirm that the patient actually has pain? The following chapter explores this relationship and clinical dilemma.

DEFINING CHRONIC PAIN SYNDROME

Chronic pain syndrome is saddled with imprecise understanding and many definitions. Thus, mastering the vocabulary is an important first step in avoiding misconception. Beecher (1957) attempted to define and quantify pain and cited 850 references, yet concluded that he could not describe pain in meaningful terms because it was a *subjective* experience. In fact, the sole unquestioned quantified element of chronic pain is its duration, with symptoms lasting longer than 6 months.

PAIN

Pain has been defined by the International Association for the Study of Pain, Subcommittee on Taxotomy (IASP, 1979), as an "unpleasant sensory and emotional experience connected with actual or potential tissue damage or described in terms of such damage." Pain is only subjective. Each individual *learns* through experience what this actually means and what secondary gains can be generated. Implicit therefore is that the definition of pain has two components. Chronic pain syndrome is by definition refractory to medical intervention. All individuals are potentially vulnerable. Although scientifically the notion that all pain should be verifiable by objective measures is valid, unfortunately at present, no biologic techniques or markers exist to measure pain. This is indeed a *subjective* complaint. However, when the neurologic examination is standardized and quantified, there is substantial correlation with observed neuropathology (Dyck et al., 1985). Ekblom (1993) believes that the IASP definition relates only to humans and is not valid in animal studies and should be excluded in the reports on animal research. He thinks it is naive to extrapolate from behavioral studies in animals to the complex sensation of pain in humans. The quantification of pain has been traditionally by self-report. The validity of these statements is based on the assumption that the patient will answer truthfully and not intentionally falsify, manipulate, or mislead. However, it is easy to fool a psychologist and pain experts (Faust et al., 1988) as well as deliberately score poorly (Bruhn and Reed, 1975; Franzen, 1991). Mersky (1993) confirmed the lack of reliability of self-report and how it can be manipulated. Patients with varying personalities have different perceptions of pain, as well as functional impairments. McFadden and Woitalla (1993) described a patient with four different personalities and four different perceptions of pain with four different results on psychological testing. It is well known that learning affects the perceived response, and this was demonstrated in the Munchausen syndrome reports of Rimon et al. (1980) and Fishbain et al. (1988). Thus, the clinician is faced with a dilemma regarding the authenticity of self-report of pain and must therefore rely on physical examination techniques to identify objective signs of organicity. Also, dependence on objective testing (i.e., magnetic resonance imaging [MRI], computed tomography [CT], electromyography [EMG], somatosensory evoked potential [SSEP], myelography, etc.) will allow for a firmer basis to corroborate the subjective complaints.

Chronic pain characteristically is regional, involving the back, neck, extremities, and head. However, when litigation is present, the location of the symptoms are not random but rather are concentrated in the functional domain of the sensory and motor systems of the injured area (Weintraub, 1988).

HYSTERICAL CONVERSION REACTION

Psychogenic musculoskeletal pain represents the most frequent presentation of hysterical conversion reaction. Traditionally, Breuer and Freud (1955) identified dissociation secondary to psychological needs as the basic cause for this presentation. A symbolic relationship existed between the symptom and the original trauma, which afforded the patient primary and secondary gain. The notion that patients playing the sick role could be an attractive and efficient means of satisfying intrapsychic conflicts and interpersonal needs was accepted for many years. However, with the surging number of claims over the past 20 years and the observation of fabrication for remuneration, a revision of thought has developed. Thus, there is a strong perception and appreciation that psychogenic pain symptoms are linked to the conscious and subconscious expectation of remuneration.

In an effort to determine the authenticity and legitimacy of complaints, there has been increasing use of videotape surveillance. It comes as no surprise that the detection of malingering and fraud in the malpractice cases of Lenahan and Matos, as well as in the New Jersey-staged "Ghost Riders Sting Operation" has raised voices for tort reform (Kerr, 1993). Hysterical conversion reaction and malingering constitute a major public health problem, and it is sobering to note how many professionals have been fooled. In the absence of biologic markers specific for hysterical conversion reaction and soft-tissue damage, the clinician's most reliable method of establishing a diagnosis is to perform a careful neurologic examination. The detection of nonanatomic and nonphysiologic findings offers the clinician a window of opportunity to explore the psychologic and financial symbolism of complaints.

TABLE 26-1. Psychogenic Sensory Findings

Variability
Sharp midline boundary to pinprick
Splitting of vibration over bones
Nondermatomal pattern
Spread to uninvolved ipsilateral areas in head, vision, hearing

Physicians are exceedingly naive about psychogenic complaints based on their traditional training to accept the history and complaints as legitimate. They routinely ignore the importance of primary and secondary gain. Hysterical conversion reaction is characterized by nonverbal communication and symbolic representation reflecting the patient's knowledge of the body (real or presumed) (Breuer). These symptoms arise because the patient wishes to obtain some gain (financial or interpersonal). The diagnosis is not confirmed by exclusion or personality traits but by the clinician demonstrating on examination that these symptoms fail to conform to known anatomic and physiologic patterns of innervation. Examination techniques have been described by Weintraub (1977a, 1977b, 1983) to assist in diagnosis. However, some authors question the reliability and validity of nonorganic sensory and motor findings (Drake, 1991; Gould et al., 1986; Merskey, 1993).

Psychogenic sensory deficits are diagnosed by their variability, sharp midline transition, and nonanatomic dermatomal distribution (Table 26-1). The use of pinpricking and vibration is extremely informative as to the specific localization of alleged abnormality. Likewise, psychogenic motor deficits are diagnosed by their variability, reserved strength, and nonanatomic distribution (Table 26-2). The dramatic hysterical conversion reaction seen in the days of Charcot (i.e. paralysis, blindness, deafness, convulsion) (Janet, 1907) has been replaced to conform to our present litigious society (Shorter, 1992). Thus is not surprising to note that psychogenic pain is the most common form of hysterical conversion reaction (Wise, 1977). Suggestion and/or intravenous saline have been used to provide confirmation of the diagnosis of pseudoseizures or psychogenic symptomatology (Cohen and Suter, 1982; Desai et al., 1982).

TABLE 26-2. Psychogenic Motor Findings

Variability
Reserve strength
Nonanatomic pattern
Spread to uninvolved areas
Absence of atrophy, trophic changes

MALINGERING

Malingering is medical lying. It is the false and fraudulent imitation or exaggeration of physical illness and/or mental symptoms to obtain financial reward. It is the behavioral pattern that is deliberate and under conscious control. The goals include financial compensation, drugs, hospitalization, or avoidance of punishment. Malingering and hysterical conversion reaction can coexist (Table 26-3). Stinnett (1987) and Evans (1992) think that malingering is relatively rare, yet most clinical neurologists managing chronic pain patients do not share this perception. For a more in-depth discussion on the topic of malingering, please see Chapter 27.

LITIGATION/COMPENSATION NEUROSIS

All pain-related litigation cannot fit neatly into a single category. In the United States, there are two distinct legal avenues: Workmen's Compensation system and civil tort litigation. Each has a distinct history that needs to be briefly reviewed if we are to more fully appreciate the current problem. Historically, the first reported case of an employee seeking compensation from an employer for a work-related injury reached the high court in England during 1837 (Mendelson, 1992). In 1879, Rigler raised the issue of compensation neurosis when he described the in-

TABLE 26-3. Hallmark Features of Combined Hysterical Conversion Reaction and Malingering

Magnitude of original trauma is *disproportionate to disability*
Refractory to *all* treatment modalities
Litigation or obvious 1 or 2 degree gain
Nonanatomic examination
Negative workup for organicity (i.e., magnetic resonance imaging/electromyogram etc)
Job dissatisfaction
Personal stress

creased incidence of post-traumatic invalidism on the Prussian railways in 1871. In 1887, Strumpell noted the role of exaggeration and embellishment related to financial compensation (Weighill, 1983). In 1888, Oppenheim popularized the concept of *traumatic neurosis.* In 1897, the Workmen's Compensation Act was formally introduced on a no-fault basis. Charcot (1880) suspected an association between litigation and psychogenic pain when evaluating cases of railway spine syndrome, which was described as "railway brain syndrome." Fabrication and embellishment of symptoms secondary to financial gain led them to doubt the authenticity of complaints when litigation was present. Foster Kennedy (1946) made the same observation that minimal observable injuries often lead to disproportionate disability. Those observations made nearly 100 years ago have relevance today. For example, it is currently estimated that 7 million workers are injured on the job yearly with most requiring limited medical attention and intervention (Pfennigstorf and Gifford, 1991). However, nearly 2 percent of the total industrial workforce suffer a compensible back injury each year, and 25 percent of these cases account for nearly 90 percent of the total cost (Leavitt et al., 1971; Snook, 1987). A current statistic suggests that disability from back pain is increasing at 14 percent of population growth (Robertson and Keeve, 1983), suggesting that back pain is an illness in search of a disease. Collie (1932) stated that "fraud is a product of the age of the Workmen's Compensation Act, of trade unions and allied clubs. There are no malingerers in countries where there is no Workmen's Compensation Act." Those observations were recently confirmed by Balla (1982) and Waddell (1987). Because the accident victim in the Workmen's Compensation system received few benefits from government entitlements, he has been made aware of the system and how to enhance awards. Thus independent lawsuits against employers or third parties for "negligence" are proliferating, thereby enabling the victim to sue for economic and noneconomic damages (pain and suffering). Claimant abuse reached a new dimension when a dozen compensation attorneys sustained a flurry of minor accidents (i.e., lifting a briefcase, inspecting a chair) that resulted in awards totaling $670,000. One attorney injured his back lifting his briefcase out of his car trunk, yet the injury did not cause him to miss any work or even miss his golf game. A Workmen's Compensation judge awarded him $95,000. In defense of the award, the senior judge stated that the lawyers were not "thieves, cheats, or exploiters, but merely aware of Worker's Compensation Laws" (Margolick, 1993). In another case, a lawyer had 30 personal lawsuits raising issues of vexatious litigant or accident-proneness (Schmidt, 1993). Thus, financial incentive and a knowledge of the system reward a significant group of abusive claimants. However, it should not be inferred that the system is without merit for most workers.

Viewing chronic pain in the context of fraudulent statements, the magnitude of the original trauma often appears disproportionate to the degree of disability. Comparisons of similar injuries in children and adults in other countries often demonstrate a marked discrepancy in length of complaints, as well as return to work (Miller, 1961, 1966; Steinbach, 1965). Some authors have concluded that the greater the financial compensation, the longer the individual remains off work (Beales, 1984; Health Insurance News, 1979; Osterweis et al., 1987; Worral and Butler, 1985). The importance of nonphysical factors such as job dissatisfaction and personal stress have also been acknowledged as important factors in return to work (Bigos and Andary, 1991).

It is difficult to calculate the degree of fraudulent behavior in the compensation system. However, the purposeful misrepresentation of claims was found acceptable in 20 percent of the Public Attitude Monitor (PAM, 1992) survey and alarmingly in 46 percent living in New York, Pennsylvania, and New Jersey. Thus, it is easy to see why the term *compensation neurosis* survives. The weight of evidence indicates that pain dysfunction syndromes exist (Amadio, 1988), triggered by three primary components: an accident that can produce pain, psychological factors, and potential for primary and secondary gain from continued disability.

Chronic Pain

Chronic pain is a common component of traumatic injuries and should be compensated. The danger of assuming that all cases of soft-tissue injury in litigation are fraudulent is a disservice to legitimate victims. Thus, how does the clinician evaluate and measure the subjective complaints and determine if they are fabricated? Pain and suffering comprise the largest element of damages, yet it is often the most difficult for the jury to convert to monetary value. Does pain and suffering exist from a medical standpoint, or is this a legal myth? These vexing questions need to be addressed if we are going to understand the current system.

Weintraub (1992) studied a cohort of 210 consecutive cases of chronic pain in tort litigation using sensitive neurologic examination techniques, as well as MRI, SSEP, CT, EMG, etc., and found that 63 percent demonstrated psychogenic findings. Citing malingering or hysterical conversion reaction as the major cause for chronic pain syndrome when litigation is involved oversimplifies this complex and poorly understood condition. In fact, Evans (1992) reaches opposite conclusions. It remains to be established how frequent fabrication of symptoms are, but the PAM survey suggests a range of 20 to 40 percent. Insurance data indicate a disproportionate number of claims from the large cities of Newark, Baltimore, New York, Detroit, and Philadelphia in comparison with their entire states. The reason for this is unclear and has been attributed to lawyer density, insurance benefits, poverty, etc. Recently, a specific type of fraud was uncovered in a New Jersey "sting" operation known as "Ghost Riders" (Kerr, 1993). In this staged bus crash, several outsiders jump on the stopped vehicle, mingle, and claim injury. Surprisingly, many individuals also submit claims even though they were not near the scene of the crash. Debunking claims for the alleged "pain and suffering" is obviously extremely difficult without a videotape (Lavin, 1991). If this problem confronts the scientific community, how valid is it that juries can easily reach a verdict? Recently, the Harvard study concluded that a solid majority of malpractice claims filed for pain and suffering and alleged injury are not valid (Weiler et al., 1993).

The notion that chronic pain, despite the absence of scientific tissue damage, was a legal entity and should be compensated was forcibly argued in 1951 by Melvin Belli (1965). He proposed a formula for compensating pain in dollars per unit of time (i.e., per diem), and subsequently the Supreme Court implicitly endorsed this per diem argument for "pain and suffering" in the *Braddock* case (1957). This issue was directly ruled on in 24 states, with 14 accepting and 10 rejecting as of 1973. Current data suggest that almost all states accept this legal premise as a means of compensation despite absence of scientific support.

Soft-Tissue Injury

Soft-tissue injury is conceptually appealing to explain the profound disability in the absence of herniated disc, spinal stenosis, denervation, fracture, etc. Various terminologies have been applied (i.e., myofascial pain syndrome, fibromyositis, etc.) (Table 26-4), but regardless of the label they cannot be confirmed by any laboratory or clinical test (Cohen, 1993; Forslind et al., 1990; Frection, 1989). Drawing firm conclusions from prior studies with heterogeneous populations, small sample size, lack of objective imaging and electrodiagnostic studies, lack of comprehensive neurologic examinations, lack of association with litigation, and lack of controls and outcome studies identifies methodologic flaws. Thus, currently there is no scientific corroboration for its existence!

Hedonic Damages

"Hedonic damages" is a concept fabricated for litigation and promoted under the guise of scientific research. It is associated with the notion that hedonic damages are intended to compensate for the "loss of enjoyment of life." The first association of this occurred with *Sherrod v. Berry*. It illustrates the liberal approaches that the courts have allowed in the direction of pseudoscientific evidence. The decline of the *Frye* rule (1974) and its outright rejection in some jurisdictions allow for the acceptance of hedonic interpretation. It remains to be seen how the recent *Daubert* decision (1994) will affect the above.

CONCLUSION

The current compensation system seems to subsidize and encourage disability as well as fraudulent behavior, whereas the current tort system rewards subjective dubious complaints of pain and suffering and hedonic loss. Inaccurate psychological conclusions, learned behavior, and hired "expert" witnesses all contribute to flaws in the system, producing not only junk science but also junk justice. Because many patients perceive themselves as medically ill and constantly seek attention, the costs of chronic pain are

TABLE 26-4. Common Syndromes Incorrectly Defined as Soft-Tissue Injury

Myofascial pain syndrome
Fibromyalgia
Chronic fatigue syndrome
Reflex sympathetic dystrophy
Repetitive stress disorder
Lyme disease

not anticipated to diminish. Although some of this behavior is legitimate, there is also clearly a fraudulent subbasis.

No permanent resolution to this problem is likely until tort reform occurs (Carlin, 1980). According to Weintraub (1992), the current system needs to be reorganized into a two-tier compensation. Claims will be heard, fault determined, and money awarded based on objective injuries and loss of future earning potential. Nonanatomic aspects of pain and suffering should also be compensated but in a manner different from that established for objective damages. Clearly, a higher settlement should be awarded for objective deficits. Until a longitudinal outcome study is completed, one must be cautious. Billions of dollars of unnecessary tests, procedures, clinical visits, and treatments would be saved by meaningful reform.

Unraveling the effects of litigation and compensation on treatment response and chronic pain syndrome is a formidable task, yet must be done due to the huge economic burden to society. Physicians must maintain a higher index of suspicion and should perform detailed analyses of the painful areas one or more times in an attempt to corroborate the subjective complaints if litigation is lurking in the background. Recovery is a multifaceted approach influenced by medical, psychologic, economic, social, and legal factors. Prospective studies are urgently needed to define more accurately the natural history of individuals with chronic pain in litigation.

REFERENCES

Amadio PC: Pain dysfunction syndrome. J Bone Joint Surg [Am] 70:944–949, 1988

Balla JI: The late whiplash syndrome: a study of an illness in Australia and Singapore. Cult Med Psychiatry 6:191–192, 1982

Beals RK: Compensation and recovery from injury. West J Med 140:233–237, 1984

Beecher HK: Review of pain. Pharmacol Rev 9:59–97, 1957

Belli M: Morris, Audio-Visual Study of Pain and Suffering in dollars-on-unit-of-time basis. 14 Def LJ 129, 1965

Bigos SJ, Andary MT: Practitioner's guide to industrial back problems. Neurosurg Clin North Am 2:868–875, 1991

Breuer J, Freud S: Studies on Hysteria. Complete Psychological Works of Freud (1893–1895). Vol. 2. Standard Ed. Hogarth Press, London, 1955

Bruhn AR, Reed MR: Simulation of brain damage on Bender-Gestalt test by college students. J Pers Assess 3:244–255, 1975

Carlin PE: Medical Malpractice Pre-Trial Screening Panels: A Review of the Evidence. Intergovernmental Health Policy Project, Washington, DC, 1980

Charcot JM: Lecons sur les Maladies du Systeme Nerveux Faites a la Salpetriere. Vol. 1. 4th Ed. Paris, 1880

Cohen ML: Fibromyalgia syndrome, a problem of tautology. Lancet 342:906–909, 1993

Cohen RJ, Suter G: Hysterical "seizures"—suggestion as a provocative EEG test. Ann Neurol aa:391–395, 1982

Collie J: Fraud in Medico-Legal Practice. 2nd Ed. Edward Arnold, London. 1932

Crane M: Malpractice Lies and Videotape. Med Econ June 13, 1994

Daubert v. Merrell Dow Pharmaceuticals, 113 S. Ct. 320 (1992)

Desai BT, Porter RJ, Penry JK: Psychogenic seizures: a study of 42 attacks in 6 patients with intensive monitoring. Arch Neurol 39:202–209, 1982

Drake ME, Jr: Conversion hysteria and dominant hemisphere lesions, abstract ed. Neurology 41:120, 1991

Dyck PJ, Karnes JL, Daube J et al: Clinical and neuropathological criteria for the diagnosis and staging of diabetic polyneuropathy. Brain 108:861–880, 1985

Ekblom A: When is "pain" appropriate? Pain 55:403, 1993

Evans RW: The postconcussion syndrome and the sequelae of mild head injury. Neurol Clin North Am 10:815–847, 1992

Faust D, Hart K, Guilmette TJ: Pediatric malingering: the capacity of children to fake believable deficits on neuropsychological testing. J Consult Clin Psychol 56:578–582, 1988a

Faust D, Hart K, Guilmette TJ, Arkes HR: Neuropsychologists capacity to detect adolescent malingerers. Prof Psychol Res Pract 14:508–545, 1988b

Fishbain DA, Goldberg M, Labbe E et al: Compensation and non-compensation chronic pain patients compared for DMS-III, operation diagnoses. Pain 32:197–206, 1968

Forslind K, Fredrikson E, Nived O: Does primary fibromyalgia exist? Br J Rheumatol 29:358–370, 1990

Frection JD: Myofascial pain syndrome. Neurol Clin 7:413–427, 1989

Frye v. United States, 293 F.2d 741 (D.C. Cir. 1974)

Franzen MD, Iverson GL, McCracken LM: The detection of malingering in neuropsychological assessment. Neuropsychol Rev 1:247–279, 1990

Gould R, Miller BL, Goldberg MA, Benson DF: The validity of hysterical signs and symptoms. J Nerv Ment Dis 174:593–597, 1986

International Association for The Study of Pain, Subcommittee on Taxonomy: Pain terms: a list with definitions and notes on usage. Pain 6:249–252, 1979

Janet P: The Major Symptoms of Hysteria. MacMillan, New York, 1907

Kennedy F: The mind of the injured worker—its effect on the disability periods. Comp Med 1:19–24, 1946

Kerr P: Ghost Riders' Are Target of an Insurance Sting. New York Times, Aug. 18, 1993, at 1

Lavin JH: Everyone believed the plaintiff except his doctor. Med Econ 34–41, 1991

Leavitt SS, Johnston TL, Beyer RD: The process of recovery patterns in industrial back injury. Part I, costs and other quantitative measures of effort. Ind Med Surg 40:7–14, 1971

Liberal payments prolong disability (editorial). Health Insurance News, August 1979

Margolick D: At the bar. New York Times, April 30, 1993a, sect. B16 (col. 1)

Margolick D: Bar group renews feud with Quayle. New York Times, Feb. 2, 1993b

McFadden IJ, Woitalla WF: Differing reports of pain perception by different personalities in a patient with chronic pain and multiple personality disorder. Pain 55:379–382, 1993

Mendelson G: Compensation and chronic pain. Pain 48:121–123, 1992

Merskey H: Regional pain is rarely hysterical. Arch Neurol 45:915–918, 1988

Merskey H: Pain and dissociation. Pain 55:281–282, 1993

Miller H: Accident neurosis. BMJ 1:19–25, 1961a

Miller H: Accident neurosis. BMJ 1:992–998, 1961b

Miller H: Accident neurosis. Proc Med Leg Soc Vic 10:71–82, 1966

Oppenheim H: Wie Sind Die Erkrankungen Des Nervensystems Aufzuffasen, Welche Sich Nach Erschutterung Des Ruckenmarks, Insbesondere, Nach Eisenbahnunfallen, Entwickeln. Berl Klin Wochenschr 25:166–170, 1888

Osterweis M, Kleinman A, Mechanic D: Pain and Disability. Clinical, Behavioral and Public Policy Perspectives. Institute of Medicine. National Academy Press, Washington, DC, 1987

Pfennigstorf W, Gifford DG: A Comparative Study of Liability Law and Compensation Schemes in Ten Countries and The United States. Insurance Research Council, 1991

Public Attitude Monitor. Insurance Research Council, 1992

Public Attitude Monitor. Insurance Research Council, 1993

Rigler J: Ueber die Verletzungen auf Eisenbahnen Insebesondere der Verletzungen des Rueckenmarks. Reimer, Berlin, 1879

Rimon R, Kampman R, Ikonen E et al: Munchausen's syndrome: a review and 2 case reports. Psychother Psychosom 33:185–192, 1980

Robertson LS, Keeve JP: Workers injuries: the effect of Workers' Compensation and OSHA inspections. Health Politics Policy Law 8:581–597, 1983

Schmidt RB: Heavy caseload: is Patricia McColm a vexatious litigant, or accident prone. Wall Street Journal, May, 1993

Seaboard Airline R. v. Braddock, 96 So. 2d 127, at 129 (Fla. 1957)

Sherrod v. Berry 629 F. Supp. 159 (M.D. Ill. 1985)

Shorter E: From Paralysis to Fatigue: A History of Psychosomatic Illness in the Modern Era. Free Press, Toronto, 1992

Snook SH: The costs of back pain in industry. State of the art review. Spine 2:1–5, 1987

Steinbach RA, Tursky B: Ethnic differences among housewives in psychophysical and skin potential responses to electric shock. Psychophysiology 1:241–246, 1965

Stinett JL: The functional somatic symptom. Psychiatr Clin North Am 10:19–33, 1987

Waddell G: A new clinical model for the treatment of low-back pain. 1987 Volvo Award in Clinical Science. Spine 12:632–644, 1987

Weighill VE: Compensation neurosis: A review of the literature. J Psychosom Res 27:97–104, 1983

Weiler PC, Hiatt HH, Newhouse JP et al: A Measure Of Malpractice: Medical Injury, Malpractice Litigation and Patient Compensation. Harvard University Press, Cambridge, MA, 1993

Weintraub MI: A Clinician's Manual of Hysterical Conversion Reactions. Interdisciplinary Communications Media, New York, 1977a

Weintraub MI: Hysteria: a clinical guide to diagnosis. Clin Symp 29:1–30, 1977b

Weintraub MI: Hysterical conversion reactions. In: A Clinical Guide to Diagnosis and Treatment. SP Medical and Scientific Books, New York, 1983

Weintraub MI: Regional pain is usually hysterical. Arch Neurol 45:914–915, 1988

Weintraub MI: Litigation—chronic pain syndrome—a distinct entity: analysis of 210 cases. Am J Pain Management 2:1989–204, 1992

Wise TN: Pain: the most common psychosomatic problem. Med Clin North Am 61:771–780, 1977

Worral JD, Butler RJ: Benefits and claim duration. In Worral JD, Appel D (eds): Workers Compensation Benefits: Adequacy, Equity & Efficiency. ILR Press, Ithica, NY, 1985

Medicolegal Aspects of Head Injury

27

Carl L. Rowley
Richard S. Cornfeld

Virtually all attorneys who prepare for and try lawsuits call on the services of experts, medical and other kinds, for advice and for testimony. Similarly, many physicians, psychologists, and other medical providers become involved in litigation in one way or another, voluntarily or not. This chapter explains the essential, typical elements of that involvement.

CONSULTATION AND TESTIMONY IN LITIGATION

Physicians, psychologists, scientists, and other experts serve two purposes in litigation: as "consultants" (providing advice to attorneys that will help them represent their client more effectively) and as witnesses (educating and drawing inferences for the judge or jury through live or recorded testimony). Experts who are retained for the purpose of testifying usually also provide consultation in the cases in which they have been retained. Experts retained exclusively for consultation are not expected to testify.

Role as Consultant Generally

In lawsuits that present comparatively simple medical and scientific issues, most attorneys can prepare adequately for trial simply by studying the applicable literature and questioning experts who already are involved in the litigation, such as treating physicians. In other cases, attorneys seek the advice of experts retained or hired specifically for the purpose of consultation because the comparative complexity of the issues renders self-study an inefficient means of preparing for trial.

Functions Served by Consultant; Importance to Attorney and Client

An expert's role as a consultant may vary from limited participation in the lawsuit or other dispute (providing a general familiarization with medical or scientific issues that are expected to arise in the case) to active, sometimes day-to-day involvement (developing evidence that may support or negate issues such as causation, injury, and extent of disability). The typical advantages of serving as a consultant as opposed to participating as a witness include likely anonymity, at least to the extent that most jurisdictions do not require a party to disclose to the opposing side its consultants' identities or even the fact that a consultant has been hired. Thus, the communications between a nontestifying consultant and an attorney can usually remain confidential with respect to opposing parties. Ironically, it frequently is the expert who has the least interest in testifying who can render the most valuable service in rebutting the testimony of the opposing experts. Experts who have no interest in giving testimony (with its often hostile cross-examination and accompanying professional scrutiny) can be indispensable in determining the truth and in helping the attorney to establish it as fact at trial or during other proceedings such as administrative hearings.

Discoverability of Consulting Expert's Work Product

Just as the identity of the consulting expert in litigation may remain confidential, the tangible results of his* efforts (e.g., notes, reports, summarizations of literature, and correspondence with counsel) usually also may remain private as between the consultant, the retaining lawyer, and his client. In the jargon of attorneys, the consultant's "work product" is not "discoverable" by the opposing side in most courts under most circumstances. By contrast, the work product of experts who are expected to testify may be compelled to be produced, to a varying extent depending on the jurisdiction, to the opposing party.

This limitation on required disclosure for nontestifying consultants can lead to a more informal (and occasionally more productive) working relationship between the lawyer and the expert because there is less need for concern that matters committed to writing might later be taken out of context during an examination at deposition or at trial or that those materials might otherwise be used to prejudice the intended beneficiary of the expert's advice.

Role as Trial Witness

Although the number of experts used in the typical lawsuit has burgeoned over the past few decades, most witnesses at trials and depositions are still "fact" or lay witnesses, not experts. Fact witnesses testify about what they saw or heard or did. Their testimony must arise from their own observations. They generally cannot give opinions even if they have them. Experts or "opinion witnesses," however, are permitted to testify to opinions that laypersons, including the jury, do not have the expertise to reach for themselves.

Functions Served; Importance to Attorney and Client

Although testifying experts usually do draw inferences and express them to the jury as professional opinions during their testimony, they may also testify as experts without rendering opinions. The rules of court that describe the circumstances under which medical evidence may be presented to the jury almost always permit experts to educate jurors on relevant scientific principles, while leaving it to the jury to reach its own conclusions by applying those principles to the evidence. When the desired inference is sufficiently obvious, this tactic can be even more effective than the more blunt approach of presenting opinion testimony.

Opinion testimony is not always permitted on every subject. The matters on which opinions may be rendered at trial differ according to the law of the jurisdiction in which the case is pending. Rule 702 of the Federal Rules of Evidence, applicable in federal courts, is representative of a standard that commonly is used to determine whether a matter can properly be the subject of expert testimony:

> **If scientific, technical, or other specialized knowledge will assist the trier of fact to understand the evidence or to determine a fact in issue, a witness qualified as an expert by knowledge, skill, experience, training, or education, may testify in the form of an opinion or otherwise.**

Thus, typically, a medical opinion, to be admissible, must be based on scientific knowledge and must assist the jury in understanding a fact or determining an issue in the case. Opinions on matters of common knowledge usually are not permitted, regardless of the identity or qualifications of the witness.

Expert testimony is essential in cases in which complex inferences must be drawn in order for the jury to decide the issues. Few lawsuits of any importance are tried today without testimony from one kind of expert witness or another.

In nearly every profession, there are now expert witnesses who are known to be willing to "say anything" for a price. Many such "experts" make their main living from testifying. The U.S. Court of Appeals for the Seventh Circuit in *Stoleson v. United States* has, in fact, observed that "there is not much difficulty in finding an expert witness to testify to virtually any

---

* Narrative illustration usually requires reference to hypothetical persons and thus to particular third-person pronouns. Because the use of masculine gender pronouns in these situations has historically been considered gender-neutral, the authors use them throughout this chapter as well.

theory of medical causation short of fantastic." Testimony by reputable, honest experts who are willing to expose these witnesses' invalid methods and conclusions is of critical importance to the just resolution of disputes in our courts.

Records and Documents from Counsel/Reports by the Expert

Participation in litigation by physicians and other professionals invariably requires the collection, generation, and exchange of written documents. Simple practicality often requires exchanges of correspondence between lawyer and witness. In a personal injury case, prior and subsequent records reflecting medical treatment, together with school, employment, and military records, must be compiled and given to the expert for his review. Unless the expert has a photographic memory, he will take notes and dictate reports on the progress of his findings and, eventually, his conclusions.

Because the opposing party may eventually attempt to use these documents in a manner that was not intended at the time of their creation, many lawyers prefer to communicate with their expert witnesses orally, by telephone or in person. They may request that their experts refrain from reducing their opinions to writing until a specified time. For example, it is usually a good idea not to express an opinion until after reviewing all the evidence; otherwise, the expert may be portrayed as biased and overly eager to jump to a conclusion.

There are legitimate reasons for these concerns. Expert witnesses are expected to come under serious attack at trial. Use of an expert's own words against him, in context or out, fairly or not, can render him ineffective. Even a seemingly innocent communication from the lawyer may be portrayed as an attempt to sway the witness's objectivity.

It therefore is prudent for opinion witnesses always to assume (absent being told otherwise by the sponsoring lawyer) that anything committed to writing in the course of consultation can be obtained by the opposing attorneys, whose job it may be to discredit the expert's opinions regardless of their validity or apparent unassailability.

Lawyers who retain experts in litigation generally do not represent one of their expert witnesses regarding events related to the litigation in which the witness is to testify; joint representation of the expert and client would create a conflict of interest. Thus, an expert witness should not think of the sponsoring lawyer as his own. If the need for legal advice arises, an independent lawyer who is not involved in the litigation should be consulted.

Physical Examinations and Reports/Disclosures of Opinions

Treating physicians often become involved in litigation not at the special request of an attorney but rather as a result of simply treating patients. Their credibility may be greater, all other things being equal, than that of a "retained" expert who has been selected by counsel. The treating physician's report may be even more persuasive to a jury if the conclusions expressed in it were reached without prior consultation with counsel or even without knowledge or anticipation of a lawsuit.

In addition to the treating physician's examination, many courts allow the defendant in a personal injury case to arrange for the plaintiff to be examined and tested by a physician of the defendant's choice. The rationale for permitting these examinations, which usually are called independent medical examinations (IMEs), is simple fairness. The plaintiff's treating physician may hold certain biases because of his relationship with the plaintiff, his family, or the plaintiff's lawyer or his law firm. Thus, the jury is permitted to hear from an independent expert to get both sides of the story.

If the independent expert's opinions are not supported by his own physical examination or tests, he may, depending on the circumstances, be at a disadvantage when rendering his testimony. Consider the likely effect on a jury of an affirmative answer to this question: "Sir, you have told the jury that Mr. Smith does not have brain damage, the opposite of what his family doctor of 25 years has said, and yet you have never talked with, met, or even laid eyes on Mr. Smith?" However, an IME may not be necessary when the scope of the expert's testimony is limited or when existing records provide an adequate basis for the opinions under the circumstances.

Defendants usually are limited to one IME of a plaintiff, unless he complains of more than one "injury" in the lawsuit. If, for example, a plaintiff claims that he suffered brain damage from head trauma and that he has depression as a result of the injury, the defendant might seek one IME regarding the supposed brain damage and another regarding the plaintiff's psychological condition.

In a typical clinical setting, absent unusual circumstances, the patient's motivation in making his complaints usually is not questioned or even considered by the physician. Most people go to a physician because they are sick and want to feel better. When, however, a patient has filed a lawsuit in which the amount of money that he will receive may depend on the existence and severity of his symptoms, motivation assumes greater importance and should be considered together with all other relevant medical factors (see Ch. 1). The IME physician may be the only physician who considers motivation in examining the plaintiff and in formulating his opinions for trial.

With respect to experts retained specifically for litigation, many courts require that a report that summarizes expected opinions and their bases be produced before they testify. Others require that "disclosures" that contain similar information, generally written by counsel, be provided in advance of depositions or trial testimony. The expert should discuss with the attorney precisely what will be required in a report generated for the litigation before he begins writing it. The safest practice is to assume that any "drafts" that are sent to counsel in advance of the "final" report may be produced to the other parties in the litigation. If changes are made in the "draft" after the attorney has reviewed and discussed it with the witness, the opposing lawyer will be in a position to argue that the changes were made at the insistence or suggestion of counsel, thereby calling into question the witness's objectivity and possibly the validity of his conclusions.

An expert's destruction of drafts, notes, or even writings such as telephone messages may lead to the inference that those documents contained entries that were unfavorable to the sponsoring party. Thus, the destruction of any document that relates to the litigation, regardless of its apparent insignificance, should be discussed with counsel before it occurs. Quite simply, it is impossible to demonstrate that the content of a document was trivial or unimportant once that document has been destroyed.

Theories of Liability

As with all testimony and other evidence, expert opinions must be relevant to an ultimate issue in the case. This means that the opinions must make it more likely than not that a proposition the jury will be asked to decide is true. There are certain prescribed propositions, called "elements," regarding which the plaintiff generally must present "substantial evidence" before his case can even be submitted to a jury. One example is the fact of negligence on the part of a defendant in a negligence case. If the plaintiff fails to present substantial evidence on any element, the defendant prevails without the necessity of presenting any of its own evidence. Generally, evidence regarding a particular element or issue is substantial when it is of sufficient force to cause reasonable minds to differ as to the proper resolution of that issue.

Many theories of recovery are available to plaintiffs in civil actions, depending on the facts of the case. The most frequently invoked theories in personal injury cases are negligence and strict liability in tort.

Negligence

In a negligence case, the elements on which the plaintiff is required to adduce substantial evidence are (1) a breach of a duty owed to the plaintiff through the defendant's failure to use the amount of care that an ordinary person in the same or similar circumstances would have used; (2) causation between the negligent act or omission and the injury; and (3) damages such as medical expenses, lost wages, or pain and suffering. Expert medical testimony usually is required on the issue of causation and typically is relevant on the issue of damages. Expert testimony from other professionals, such as engineers, may be relevant to the issue of liability or negligence.

Strict Liability

Briefly, the doctrine of strict liability in tort allows plaintiffs to recover damages in cases without demonstrating negligence (the failure to use ordinary care) on the part of the defendant. Strict liability cases usually are predicated on proof that the defendant marketed a product that was "defective" in that it was "unreasonably dangerous" when used as intended. As in negligence cases, plaintiffs in strict liability lawsuits must present substantial evidence regarding causation and damages, both of which usually involve expert testimony. Other professionals typically testify on the issues of product defect (engineers, human factors experts), the dollar value of plaintiff's financial losses (economists), and the like.

Depositions and Trial Testimony

Although their purpose often is the same, the experiences of deposition and trial testimony differ dramatically. One might think that because depositions are held outside of the courtroom (usually in a private office), typically with fewer people present, they might provide a more relaxed atmosphere for a witness's testimony. During depositions, however, particularly those that are not videotaped, lawyers sometimes engage in behavior that they would not exhibit while in the presence of a judge and jury at trial. Occasionally, "special masters" (temporary judges of sorts) are appointed to observe and keep order during depositions. These aberrations are unfortunate but infrequent.

Depositions

A deposition is a formal session held outside of the courtroom, almost always in advance of trial, during which a witness's sworn answers to an attorney's questions are recorded stenographically by a court reporter and, under some circumstances, on videotape (Ziskin and Faust, 1988).

It may be helpful to consider depositions as being of two general types: those taken for "discovery" purposes, and those taken for "evidentiary" purposes. Discovery depositions, as their name implies, are examinations of an opposing party's expert, conducted at least in part to gather information regarding his opinions. Evidentiary depositions are taken by the party who has endorsed or identified the witness as an expert. They serve the purpose of preserving the witness's testimony for later presentation to the judge or jury.

In some jurisdictions (Illinois, for example), the rules of court draw a clear distinction between the two types of depositions, with different permissible uses for each. In other jurisdictions (such as the federal courts), the distinction is not a formal one but instead is simply a shorthand way of identifying the party who will conduct the primary examination of the witness and his main purpose in doing so.

Discovery Depositions

Attorneys take discovery depositions of experts to learn the bases of their opinions and to lay a foundation for rebuttal of those opinions at trial. In most courts in the United States, an attorney who has retained an expert for the purpose of giving testimony must identify the witness to the other parties in the lawsuit in writing within a prescribed period before trial. This "disclosure" or "endorsement" typically also must provide at least some information regarding the substance of the expert's opinions. Thus, in most lawsuits, the examining lawyer already has learned, long before the discovery deposition of the expert, the substance of the opinions that are expected to be rendered. Also, many jurisdictions require that the documents (medical records, literature, and the like) on which the expert has relied in forming his opinions be identified or produced before the deposition takes place.

Obtaining a Discovery Deposition. A competent attorney in an important case will have very little "discovering" of the expert's opinions and their bases to perform by the time the expert's discovery deposition is taken. He already will know what opinions will be rendered, the general bases for those opinions, and how he intends to rebut them. The main purpose in taking so-called discovery depositions in many cases is to force the witness to commit to his testimony (i.e., to "lock him in" or "tie him down")—and to obtain what seemingly are inconsequential admissions or concessions for later use, perhaps in ways that are unforeseen by the witness, at trial.

Preparation for Discovery Depositions. An expert witness should be as prepared for a discovery deposition as he is for trial testimony or a deposition taken for evidentiary purposes. In fact, if the examining lawyer does his job, the expert's trial testimony, including his opinions and their weaknesses, will be set in stone at the conclusion of the discovery deposition.

Scope of Testimony. The scope of the opinions that an expert is expected to render must be determined in advance of the discovery deposition and adhered to during it. Will you simply teach the important medical and scientific principles to the jury, or will you render opinions? Will you testify regarding the existence or extent of plaintiff's injuries or solely as to diagnosis? Or causation? If an expert witness testifies regarding an issue to which he has not given sufficient thought or analysis, the other opinions that he gives may be rendered suspect by implication.

Adequacy of Foundation for Opinions. Although lawyers occasionally forget it, jurors tend to expect a certain degree of civility between professionals, including testifying experts and the lawyers who cross-examine them. Both presumably have been the beneficiaries of valuable educations and have been fortunate in their professional lives. Thus, direct, personal attacks on expert witnesses by cross-examining lawyers are rarer than one might expect, although they are used both legitimately and effectively against some "experts.'' On balance, it is far less risky for an attorney to attack the foundation of an expert's opinions rather than the expert himself.

Examination of All Relevant Evidence and Other Materials. One of the simplest and frequently most effective means of challenging an expert's conclusions consists of demonstrating, through the witness's own testimony, that, at the time he reached his conclusion for the litigation, he was misinformed or was given only half the facts (McQueen, 1979). The examining witness may even seek to imply through his questions and the answers that they evoke that information was purposefully withheld from the expert by the opposing lawyer solely because it was detrimental to his case. To avoid embarrassment, an expert witness must assure himself that he has been provided with all records and information that could conceivably affect the opinions he expects to give. This must be done before he commits his opinions to writing and before his discovery deposition commences.

Prior medical records and reports of other examinations in the litigation. When purported victims of personal injuries file lawsuits seeking money damages for those injuries, they place their medical condition at issue and thus, to some extent, compromise the confidentiality afforded by the physician-patient privilege. The extent to which the privilege is waived varies among jurisdictions. At a minimum, counsel for the defendant is entitled to obtain records of examination and treatment that are related to the injury at issue. The ''discoverability'' of records, however, may vary, depending on their type (APA, 1992; Tranel, 1994).* In some jurisdictions, the privilege is lost completely or ''waived'' with respect to typical, clinical records, allowing the opposing lawyer to contact and communicate with treating physicians and other medical providers concerning the injury or condition at issue.

One of the first things that lawyers who litigate personal injury lawsuits do in preparing cases for trial is to compile every medical record they can find that reflects examination or treatment of the plaintiff, regardless of the reason for that examination or treatment. The importance of a review of all those records by any expert who expects to provide opinions on diagnosis, causation, or other issues cannot be overstated.

In a recent lawsuit that we defended, the plaintiff claimed that he had suffered hearing loss and intolerable tinnitus while working for the defendant. His causation expert testified that virtually all the plaintiff's hearing loss and tinnitus was caused on the job. With some persistence, we obtained old records from an out-of-town Veteran's Administration Hospital that reflected the plaintiff's admission for psychiatric observation because ''this constant ringing in my ears is making me crazy. I need to be on disability.'' That hospitalization occurred more than 4 years before the plaintiff first worked for the defendant. It was not necessary to question the plaintiff's causation expert, who was unaware of the prior hospitalization, about that record specifically during his discovery deposition. He did admit, in the abstract, that no accident can cause symptoms to manifest themselves 4 years earlier, but even that self-evident proposition need not have been established to lay a sufficient foundation for cross-examination at trial.

School and employment records. School and employment records are no less important than medical records, particularly in cases that involve claims of brain injuries (see Ch. 25). If, for example, a plaintiff claims that he is ''unemployable'' because he is no longer able to perform his most recent ''heavy industrial labor,'' prior successful work in a sedentary occupation may disprove that claim. Standardized tests that may have been administered in advance of or during the plaintiff's primary, secondary, technical, or college education may be the best indicator of employability in the light of his claimed injury, particularly when those results are combined with other evaluations contained in his school records.

Our firm defended what remains the longest jury trial in U.S. history, involving injuries that were alleged to have been caused by dioxin exposure. One of the plaintiffs' medical experts testified that one plaintiff, a high school student, had been rendered ''a markedly and pervasively deviate child.'' Investigation revealed that the plaintiff's accomplishments included his election as president of his class and as a member of the National Honor Society (presumably the deviate wing). The expert had not bothered to look at the plaintiff's high school yearbook, and plaintiff's lawyer had not thought to get it for him.

Depositions of other witnesses, including plaintiff and treating physicians. Physicians nearly always rely on a plain-

* Care should be taken in the release of any patient records, even when an authorization for release is executed by the patient. This is particularly important with respect to ''raw'' psychological data and other sensitive materials.

tiff's medical history in rendering a diagnosis and opinions on such matters as causation. Just as statements made by the plaintiff before and during examination yield information about that history, so does his deposition. It should be considered no less important than the history that he gave to other physicians. In fact, because depositions are recorded in the plaintiff's own words, under oath and with counsel present, they make a more reliable source of historical data than notes made by a physician incident to examination or treatment.

Similarly, just as review of the plaintiff's prior medical records and his deposition may be indispensable in rendering valid opinions, the depositions of his treating physicians and other experts may be just as valuable.

Use of Authoritative Literature and "First-Hand" Experts. Attorneys frequently ask experts if certain literature is "authoritative" or relied on by members of the expert's specialty or field in carrying out their profession. Literature that is sufficiently reliable and established and that contradicts statements made by an expert in a lawsuit generally may be used to confront him during cross-examination (Perr, 1977). Some expert witnesses attempt to avoid impeachment by authoritative literature by refusing to admit that any literature is authoritative; that approach may detract from their credibility, depending on how widely known the literature is and what the other experts in the case say about it. It would seem odd, even to the average juror, for a medical expert to testify that he does not know whether the *Journal of the American Medical Association* or the *New England Journal of Medicine* are authoritative and relied on. The expert should remember that, by conceding that literature is authoritative, he is not vouching for everything in it. If confronted by literature that seems to contradict his testimony, the expert should be prepared to explain the reason for the apparent contradiction and perhaps to present other literature that agrees with him.

In brain damage cases, various diagnostic studies and tests, including neuropsychological batteries, often are administered by medical experts who seek to establish or rebut issues such as medical causation. The tests sometimes are administered, scored, or interpreted erroneously. The physicians, psychologists, neuropsychologists, and other scientists who actually developed the various tests occasionally are called on to testify in cases in which one of the opposing experts seeks to use the developer's testing methods improperly or for purposes that were not intended. Thus, it is imperative in litigation for the expert to assure himself that any tests on which he plans to rely have been administered precisely as prescribed, scored correctly, and used solely for the purpose for which they were developed.

In one case, a testifying expert had arranged for blood tests to be performed by a national laboratory. He then misinterpreted the results and claimed that the plaintiff was deathly ill: "The plaintiff's muscle damage is revealed by his abnormally low CPK." The pathologist at the well-known laboratory who had actually performed the test testified during his deposition that there was no disease known to medical science that results in a "low CPK" and that a low CPK was a "sign of good health." After a similar experience with another national laboratory, the expert stopped testifying against that defendant.

Inadequacy of Foundation for Opinions. Federal Rule of Evidence 703, which relates to the permissible bases of an expert's opinions, provides that

> **The facts or data in the particular case upon which an expert bases an opinion or inference may be those perceived by or made known to him at or before the hearing. If of a type reasonably relied upon by experts in the particular field in forming opinions or inferences upon the subject, facts or data need not be admissible in evidence.**

Also, the Supreme Court (*Daubert v. Merrell Dow Pharmaceuticals, Inc.*), requires courts to examine the validity of the methodology used in reaching the opinion:

> **The inquiry envisioned by Rule 702 is, we emphasize, a flexible one. Its overarching subject is the scientific validity—and thus the evidentiary relevance and reliability—of the principles that underlie a proposed submission. The focus, of course, must be solely on principles and methodology, not on the conclusions that they generate. . . .**
>
> **We recognize that in practice, a gatekeeping role for the judge, no matter how flexible, inevitably on occasion will prevent the jury from learning of authentic insights and innovations. That, nevertheless, is the balance that is struck by Rules of Evidence designed not for the exhaustive search for cosmic understanding but for the particularized resolution of legal disputes. . . .**
>
> **To summarize: "general acceptance" is not a necessary precondition to the admissibility of scientific evidence under the Federal Rules of Evidence, but the**

Rules of Evidence—especially Rule 702—do assign to the trial judge the task of ensuring that an expert's testimony both rests on a reliable foundation and is relevant to the task at hand. Pertinent evidence based on scientifically valid principles will satisfy those demands.

Attorneys would prefer to render all adverse opinion testimony in their cases inadmissible—or at least neutralize it in the jury's eyes—on the basis of inadequate foundation. Unless there are favorable entries in their records (e.g., "I think Mr. Smith is malingering"), the depositions of treating physicians, for example, often are taken by defendants as a "preemptive strike." The attorney hopes to demonstrate that the physicians are not qualified to give causation testimony or that their bases for reaching their conclusions on causation are inadequate (Ziskin and Faust, 1988). The latter objective may be preferable in some cases, because it appears less like an attack on the physician himself. The former objective usually is reserved for the expert who flaunts his disrespect for science, law, or both.

In a recent case defended by our firm, analysis of the medical literature on which the plaintiff's expert claimed to rely in reaching his causation opinions revealed that the literature did not support those opinions. During his discovery deposition, taken after he had formed and expressed his causation opinions in a formal disclosure, the expert testified that he did not know whether the first article on which he claimed to rely "would indicate one way or the other whether" the occurrences "would be capable of causing long-term brain or nerve effects," the injury claimed by the plaintiff. The second study was insufficient to support his opinions, because "they didn't look at chronic effects," such as those allegedly suffered by the plaintiff. Similarly, the third study on which he said he relied did not deal with "long-term brain or nerve effects." As it turned out, none of the literature was applicable.

Inaccuracy of Foundation for Opinions. To avoid embarrassment, the assumptions or foundation for the opinions that an expert expects to provide should be verified to the extent possible by the expert himself, through a review of all available written documentation. If important assumptions are shown at trial to be inaccurate, the soundness of the reasoning applied to them will not matter.

In a case in which the plaintiff sought to recover for purported brain damage, his expert witness testified that the plaintiff's score on a neuropsychological test (a test called the "Writing to Dictation Test") was abnormal. In the sentence "Do you want to go out for a walk?" the plaintiff wrote his U's backward. Implicit in the conclusion that this response was caused by the occurrence at issue in the lawsuit was the assumption that the plaintiff began writing his U's backward after the occurrence. Examination of his school records, however, revealed backward U's on a form that he had filled out in college, 25 years before his supposed brain injury. The expert had not bothered to ask that those records be obtained before he formed and formally expressed his opinions.

Purpose and Propagation of Evidentiary Depositions

Evidentiary depositions are the equivalent of trial testimony, except that they are taken outside of the courtroom, usually in the same setting as discovery depositions, and are recorded stenographically for later presentation to the jury.

Evidentiary depositions are generally conducted by the lawyer who retained the witness and who seeks to preserve the testimony of that witness because of his unavailability for trial or for some other reason. These depositions frequently are videotaped so that the presentation at trial will be closer in character to live testimony, with the jury observing the witness's demeanor, hearing his tone of voice, and so on.

The previous discussion regarding discovery depositions as well as the following discussion on trial testimony should be kept in mind when preparing to give an evidentiary deposition.

Trial Testimony

It is generally accepted that "live" witnesses, ones who personally appear in the courtroom, are more effective than those who appear on videotape or whose testimony is read to the jury by one of the lawyers (Balabanian, 1980). Although the quality of videotaped depositions, and therefore their effectiveness, has improved throughout the years, the jury obviously is still in a better position to observe the witness when he is present. The witness can direct his testimony straight to the jury, can observe them, and in turn, can respond to their reactions. The purposes of live testimony are identical to those served by evidentiary depositions. Thus, all the matters discussed in this chapter regarding discovery and evidentiary depositions should be considered in preparing for live testimony at trial.

What to Expect

The stage of litigation at which an expert can expect to testify depends on whether he will be called as a witness by the plaintiff or the defendant. At the very least, by the time the expert is called to testify, the jury will have heard a summary of the most important aspects of the evidence from counsel for each party delivered in the form of opening statements. If the expert's testimony is sufficiently important, counsel will describe during opening statement the opinions he expects to elicit from the expert. Thus, in most cases, the jury already will be familiar, if only in a general way, with how the testimony or opinions relate to the issues in the case and to the other evidence that the lawyers expect to adduce.

Direct Examination

"Admissibility" of Opinions. The "admissibility" of medical and scientific opinions (i.e., the determination, made by the judge, as to whether the jury will be permitted to hear them) often is challenged in lawsuits, particularly when the theory on which the opinion is based is novel or controversial. One objective of discovery depositions may be to elicit testimony from the expert witness that will support an argument to the judge that the jury should not be allowed to hear his opinions. Thus, an expert who is expected to provide opinions during his testimony should be familiar with the standard by which their admissibility will be measured. Unfortunately, this standard also differs from court to court.

One widely used standard examines whether the scientific principle or methodology "from which the deduction is made" is "sufficiently established to have gained general acceptance in the particular field in which it belongs" (*Frye v. United States*). This standard questions the dependability, trustworthiness, certainty, scientific precision, or accuracy of the principle on which the inference to be presented to the jury is based.

With the increasing number of experts who seek to render scientifically questionable opinions at trial, the courts are increasingly willing to examine the validity or reliability of those opinions and to exclude from the evidence questionable or unsupported opinions. However, the U.S. Supreme Court recently held that, in the federal courts, scientific opinions are not necessarily limited to evidence that is "generally accepted" in the fields to which they belong (*Daubert v. Merrell Dow Pharmaceuticals*).

Testifying experts should be prepared for questions, particularly during discovery-type depositions, whereby the attorney will seek to establish that the methodology used in forming the opinions were unreliable, unscientific, or speculative. When the expert relies on epidemiologic studies in determining whether a causal connection exists between an accident or exposure and a particular condition or symptom, questioning may seek to establish the following for purposes of attempting to persuade the court that the opinions are not admissible because their bases are unreliable:

1. Even the most scientifically valid study can establish only an association between a disease and an exposure or occurrence, not a causal relationship. The proof required in a civil case is of causation, not mere association. The relative risks evinced by the studies relied on by the expert are not statistically significant or sufficiently strong to warrant an inference of causation. (A relative risk that includes a number close to one, for example, or a confidence interval of less than 95 percent would render the study subject to plausible challenge.)
2. There are persuasive, valid studies that show no statistically significant elevated relative risk.
3. The designs of the studies that show no statistically significant relative risk were better than the designs of the studies that the expert claims show such a relative risk.
4. The studies on which the expert relies were poorly designed in that inappropriate control group data were used when either a more appropriate data set was available or no sufficient control data existed.
5. The studies do not demonstrate a dose response and thus cannot be shown to be relevant to the plaintiff's exposure.
6. The studies did not account for variations in individual susceptibility to the condition at issue.
7. The studies were not peer-reviewed or otherwise held out for critical comment.

Even if the expert's testimony on these points does not result in the exclusion of his opinions at trial, they often will provide an effective basis for cross-examination.

Form of Questions. Lawyers conducting trials are not permitted to testify for their witnesses. They are not permitted, on direct examination of their own witness, to "lead" that witness's testimony with questions that suggest the response sought by the lawyer. Although cross-examination is said to be more difficult, many trial lawyers prefer it to direct examination precisely because "leading" questions, and the control that they provide over the interrogation, are allowed during cross but not during direct (Costello, 1981).

There are essentially two methods of conducting direct examinations, both of which involve different forms of questions. Before he testifies, as part of the preparation process, an expert witness should be told which method the interrogating attorney plans to use in asking his questions on direct examination.

The first method of conducting direct examinations uses questions that call for mostly unguided "narrative" responses by the witness. Attorneys prefer this method when conducting a direct examination of a witness in whom they have confidence, usually one who has experience on the witness stand or who has been prepared extensively. General questions such as "what was the next step?" or "what happened next?" call for narrative responses. When this method is used, a persuasive witness's testimony can be rendered even more convincing, because it goes unguided and therefore does not appear manipulated or controlled by the lawyer.

The second method of conducting direct examination uses fact-specific questions ("what, if any, weight did you give the Taylor study in reaching your opinion?") and gives the witness less control over the presentation of his testimony. This method may result in a more complete and better-structured examination. During actual examinations of witnesses, most lawyers blend the two methods, relying more heavily on one or the other depending on the strength of the witness and his familiarity with the issues in the lawsuit.

Diagnosis and Causation. A plaintiff in a lawsuit involving bodily injury is required to prove that a causal connection existed between the conduct at issue (e.g., negligence) or the condition at issue (e.g., defect in a product that renders it unreasonably dangerous) and the injuries for which he seeks compensation. He must, of course, first establish that he suffers from the condition complained of, which also usually involves expert testimony in the form of a medical diagnosis.

In all but the simplest of cases and in virtually all American jurisdictions, expert medical testimony is required to support the inference of causation. One exception is the so-called sudden onset rule whereby the jury may infer a causal connection between a defendant's conduct or defective product and an injury based on common experience and a showing of a temporal relationship (when, for example, the plaintiff is hit in the arm with a baseball bat, testifies that he felt pain immediately afterward, that there was no pain before the incident, and when a diagnosis of fracture is made shortly thereafter with no intervening trauma).

Causation opinions usually must come from a physician (or, in some cases, another professional who by training or experience is qualified to render a diagnosis and exclude, in a scientifically valid way, other possible causes) and usually must be expressed "to a reasonable degree of certainty" within the expert's field. The definition of that phrase can differ from jurisdiction to jurisdiction, depending on the circumstances, and may include opinions that basically are meaningless ("might or could") or essentially speculative ("greater than 50 percent probability"). Some experts assume, often incorrectly, that the standard for "reasonable degree of medical certainty" in the context of testimony in a lawsuit always is "more probable than not." An expert who expects to provide causation testimony in support of a plaintiff's claim should always consult with counsel who retained him regarding the extent of certainty on the issue of causation that will be required in that particular case, given the condition at issue and the law of the jurisdiction in which the lawsuit is pending.

Damages. Medical experts are in a unique position to provide evidentiary support for the dollar amount of a plaintiff's damage claim. Physicians, for example, often testify regarding the likelihood that future surgery or other treatment will be required and of its cost. They describe the extent to which the plaintiff's pain or discomfort is expected to improve or worsen. Also, medical experts frequently testify regarding a plaintiff's ability to hold gainful employment, thereby providing a basis for an award of future lost wages and benefits.

As with all other issues, the expert witness should not stray from the area of his expertise in giving testimony that relates to damages. It is, for example, one thing for a physician to opine that a plaintiff's injuries prevent him from returning to his previous employment (if a sufficient foundation on which to base that opinion is provided) but quite another to state that he is "unemployable." Expression of the latter opinion would require expertise in such matters as vocational rehabilitation and training, the prevailing job market, and other matters that are likely to be far outside the scope of a physician or other provider's discipline.

Cross-Examination

There are two principles of cross-examination with which most nonlawyers are familiar: ask leading questions, and never ask a question to which you do not know the answer. An expert testifying at trial or during an evidentiary deposition should expect a competent cross-examiner to adhere, more or less, to these principles.

Form of Questions

Questions on cross-examination typically are not questions at all but statements. ("You were denied board certification seven times because you failed the test, am I right?" "Doctor, you reached your opinions in this case without even having seen this record, didn't you?") The ability to respond effectively and appropriately to cross-examination often is the difference between a good witness and a bad one.

Jurors usually are able to discern when a witness is being evasive and do not like witnesses who refuse to answer questions. Argument and advocacy by an expert witness during cross-examination may call his objectivity into question, showing that he is biased to such an extent that he does not want the jury to know the truth. Also, attempts to argue with essentially correct statements posed during cross-examination based on the implications that they might raise can backfire by underscoring both the statement and the inference. Thus, the best option often is to simply acknowledge that the statements are correct during cross and then to explain during redirect examination why, notwithstanding their accuracy, those things do not matter.

Use of Discovery Deposition at Trial

Lawyers take discovery depositions with later cross-examination in mind. If, during trial, the expert contradicts his deposition testimony, he can expect to be confronted with that testimony, in the most dramatic fashion possible, in front of the jury. It therefore is of critical importance that the expert be thoroughly familiar with all his prior testimony, including testimony rendered on similar issues in other cases, before he testifies at trial.

QUALIFICATIONS FOR EXPERT TESTIMONY

Plaintiff's lawyers often hope to obtain their expert testimony regarding diagnosis, causation, prognosis, and damages from one of plaintiff's treating physicians whom plaintiff saw before he filed his lawsuit. In contrast with an expert who has been selected by the plaintiff's lawyer, the treating physician is likely to appear more independent and trustworthy.

Similarly, defense lawyers prefer to elicit opinion testimony favorable to their clients from treating physicians rather than from their own experts. In fact, favorable testimony from a treating physician for the defendant can be even more persuasive than favorable testimony for the plaintiff, because treating physicians often are seen as having developed some loyalty, albeit in a clinical context, to their patients. If a treating physician supports a defense lawyer's case, he may be the most important defense witness in the lawsuit.

Even when favorable opinions are not likely, experienced defense lawyers often take the treating physician's deposition to eliminate him as a potential causation witness before the plaintiff's lawyer has a chance to adduce the testimony. Before the doctor states his opinions (and perhaps before he has even formed them), defense counsel may seek to convince him that he does not know enough to support a causation or even a diagnostic opinion to a reasonable degree of medical certainty (often the standard that those opinions must meet to be presented to the jury).

In one of our recent cases, plaintiff claimed that he developed leukemia from exposure to benzene. It was possible that if his treating oncologist's deposition were taken by the plaintiff's lawyer first, he might testify as to a causal connection between the exposure and the pathology. Thus, we sought to eliminate this physician as a causation witness through a discovery deposition. This abbreviated version of the testimony is representative of what is asked when this tactic is used:

Q: Doctor, you are an oncologist. Do you have a background in toxicology?

A: Nothing in particular except for medical school.

Q: Do you have a background in epidemiology?

A: Again, I studied it in medical school 30 years ago and I read studies in journals.

Q: Do you attend seminars in toxicology or epidemiology?

A: Not specifically, no.

Q: Are you familiar with the principles that scientists use in evaluating toxicologic and epidemiologic studies?

A: As I said, I read studies in the journals, but I cannot say that I am an expert in evaluating them in those fields more than most others.

Q: For example, do you know what they mean when they talk about an "odds ratio?"

A: I think it relates to risk, but I would have to check the books to be more precise.

Q: And regarding animal studies, do you know which animal species are most like humans when it comes to causation of acute lymphoblastic leukemia?

A: All I know is that they usually study it in rats and mice.

Q: So if a chemical causes leukemia in rats but not in mice, do you know whether that would be better than if it caused it in mice and not in rats in terms of risk to humans?

A: I don't know.

Q: Do you know what scientific flaws in the benzene literature have drawn criticism, or whether there even has been such criticism?

A: I am not familiar enough with it to say.

Q: Are the benzene levels that are discussed in the literature more or less than the plaintiff claims to have had?

A: I don't know.

Q: Do you keep up with the literature pertaining to the toxic effects of benzene?

A: No.

Q: I take it then, Doctor, that the determination of whether benzene had caused any particular person's leukemia would be a matter for a different specialty than yours and that you would not be able to express an opinion to a reasonable degree of medical certainty that benzene had caused someone to develop leukemia?

A: No, I couldn't do that. I can only give a diagnosis of leukemia; I don't know for sure what caused it.

Q: Determining whether benzene caused someone's leukemia would be a matter for someone of a different specialty than yours?

A: Yes.

Had the last two questions been asked first instead of last, the attorney would run the risk of this response:

> **I am not a toxicologist or an epidemiologist, but I am a medical doctor and I know that exposure to benzene is a risk factor for leukemia from literature that I have reviewed. I know that Mr. Smith has leukemia and apparently he was exposed to quite a dose of benzene, at least that's what he told me. Since I am not aware of any other risk factors from Mr. Smith's history, it was likely the benzene that caused the leukemia.**

This type of reasoning can be challenged quite easily, but the point is that the first set of answers rendered challenge unnecessary because the expert disqualified himself from giving any opinions as to causation.

Technical Requirements/Challenges to Credentials

The general technical qualifications that are necessary to render expert testimony are usually that the witness is qualified as an expert by knowledge, skill, experience, training, or education. The type and amount of knowledge, skill, etc., required depends on the subject matter of the opinion and the facts of the lawsuit.

The expert should expect the opposing attorneys to investigate the accuracy of every credential he claims. They do so not only for the purpose of laying a foundation for the exclusion of his opinions but for use during cross-examination at trial if the opinions are admitted into evidence. Experts who exaggerate their credentials risk their credibility. In one of our cases, an expert for the opposing party claimed on his C.V. to have been an adjunct professor at a community college. That is obviously a credential of only marginal importance, but it became significant when we took the deposition of the registrar of the college, who testified that the expert had taught only one class for 3 hours on one night a decade before and was not considered a member of the faculty.

The "Jack of All Trades" Problem

Some witnesses will claim to be experts on almost any topic. One expert in St. Louis frequently is cross-examined with a list of 26 largely unrelated subjects on which he has testified. The list is reviewed one item at a time, with a different subject for each of the letters "A to Z."

We know from reviewing prior deposition transcripts that one of the experts we have encountered has changed his area of specialization to fit the current lawsuit. In a case that involved immunology, he said that he held a Ph.D. in microbiology, was a professor of immunology and ran a university laboratory called the "Laboratory of Immuno-Parasitology." In an earlier case, where the issues related to biochemistry, he testified that his Ph.D. was in biochemistry, that he was a professor of biochemistry, and that he headed a university laboratory called, not surprisingly, the "Laboratory of Biochemical-Parasitology." Jurors, of course, do not react favorably to such revelations.

FEES

Experts who are perceived by jurors as "hired guns" are less likely to persuade them than experts who have been paid primarily for treatment or for other reasons unrelated to litigation. Every expert should expect to be questioned about the amount of time that he has spent on the case and the dollar amount that he charged. Furthermore, the inquiry is not always limited to fees paid in the case for which the deposition is being taken.

Excessive hourly fees may give the appearance that the witness is interested mainly in money and that he has been "bought off." Also, reluctance on the part of litigants to pay excessively high fees has led to the practice of requesting that the court place reasonable limits on the hourly rate that an opposing expert can charge for his time during his discovery deposition. These and similar requests frequently are granted by the courts, even when the request is made after the deposition has been concluded.

How much should an expert witness charge for his time? One reasonable and relatively safe means of setting a fee is to determine the opportunity cost of testifying. If the expert can legitimately say that for every hour he spends on a litigation-related matter he loses a certain number of dollars from his clinical practice, a jury is likely to accept that hourly rate as reasonable under the circumstances. Experts who do nothing professionally but testify obviously cannot use this method. Jurors may be prone to conclude that an expert who testifies for a living was overpaid for his time (regardless of the amount that he charged) and that his opinions are biased, simply because he has no real job.

Some institutions, including several universities, are now issuing standardized guidelines for use by their faculties and staffs in setting hourly rates for consultation. Rates calculated pursuant to such guidelines may be easier to justify to a jury than some arbitrary hourly fee that bears no relationship to the opportunity cost of testifying.

Many experts believe that the hostility that they may be required to endure as a witness justifies an hourly rate in excess of the amount that they earn pursuing the typical activities of their profession. Jurors are unlikely to accept this justification unless they actually observe in the courtroom the hostility that serves as the basis for the fee. As we discuss above, that circumstance is rarer than one might expect.

It would be unethical for an attorney to pay an expert in litigation a percentage of the plaintiff's recovery or to otherwise link the expert's fee to the "result" in the case, even though that result may have been obtained in part as a consequence of the expert's testimony. This ethical principle is probably superfluous because such a fee arrangement, once disclosed, would destroy any expert's credibility in the eyes of reasonable jurors. Similarly, attempting to justify an inflated hourly rate by reference to the comparative "size" or "importance" of the particular litigation in which the expert is involved is likely to have the same undesired effect on the jury.

CONCLUSION

When an expert chooses to become involved in lawsuits by rendering testimony, the importance of preparation and investigation, which must be fully completed before any opinions are committed to writing in any form, cannot be overstated. He must be sure that the foundation for his opinions is solidly based in the scientific method, and he must anticipate, in advance of presenting his testimony, the bases on which those opinions will be challenged. Also, the expert must understand fully the scope of his expected testimony and limit his opinions to the subjects on which he has been designated to testify.

Expert testimony can be indispensable to the just resolution of lawsuits. The increasing willingness on the part of a few witnesses to "say anything" for a price (and the continued willingness on the part of many courts to allow them to do so) merely underscores the critical importance of involvement in litigation by reputable, honest experts who base their testimony on generally accepted medical and scientific principles and on strict adherence to scientifically valid methodologies. Experts who do not wish to subject themselves to the hostility and professional scrutiny that testifying occasionally entails can still contribute to keeping the process "honest" by participating in litigation on a consulting basis.

REFERENCES

American Psychological Association: Ethical principles of psychologists and code of conduct. Am Psychol 47:1597, 1992

Balabanian E: Medium v. tedium: video depositions come of age. Litigation 6:26, 1980

Costello JM: The direct examination of the expert witness. For Defense 23:21, 1981

Daubert v Merrell Dow Pharmaceuticals, Inc., 113 S Ct 2786, 125 L Ed 469 (1993)

Fed R Civ P, 702

Fed R Evid, 703

Frye v United States, 293 F 1013 (DC Cir 1923)

McQueen R: The psychologist to the witness stand. Clin Psychol 32:4, 1979

Perr IN: Cross-examination of the psychiatrist using publications. Bull Am Acad Psychiatry Law 5:237, 1977

Stoleson v United States, 708 F2d 1217, 1222 (7th Cir 1983)

Tranel D: The release of psychological data to nonexperts: ethical and legal considerations. Prof Psychol Res Pract 25:33, 1994

Ziskin J, Faust D: Coping with psychiatric and psychological testimony. 2nd Ed. Vol. 1–2. Law and Psychology Press, Marina del Ray, CA, 1988

SUGGESTED READINGS

Doerr HO, Carlin AS: Forensic Neuropsychology. Guilford Press, New York, 1991

Pappas EH: Preparing your witness for deposition. For Defense 29:8, 1987

Postol LP: A legal primer for expert witnesses. For Defense 29:21, 1987

Waitzkin H: Doctor-patient communication. JAMA 225:2441, 1984

Weiner IB, Hess AK: Handbook for forensic psychology. Wiley, New York, 1987

Index

Page numbers followed by f *indicate figures; those followed by* t *indicate tables.*

B

C

D

E

I

O

T

U